# Complementary and Alternative Medicine: A Case-Based Approach

# Complementary and Alternative Medicine: A Case-Based Approach

Edited by Penelope Higgins

AMERICAN
MEDICAL PUBLISHERS
www.americanmedicalpublishers.com

American Medical Publishers,
41 Flatbush Avenue,
1st Floor, New York,
NY 11217, USA

Visit us on the World Wide Web at:
www.americanmedicalpublishers.com



ISBN: 978-1-63927-046-0



**Cataloging-in-Publication Data**

Complementary and alternative medicine : a case-based approach / edited by Penelope Higgins.
p. cm.
Includes bibliographical references and index.
ISBN 978-1-63927-046-0
1. Alternative medicine. 2. Alternative medicine--Case studies. 3. Integrative medicine.
4. Medicine. I. Higgins, Penelope.

R733 .C66 2022
615.5--dc23

# Table of Contents

# Preface

Over the recent decade, advancements and applications have progressed exponentially. This has led to the increased interest in this field and projects are being conducted to enhance knowledge. The main objective of this book is to present some of the critical challenges and provide insights into possible solutions. This book will answer the varied questions that arise in the field and also provide an increased scope for furthering studies.

Complementary medicine refers to the use of alternative medicine with functional medical treatment, for the purpose of improving the effects of the treatment. Alternative medicine involves the use of such practices, which are not proven to relieve the pain or to achieve other healing effects of medicine. Naturopathy and homeopathy are the two most common forms of alternative medicine. Naturopathy is a natural and non-invasive therapeutic treatment method based on the belief that the body heals itself by using a vital energy, which guides the bodily processes. The belief, that the substances, which cause the symptoms of a disease in healthy people, cure similar symptoms in sick people, forms the roots of homeopathy. Some other common complementary and alternative medicine practices include ayurveda, chiropractic, traditional Chinese medicine, reiki, etc. This book unfolds the innovative aspects of complementary and alternative medicine which will be crucial for the readers and medical practitioners. It unravels the recent studies in the area of complementary and alternative medicine. Those in search of information to further their knowledge will be greatly assisted by this book.

I hope that this book, with its visionary approach, will be a valuable addition and will promote interest among readers. Each of the authors has provided their extraordinary competence in their specific fields by providing different perspectives as they come from diverse nations and regions. I thank them for their contributions.

**Editor**

# Attitudes of Hungarian Healthcare Professionals (Mds, Nurses) According to Cam Homeopathy: A Cross-Sectional, Qualitative Accumulated Survey's Data

**Hegyi Gabriella**[1*], **Csütörtöki Krisztina**[1], **Pfeifenróth Anna**[1], **Göbölyös Ildiko**[1], **Roberti di Sarsina Paolo**[2*]

[1]*Department of Dietetic and CAM, Pecs University, Hungary*

[2]*Observatory and Methods for Health, University of Milano-Bicocca, Italy*

[*]Corresponding authors: Hegyi Gabriella, Department of Dietetic and CAM, Pecs University, Vörösmarty u.4 , Pecs, Baranya 7646, Hungary, Email: drhegyi@hu.inter.net

**Abstract**

**Aim of the study:** In Eastern-Central Europe, homeopathy has a long history starting from XIXth century which has however been interrupted and later renewed in 1997. A large number of physicians and pharmacists have been trained in homeopathy since. This survey is aimed to measure attitudes to homeopathy in Hungarian GPs and nurses for pediatric and adult population.

**Materials and methods:** An identical original self-administered questionnaire was submitted in 2012 to 550 general physicians's nurses. 536 (98.9%) women and 6 (1.1%) men replied. Results: Approximately one third of GPs is using homeopathy. The usage of homeopathy is quite similar to other European countries in spite of the controversal and refusal habit of academic medicine. Effects of gender, age and location are weak and inconsistent.

**Discussion/Conclusions**: Homeopathy has firmly been integrated into the Hungarian health care system and has sustained despite the worse economic conditions of the population and no public support from the official health insurance system (only private health insurance companies accepted it). Accumulated survey data were concluded with future achievements of harmonization in this CAM field. The life-style advice given by nurses can influence homeopathic usage among patients; further education is necessary for the ethical application of homeopathy and remedies after CEU-courses at University. We emphasize the ethical application of any CAM method, such as homeopathy for patients. CAM courses should be involved into curricula of nurses and MDs according to interest either in basic or in further education

**Keywords:** CAM; Homeopathy; Legislation of CAM-Homeopathy; Usage of CAM; Usage of homeopathy; Nurse-education; Curriculum

## Abbreviations:

CAM: Complementary and Alternative Medicine; NADA: National Acupuncture Detoxification Association; SPSS: Frequently used Evaluating Software for Statistical Analysis; CAMbrella: Mosaic-Word Originated form "CAM" and "Umbrella", for Pan-European Project on CAM, international research for 31 countries in EU, 2010-2013, Frame Work 7, European Union Tender; CME: Continuous Medical Education (credit); CEP: Continuous Education Point (credit); UV: Ultraviolet

## Introduction- background

The study was completed in Hungary (country situated on eastern part of Europe). Homeopathy being one amongst so called complex systems sorted in CAM therapies. Our aim was to investigate different attitudes of health care professionals using this therapy including their opinion on usage, education level, indication for usage, study they participated in past.

The comprehensive CAM legislation came into force on 1 July 1997. The Act CLIV of 1997 on Health Care institutionalized the "National health care promotion program" with the principles "health for all" and "equal access to health care services" [1]. The Act on Health, the Governmental Decree on CAM [1,2] and the Decree of the Ministry of Social Welfare on the practice of CAM [1,2] confirm a definition of CAM treatment, regulate the scope of CAM treatments, and state that "non-conventional procedures that substitute conventional therapy shall only be applied under the supervision of a physician". The non-medical practitioners have to be officially registered members of the public health system. The recent Hungarian CAM law is under reconstruction by the Ministry of Health and the revised version is expected to come out in the last months of 2014 to be more rigorous. Hungary follows the tradition of detailed regulation of practitioners and treatments; consequently each CAM treatment has been included in the public health system and legislation with regulation of education, licenses, authorization etc. [3]. Act XXVIII of 1994 made membership of the Hungarian Medical Chamber compulsory for practicing physicians and dentists. The Chamber of Non-medical Health Professionals (2003/13) was established to extend professional self-regulation to other qualified health care workers. The Chambers are responsible for the follow-up of CAM regulations. There are three categories of authorized medical practitioners in Hungary; physicians, practitioners with a non-academic higher health qualification and other practitioners. In 2011 a wide range of CAM treatments were regulated in detail and most medical universities and schools offer training courses. Only physicians are allowed to practice acupuncture, anthroposophy medicine, Ayurveda medicine, chiropractic, homeopathy, manual medicine, Traditional Chinese

Medicine (TCM), Traditional Tibetan Medicine and Kneipp practices. Acupressure, kinesiology, shiatsu (in complementary moving and massage therapies), phytotherapy and reflexology may be provided by practitioners (non- medical doctors). The University of Pécs is the unique CAM educational institution for medical doctors in Hungary. All providers of CAM in Hungary must take a 2-year education in CAM and pass a license exam. Medical doctors are offered continuing medical education (CME) mostly at universities; non-MD practitioners take courses mostly at the Institute of Continuing Education for health workers in registered evaluated courses. Use of Homeopathy: Only medical doctors may practice homeopathy in Hungary. The "Magyar Homeopata Orvosi Egyesület" (Hungarian Homeopathic Medical Association) was founded in 1991).

## Materials and Methods

The works described in this article have been carried out in accordance with The Code of Ethics of the World Medical Association (Declaration of Helsinki) for experiments involving humans.

We composed a special questionnaire (Homeo-CAMQ), sharing in more province in Hungary among health care providers (nurses) and collecting answers finally we made a statistical analysis for data forming recent data on usage of homeopathy. Criteria definition of Homeo-CAMQ was the following: trial type was exploratory, descriptive, cross-sectional and qualitative. Our target groups were the follows: Health Care employees: GPs, pharmacists, pharmaceutical assistants, nurses. The Qualification criteria were the selection of healthcare employees was carried out using layered sampling, the further selection was done by random sampling. Exclusion criteria were: missing medical qualification. Sampling process was: amongst leading health visitors, pharmacists, chief physicians of the counties-provincial (10 of 18) were requested to participate in the sampling survey.

### Sample quantity definition

The originally planned sample quantity was 550 from which 544 Homeo-CAMQs have been distributed, processed and assessed. Within this study we are trying to set a comparison to a survey carried out in 2011 which studied laymen, people buying homeopathic substances in pharmacies with the sample quantity n=386. The survey was carried out in 10 counties (Heves, Nógrád, Borsod-Abaúj-Zemplén, Hajdú, Jász-Nagykun-Szolnok, Békés by doctors, health visitors, pharmacists, pharmaceutical assistants at pharmacies and doctors' offices. Survey duration: The survey lasted 5 months: June – October of 2012.

Contains of Homeo-CAMQ: For the data gathering a self-composed survey was used. An anonym, self-filling survey method was chosen. The questionnaire contained 21 questions, which were multiple choice, half-closed, ranking (Likert), evaluating, index- and scale type and focused mainly on the opinion of the subject. During the definition of the types of questions asked the following considerations were made: topic of the survey, particularities of healthcare employees and the planned processing and analyzing methods. Using the questionnaire we gathered following types of information:

a. Socio-demographic data (age, highest degree of education, pharmaceutical purchasing habits, usage of pharmaceuticals)

b. cognition (definitions, rules)

c. health-disease behavior study (pharmaceuticals used for acute and chronic diseases)

d. attitude questions (opinions, attitudes, feelings, explanations, beliefs, satisfaction)

Definition of studied variables pending variables: Purchased homeopathic medicine and its characteristics (price, way of purchase) subjective medical effect, homeopathic knowledge, sources of knowledge, independent variables: sociodemographic data, usage of homeopathic medicine, qualification of healthcare employees

### Methods of statistical analysis

Software used: Microsoft Word for gathering the data, SPSS v. 18 for processing and Microsoft Excel for creating tables and diagrams. The following statistical methods and tests are included in this article: base-frequency, partial correlation, cross-table analysis, chi square test. During the statistical analysis a significance level of $p<0.05$ was used.

## Results

The results of the primary study conclude that the distribution of healthcare employees by sex is as previously expected, 536 (98.9%) women and 6 (1.1%) men completed the questionnaire. Main age of the subjects: 49 years. Study range: the youngest subject was a woman from Budapest born in 1990 (22 years of age), while the oldest subject was a health visitor born in 1940 (62 years of age).

The oldest healthcare employees were found in county Nógrád where the main year of birth was 1966 (46 years of age, n=66), while the youngest were found in county Szabolcs-Szátmár-Bereg with the mean year of birth 1972 (40 years of age, n=18). According to the hypothesis of knowledge about homeopathic methods the younger age groups (25-40 years) were aware of homeopathic methods, according to the data however it can be concluded that the 5-10 years older age group is also familiar with it. The following results are displayed using the circle diagram (Figure 1) below.

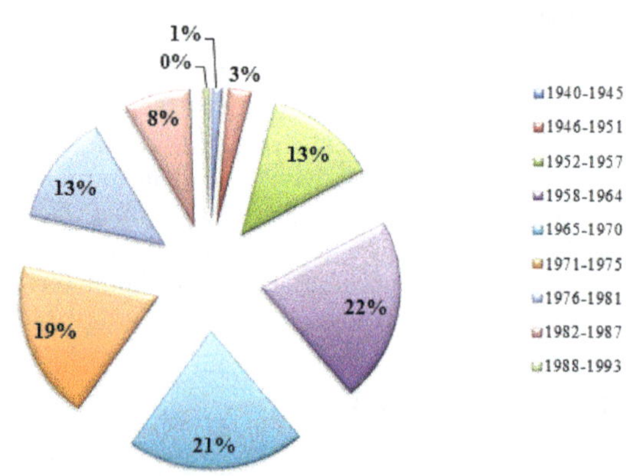


Figure 1: Data of birth of Health Care providers (n=544)

Counties found the most active subjects in Budapest (n=81). In the capital 81 questionnaires were completed, but the healthcare employees in county Pest were very cooperative as well (n=71). The distribution between the capital and the counties is displayed by the diagram (Figure 2) below.

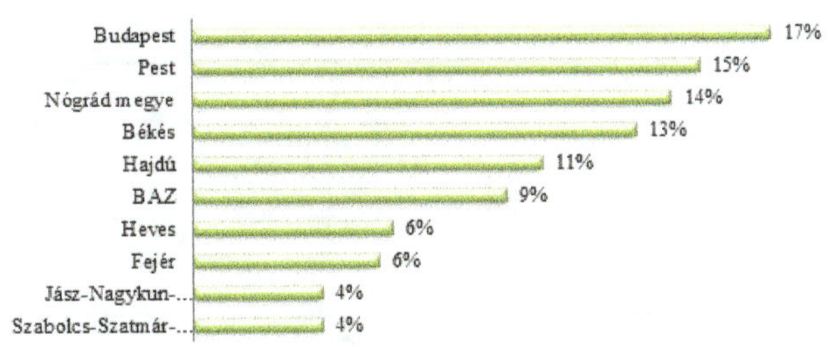


Figure 2: Responsers in different provinces of Hungary (n=544)

We concluded the following results by highest degree of the subjects: 58% (n=310) have an academic degree or higher (university). Within the category „other" we have experienced a variety of other types of health care qualifications: psychologist, nurse, social caretaker, laboratory assistant, masseur, physiotherapeutic assistant, etc. (Figure 3).

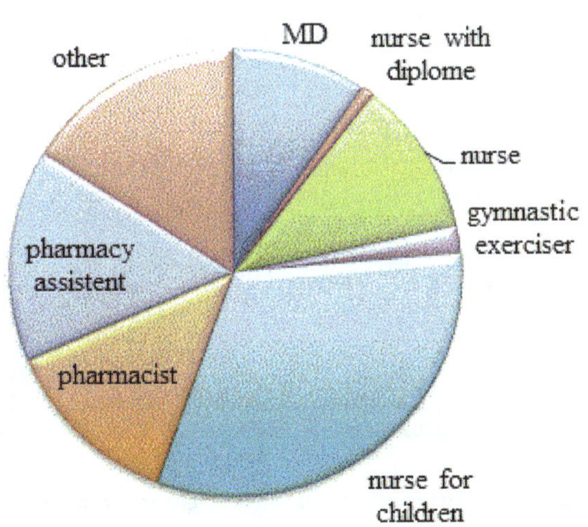


Figure 3: Distribution according qualification degree (n=544)

99.8% (n=543) of the healthcare employees completing the questionnaire have already heard of the method, only one woman from county Nógrád did not know homeopathy. According to the answers almost half of the subjects (48%, n=266) received the knowledge by postgraduate courses, 30 % (n=163) from medical literature and only 67 – which amounts to 12 percent - claimed to have received their knowledge from the press. Nurses for children have formed a big group (Figure 4).

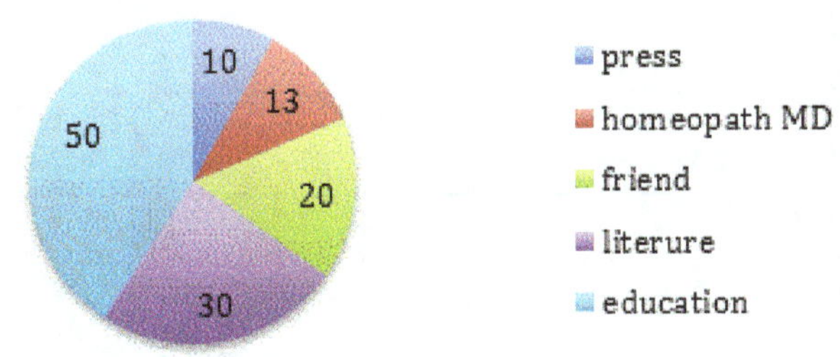


Figure 4: Where do you have got knowledge on Homeopathy from?

The above 4th figure shows that 83% (n=449) of the subjects does have a book on homeopathy in possession while 17 percent does not possess such literature. It is remarkable that a very high percentage (94.5%, n=514) of the subjects has already used homeopathic medicine while 30 of them (6%, n=30) have claimed not having used any. Within the acute diseases the first places were taken by illnesses presenting symptoms of the cold and influenza. Two thirds (70.6%, n=489) of the subjects have marked an illness presenting with these symptoms in their answers.

Homeopathy as a method of treatment was most often used against coughing (n=265) and for increasing milk production (n=167). Concerning acute diseases 55 of the 544 subjects (which amounts to 10.1%) have not answered this question. We need to mention that not all subjects having marked acute diseases (n=489) have not always marked chronic diseases (n=405) and vice versa, a sum of 84 subjects – 15%- have only marked either acute or chronic diseases (Figure 5).

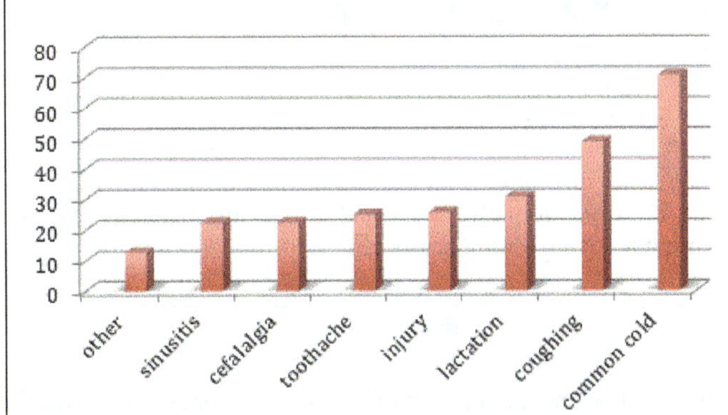


Figure 5: Usage of homeopathic remedy in acute problems (y axis: number of answering health care professionals)

Within chronic diseases 25,75% of the subjects has not named any disease. The other 405 have named 822 answers. This averaged two naming's. The patients have mostly used homeopathic medicine for allergies, stress and symptoms of joint problems (Figure 6).

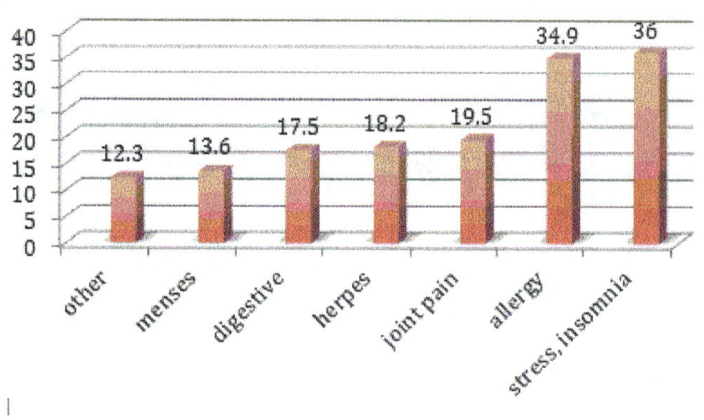


We have also asked questions regarding the usage of pharmaceuticals concerning treatment of both acute and chronic diseases. In both cases the subjects could choose on a scale of five where the meaning of the lowest value was: "I have experienced no change whatsoever" and the highest value meant: "I have soon experienced the effect and felt a definitive improvement, were healed".

While evaluating the answers concerning cases of acute illness we have found that 85,8% (n=415) have given the evaluation excellent or good. Average: 4.15 (Figure 7).

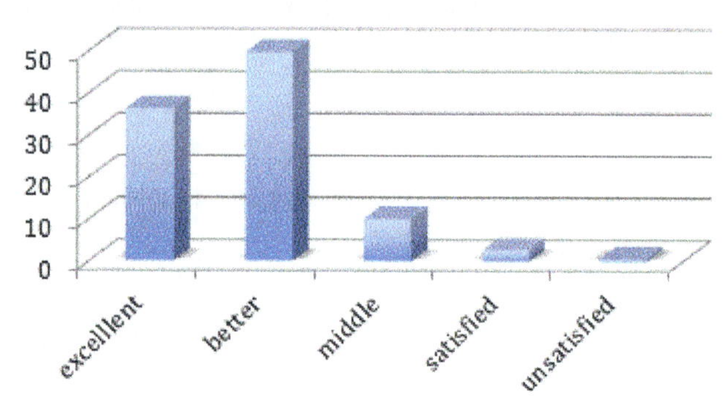


Figure 7: Satisfaction with homeopathy in acute cases (n=484) (y axis: number of answering professionals)

The result is intriguing even if we assume some degree of the placebo effect in some of these cases. Based on these answers a serious re-thinking of opinion towards homeopathic treatment should be concluded involving their stronger recommendation to patients for their own good.

In the usage of homeopathic medicine for chronic diseases 74,4% of the subject have given good or excellent evaluation. The average was 3,94 (Figure 8). Only 6 subjects who have marked chronic diseases for which they used homeopathic medicine have not given an answer to its results.

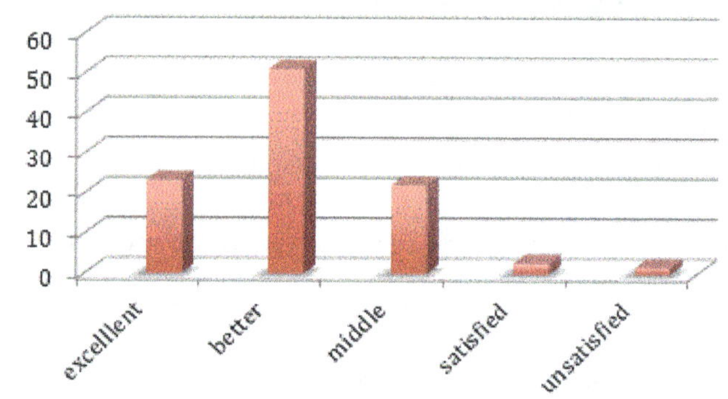


Figure 8: Satisfaction feeling in chronic cases (y axis: number of answering professionals)

The next, Figure 9 compares the results of taking homeopathic remedies in acute and chronic cases.

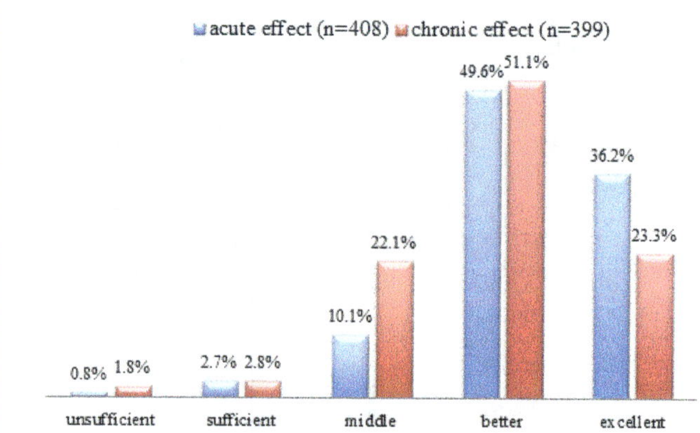


Figure 9: Comparing effect in acute and chronic problems.

Aside of the positive effects of the medication we also asked about eventual side effects. 95,3% (n=482) of the subject has not noticed any unwanted side effects (Figure 10). The other 24 who represent 5 percent of the subjects mainly mentioned the following effects: "allergic to sugar of milk", "symptoms have increased in intensity".

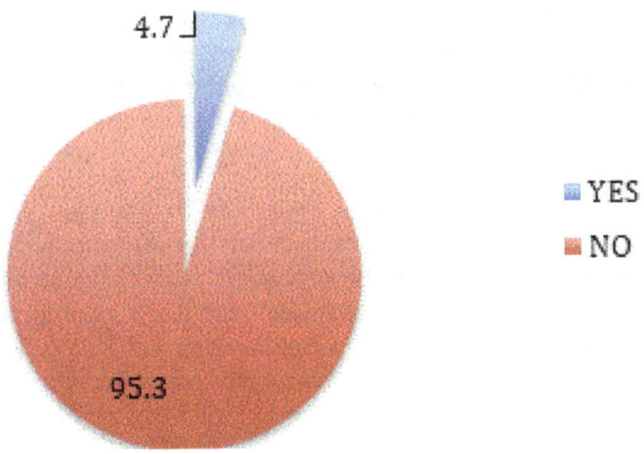


Figure 10: Have you experienced any side effect in homeopathy?

It is a well-known occurrence in related medicine that the patients' symptoms may increase in intensity temporarily. This is explained to the patient by the homeopath, furthermore this is described as a warning in the usage recommendation of homeopathic complexes. The unwanted effects of homeopathic substances are – according to the received answers – minimal, compared for example with the side-effects of non-steroidal anti-inflammatory drugs, drugs containing herbal agents or prescription-free substances available at pharmacies - used for similar indications. The preference list (Figure 11) in medical treatment of the sampled health care employees was the following:

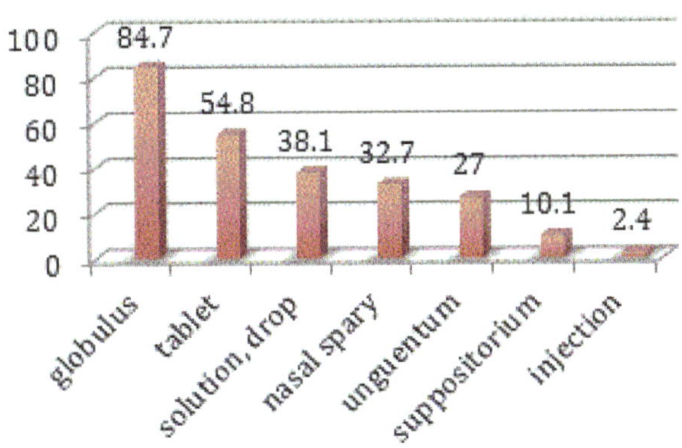


Figure 11: Used forms in homeopathy by health care providers (y axis: number of answering professionals)

The 520 subjects who answered the question could name multiple forms of medication – used and tested by them. This amounted to a total of 1359 naming's with an average of 2,61. 22 of them gave no answer to the question, which is 4%.

83% of the ones answering the question have no problems taking the medication (Figure 12). 89 of the subjects had difficulties with following the recommendations of taking the medicine. They gave the following answers to this half-closed question: "I smoke", "I forget to take it", "menthol, chewing gum", "I forget it during work".

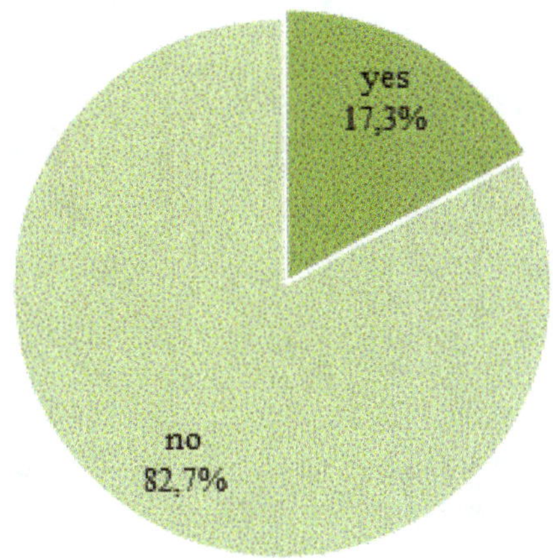


Figure 12: Was any difficulties with taking homeopathic remedies-(according taking-law)? (n=516)

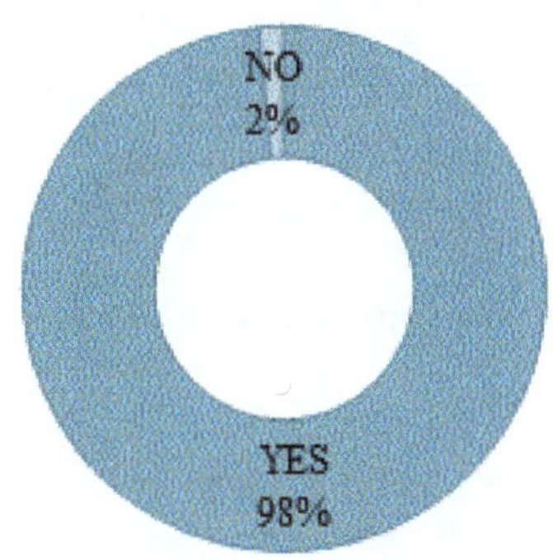


Figure 13: Do you suggest to introduce in common usage homeopathy? (n=528)

The above circle diagram (Figure 13) shows that 98% of the subjects would welcome the therapy every day, 8 subjects would not welcome this one person gave no answer. Those who "do not want the solid therapy to become general" unfortunately gave no further explanation. Those who would welcome homeopathy to become general and gave further explanations gave the following common reasons: natural, free of chemicals, does not harm the intestinal flora, humane, easy on antibiotics, free of side-effects, easy to use, organism-friendly, quick and easy, especially important when treating children, the best medicine from an ecological point of view. A further question was: concerning the profession of healthcare, which medical fields could you put homeopathy in? The next 14th Figure talks on medical professions, which should to be built Homeopathy in:

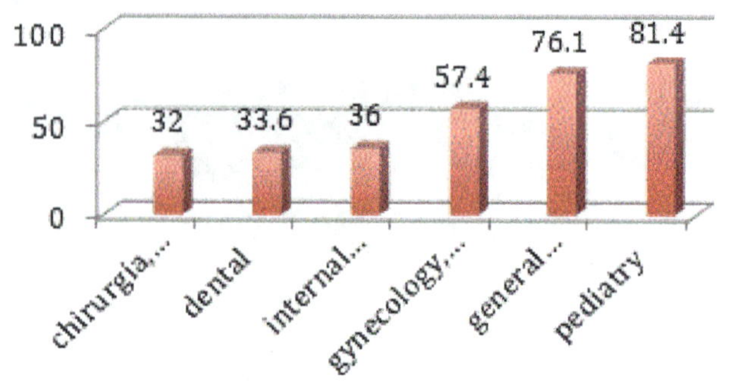


Figure 14: Medical professions for homeopathy could be built in (y axis: number of answering professionals)

The graph shows quite well that the subjects mostly see the role of the solid treatment within the base-services in health care, but more than half of them would also apply it within obstetrics and gynecology. The 524 subjects who gave answers provided 1773 nominations. Average nominations per subject: 3.38. 20 gave no answer.

A further question was whether patients already enquired about the treatment method by the health care professional. The results to this question show that in 66% of the subjects there already have been enquiries. Also two thirds of the answering subjects have already participated in postgraduate courses in the field of homeopathy (Table 1).

| | | Frequency | % | Real % | Cumulative % |
|---|---|---|---|---|---|
| | yes | 508 | 93% | 97,1 | 97,1 |
| | no | 15 | 3% | 2,9 | 100,0 |
| | total | 523 | 96,1 | 100,0 | |
| Missing values | 99 | 21 | 3,9 | | |
| Totally | | 544 | 100,0 | | |

Table 1: Would you like to participate on homeopathy courses?

The above 15th Figure shows answers to the question if nurses would like to participate. 93% of the subjects would like to participate in homeopathy courses while only 3 percent would not. We think the high proportion of positive answers could be an indication to the open mindedness of the subjects, the popularity of the healing method, changes in attitude. After analyzing the answers received regarding the solid therapy we can conclude that this field of complementary medicine divides the trade. The subjects selected 1 for "absolutely not recognized" and 10 for "absolutely recognized". The diagram (Figure 15) below shows that only 0,2% (n=1) of the subjects thinks this method is absolutely not recognized. More than half of the subjects (57%) evaluated the method at a value of 5-moderately recognized-or higher. The average was 4,9, which concludes that healthcare professionals evaluate the recognition of homeopathy as moderate. The above results are shown by the diagram below on scale 1-9 (Figure 16).

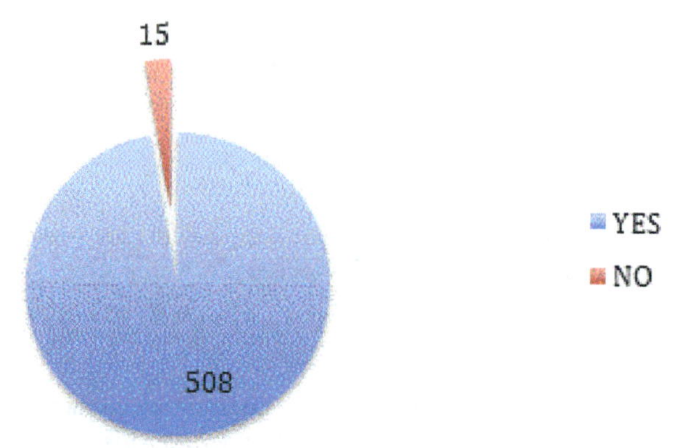


Figure 15: Would you like to participate on any further courses regarding homeopathy?

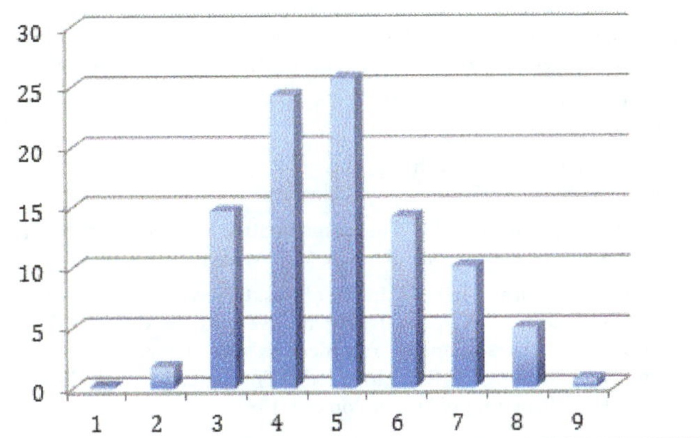


**Figure 16**: Scale from 1-9 believing of acceptance according homeopathy, (1: not accepted totally, 9: well accepted totally.) (y axis: number of answering professionals)

Around half (49.2%) of the subjects purchasing pharmaceuticals found the price of these substances similar to other medicine. The other half (47.1%) found these substances cheaper than other medicine. Only 19 persons, which are 3.7 percent of the ones who gave an answer, found these substances more expensive than other OTC medicine. 24 subjects (4%) did not provide an answer to the question (Figure 17).

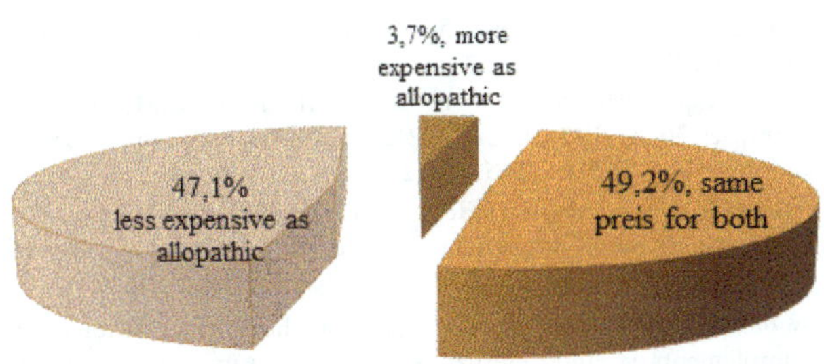


**Figure 17**: Price of homeopathic remedies according to opinion of health care providers (N=518)

In 33% of the cases they never had any difficulties acquiring the medicine, in 40% there is no difficulty anymore since they know where to purchase them now. 90 (16.5%) subjects could acquire the medicine after one day, while 6 (1,1%) of them could only get the medicine within a few weeks. This can be explained by the fact that in cases of some rare constitutional (chronic) diseases even the pharmacist faces difficulties acquiring the homeopathic remedy which might have to be imported privately from abroad, while other more often used homeopathic remedies can be kept in stock within the pharmacy. 18th figure shows a summary on legislation of homeopathy in EU.

## Conclusion

Homeopathy is sorted to “whole medical systems” that originated in German, widely officially used in Hungary (1.17). The fundamental idea of homeopathy is the “Similarity Principle”, which implies that remedies capable of causing disorder in healthy subjects are used as medicines to treat similar patterns of disorder experienced by ill people [4,5]. Homeopathic medicines are aimed to direct and stimulate the body’s self-regulatory mechanisms. Homeopathy is highly individualized while taking into account the symptoms and signs of the disease, patient’s physical attributes, personality, temperament and genetic predispositions. Apart from homeopathic medication, advice on change of lifestyle, diet and remedies abuse behaviors, acquisition of stress-reduction techniques and exercise are part of the package of care provided by the nurses working close together in praxis. Number of patients and medical, paramedical employers tend to use homeopathy as in Europe, as in Hungary [4-11].

## Discussion

According to increasing demand of patient and nurses, doctors, homeopathy is accepted in Hungary by health care providers as an additional part of health care profession in spite of negative attitude of academic medicine schools [1-3]. The health care professionals in Budapest -being the capital of Hungary- are more interested and involved in newer complementary therapies, they visited more frequently on courses jointed to topic and introduced knowledge sooner into daily use.

The unified “education-teaching system-control” is necessary to achieve safety of patients who wanted to be cured with homeopathy [3]. It is necessary to organize further education for nurses at Health Science Faculties of Universities. They have a closer connection to patients in their daily practice. The demand for CAM therapies is getting larger by patients. This generates more interest by the following practitioners. This recent situation according to international trends in EU has a similarity in Hungary too [12]. Additionally we recognized some negative attitudes of medical universities for introducing of Homeopathy into medical curriculums of medical students with arguments of skeptical opinions.

To summarize the recent situation in the European Union in relation of Homeopathy and university: Postgraduate training courses in homeopathy for doctors are provided at universities in Bulgaria, France, Germany (five universities), Greece (some universities), Italy (one university), Lithuania, Poland (eight universities), Romania (eight universities) and Spain (three universities), in other countries at private teaching centers only, but the final exam after the courses is provided in Hungary et University Pécs, CAM Department (one only in Hungary) [12-14]. Homeopathy is an official part of the Continuous Education Program for doctors in Hungary and Romania. CAM has, however, not been given a similar degree of attention despite its widespread and advised use [8]. A lectureship specifically for homeopathy exists only in the Netherlands (Amsterdam), a professorial chair of CAM including homeopathy in Hungary (Pécs) and Switzerland (Bern) [15].

Despite of recent bad economic situation in Europe (and Hungary), (it means there is no reimbursement by state insurance) health care professional nurses use homeopathy more frequently. Furthermore, they have more knowledge and homeopathy has implanted into their daily practice in the last two decades [4,5,16].

According to old proverb: "What you cannot arrest, you should lead...", we propose scientific explanation, more research on effectiveness and efficacy in the frame of University. Further advice is to address organizers additional Homeopathic courses for nurses as a part of obligatory further education, which could be useful for ethical application for shake of patient' safety they want to use homeopathic remedies [17,18]. Health care professionals meet patients frequently giving them "life style advises" including not only use of medicaments, they should know indications and contraindications of different natural healing methods like Homeopathy.

It seems to be useful application of CAM therapies like homeopathy because easy medication of antibiotics became less for unnecessary reason ("preventive") in pediatric profession where practitioner was educated in Homeopathy too.

Declaration: There is no conflict of interest of any authors, (including pharmaceutical companies existing in Europe, Hungary)

## Supplement

The CAM Department of the University of Pécs (established 1367) provides education, controls and exams. Studies are offered for MDs only, and the following treatments are examples of courses provided: acupuncture, TCM, manual medicine (chiropractic, osteopathy), neural therapy, anthroposophy medicine, life-style adviser. Courses at other educational institutions offer studies for non-medical professionals (= natural healers, additionally part of the health care system) for courses like acupressure, reflexology, NADA (detoxification), eye training, herbal medicine, kinesiology, complementary moving and massage therapies, complementary physiotherapies (Kneipp courses, electro, magneto, UV e.t. practice) [1-3]. Health care practitioners (non-medical educated practitioners: nurses and natural healers) may offer CAM treatments like; acupressure, reflexology, NADA (special acupuncture techniques of detoxification), eye training, herbal medicine, kinesiology, complementary moving and massage therapies, complementary physiotherapies (Kneipp courses, electro, magneto, UV e.t.) practice after state exam [1-3]. National CAM legislation regulates health products and the use, practice and education of CAM (Homeopathic remedies are regulated by the pharmaceutical law). However, CAM non-medical practitioners (herbalist, many non-MDs, and acupressure therapist and others) are not regulated by the state. The Provincial and Territorial Government Agency regulates and controls regional health care practitioners. This public health system constitutes a heterogeneous regulation system in Hungary and challenges the CAM legislation. Legislative review and re-organization in several provinces have resulted in the establishment of permanent mechanisms for regulation of CAM practitioners including possible statutory self-regulation as health care practitioners in the future. The governmental supervision of CAM Practices: The national government of Hungary exercise statutory supervision of health services, including the Health Insurance Fund (HIF). The National CAM Supervisor Committee has the right to control and punish. Regulated CAM providers are included in the governmental supervisor Head Physician-system [1-3]. The University of PÉCS (Faculty of Health Science, CAM Department) offers a 3-year educational program for homeopathy with CME, CEP points only for medical doctors. Homeopaths have to be registered in a statutory register for legal practice. Pharmacists can be involved into courses without personal practice [19-22].

## References


1. Decree of the Ministry of Social Welfare on the practice of CAM), the government of Hungary (1997). 11/1997(V.28.) NM. –"Rendelet a természetgyógyászati tevékenység gyakorlásának egyes kérdéseiről"
2. Governmental Decree on CAM), The Parliament of Hungary (1997), 40/1997(III.5.)
3. http://net.jogtar.hu/jr/gen/hjegy_doc.cgi?docid=99700040.KOR&celpara=#xcelparam
4. Hahnemann, Samuel (1833). The Homœopathic Medical Doctrine, or "Organon of the Healing Art". Dublin: W.F. Wakeman. pp. iii, 48–49
5. Hippocrates, (born c. 460 BC , Island of Cos, Greece—died c.375 , Larissa, Thessaly), ancient Greek physician who lived during Greece's Classical period and is traditionally regarded as the father of medicine): Hippocratic Writings, G.E.R. Lloyd (ed.), Translated by J. Chadwick and W.N. Mann, Penguin Books, London etc., 1983.
6. Ernst E (2002) A systematic review of systematic reviews of homeopathy. Br J Clin Pharmacol 54: 577-582.
7. Ernst E, Pittler MH (1998) Efficacy of homeopathic arnica: a systematic review of placebo-controlled clinical trials. Arch Surg 133: 1187-1190.
8. Walach H (1999) Magic of signs: a non-local interpretation of homeopathy. Journal of Scientific Exploration 13: 291-315.
9. Pfeiffer H, Drescher M, Hirte M (2012) Homöopathie in der Kinder- und Jugendmedizin, Verlag Urban & Fischer 2007, ÄrzteWoche, SpringerMedizin-Verlag.
10. Fischer FH, Lewith G, Witt CM, Linde K, Ammon KV, et al. (2014) High prevalence but limited evidence in complementary and alternative medicine: guidelines for future research. BMC Complementary and Alternative Medicine 14: 46.
11. Ammon KV, Frei H, Kaufmann F, Schmitz SFH, Steinlin M, et al. (2010) Homoeopathic RCT embedded in an observational study of children with attention deficit hyperactivity disorder - a successful model of whole-systems CAM research. Focus on Alternative and Complementary Therapies 12: 5-5.
12. The Medicines and Healthcare products Regulatory Agency (MHRA). Department of Health announcement about the regulation of herbal practitioners - including questions and answers: News 18 February 2011. London: MHRA.
13. CAMbrella Deliverable 9–WP2 report no.1–CAM in European countries-30 April 2012, FP7- HEALTH-2009, GA No. 241951-Project duration: 01/01/2010 – 31/12/2012.
14. Wiesener S, Falkenberg T, Hegyi G, Hök J, Roberti di Sarsina P (2012) Legal status of Complementary Medicine in Europe, Forschende Komplementärmedizin/Research in Complementary Medicine.
15. Bodeker G, Kronenberg F (2002) A public health agenda for traditional, complementary, and alternative medicine. Am J Public Health 92: 1582-1591.
16. White AR, Resch KL, Ernst E (1997) Complementary medicine: use and attitudes among GPs. Fam Pract 14: 302-306.
17. CAMbrella Project Reports, WP1-8. www.cambrella.eu
18. Wetzel MS, Kaptchuk TJ, Haramati A, Eisenberg DM (2003) Complementary and alternative medical therapies: implications for medical education. Ann Intern Med 138: 191-196.
19. von Ammon K, Frei-Erb M, Cardini F, Daig U, Dragan S, Hegyi G, et al. (2012) Complementary and alternative medicine provision in Europe--first results approaching reality in an unclear field of practices. Forsch Komplementmed 19: 37-43.
20. Eardley S, Bishop FL, Cardini F, Santos-Rey K, Jong MC, et al. (2012) A pilot feasibility study of a questionnaire to determine EU wide Complementary and Alternative Medicine (CAM) use. Forsch Komplementmed 19: 14-27.

21. Eardley S, Bishop FL, Prescott P, Cardini F, Brinkhaus B, et al. (2012) A systematic literature review of Complementary and Alternative Medicine (CAM) prevalence in EU. Forsch Komplementmed 19:18-28.

22. Wiesener S, Falkenberg T, Hegyi G, Hök J, Roberti di Sarsina P, et al. (2012) Legal status and regulation of complementary and alternative medicine in Europe. Forsch Komplementmed 19 Suppl 2: 29-36.

2

# Bufadienolides Overcome TRAIL Resistance in Breast Cancer Cells via JAK-STAT Pathway

**Lia Hafiyani, Satoru Yokoyama, Sherif Abdelhamed, Yoshihiro Hayakawa and Ikuo Saiki***

*Division of Pathogenic Biochemistry, Institute of Natural Medicine, University of Toyama, Toyama, Japan*

**Abstract**

**Aim and objective:** Although the clinical significance of tumor necrosis factor-related apoptosis-inducing ligand (TRAIL) has been elucidated, primary or acquired resistance to TRAIL limits its efficacy in cancer patients. This study aimed to investigate bufadienolides as promising candidates to combine with TRAIL and to determine the pathway involved in overcoming TRAIL resistance in breast cancer cells.

**Methods:** The effects of bufadienolides, cinobufagin and cinobufotalin, in combination with TRAIL were examined in TRAIL-sensitive and TRAIL-resistant breast cancer, MDA-MB-231 and MDA-MB-468 cells, respectively. Cell viability was determined using count and viability assays. Apoptotic cell death was detected by annexin-V/7-AAD staining. Silencing of MCL-1 expression was established using MCL-1 siRNA and protein expression was assessed by Western blot analysis. STAT3 localization was determined using immunofluorescence staining.

**Results:** The combination of bufadienolides with TRAIL significantly reduced cell viability in both TRAIL-sensitive and TRAIL-resistant breast cancer cells *in vitro*. Bufadienolides overcame TRAIL resistance by downregulating MCL-1, an anti-apoptotic protein, through the JAK-STAT pathway. The combination of TRAIL with knock down of MCL-1 or JAK-STAT inhibitor, JSI-124, could synergistically induce apoptosis similar to bufadienolides.

**Conclusion:** Bufadienolides enhance TRAIL-induced apoptosis in breast cancer cells through Mcl-1 downregulation via JAK-STAT pathway. Targeting MCL-1 or JAK2 could be one of the strategies to overcome breast cancer cell resistance to TRAIL. Bufadienolides, through JAK2/STAT3/MCL-1 inhibition, could be considered as promising cancer therapy agents in combination with TRAIL.

**Keywords:** Bufadienolides; MCL-1; Breast cancer; JAK-STAT pathway

## Introduction

Breast cancer is the most frequently diagnosed cancer and the leading cause of cancer death in women in both economically developed and developing countries, accounting for 23% of total new cancer cases and 14% of total cancer deaths in 2008 [1]. According to the molecular markers to determine prognosis and treatment, breast cancers can be classified into estrogen receptor (ER)-positive tumors, progesterone receptor (PR)-positive tumors, overexpress one of the members of the epidermal-growth-factor receptor family (HER2/Neu)-positive tumors, or none of these; known as triple-negative breast cancer (TNBC) [2]. Due to its lack of three receptors, TNBC therapy is a difficult clinical challenge because of its unresponsiveness to endocrine therapy or other available targeted therapy.

While endocrine therapy cannot help in the management of TNBC, a promising therapy for various types of cancers including TNBC is tumor necrosis factor-related apoptosis-inducing ligand (TRAIL) because of its high selectivity for various carcinomas over normal cells [3]. TRAIL has been shown to induce apoptosis via both extrinsic (non-mitochondrial) and intrinsic (mitochondrial) pathways [4-6]. Even though the clinical significance of TRAIL has been investigated [7], primary or acquired resistance to TRAIL limits its clinical efficacy in cancer patients [8,9]. Several molecules are involved in TRAIL resistance, including the involvement of anti-apoptotic mechanisms (BCL-2, MCL-1, BCL-XL, etc), defects in death receptor signaling (death receptor 4 and death receptor 5), and overexpression of Six1 [8-12]; however, even though the antitumor effect of TRAIL as a single agent is limited, TRAIL exerts marked antitumor activity upon combination with various cytotoxic drugs [6,10].

It has been reported that chemical compounds from natural products could overcome TRAIL resistance, such as chrysin, curcumin, and wogonin [13-18]. Among these natural products, we focused on two bufadienolides, cinobufagin and cinobufotalin, which are known as cardiotonic steroids, because their antitumor activities as single agents in a wide type of tumors have been previously shown [19-21]. Bufadienolides are the major constituents of cinobufacini extracted from the skin and parotid venom glands of the giant toad *Bufo bufo gargarizans Cantor,* which has been widely used for thousands of years in China as a cardiotonic, antimicrobial, local anesthetic, and anti-neoplastic agent in clinical practice [21].

In this study, we demonstrate bufadienolides as promising candidates to TRAIL-based combination therapy, and investigate the molecular pathway involved in its effect to overcome TRAIL resistance in MDA-MB-468 breast cancer cells.

## Materials and Methods

### Drugs and reagents

Cinobufagin and cinobufotalin were purchased from Wako Pure

***Corresponding author:** Dr. Ikuo Saiki, Division of Pathogenic Biochemistry, Institute of Natural Medicine, University of Toyama, 2630 Sugitani, Toyama 930-0194, Japan, E-mail: byosei@inm.u-toyama.ac.jp

Chemical Industries, Ltd. (Osaka, Japan). Recombinant human TRAIL was purchased from PeproTech (PeproTech, London, UK).

## Cell culture

MDA-MB-231 and MDA-MB-468 (ATCC, Rockville, MD, USA) were cultured in Dulbecco's modified eagle's medium (DMEM) supplemented with 10% heat-inactivated fetal calf serum, 2 mM L-glutamine, 100 U/ml penicillin, and 10 μg/ml streptomycin. Cells were maintained at 37°C in a humidified atmosphere of 5% $CO_2$/95% air.

## Count and cell viability assay

Viability of the cells following treatment was determined using the MUSE Count and Viability Kit (Merck KGaA, Darmstadt, Germany) according to the manufacturer's instructions. Briefly, cinobufagin- or cinobufotalin-containing medium was added at a final concentration of 10, 25, and 50 μM and, after 30 min, TRAIL was added. After 24 h further incubation, all cells were collected and diluted with phosphate buffered saline (PBS) to a concentration of $2 \times 10^5$ cells/ml. 50 μl of cell suspension was then added into 450 μl MUSE Count and Viability reagent (10x dilution), incubated for 5 min at room temperature, and analyzed using the MUSE Cell Analyzer. Relative cell viability and synergistic effects were determined as previously described [22,23].

## Annexin V & dead cell assay

Apoptotic cell number was determined using the MUSE Annexin V & Dead Cell Kit (Merck KGaA) according to the manufacturer's instructions. Briefly, after cells were incubated for 24 h, cinobufagin- or cinobufotalin-containing medium was added, cells were incubated for 30 min, and then stimulated with TRAIL. After 12 h further incubation, all cells were collected and diluted with PBS containing 1% bovine serum albumin (BSA) as a dilution buffer to a concentration of $5 \times 10^5$ cells/ml. 100 μl of cell suspension was then added to 100 μl MUSE Annexin V & dead cell reagent (2 × dilution), incubated for 20 min at room temperature, and analyzed using the MUSE Cell Analyzer.

## Western blot analysis

After treatment, whole cell lysates, cytoplasmic extracts, and nuclear extracts were collected as described previously [23]. Equal amounts of protein were resolved by electrophoresis on acrylamide gels. Primary antibodies specific to caspase-3, poly (ADP-ribose) polymerase (PARP), XIAP, MCL-1, BCL-XL, BCL-2, BAX, FLIP, TRAF2, TRAF5, STAT3 and the phosphorylated form of STAT3 (Tyr705 and Ser727), AKT (Ser473), ERK1/2 (Thr202/Tyr204), p65 NF-κB (Ser536) were purchased from Cell Signaling Technology (MA, USA). Primary antibodies specific to β-actin, AKT, ERK1/2, and p65 NF-κB were purchased from Santa Cruz Biotechnology (Santa Cruz, CA, USA).

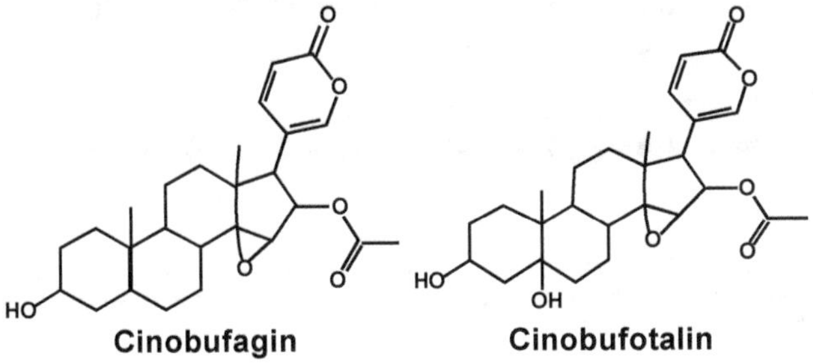


**Figure 1a:** Chemical structure of cinobufagin and cinobufotalin. Bufadienolides synergistically induce apoptosis with TRAIL in human TNBC cells.

## Transfection of small interfering RNAs

Silencing of MCL-1 expression in MDA-MB-468 cells was performed as described previously [13]. Human MCL-1 Stealth RNAi siRNA (HSS181042) was purchased from Invitrogen, (Carlsbad, CA, USA). Firefly luciferase siRNA was obtained from Hokkaido System Science Co. Ltd. (Sapporo, Japan) and used as control siRNA. MDA-MB-468 cells were transfected with each siRNA at a final concentration of 20 nM, using Lipofectamine RNAiMax (Invitrogen, Carlsbad, CA, USA).

## Immunofluorescence staining

After 12 h bufadienolide treatment, cells were washed with warm PBS, fixed with 4% paraformaldehyde for 10 min at room temperature, permeabilized with 0.1% Triton-X/PBS for 10 min at RT and blocked with 1% BSA/0.1% Triton-X solution for 1 hr at RT. For the detection of STAT3, cells were incubated with the primary antibody (x100) for 12 h at 4°C. After washing, cells were treated with secondary antibody (x30) using Rhodamine-conjugated swine anti-rabbit IgG (DakoCytomation, Glostrup, Denmark) for 1 h at RT. Finally, cells were mounted using VECTASHIELD mounting medium containing 4',6-diamidino-2-phenylindole (DAPI) (Vector Laboratories, Burlingame, CA). Confocal fluorescence images were observed by LSM700 microscopy and ZEN software (Carl Zeiss, Oberkochen, Germany).

## Statistical analysis

The results are expressed as the mean ± standard deviation. Statistical significance ($p<0.05$) was evaluated by either Student's two-tailed t-test or one-way ANOVA followed by the Bonferroni post hoc test, comparing the results to the control.

# Results

## Combination with bufadienolides enhances TRAIL-induced apoptosis in triple-negative breast cancer cells

To evaluate the cytotoxicity of bufadienolides, cinobufagin and cinobufotalin (Figure 1a), and their combination with TRAIL to TNBC cells, we chose TRAIL-sensitive or -resistant TNBC cells, MDA-MB-231 or MDA-MB-468, respectively [22]. Even though bufadienolides have been shown to be anti-tumor agents [19-21], these compounds showed limited cytotoxicity in both TNBC cell lines (Figure 1b). Interestingly, both bufadienolides could significantly increase TRAIL-induced cytotoxicity in TNBC cells, even in TRAIL-resistant cells, MDA-MB-468 cells, compared to single therapy with TRAIL or bufadienolides alone.

We next examined whether bufadienolides overcome TRAIL resistance in TRAIL-resistant cells through apoptosis, because only the combination of bufadienolides with TRAIL could show cytotoxicity even in MDA-MB-468 cells, without any cytotoxicity by either bufadienolides or TRAIL alone. Annexin-V-positive cells were increased in TRAIL/bufadienolide-treated cells compared with non-treated, TRAIL-treated, or bufadienolide-treated cells (Figure 1c). In addition, the cleavage of pro-caspase-3, and poly (ADP-ribose) polymerase (PARP) protein were detected as hallmarks of apoptosis only in TRAIL/bufadienolide-treated cells (Figure 1d). These data suggest that bufadienolides could overcome TRAIL resistance in TRAIL-resistant TNBC cells.

## Bufadienolides suppress MCL-1 expression

To identify the mechanisms by which bufadienolides overcome TRAIL resistance, we further examined several proteins related to

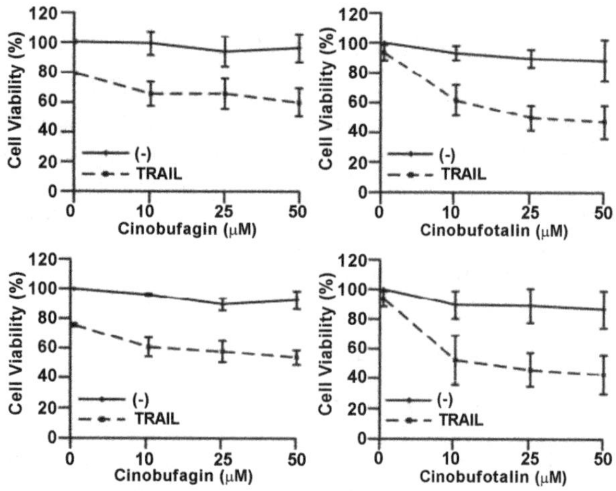


**Figure 1b:** MDA-MB-231 and MDA-MB-468 cells were pretreated with cinobufagin or cinobufotalin at various concentrations (10 μM, 25 μM, and 50 μM) for 30 min, followed with or without TRAIL (50 ng/mL) for 24 h. Cell viability was determined by count and cell viability assays.

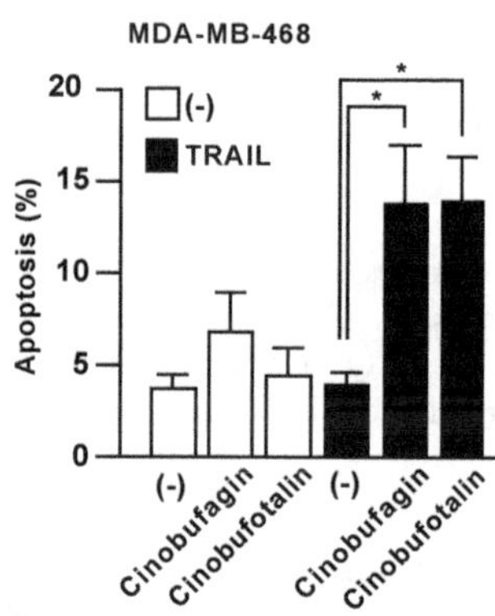


**Figure 1c:** MDA-MB-468 cells were pretreated with 25 μM cinobufagin or cinobufotalin for 30 min, followed with or without TRAIL (50 ng/mL) for 12 h. Total apoptotic cells were determined by Annexin V and dead cell assays. *p <0.01 vs. non-treated cells by one-way ANOVA followed by the Bonferroni test, n = 3.

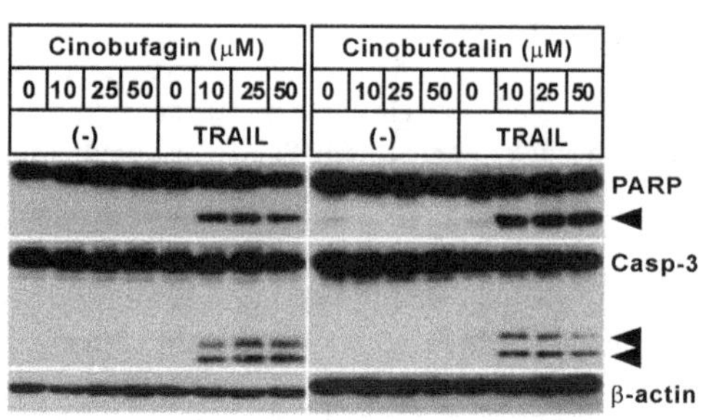


**Figure 1d:** MDA-MB-468 cells were pretreated with cinobufagin or cinobufotalin at various concentrations (10 μM, 25 μM, and 50 μM) for 30 min, followed with or without TRAIL (50 ng/mL) for 12 h. Whole cell extract was subjected to Western blot analysis using antibodies against the indicated proteins. Arrows indicate cleaved forms of caspase-3 and PARP.

either intrinsic (BCL-2, BCL-XL, MCL-1, BAX) or extrinsic (TRAF2, TRAF5, XIAP, FLIP) pathways of TRAIL in MDA-MB-468 cells [4-6]. Both cinobufagin and cinobufotalin could selectively suppress MCL-1 expression with either bufadienolide alone or in combination with TRAIL (Figure 2a). We also confirmed the time- and dose-dependent MCL-1 suppression in concert with the induction of apoptotic markers (Figure 2b), suggesting that MCL-1 could be involved in overcoming TRAIL resistance.

## Silencing MCL-1 expression is sufficient to overcome TRAIL resistance in MDA-MB-468 cells

To investigate its role in overcoming TRAIL resistance, MCL-1 was knocked down in MDA-MB-468 cells using siRNA against MCL-1 (siMCL-1). The cleavage of caspase-3 and PARP could be detected only in siMCL-1-transfected cells with TRAIL (Figure 3a). Consistently, we could also detect apoptosis by using annexin V staining in siMCL-1-transfected cells treated with TRAIL (Figure 3b). Taken together, MCL-1 downregulation is sufficient to overcome TRAIL resistance in MDA-MB-468, and to induce apoptosis with TRAIL.

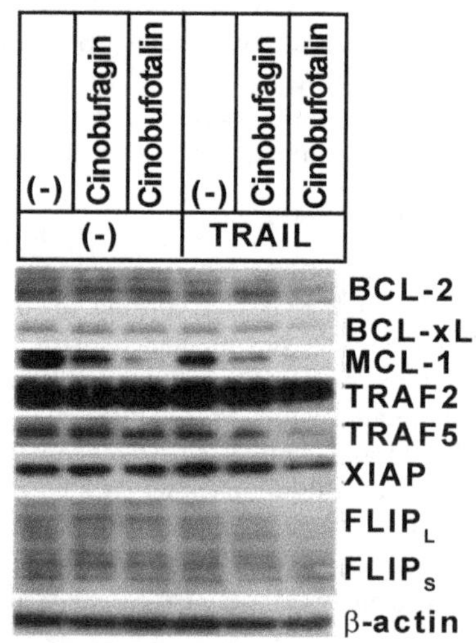


**Figure 2a:** Bufadienolides suppress MCL-1 expression. Whole cell extract was subjected to Western blot analysis against the indicated proteins related with the intrinsic and extrinsic death pathways of TRAIL. Arrows indicate two forms of FLIP. Other conditions were similar to figure 1c.

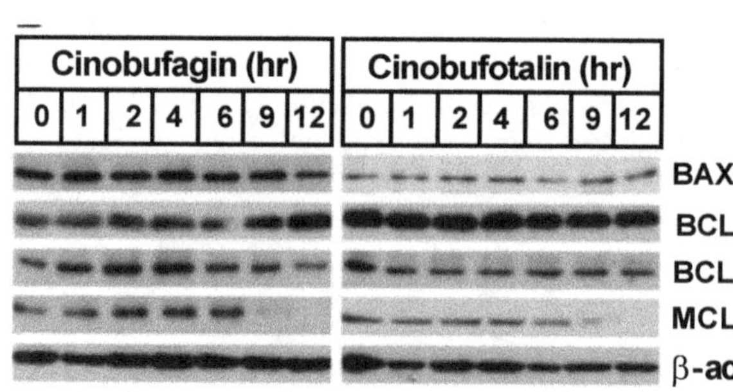


**Figure 2b:** MDA-MB-468 cells were treated with 25 μM cinobufagin or cinobufotalin for the indicated time. Whole cell extract was subjected to Western blot analysis.

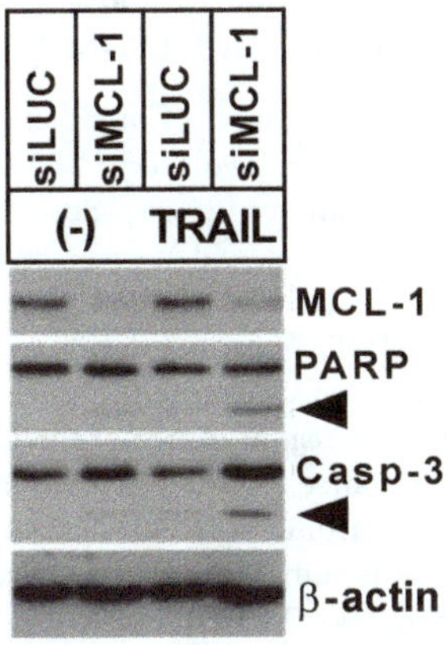


**Figure 3a:** Silencing MCL-1 expression is sufficient to overcome TRAIL resistance in MDA-MB-468 cells. MDA-MB-468 cells were transfected with siRNA against luciferase and MCL-1 for 24 h, followed with or without TRAIL (50 ng/mL) for 12 h. Whole cell extract was subjected to Western blot analysis using antibodies against the indicated proteins.

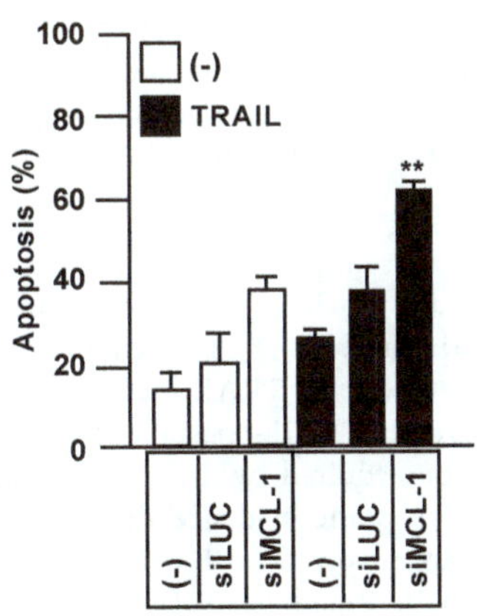


**Figure 3b:** The cells were subjected to Annexin V and dead cell assays. Other conditions were similar to figure 3a.

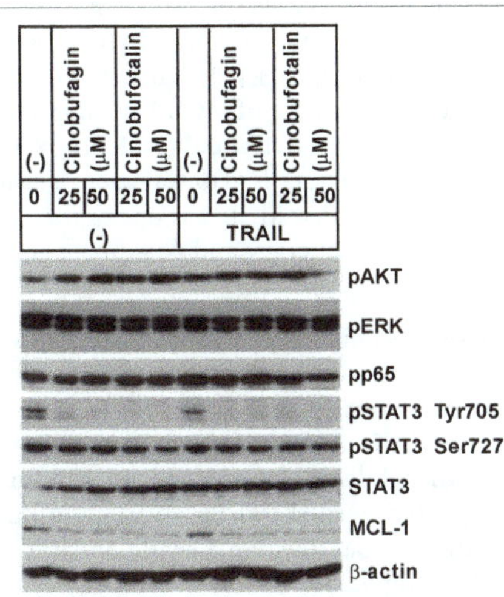


**Figure 4a:** Inhibition of STAT3 Tyr705 phosphorylation and nuclear translocation mediates MCL-1 downregulation by bufadienolides in MDA-MB-468 cells. MDA-MB-468 cells were pretreated with cinobufagin or cinobufotalin at 25 μM and 50 μM for 30 min, followed with or without TRAIL (50 ng/mL) for 12 h. Whole cell extract was subjected to Western blot analysis using antibodies against the indicated proteins.

## Inhibition of STAT3 phosphorylation and nuclear translocation mediate MCL-1 downregulation by bufadienolides in MDA-MB-468 cells

We further examined the effects of bufadienolides on several MCL-1 upstream proteins related to AKT, ERK, NF-κB, and STAT pathways [24]. Amongst these proteins, bufadienolides markedly suppressed constitutive STAT3 tyrosine phosphorylation (Tyr705), which is necessary for STAT3 translocation to the nucleus and its transcriptional activity in the targeted genes, including MCL-1 [25,26]. The downregulation of pSTAT3 Tyr705 by bufadienolides was highly correlated to the decrease of MCL-1 protein in a dose- and time-dependent manner (Figures 4a and 4b). The phosphorylation at Ser727 of STAT3 could not be inhibited by bufadienolides, indicating that its inhibitory activity is specific to tyrosine kinases but not to serine/threonine kinases. To check the STAT3 nuclear localization, we performed immunofluorescence staining and Western blot analysis (Figures 4c and 4d). After bufadienolide treatments, STAT3 showed a ring-like appearance, indicating its localization in cytoplasm, while it was distributed evenly and diffusively both in the nucleus and cytoplasm of non-treated cells (Figure 4c). Similar to immunofluorescent staining, we could detect the suppression of nuclear STAT3 by Western blot

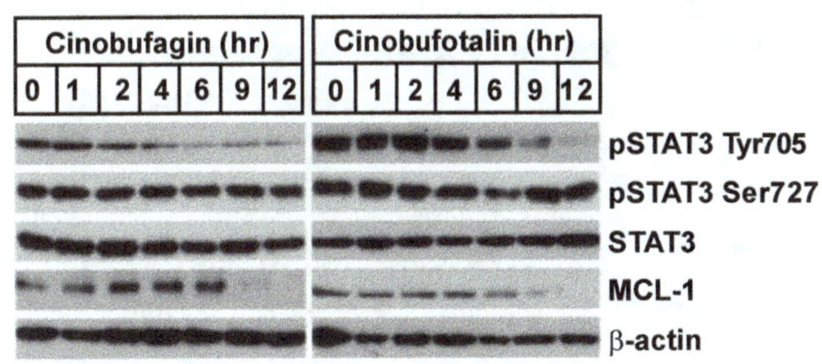


**Figure 4b:** Whole cell extract was subjected to Western blot analysis. Other conditions were similar to figure 2b.

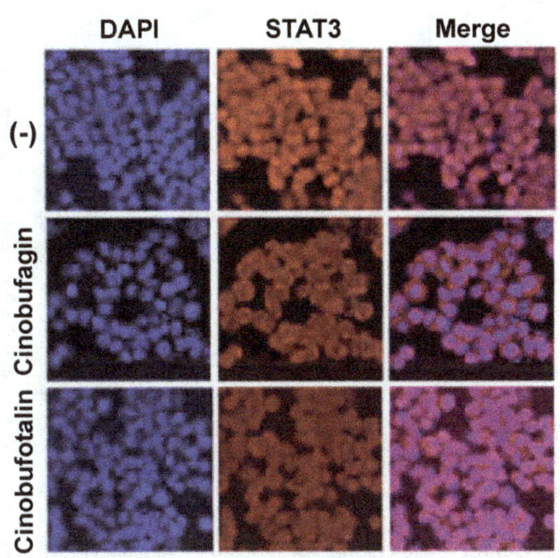


**Figure 4c:** MDA-MB-468 cells were treated with 25 μM cinobufagin or cinobufotalin for 12 h and subjected to immunofluorescence staining using STAT3 antibody and Rhodamine-conjugated swine anti-rabbit IgG.

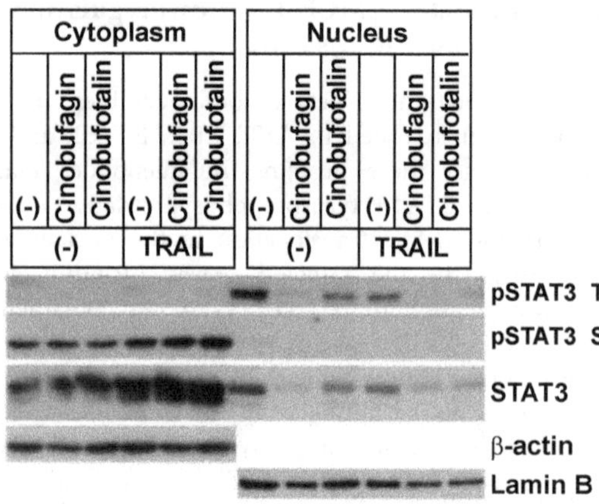


**Figure 4d:** Cytoplasmic fraction and nuclear fraction were prepared and subjected to Western blot analysis. Other conditions were similar to figure 2a.

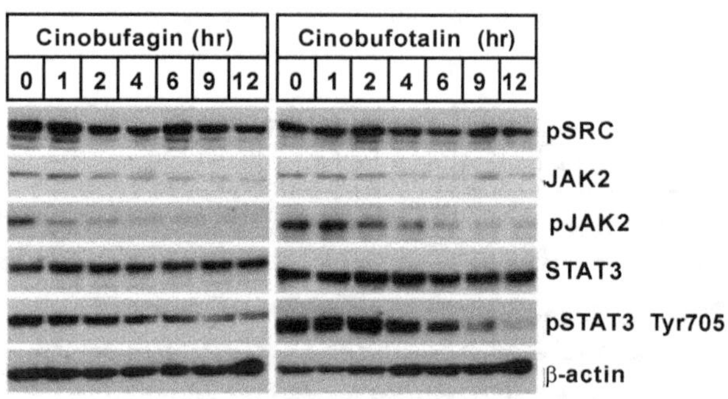


**Figure 5a:** JAK2 inhibition is sufficient for synergistic effects of bufadienolides with TRAIL in MDA-MB-468 cells. MDA-MB-468 cells were treated with 25 mM cinobufagin or cinobufotalin for the indicated time. Whole cell extract was subjected to Western blot analysis using antibodies against the indicated proteins

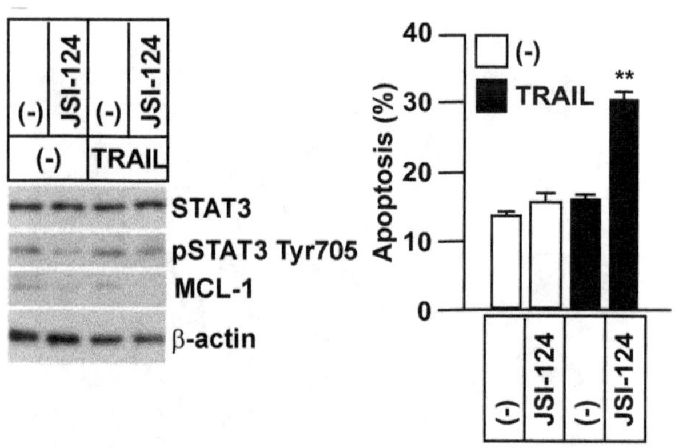


**Figure 5b:** MDA-MB-468 cells were treated with 1 μM JAK-STAT inhibitor, JSI-124, and TRAIL (50 ng/ml) for 12 h and subjected to Western blot analysis (left) and annexin V and dead cell assays (right).

analysis without any change of phosphorylated STAT3 at Ser727 (Figure 4d). Collectively, these data suggested that the phosphorylation at Tyr705 of STAT3 was the target of bufadienolides, leading to the inhibition of the nuclear translocation and transcriptional activity of STAT3 in MDA-MB-468 cells.

### JAK2 inhibition is sufficient to show synergistic effects of bufadienolides with TRAIL in MDA-MB-468 cells

To identify the upstream target of bufadienolides, we focused on the two major tyrosine kinases involved in STAT3 phosphorylation in breast cancer cells: JAK2 and Src [25-29]. Both the protein expression and phosphorylation of JAK2 were decreased by bufodienolides, while phosphorylation of Src remained unaffected (Figure 5a), suggesting that the downregulation of STAT3 phosphorylation by bufadienolides might be caused by suppression of JAK2 protein expression in MDA-MB-468 cells. Finally, to confirm the significance of the JAK-STAT pathway in overcoming TRAIL resistance, we inhibited the JAK-STAT pathway by using 1 μM JSI-124 (Cucurbitacin I) [30]. Strikingly, the combination of JSI-124 and TRAIL was sufficient to sensitize cancer cells to TRAIL, even though either JSI-124 or TRAIL alone could not induce apoptosis (Figure 5b). These results suggest that overcoming TRAIL resistance by bufadienolides could be mediated through inhibition of the JAK2-STAT3 pathway.

## Discussion

Our study showed that the combination of TRAIL and bufadienolides synergistically induced apoptosis in TRAIL-sensitive and even in TRAIL-resistant TNBC cells *in vitro*. Furthermore, bufadienolides enhanced apoptosis by decreasing MCL-1 expression, which is mediated through JAK2/STAT3 Tyr705 phosphorylation pathways.

Although TRAIL-based therapies, including anti-death receptor 5 agonistic antibody, have provided a significant clinical benefit in some cancer patients in clinical trials [7], the acquisition of drug resistance is known to limit the efficacy of TRAIL-based therapy [8,9]. Moreover, there are some inherently TRAIL-resistant breast cancers, and TRAIL resistance can also be acquired by cells that were originally TRAIL sensitive [10]. There is some evidence that BCL-2 family members containing MCL-1 are involved in TRAIL-resistance in cancer cells by enhancing the intrinsic pathways of TRAIL [31-35]. Consistently, we showed that knocking down MCL-1 is sufficient to overcome TRAIL resistance in MDA-MB-468 cells (Figure 3), regardless a lack of change in the caspase-8 or other extrinsic and intrinsic pathway-related proteins (Figure 2). Similar to MDA-MB-468 cells, MCL-1 downregulation is sufficient to overcome TRAIL resistance in A549 human lung adenocarcinoma cells [13]. Further investigation is still needed to confirm the significance of MCL-1 in other types of TRAIL-resistant cancers and its role in determining TRAIL-resistant cell lines compared to TRAIL-sensitive cells. However, our results and those reported previously suggest that MCL-1 is one of the most important molecules for TRAIL-based therapy and could be a good therapeutic target to overcome TRAIL resistance.

Although an MCL-1 inhibitor is a good candidate for combination therapy with TRAIL, it has been difficult to target only MCL-1 itself by BCL-2 family inhibitors. In addition to MCL-1, we identified the significance of the JAK2-STAT3 pathway in overcoming TRAIL resistance by bufadienolides (Figure 4 and 5). Clinically, persistent activation of STAT3 has been shown in a variety of human cancers, including pancreatic, prostate, ovarian, hepatic, and breast carcinomas, as well as in hematopoietic tumors, including lymphomas and leukemia [36-42], and also has been correlated with a poor prognosis [36,43]. In addition to constitutive active STAT3, IL-6 production in primary breast cancers plays a critical role in activating the JAK-STAT pathway and is widely known to be highly correlated with tumor cell proliferation, advanced stage breast cancers, and poor prognosis [44].

Given that human breast cancers produce more IL-6, which activates the JAK/STAT pathway, than matched healthy breast tissue, inhibition of the JAK-STAT pathway could be a promising target for breast cancer therapy.

We determined that bufadienolides suppressed MCL-1 expression via the JAK-STAT pathway; however our study could not exclude the possibility that other pathways were also involved in its effect on TRAIL sensitization. Previously, Bufadienolides have been shown to be cardiac glycosides, potent Na+ K+-ATPase inhibitors. Ouabain, also a cardiac glycoside, could suppress MCL-1 through ROS-mediated proteasomal degradation [45]. Another cardiac glycoside, thevefolin, overcomes TRAIL-resistance through enhancing the expression of TRAIL receptors in gastric cancer [46]. In addition to their role in TRAIL-induced apoptosis, inhibition of Na+ K+-ATPase by cardiac glycosides is important for overcoming multi-drug resistance and promoting anoikis [47,48], suggesting another possible role for cardiac glycosides in cancer therapy.

Taken together, pending further in vivo and clinical experiments to determine safe and optimal doses, bufadienolides or JAK inhibitors can be considered not only as adjuvants with TRAIL but also as single agents for triple-negative breast cancer therapy.

## Acknowledgement

We thank all members of the Saiki laboratory for discussions and suggestions. This study was supported in part by a Grant-in-Aid for Young Scientists (B) (No.24700971) (S.Y.), by Grant-in-aid for Challenging Exploratory Research 24659348 (I.S.) from the Ministry of Education, Culture, Sports, Science, and Technology (Japan), by The YASUDA Medical Foundation (S.Y.), by a Grant-in- Aid for the Cooperative Research Project (I.S.) from Joint Usage/Research Center (Joint Usage/Research Center for Science-Based Natural Medicine), Institute of Natural Medicine, University of Toyama in 2013.

## References

1. Jemal A, Bray F, Center MM, Ferlay J, Ward E, et al. (2011) Global cancer statistics. CA Cancer J Clin 61: 69-90.
2. Perou CM (2010) Molecular stratification of triple-negative breast cancers. Oncologist 15 Suppl 5: 39-48.
3. Keane MM, Ettenberg SA, Nau MM, Russell EK, Lipkowitz S (1999) Chemotherapy augments TRAIL-induced apoptosis in breast cell lines. Cancer Res 59: 734-741.
4. Ashkenazi A, Pai RC, Fong S, Leung S, Lawrence DA, et al. (1999) Safety and antitumor activity of recombinant soluble Apo2 ligand. J Clin Invest 104: 155-162.
5. Johnstone RW, Frew AJ, Smyth MJ (2008) The TRAIL apoptotic pathway in cancer onset, progression and therapy. Nat Rev Cancer 8: 782-798.
6. Walczak H, Miller RE, Ariail K, Gliniak B, Griffith TS, et al. (1999) Tumoricidal activity of tumor necrosis factor-related apoptosis-inducing ligand in vivo. Nat Med 5: 157-163.
7. Bellail AC, Qi L, Mulligan P, Chhabra V, Hao C (2009) TRAIL agonists on clinical trials for cancer therapy: the promises and the challenges. Rev Recent Clin Trials 4: 34-41.
8. Dyer MJ, MacFarlane M, Cohen GM (2007) Barriers to effective TRAIL-targeted therapy of malignancy. J Clin Oncol 25: 4505-4506.
9. Tolcher AW, Mita M, Meropol NJ, von Mehren M, Patnaik A, et al. (2007) Phase I pharmacokinetic and biologic correlative study of mapatumumab, a fully human monoclonal antibody with agonist activity to tumor necrosis factor-related apoptosis-inducing ligand receptor-1. J Clin Oncol 25: 1390-1395.
10. Thorburn A, Behbakht K, Ford H (2008) TRAIL receptor-targeted therapeutics: resistance mechanisms and strategies to avoid them. Drug Resist Updat 11: 17-24.
11. Behbakht K, Qamar L, Aldridge CS, Coletta RD, Davidson SA, et al. (2007) Six1 overexpression in ovarian carcinoma causes resistance to TRAIL-mediated apoptosis and is associated with poor survival. Cancer Res 67: 3036-3042.
12. Wagner KW, Punnoose EA, Januario T, Lawrence DA, Pitti RM, et al. (2007) Death-receptor O-glycosylation controls tumor-cell sensitivity to the proapoptotic ligand Apo2L/TRAIL. Nat Med 13: 1070-1077.
13. Lirdprapamongkol K, Sakurai H, Abdelhamed S, Yokoyama S, Athikomkulchai S, et al. (2013) Chrysin overcomes TRAIL resistance of cancer cells through Mcl-1 downregulation by inhibiting STAT3 phosphorylation. Int J Oncol 43: 329-337.
14. Deeb D, Jiang H, Gao X, Hafner MS, Wong H, et al. (2004) Curcumin sensitizes prostate cancer cells to tumor necrosis factor-related apoptosis-inducing ligand/Apo2L by inhibiting nuclear factor-kappaB through suppression of IkappaBalpha phosphorylation. Mol Cancer Ther 3: 803-812.
15. Ding J, Polier G, Kohler R, Giaisi M, Krammer PH, et al. (2012) Wogonin and related natural flavones overcome tumor necrosis factor-related apoptosis-inducing ligand (TRAIL) protein resistance of tumors by down-regulation of c-FLIP protein and up-regulation of TRAIL receptor 2 expression. J Biol Chem 287: 641-649.
16. Hasegawa H, Yamada Y, Komiyama K, Hayashi M, Ishibashi M, et al. (2006) Dihydroflavonol BB-1, an extract of natural plant Blumea balsamifera, abrogates TRAIL resistance in leukemia cells. Blood 107: 679-688.
17. Jeon KI, Rih JK, Kim HJ, Lee YJ, Cho CH, et al. (2003) Pretreatment of indole- 3-carbinol augments TRAIL-induced apoptosis in a prostate cancer cell line, LNCaP. FEBS Lett 544: 246-251.
18. Szliszka E, Sokol-Letowska A, Kucharska AZ, Jaworska D, Czuba ZP, et al. (2013) Ethanolic Extract of Polish Propolis: Chemical Composition and TRAIL-R2 Death Receptor Targeting Apoptotic Activity against Prostate Cancer Cells. Evid Based Complement Alternat Med 2013: 757628.
19. Emam H, Zhao QL, Furusawa Y, Refaat A, Ahmed K, et al. (2012) Apoptotic cell death by the novel natural compound, cinobufotalin. Chem Biol Interact 199: 154-160.
20. Ma L, Song B, Jin H, Pi J, Liu L, et al. (2012) Cinobufacini induced MDA-MB-231 cell apoptosis-associated cell cycle arrest and cytoskeleton function. Bioorg Med Chem Lett 22: 1459-1463.
21. Qi F, Li A, Inagaki Y, Kokudo N, Tamura S, et al. (2011) Antitumor activity of extracts and compounds from the skin of the toad Bufo bufo gargarizans Cantor. Int Immunopharmacol 11: 342-349.
22. Abdelhamed S, Yokoyama S, Hafiyani L, Kalauni SK, Hayakawa Y, et al. (2013) Identification of plant extracts sensitizing breast cancer cells to TRAIL. Oncol Rep 29: 1991-1998.
23. Sakurai H, Suzuki S, Kawasaki N, Nakano H, Okazaki T, et al. (2003) Tumor necrosis factor-alpha-induced IKK phosphorylation of NF-kappaB p65 on serine 536 is mediated through the TRAF2, TRAF5, and TAK1 signaling pathway. J Biol Chem 278: 36916-36923.
24. Akgul C (2009) Mcl-1 is a potential therapeutic target in multiple types of cancer. Cell Mol Life Sci 66: 1326-1336.
25. Berclaz G, Altermatt HJ, Rohrbach V, Siragusa A, Dreher E, et al. (2001) EGFR dependent expression of STAT3 (but not STAT1) in breast cancer. Int J Oncol 19: 1155-1160.
26. Berishaj M, Gao SP, Ahmed S, Leslie K, Al-Ahmadie H, et al. (2007) Stat3 is tyrosine-phosphorylated through the interleukin-6/glycoprotein 130/Janus kinase pathway in breast cancer. Breast Cancer Res 9: R32.
27. Garcia R, Bowman TL, Niu G, Yu H, Minton S, et al. (2001) Constitutive activation of Stat3 by the Src and JAK tyrosine kinases participates in growth regulation of human breast carcinoma cells. Oncogene 20: 2499-2513.

28. Rawlings JS, Rosler KM, Harrison DA (2004) The JAK/STAT signaling pathway. J Cell Sci 117: 1281-1283.

29. Seavey MM, Dobrzanski P (2012) The many faces of Janus kinase. Biochem Pharmacol 83: 1136-1145.

30. Blaskovich MA, Sun J, Cantor A, Turkson J, Jove R, et al. (2003) Discovery of JSI-124 (cucurbitacin I), a selective Janus kinase/signal transducer and activator of transcription 3 signaling pathway inhibitor with potent antitumor activity against human and murine cancer cells in mice. Cancer Res 63: 1270-1279.

31. Dong Y, Yin S, Li J, Jiang C, Ye M, et al. (2011) Bufadienolide compounds sensitize human breast cancer cells to TRAIL-induced apoptosis via inhibition of STAT3/Mcl-1 pathway. Apoptosis 16: 394-403.

32. Kim SH, Ricci MS, El-Deiry WS (2008) Mcl-1: a gateway to TRAIL sensitization. Cancer Res 68: 2062-2064.

33. Qi F, Inagaki Y, Gao B, Cui X, Xu H, et al. (2011) Bufalin and cinobufagin induce apoptosis of human hepatocellular carcinoma cells via Fas- and mitochondria-mediated pathways. Cancer Sci 102: 951-958.

34. Su CL, Lin TY, Lin CN, Won SJ (2009) Involvement of caspases and apoptosis-inducing factor in bufotalin-induced apoptosis of Hep 3B cells. J Agric Food Chem 57: 55-61.

35. Waiwut P, Inujima A, Inoue H, Saiki I, Sakurai H (2012) Bufotalin sensitizes death receptor-induced apoptosis via Bid- and STAT1-dependent pathways. Int J Oncol 40: 203-208.

36. Al Zaid Siddiquee K1, Turkson J (2008) STAT3 as a target for inducing apoptosis in solid and hematological tumors. Cell Res 18: 254-267.

37. Trevino JG, Gray MJ, Nawrocki ST, Summy JM, Lesslie DP, et al. (2006) Src activation of Stat3 is an independent requirement from NF-kappaB activation for constitutive IL-8 expression in human pancreatic adenocarcinoma cells. Angiogenesis 9: 101-110.

38. Abdulghani J, Gu L, Dagvadorj A, Lutz J, Leiby B, et al. (2008) Stat3 promotes metastatic progression of prostate cancer. Am J Pathol 172: 1717-1728.

39. Burke WM, Jin X, Lin HJ, Huang M, Liu R, et al. (2001) Inhibition of constitutively active Stat3 suppresses growth of human ovarian and breast cancer cells. Oncogene 20: 7925-7934.

40. Kortylewski M, Kujawski M, Wang T, Wei S, Zhang S, et al. (2005) Inhibiting Stat3 signaling in the hematopoietic system elicits multicomponent antitumor immunity. Nat Med 11: 1314-1321.

41. Cheng F, Wang HW, Cuenca A, Huang M, Ghansah T, et al. (2003) A critical role for Stat3 signaling in immune tolerance. Immunity 19: 425-436.

42. Li Y, Du H, Qin Y, Roberts J, Cummings OW, et al. (2007) Activation of the signal transducers and activators of the transcription 3 pathway in alveolar epithelial cells induces inflammation and adenocarcinomas in mouse lung. Cancer Res 67: 8494-8503.

43. Yu H, Pardoll D, Jove R (2009) STATs in cancer inflammation and immunity: a leading role for STAT3. Nat Rev Cancer 9: 798-809.

44. Sullivan NJ (2011) Interleukin-6 in the Breast Tumor Microenvironment: Breast Cancer - Focusing Tumor Microenvironment, Stem cells and Metastasis. InTech, Rijeka, Croatia.

45. Chanvorachote P, Pongrakhananon V (2013) Ouabain downregulates Mcl-1 and sensitizes lung cancer cells to TRAIL-induced apoptosis. Am J Physiol Cell Physiol 304: C263-272.

46. Miyagawa T, Ohtsuki T, Koyano T, Kowithayakorn T, Ishibashi M (2009) Cardenolide glycosides of Thevetia peruviana and triterpenoid saponins of Sapindus emarginatus as TRAIL resistance-overcoming compounds. J Nat Prod 72: 1507-1511.

47. Mijatovic T, Jungwirth U, Heffeter P, Hoda MA, Dornetshuber R, et al. (2009) The Na+/K+-ATPase is the Achilles heel of multi-drug-resistant cancer cells. Cancer Lett 282: 30-34.

48. Simpson CD, Mawji IA, Anyiwe K, Williams MA, Wang X, et al. (2009) Inhibition of the sodium potassium adenosine triphosphatase pump sensitizes cancer cells to anoikis and prevents distant tumor formation. Cancer Res 69: 2739-2747.

# 3

# Abri Cantongnesis Modulates Detoxifying Enzymes to Ameliorate Hepatotoxicity in Rats

**Jing Zheng Song and John WS Ho***

*Biochemistry Programme, School of Life Sciences, The Chinese University of Hong Kong, Shatin, Hong Kong*

**Abstract**

Abri cantongnesis in combination with herbs are used for treatment of diseases. However, the detail of its pharmacological activities is lacking. In this study, the chemoprotective effects of the active fraction of Abri cantongnesis on toxicant-induced liver toxicity in rats were studied. The Abri cantongnesis extract was orally administered to SD rats for three days before treatment of rats with trichloroethylene once for two days. Rat urines and hepatic enzymes were collected for analysis. The results showed that CYP 1A and CYP 2E1 and glutathione transferase increased over 45% while the activity of diaphorase increased by 30%. These enzyme activities were increased with the extract concentration. However, only UGT showed a decrease in activity upon treatment with Abri cantongnesis. The treatment of rats with Abri cantongnesis caused an increase in catalytic activities of CYP 1A and CYP 2E1, GST and diaphorase in the rat. The results show that Abri cantongnesis enhanced elimination of trichloroethylene and its metabolites; thus the treatment of Abri cantongnesis can reduce liver toxicity in rats. The findings suggest that Abri cantongnesis has chemopreventive effects on toxicants-induced hepatotoxicity in rats. The Abri cantongnesis can be used as a chemo-protective agent for the liver.

**Keywords:** Abri cantongnesis; Trichloroethylene; Carcinogenesis; Cytochrome P450s

## Introduction

The composition of herbal medicines for treatment of liver disorders contains Abri cantongnesis. However, the detail pharmacological activity of Abri cantongnesis is lacking. Abri cantongnesis is a member of the family Leguminosae of which active saponins are commonly found. Though the combination of Abri cantongnesis and other herbs has been used for treatment of liver disorders, it has not been used alone for treatment of disease. Ingestion of appropriate quantities of Abri cantongnesis can enhance hepatic functions in man and experimental animals [1,2]. Hepato-protective properties of Abri cantongnesis have been reported [3]. However, the pharmacological activity of Abri cantongnesis in the liver remains unclear. Trichloroethylene (TCE) is known to cause toxic effects in the liver. It was reported that TCE undergoes metabolism by two major pathways, namely, cytochrome P450-mediated oxidation and conjugation with glutathione (GSH) [4-6]. Differing rates and extent of TCE metabolism have been implicated as being responsible for the hepato-carcinogenic effects of TCE in mice and rats. Previous study reported that the metabolites of TCE, trichloroacetate (TCA) and/or dichloroacetate could induce hepatic tumors in mice [7-9]. If the formation of these metabolites can be attenuated, tumor formation can be inhibited. Several P450s have been implicated in TCE bio-activation, including CYP2E1 and CYP1A2 in man and lab animals [4,10,11]. In animal studies, the administration of TCE produced liver toxicity in the rat and its toxicity may be potentiated by alcohol consumption [12].

The aim of present study was to investigate effects of Abri cantongnesis on the trichloroethylene toxicity in the rat.

## Methods and Materials

### Chemicals

Trichloroethylene, trichloroacetic acid, trichloroethanol, *p*-nitrophenol (*p*-NP), β-nicotinamide adenine dinucleotide phosphate tetrasodium salt (NADPH), 2,6-dichlorophenol-indophenol (DCPIP), glutathione (GSH), uridine 5'-diphosphoglucuronic acid trisodium salt (98%, UDPGA), were purchased from Sigma Chemical Co (St. Louis, MO). Other chemicals and solvents were of analytical reagent grade.

### Animals, dosing and sample collection

Male Sprague-Dawley rats (150-180 g) were obtained from the Laboratory Animal Service Center of the Chinese University of Hong Kong. Rats were housed under controlled conditions (12 h light-dark cycles, 22°C, 60% humidity). They were fed a standard rodent chow and had water *ad libitum*. Rats were administered orally with Abri cantongnesis extract for three days, followed by TCE (2.4 g/kg) for two days. Urinary samples were collected at 24 and 48 h after TCE administration. The liver and blood were used for enzyme assays after rats were sacrificed. The serum was used for measurement of the activity of Glutamic Oxalacetic Transferase (GOT) and Glutamic Pyruvic Transferase (GPT).

### Preparation of microsomal fractions

The liver homogenate 20% (w/v) in 0.1M tris-sucrose buffer (pH 7.4) was centrifuged at 10,000 g for 20 min. The supernatant was centrifuged at 105,000 g for 60 min. The pellets were resuspended in 0.1 M tris-sucrose buffer (pH 7.4) and centrifuged again at 105,000 g for 60 min. The microsomes were resuspended in 50 mM phosphate buffer containing 1 mM EDTA and 10% glycerin (pH 7.4) and stored frozen at -70°C until use. The protein content of rat liver microsomes was measured by Bradford's method [13].

***Corresponding author:** John WS Ho, Biochemistry Programme, School of Life Sciences, The Chinese University of Hong Kong, Shatin, Hong Kong, E-mail: ws203ho@cuhk.edu.hk

### EROD assay (CYP 1A)

The microsomal P450 content was quantified according to the described method with modifications [14]. The reactions were done in 96-well plate. The fluorescent intensity was measured by the Cytfluor instrument for resorufin [15]. The reaction assay contained microsomal protein (20 μg), the substrate 7-ethoxyresorufin (2 μM), Tris-NaCl buffer (50 mM Tris base and 0.1 M NaCl, pH 7.8), and was started by the addition of NADPH 100 μM. The fluorescence of the assay was measured at an excitation wavelength of 590 nm and emission wavelength at 530 nm for 10 min at 2-minutes interval. The blank contained no enzyme. The reaction rate was determined based on standard curve using 1.25 nmol to 250 nmol resorufin in the reaction medium. The specific activity of the reaction was expressed in nmol resorufin formed/min/mg protein.

### p-Nitrophenol assay (CYP 2E1)

The *p*-nitrophenol hydroxylation activity was measured according to the previous method with modifications [16]. A total of 500 μl of the assay mixture contained 100 mM potassium phosphate buffer pH 7.4, 100 μM *p*-nitrophenol, 1 mM NADPH and micirosomal protein (200 g/ml). The assay was performed at 37°C for 0, 5, 10 and 20 min in the dark and terminated by the addition of 100 μl of 20% (w/v) tricholoroacetic acid. After centrifugation at 10,000 g for 5 min, 0.5 ml of the supernatant was mixed with 0.25 ml of 2M NaOH. The absorbance of *p*-Nitrocatechol was determined at 546 nm. All experiments were performed in triplicate.

### Glutathione S-transferase assay

The GST activity was measured with 1-Chloro-2,4-Dinitrobenzene (CDNB) according to the described method [17]. The reaction mixture contained 100 mM phosphate buffer (pH 6.5) and 1 mM GSH, and started by the addition of 1 mM CDNB.

### UDP-glucuronosyl transferase assay

The UGT activity was determined with *p*-nitrophenol as substrate by the established methods [18,19]. Microsomes (0.8 mg) were treated with 560 μg Emulgen 911 in 75 mM Tris-HCl buffer, pH 7.3; 5 mM $MgCl_2$, 2 mM UDP-glucuronic acid and 0.6 mM *p*-nitrophenol in a total volume of 0.4 mL and stirred continuously at 4°C for 30 min. The reaction was incubated at 37°C for 0, 5, 10 and 20 min in the dark, and was terminated by the addition of 20% (w/v) trichloroacetic acid to a final concentration of 3% (w/v). After centrifugation, 70 μL of supernatant was transferred to 1 mL of 0.5 M NaOH solution. The *p*-nitrophenol glucuronidation was measured by the change in absorbance at 400 nm with respect to time.

### DT-diaphorase assay

DT-diaphorase activity was measured according to the described method [20]. The reaction mixture contained 50 mM Tris-HCl, pH 7.5, 0.08% Triton X-100, 0.05 mM NADPH and 40 μM DCPIP. The assay was started by the addition of 100 μg protein of rat liver microsomes. The reduction of DCPIP was measured at 600 nm. An extinction co-efficient of 21.0 $mM^{-1}cm^{-1}$ at 600 nm for DCPIP was used. The DT-diaphorase activity was expressed as nmol $min^{-1}$ $mg^{-1}$ protein.

### Glutamic oxalacetic transferase (GOT) and glutamic pyruvic transferase (GPT) assay

The assay methods were the same as those described by Reiman and Frankel in the Sigma Diagnostics Transaminase reagents.

### Preparation of Abri cantongnesis

Small pieces (1 kg) of dried *Abri Cantongnesis* (SIPI-12-008-AC) were boiled in water (2000 mL) for 2 h. The mixture were filtered and concentrated under reduced pressure. The concentrated extract was dried with freeze dryer. About 85 g of the crude extract was obtained and extracted in a small volume (40 ml) of absolute ethanol.

### Analysis of the metabolites of TCE in rat urine

GC/MS analysis was conducted to determine the metabolites of TCE in rat urine. The GC-MS system consisted of a Hewlett-Packard (Palo Alto, CA, USA) HP6890 gas chromatography, a 5973 series mass selective detector, a HP 6890 auto-injector, a G1512A auto sampler controller and a Vectra XM series 45/166 computer using HP G1701AA MS Chem Station software (Version A.01.00). The capillary column was an HP-5 5% phenyl methyl siloxane (30 m x 0.25 mm I.D) with 0.50 μm film thickness. The carrier gas was set at a flow rate of 1.0 ml/min and a head pressure of 13.8 psi on the column. One μl of the sample in hexane-dichloromethane (1:1) was injected using splitless mode. Temperature of the injection port and mass selective detector interface were set at 150°C and 280°C, respectively. The temperature gradient of the GC oven was programmed to start at 60°C for 4 min, raised to 200°C at 50°C/min and held at the final temperature for 2 min. An Electron Impact (EI) ionization mode with the ionization of 70 eV was used. Perfluoro tributylamine was used for the calibration of the MS detector.

The derivatization procedure was done according to the published method [21] with modifications. Urine sample (200 μL) and internal standard (DCA, 200 mM in methanol, 5 L) were mixed with 500 μL of water-sulfuric acid-methanol (6:5:1) in tightly-capped glass tube. The mixture was heated at 70°C for 10 min. After cooling to room temperature, 500 μL of hexane-dichloromethane (1:1) was added to the mixture and vortexed for 10 min before centrifugation at 600 g for 5 min. The organic layer was used for GC-MS analysis. Chemical structures of the metabolites of TCE were identified using a full mass spectra scan mode in comparison with the authentic compounds.

## Results

### Hepatic enzyme activity

The TCE metabolites were measured by GC-MS. Treatment of rats with different concentrations of Abri cantongnesis produced significant effects on both cytochrome P450s and Phase II enzymes (Figure 1). Abri cantongnesis treatment produced a remarkable increase in the enzyme activity in the liver. CYP 2E1 and CYP1A1 exhibited a considerable increase ($P < 0.01$). The GST activity was considerably elevated while diaphorase was increased noticeably. The relative changes in enzyme activity were summarized in Table 1. Abri cantongnesis treatment decreased the GOT (Figure 2) and GPT (Figure 3) levels of TCE-treated rats. The activity of CYP 1A1 and CYP 2E1 increased up to 53% and 45% in Abri cantongnesis treated rats relative to those in the un-treated groups (Table 1). The increase was dose-dependent but represented a downward change in activity at dose > 5 kg.

### TCE metabolites

The ability of Abri cantongnesis to influence the activities of hepatic drug-metabolizing enzymes was recognized by the change in metabolite level. Trichloroethanol (TCEOH) and Trichloroacetate (TCA) were increased after Abri cantongnesis treatment (Figure 4).

However, no conjugated forms of TCE metabolites were observed. The levels of TCEOH and TCA in the urine from both the treated and un-treated rats were compared. Figure 4 showed the treatment of rats with the extract on the metabolite formation. The concentration of Abri cantongnesis affected the production of metabolite (Figure 5). Considerable changes were observed in the liver weight between the two groups (Figure 6).

## Discussion

The effects of Abri cantongnesis on TCE-induced liver toxicity in the rat were demonstrated in the study. Abri cantongnesis reduced the level of metabolite formation in the rat liver. The active fraction of Abri cantongnesis ameliorated the enzyme activity in the liver. Previous studies of TCE toxicity in animal and human livers showed that CYP 2E1 was more important isoform in TCE-induced carcinogenicity in rats and mice, although CYP 1A1 may also contribute. It is therefore believed that TCE activation by P450s and its toxicity can be attenuated by herbal medicines. In this study, CYP 2E1 and CYP 1A1 were both found to be responsible for the conversion of TCE to TCEOH and TCA. The activities of P450s were significantly enhanced by the Abri cantongnesis treatment (Table 1). The severity of TCE-induced hepato-toxicity in the rat can be abrogated by the treatment of rats with the active fraction. In as much as the difference between the treated and the un-treated rats with Abri cantongnesis is the biologic action of Abri cantongnesis on CYP 1A1, CYP 2E1 and the other hepatic enzymes, among which only UGT decreased in activity (P < 0.01) [4,5]. The present findings provide supporting experimental evidence that Abri cantongnesis can reduce liver toxicity related to TCE metabolism compared with the un-treated rats, which showed physiological changes in the liver manifested as increased plasma concentrations of the liver enzymes, GOT and GPT.

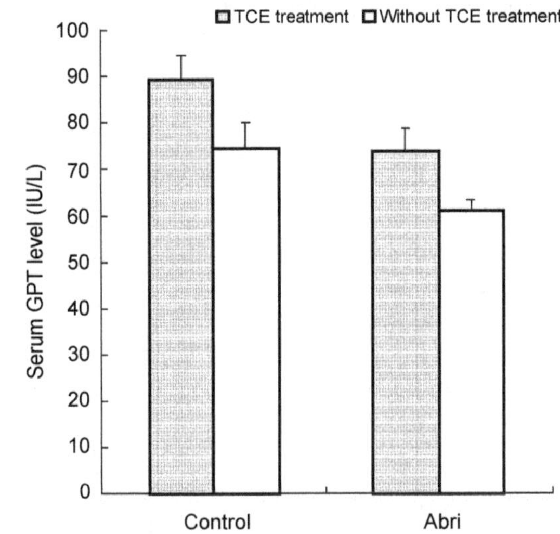


**Figure 3:** Effects of Abricantongnesis extract on GPT in rats.

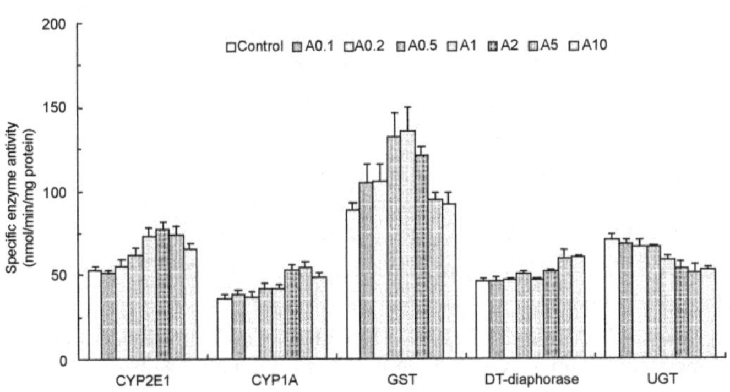


**Figure 1:** Effects of pre-treatment of rats with Abricantongnesis extract (g/kg) on the enzyme activity. Values represent the mean activity (n = 5). CYP 2E1 is 100-fold less than the specified value as indicated in the graph.

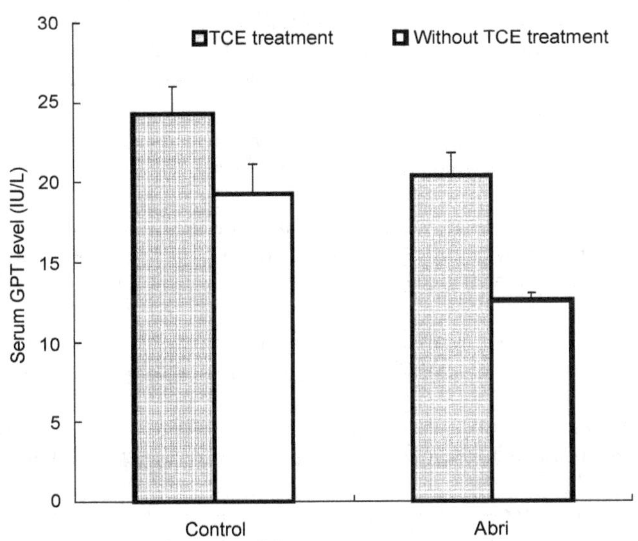


**Figure 2:** Effects of Abricantongnesis extract on GOT in treated and untreated rats.

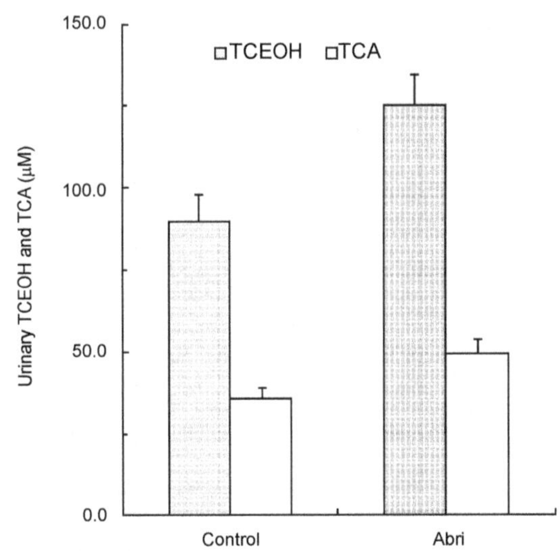


**Figure 4:** Effects of pre-treatment of rats with Abricantongnesis extract on metabolite production in the rat urine.

Early studies have demonstrated that P450-mediated TCE metabolism produced TCEOH and TCA, which are believed to be responsible for the subsequent TCE-induced carcinogenicity. Selective hydroxylation of TCE is more closely associated with TCE-induced hepato-toxicity than GST-mediated metabolic pathway. Treatment of

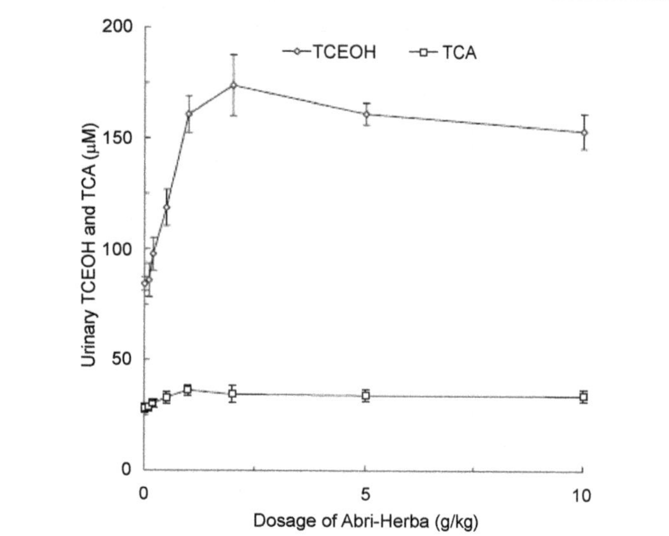


**Figure 5:** Changes of the metabolite level with the dosage of Abricantongnesis.

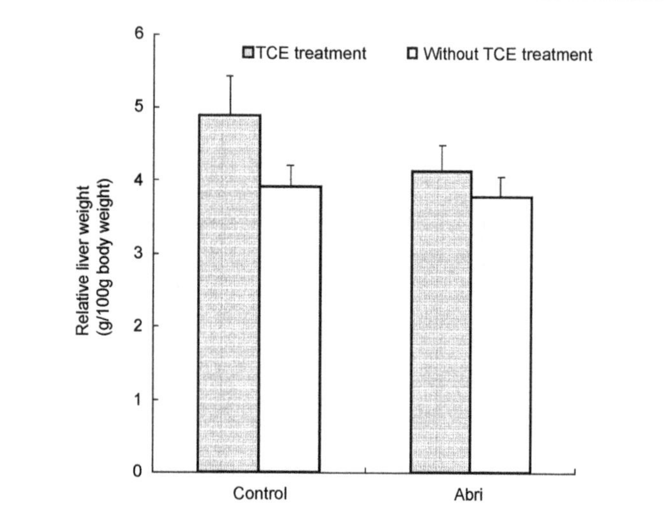


**Figure 6:** Effects of pre-treatment of rats with Abricantongnesis extract on the rat liver weight.

the rat with the Abri cantongnesis extract ameliorated the detoxifying enzyme activities. The increase of the drug-metabolizing enzyme activity in the treated group of rats suggest that the chemo-protective roles of Abri cantongnesis in reduction of toxicant-induced liver toxicity. The studies also demonstrated that these enzymes were responsible for activating TCE. Besides detoxifying enzymes, previous studies reported that GSH is important in TCE detoxification [22,23]. After treatment of rats with Abri cantongnesis, the increase in GST activity contributed to the elimination of toxic metabolites of TCE through conjugation reaction; thus, TCE-induced hepato-toxicity can be reduced in the rat. It is possible that the activation of TCE could be mediated to some extent by both GST and CYP 1A1 and CYP 2E1 which are the major enzymes associated with TCE metabolism.

In summary, the present studies demonstrate the therapeutic benefits of Abri cantongnesis in TCE-induced liver toxicity in rats through activation of enzymes in the rat. The findings suggest a functional significance of CYP 2E1 and CYP 1A1 in TCE-induced

| Dosage (g/kg) | CYP2E1 | CYP1A | GST | DT-diaphorase | UGT |
|---|---|---|---|---|---|
| 0.1 | -3.78 ± 0.20 | 7.06 ± 0.58 | 17.99 ± 0.74 | 0.22 ± 0.01 | -4.11 ± 0.19 |
| 0.2 | 3.78 ± 0.11 | 3.95 ± 0.32 | 18.78 ± 1.95 | 1.97 ± 0.13 | -5.52 ± 0.23 |
| 0.5 | 17.15 ± 1.27 | 17.80 ± 1.41 | 49.32 ± 4.00 | 10.28 ± 0.22 | -5.52 ± 0.36 |
| 1 | 38.67 ± 2.53 | 18.64 ± 1.35 | 53.17 ± 5.42 | 2.41 ± 0.08 | -16.29 ± 0.18 |
| 2 | 45.94 ± 3.02 | 49.15 ± 2.51 | 36.20 ± 4.30 | 13.35 ± 0.27 | -24.22 ± 1.17 |
| 5 | 40.31 ± 2.38 | 52.82 ± 3.42 | 7.24 ± 0.43 | 30.63 ± 0.62 | -27.05 ± 2.36 |
| 10 | 23.55 ± 1.64 | 36.16 ± 2.70 | 4.07 ± 0.19 | 33.04 ± 2.61 | -24.93 ± 2.21 |

**Table 1:** Relative percentage change in enzyme activity in rats after pre-treatment with Abri extract compared with the control.

toxicity. Comparison of the treated with the un-treated rats, Abri cantongnesis provides an alternative medicine for prevention and treatment for toxicant-induced liver toxicity. The results show experimental evidence of the pharmacological activities of Abri cantongnesis as a potential chemo-protective agent for the liver.

## Acknowledgement

This work was supported by a grant no. 6903088.

## References

1. Miyao H, Arao T, Udayama M, Kinjo J, Nohara T(1998) Kaikasaponin III and soyasaponin I, major triterpenesaponins of Abruscantoniensis, act on GOT and GPT: Influence on transaminase elevation of rat liver cells concomitantly exposed to CCl4 for one hour.Planta Med 64: 5-7.
2. Jürgenliemk G, Nahrstedt A (2002) Phenolic compounds from Hypericumperforatum. Planta Med 68: 88-91.
3. Kinjo J (1996) Studies on bioactive compounds from leguminous plants; structures, activities, HPLC profiles and functional importances of sugar moiety for oleaneneglucuronides. Nat Med 50: 79-85.
4. Lash LH, Fisher JW, Lipscomb LC, Parker JC (2000) Metabolism of trichloroethylene," Environ. Health Perspect 108:177-200.
5. Channel SR, Pravecek TL (1998) Metabolism of trichloroethylene in B6C3F1 mouse and human liver slices. Drug ChemToxicol 21: 275-289.
6. Lipscomb JC, Fisher JW, Confer PD, Byczkowski JZ (1998) In vitro to in vivo extrapolation for trichloroethylene metabolism in humans. ToxicolApplPharmacol 152: 376-387.
7. Larson JL, Bull RJ (1992) Species differences in the metabolism of trichloroethylene to the carcinogenic metabolites trichloroacetate and dichloroacetate. ToxicolApplPharmacol 115: 278-285.
8. Bull RJ, Sanchez IM, Nelson MA, Larson JL, Lansing AJ (1990) Liver tumor induction in B6C3F1 mice by dichloroacetate and trichloroacetate. Toxicology 63: 341-359.
9. DeAngelo AB, Daniel FB, Stober JA, Olson GR (1991) The carcinogenicity of dichloroacetic acid in the male B6C3F1 mouse. FundamApplToxicol 16: 337-347.
10. Walgren JE, Kurtz DT, McMillan JM (2000) The effect of the trichloroethylene metabolites trichloroacetate and dichloroacetate on peroxisome proliferation and DNA synthesis in cultured human hepatocytes. Cell BiolToxicol 16: 257-273.
11. Steel-Goodwin L, Pravecek TL, Carmichael AJ (1996) Trichloroethylene metabolism in vitro: an EPR/SPIN trapping study. Hum ExpToxicol 15: 878-884.
12. Watanabe M, Takano T, Nakamura K (1998) Effect of ethanol on the metabolism of trichloroethylene in the perfused rat liver. J Toxicol Environ Health A 55: 297-305.
13. Bradford MM (1976) A rapid and sensitive method for the quantitation of microgram quantities of protein utilizing the principle of protein-dye binding. Anal Biochem 72: 248-254.

14. Klotz AV, Stegeman JJ, Walsh C (1984) An alternative 7-ethyoxyresorufin O-deethylase activity assay: a continuous visible spectrophotometric method for measurement of cytochrome P-450 monooxygenase activity. Anal Biochem140: 138-145.

15. Kennedy SW, Jones SP (1994) Simultanous measurement of cytochrome P450 1A1 catalytic activity and total protein concentration with a fluorescence plate reader. Anal. Biochem 222: 217-2234.

16. Ho JW, Leung YK, Chan CP (2002) Herbal medicine in the treatment of cancer. Curr Med Chem Anticancer Agents 2: 209-214.

17. Habig WH, Pabst MJ, Jakoby WB (1974) Glutathione S-transferases. The first enzymatic step in mercapturic acid formation. J BiolChem 249: 7130-7139.

18. Mulder GJ (1971) The heterogeneity of uridinediphosphateglucuronyltransferase from rat liver. Biochem J 125: 9-15.

19. Neumann CM, Zannoni VG (1990) Ascorbic acid deficiency and hepatic UDP-glucuronyltransferase. Qualitative and quantitative differences. BiochemPharmacol 39: 1085-1093.

20. Lind C, Cadenas E, Hochstein P, Ernster L (1990) DT-diaphorase: purification, properties, and function. Methods Enzymol 186: 287-301.

21. Muralidhara, Narasimhamurthy K, Viswanatha S, Ramesh BS (1999) Acute and subchronic toxicity assessment of debitterized fenugreek powder in the mouse and rat. Food ChemToxicol 37: 831-838.

22. Hinson JA (1983) Reactive metabolites of phenacetin and acetaminophen: a review. Environ Health Perspect 49: 71-79.

23. Cohen SD, Khairallah EA (1997) Selective protein arylation and acetaminophen-induced hepatotoxicity. Drug Metab Rev 29: 59-77.

4

# The Impact of Hatha Yoga Practice on Flexibility

**Maja Petrič**[*]**, Renata Vauhnik and Miroljub Jakovljević**

*Cesta v log 24, Ljubljana, Slovenia*

[*]**Corresponding author**: Maja Petrič, Cesta v log 24, Ljubljana, Slovenia 1351,Slovenia, E-mail: maja.53c@gmail.com

**Abstract**

**Background:** In modern times people have to cope daily with various challenges that can leave an impact on their body flexibility. Physical inactivity is one of the reasons for the diminishment of our natural body flexibility. The consequence of physical inactivity is decreased flexibility of soft tissues surrounding joints. Simple yoga techniques including body postures and breathing techniques can restore natural body flexibility.

**Methods:** Our study involved 9 young healthy females (mean age 23.8 ± 2.9 years). The training program was held twice a week over a period of five months. The program included therapeutic yoga exercises, with the aim of increasing joint mobility as well as stretching shortened skeletal muscles. We used goniometric measurement procedures for measuring joint mobility (for shoulder, hip and ankle joints), linear measurement procedures for measuring the active mobility of the thoracolumbar part of the spine and specific assessing tests for evaluating skeletal muscle shortness. Measurements of body flexibility were taken three times over the five months period.

**Results:** The results obtained by measuring joint mobility showed significant increase of mobility in elevation through abduction, shoulder retroflexion, hip flexion, internal and external hip rotation, dorsal flexion and inversion of the ankle. The mobility of the thoracolumbar part of the spine was increased in all the measured movements: flexion, extension, lateral flexion and rotation of the spine. There was also a significant improvement in the flexibility of m. Soleus, m. Gastrocnemius, m. Rectus femoris, knee flexors and m. Pectoralis major. A significant improvement in body flexibility was also confirmed by the "Back Scratch Test" and the "Sit and Reach Test".

**Conclusion:** Improved body flexibility is one of the most obvious and quickly achieved effects of regular hatha yoga practice. The results of this study confirm that regular practice of yoga has a significant effect on body flexibility in young healthy women, which is particularly obvious in measurements of the increase of the flexibility of skeletal muscles.

**Keywords:** Yoga; Flexibility; Therapeutic effects

## Introduction

Regular physical activity is one of the bases of a healthy lifestyle. It creates and maintains general well-being, physical and mental health, as well as promoting human performance in all areas of life. Physical inactivity is one of the reasons for the diminishment of our natural body flexibility and strength; it dulls our senses and generally reduces the awareness of our own body. Eventually, all this results in poor posture, which, by it, can lead to pain and injury. In addition to reduced physical activity, stress has a large and equally negative impact on health, and stress is becoming quite common nowadays. We are not always able to influence the external environment, but we can control our body, breathing, mind and emotions, and thus can prevent or at least mitigate the negative effects of stress on our health. This is probably the most common reason why yoga and other similar forms of exercise are so accepted and popular in modern societies. Yoga enables us to reconnect the body, breath and mind into a whole and thus improve awareness of our own body [1].

Mobility is defined as the ability to move body structures or parts of the body through the existing range of motion for a functional activity (functional range of motion) [2]. Mobility referring to the functional range of motion is strongly associated with joint integrity as well as flexibility. The term flexibility in this context means the elasticity of soft tissues that cross or surround joints (muscles, tendons, fascia, articular capsule, ligaments, nerves, blood vessels, skin), and is absolutely necessary for painless movement of the body [2]. In most situations flexibility does not depend solely on the actual length of soft tissues, for example muscle or muscle fibers forming the muscles. The length of an active muscle, its tone and the length of its stretch also depend on proprioceptive nerve endings in the muscle [3]. The length of stretch, regarding the adequacy, safety and functionality of stretch, is therefore controlled by the nervous system, which consequently affects the range of motion of the joint surrounded by the soft tissue [3].

There can be many different reasons for reduced range of motion, but one of them definitely is muscle shortness, which occurs as a result of physical inactivity and putting irregular or excessive pressure on muscles and other soft tissues crossing or surrounding joints. However, not all the muscles respond to the above-mentioned pathological stimuli with shortening. This response is typical for predominantly tonic, postural muscles whose main function is to maintain the posture [4]. Another group of muscles, mainly phasic muscles, is involved in carrying movements in daily activities. Those muscles respond by weakness under incorrect or excessive pressure [4]. If there is shortness of tonic muscles, this aggravates the weakness of phasic muscles, and vice versa. Therefore there has to be a balanced and coordinated action of both muscle groups for the normal functioning of the musculoskeletal system.

Improved flexibility is one of the most obvious and quickly achieved effects of regular yoga practice, since this is based on gradual stretching of muscle and connective tissue around bones and joints [5], static retention of yoga poses and movements of joints throughout the entire existing range of motion [6]. The latter provide straight-line compression and lubrication of articular cartilage by the synovial fluid, thereby bringing fresh nutrients and oxygen to those parts of joint cartilage which are rarely used in everyday activities [6].

In this research we examine the quantitative impact of regular yoga practice on body flexibility in young healthy females. Most of the published studies of the impact of yoga practice on flexibility only measure the general flexibility of the upper and/or lower part of the body. The most commonly used tests are versions of the "Sit and Reach Test" [7-10] and the "Back Scratch Test" [8]. Among the studies taken into consideration none observes changes in mobility of individual joints by goniometric measurement procedures, isolated flexibility of the spine or the impact of yoga practice on the flexibility of individual skeletal muscles.

## Materials and Methods

Healthy, young subjects were recruited by flyer from our local community. No incentives were offered other than the yoga classes and physiotherapeutic testing. Following approval of The National Medical Ethics Committee of the Republic of Slovenia, written informed consent was obtained from 10 young healthy females who volunteered to participate. All participants were healthy, and did not present recent skeletal or muscle injuries. Furthermore, all participants fulfilled the condition for participation in this study, namely that they had not participated in yoga or any other activities aimed at increasing flexibility for a period of 6 months prior to the start of our training program. Nine females (mean age 23.8 ± 2.9 years) completed the study; one subject dropped out during the second half of the study and declined to perform last testing.

In present study we performed the so-called hatha yoga. The training program of hatha yoga was held twice a week (in 75 minutes sessions) over a period of five months, performed solely for the purposes of this study. The training was led by certified yoga teachers. The program included therapeutic yoga exercises aimed at increasing joint mobility as well as stretching shortened skeletal muscles. Each training session consisted of 10 minutes of pranayama (controlled breathing exercises), 10 minutes of warm-up exercises, 45 minutes of asana practice (yoga poses) and 10 minutes of relaxation.

We used goniometric measurement procedures [11] for measuring joint mobility. An universal goniometer (Baseline measurement instruments, ZDA) was used to measure the range of motion at the shoulder (elevation through anteflexion, elevation through abduction, retroflexion, internal and external rotation), hip (flexion, extension, abduction, adduction, internal and external rotation) and ankle joints (dorsal/plantar flexion, eversion and inversion) bilaterally. All goniometric measurements were passive, performed by examiner [11].

The active mobility of the thoracolumbar part of the spine was measured by linear measurement procedures [11]. Flexion, extension and lateral flexion range of motion recorded was difference between initial and final measurement of distance between the spinous process of C7 and S1 vertebra in an erect posture and final flexion/extension/lateral flexion of the spine. For measuring rotation of the thoracolumbar spine a measuring tape was aligned with 0 cm at acromion and maintained against subject's back to pelvic opposite spina iliaca anterior superior. Rotation range of motion was difference between length measured at erect sitting posture (initial measurement) and length measured at end of rotation motion (final measurement) [11].

Specific muscle length tests were used for evaluating skeletal muscle shortness [4,11]. For measurement of m. Soleus length the ankle dorsal flexion with the knee flexed was performed [11]. Same motion, but with the knee extended, was used for measuring the length of m. Gastrocnemius. The shortness of m. Rectus femoris was assessing by knee flexion while hip was extended in supine position [11]. Hamstring muscles (m. Semimembranosus, m. Semitendinosus and m. Biceps femoris) shortness were assessing with maximal hip flexion maintaining the knee extended [11]. With shoulder elevation through abduction we tested the flexibility of m. Pectoralis major [11]. For subject all motions at muscle length testing were passive, performed by examiner [11].

We also used the "Back Scratch Test" [11,12] for evaluating overall shoulder flexibility, and the "Sit and Reach Test" [11,13,14] for low back and hamstring flexibility. The "Back Scratch Test" involves reaching behind the head with one hand and behind the back with the other. We measure the distance between (or overlap of) the middle fingers behind the back [12]. The "Sit and Reach Test" was performed by having the subject assume the long sitting posture and reach forward with both hands as far as possible, not allowing the knees to flex. A score was given based on the most distant point reached by both hands [14].

All the above-mentioned measurements of body flexibility were taken three times over the five months period; first at the beginning of the training program, next after 2 months of training and finally, at the end of the 5 months training program. All the measures were taken prior the yoga session or at least one day after it. Since the flexibility of soft tissues in women is subject to minimal changes in relation to the phase of the menstrual cycle [15], we measured all participants in the same phase of the cycle, on the 6th day of the ovulation.

The results are presented with descriptive statistics (mean range of motion ± standard deviation (SD)). We compared baseline measurements to the results obtained after two months of training, and after five months of training (change of motion in °/cm). Clinically significant changes in flexibility were ≥ 5°. To analyze the differences between periods we used the analysis of variance for repeated measurements (ANOVA, $p \leq 0.05$) and Student's »post hoc« t test with Bonferroni correction ($p \leq 0.05$). The analysis was performed with the statistical program MedCalc (version 11.1.0.0).

## Results

The average attendance at the training was 77.5% (27.9 ± 4.0 hours of a total of 36 hours of yoga practice). The attendance was higher in the first part of the training program (before the 2nd measurement).

As shown by the first measurement, all participants had some deviations from the normal range of motion [11] at the beginning of the training program (Table 1). For most of the measurements the flexibility increased steadily on both measured sides and there was a reduction in the differences between the range of motion on the left and right measured side through the research.

The results obtained by measuring joint mobility showed significant increase of mobility in elevation through abduction, shoulder retroflexion, hip flexion, internal and external hip rotation, dorsal flexion and inversion of the ankle (Table 1).

| Joint mobility (°) | 1. | 2. | 3. |
|---|---|---|---|
| Shoulder elevation through abduction | 164.4 ± 6.2 | 167.5 ± 8.5 | 172.5 ± 5.8* |
| Shoulder retroflexion | 44.7 ± 5.4 | 47.8 ± 4.5 | 50.0 ± 4.4* |
| Hip flexion | 107.8 ± 7.9 | 112.8 ± 5.3 | 114.4 ± 6.4* |
| Internal hip rotation | 38.6 ± 4.3 | 42.2 ± 5.1 | 43.9 ± 6.6* |
| External hip rotation | 31.1 ± 3.9 | 35.0 ± 6.0 | 36.1 ± 4.9* |
| Ankle dorsal flexion | 7.8 ± 3.0 | 12.5 ± 6.3* | 17.2 ± 6.3* |
| Ankle inversion | 20.0 ± 6.0 | 24.7 ± 6.8 | 26.7 ± 6.2* |

**Table 1:** Improvements in mobility (mean values ± SD) of shoulder, hip and ankle joints before training (1. measurement), after two months of training (2. measurement) and at the end of the 5 months training program (3. measurement).

The mobility of the thoracolumbar part of the spine was increased in all the measured movements: flexion, extension, lateral flexion and rotation of the spine (Table 2).

| Spine mobility (cm) | 1. | 2. | 3. |
|---|---|---|---|
| Flexion | 11.1 ± 1.5 | 12.0 ± 1.8 | 12.7 ± 1.6* |
| Extension | 6.9 ± 2.6 | 7.7 ± 2.0 | 8.4 ± 2.8* |
| Lateral flexion | 1.2 ± 0.5 | 1.7 ± 0.6* | 2.3 ± 0.7* |
| Rotation | 6.2 ± 1.6 | 6.9 ± 1.2* | 7.2 ± 1.0* |

**Table 2:** Improvements in mobility (mean values ± SD) of thoracolumbar part of the spine before training (1. measurement), after two months of training (2. measurement) and at the end of the 5 months training program (3. measurement).

There was a significant improvement in the flexibility of m. Soleus, m. Gastrocnemius, m. Rectus femoris, knee flexors and m. Pectoralis major (Table 3).

| Muscle flexibility (°) | 1. | 2. | 3. |
|---|---|---|---|
| *m. Soleus*<br>(ankle dorsal flexion with the knee flexed) | 7.8 ± 3.0 | 12.5 ± 6.3* | 17.2 ± 6.3* |
| *m. Gastrocnemius*<br>(ankle dorsal flexion with the knee extended) | 0.6 ± 2.8 | 3.9 ± 4.9* | 7.2 ± 6.3* |
| *m. Rectus femoris*<br>(knee flexion with the hip extended) | 55.6 ± 9.7 | 58.6 ± 8.1 | 63.6 ± 6.2* |
| *knee flexors*<br>(hip flexion with the knee extended) | 80.3 ± 7.9 | 93.9 ± 8.1* | 102.5 ± 12.7* |
| *m. Pectoralis major*<br>(shoulder elevation through abduction) | 164.4 ± 6.2 | 167.5 ± 8.5 | 172.5 ± 5.8* |

**Table 3:** Improvements in flexibility (mean values ± SD) of skeletal muscles before training (1. measurement), after two months of training (2. measurement) and at the end of the 5 months training program (3. measurement).

A significant improvement in body flexibility was also confirmed by the "Back Scratch Test" for the upper body and the "Sit and Reach Test" for the lower body (Table 4).

| General flexibility (cm) | 1. | 2. | 3. |
|---|---|---|---|
| Back Scratch Test | 4.9 ± 7.5 | 6.2 ± 6.7* | 7.4 ± 6.3* |
| Sit and Reach Test | 0.1 ± 10.0 | 7.8 ± 8.0* | 12.9 ± 6.6* |

**Table 4:** Improvements in general flexibility (mean values ± SD) of the upper and lower part of the body before training (1. measurement), after two months of training (2. measurement) and at the end of the 5 months training program (3. measurement).

## Discussion

Improved body flexibility is one of the most obvious and quickly achieved effects of regular hatha yoga practice, which was confirmed also by the results of our study. As found in previous studies, regular yoga practice helps to increase joint mobility primarily in older people [16]. Thus in our study, focusing on young and healthy participants, a significant improvement in joint mobility had not been expected. However, the mobility of some joints did increase significantly. Given that the participants were young, healthy persons with no recent skeletal or muscle injuries, we may assume that the cause of initially limited joint mobility was not reduced sliding of articulating surfaces. The reasons can be found in the shortness of the soft tissues surrounding the joints, especially in reduced skeletal muscle flexibility.

Among all the forms of yoga, hatha yoga is the one that gives the most priority to the importance of physical fitness. Based on the interpretation of the word hatha – in Sanskrit the syllable "ha" means the sun, male energy, strength, and "tha" means the moon, female energy, flexibility [1] – it can be summarized that hatha yoga is a dynamic balance between strength and flexibility, which concerns the physical, mental and also emotional level [1].

Some of the published research papers studied the effect of regular yoga practice on the general flexibility of the upper and/or lower body. Some of these studies lasted for 8 weeks [7-9], so their results can be compared with the results of our first mid-term measurement, which was also carried out after 8 weeks of practicing yoga. In the above-mentioned studies lower body flexibility improved by 4.1 cm [7], 0.9 cm (used test version: "Chair Sit and Reach Test") [8] and 10.0 cm [9] after 8 weeks of training program. One study also measured flexibility of the upper body by "Back Scratch Test" and there the increase of flexibility was 1.3 cm [8]. Our results at the 2nd measurement (after 8 weeks training program) showed for 7.7 ± 5.4 cm greater flexibility in "Sit and Reach Test" and by 1.3 ± 1.5 cm greater flexibility in "Back Scratch Test". We found no other similar research monitoring the impact of regular yoga practice on joint and spine mobility or specific skeletal muscle flexibility, to compare with the results obtained in this study.

With yoga practice we can relax many physical dysfunctions and improve the flexibility of the body. Compared to physiotherapy procedures, yoga, with its static-dynamic procedures, can also be discussed as a means of "self-mobilization" of the nervous system and joints of spine and extremities [17]. In general yoga practice is performed slowly and gradually, in a closed kinetic chain (specific poses or static postures), which may include active stretching, isometric muscle contractions, enhancing concentration and proper breathing patterns. Conceptually, we can conclude that both physiotherapy and yoga, each through its own procedures, improve muscle strength, increase joint mobility and soft tissue flexibility, mobilize the nervous system, improve body posture, improve proprioception and thereby encourage better awareness of the body, releasing trigger points and relieving pain [17]. The National Institutes of Health (NIH) and the National Center for Complementary and Alternative Medicine (NCCAM) acknowledged yoga as a form of complementary and alternative medicine in the category of "Mind and Body Practices" [18]. According to the NCCAM's definition yoga therapy is defined as a process of empowering individuals to progress toward improved health and well-being through the application of the philosophy and practice of yoga [19].

In recent years there have been a growing number of studies showing that regular exercise of hatha yoga increases muscle strength and flexibility [20]. Of course, various styles of yoga can differ greatly. And depending on the intensity of each yoga style the effects (e.g. increase of mobility) can be very different as well. One study compares the effects of two different styles of yoga: ashtanga and hatha yoga [21]. Ashtanga yoga is a physically demanding form of yoga in which the majority of poses are dynamically linked in sequences, such as Sun Salutation, also used in hatha yoga [22]. The study used the "Sit and Reach Box" test for measuring the flexibility. A group which had practiced ashtanga yoga improved the flexibility of the body by 20 percent, while a group which had practiced hatha yoga improved it by 14 percent.

Most of the measurements in our study showed greater improvement in the first part of the training program compared to the period between the intermediate and the final measurements. There may be several reasons for that. Most participants in the study practiced yoga for the first time. Therefore a possible explanation for the difference in the progress between the periods is that the participants' bodies responded better and more quickly to stretching and relaxation in yoga practice in the first weeks of training, and then at some point their bodies got used to this kind of exercise and the progress slowed. Another reason may be higher attendance in the first part of the training program (8 percent higher attendance). And the third reason could be a few days break of guided exercise in the second part of the research program, because of the holidays.

In terms of increasing flexibility the aim of yoga is not hypermobility but an adequate level of flexibility enabling us to easier and better use our muscles in everyday activities. For this we need appropriate flexibility of muscles that maintain posture (tonic muscles) and adequately strengthened muscles which are responsible for the movement of the distal segments of the body (phasic muscles) [4]. In our study yoga proved an effective form of exercise, at least from the viewpoint of the postural muscles.

The disadvantages of the majority of research of the effects of yoga on the body (including ours) are a small sample of subjects, varying duration of the research and different methods of measuring body flexibility. Therefore it would be important to explore this area through studies of standard duration using standard measurement procedures, especially on a larger sample of subjects. It would also be meaningful to further explore the effects of regular yoga practice on flexibility as well as its impact on stability and protection of the joints in which mobility is increasing. Further research into the effects of yoga practice in various pathologies and injuries meant to enhance the usefulness of yoga techniques in physiotherapy would also be welcome.

## Conclusion

The results of this study confirm that regular practice of hatha yoga has a significant effect on body flexibility in young healthy women. This is particularly obvious in measurements of the increase of the skeletal muscles flexibility.

## Acknowledgements

The author thanks to the Faculty of Health Sciences Ljubljana, Miroljub Jakovljević, PhD, PT, and Renata Vauhnik, PhD, PT, for inspiring attitude and professional assistance in the creation of this research. Special thanks are due to yoga teacher Blaž Bertoncelj who has enabled the implementation of the training program and take care of the professional conducting of yoga practice.

## References

1. Schöps I (2010) Yoga: Theory and practice for beginners and advanced students. Bath: Parragon Book Service Ltd.
2. Kisner C, Colby LA (2007) Therapeutic exercise: foundations and techniques. (5thedn), Philadelphia: F. A. Davis Company.
3. Kaminoff L, Matthews A (2012) Yoga anatomy. (2ndedn), Campaign (IL): Human Kinetics.
4. Schneider W, Spring H, Tritschler T (1992) Mobility: theory and practice. New York: Thieme Medical Publishers.
5. Woodyard C (2011) Exploring the therapeutic effects of yoga and its ability to increase quality of life. Int J Yoga 4: 49-54.
6. McCall (2007) Yoga as medicine: the yogic prescription for health & healing. New York: Random house, Inc.
7. Tran MD, Holly RG, Lashbrook J, Amsterdam EA (2001) Effects of Hatha Yoga Practice on the Health-Related Aspects of Physical Fitness. Prev Cardiol 4: 165-170.
8. Van Puymbroeck M, Payne LL, Hsieh PC (2007) A phase I feasibility study of yoga on the physical health and coping of informal caregivers. Evid Based Complement Alternat Med 4: 519-529.
9. Telles S, Dash M, Naveen KV (2009) Effect of yoga on musculoskeletal discomfort and motor functions in professional computer users. Work 33: 297-306.
10. Cowen VS (2010) Functional fitness improvements after a worksite-based yoga initiative. J Bodyw Mov Ther 14: 50-54.
11. Berryman Reese N, Bandy WD (2002) Joint range of motion and muscle length testing. Philadelphia, Pa: W.B. Saunders Company.
12. Rikli RE, Jones CJ (2013) Development and validation of criterion-referenced clinically relevant fitness standards for maintaining physical independence in later years. Gerontologist 53: 255-267.
13. Wells KF, Dillon EK (1952) The sit-and-reach. A test of back and leg flexibility. Res Q 23: 115-118.
14. Ayala F, Sainz de Baranda P, De Ste Croix M, Santonja F (2012) Reproducibility and criterion-related validity of the sit and reach test and toe touch test for estimating hamstring flexibility in recreationally active young adults. Phys Ther Sport 13: 219-226.
15. Melegario SM, Simao R, Vale RGS, Batista LA, Novaes JS (2006) The influence of the menstrual cycle on the flexibility in practioners of gymnastics at fitness centers. Rev Bras Med Esporte 12: 114-117.
16. Gonçalves LC, Vale RG, Barata NJ, Varejão RV, Dantas EH (2011) Flexibility, functional autonomy and quality of life (QoL) in elderly yoga practitioners. Arch Gerontol Geriatr 53: 158-162.
17. Posadzki P, Parekh S (2009) Yoga and physiotherapy: a speculative review and conceptual synthesis. Chin J Integr Med 15: 66-72.
18. National Center for Complementary and Alternative Medicine (2008) What is complementary and alternative medicine?
19. Taylor MJ (2007) What is yoga therapy? IAYT offers a definition for the field. YTIP, 3: 3.
20. Raub JA (2002) Psychophysiologic effects of Hatha Yoga on musculoskeletal and cardiopulmonary function: a literature review. J Altern Complement Med 8: 797-812.
21. Cowen VS, Adams TB (2005) Physical and perceptual benefits of yoga asana practice: results of a pilot study. J Bodywork Movement Ther 9: 211-219.
22. Broad WJ (2012) The science of yoga: the risks and the rewards. New York: Simon & Schuster.

# 5

# Can Standardized Plant Extracts Induce Complete Remission in Patients with Metastatic Tumors?

**Tibor Hajtó[1*], András Adámy[1], Lilla Baranyai[1], Zoltán Langmár[2], Angelika Kirsch[3], Monika Kuzma1, Lajos Ábrahám[4] and Perjési Pál[1]**

[1] *Institute of Pharmaceutical Chemistry, Medical University Pecs, Hungary*

[2] *Semmelweis University, 2nd Department of Gynecology, Budapest*
[3] *Private practice, Arlesheim, Switzerland.*

[4] *Surgical Department of Szent János Hospital Budapest, Hungary*

***Corresponding author:** Tibor Hajtó, MD, PhD, Károly krt. 3/C, H-1075 Budapest, Hungary, E-mail: drhajtot@t-online.hu

**Abstract**

**Background:** The prognostic significance of malignant tumor-induced imbalance in the innate immune system is well known. The innate system uses a limited number of Pattern Recognition Receptors (PRR) to recognize conserved Pathogenic Associated Molecular Pattern (PAMP) structures expressed by microbes but not by host. PRR engagement often leads to the activation of natural immune cells which are important in the tumor defense. Growing evidence supports the hypothesis that similar to microbes various plant extracts can also contain PAMP-like structures which can activate cellular immune functions. Since the chemical production of PAMP structures is hardly accomplishable, the phytotherapy may be promising for the future tumor therapy. Objectives: The aim of this article is to present and discuss several favorable clinical responses of tumor patients treated with immunologically effective and standardized plant extracts (containing PAMP-like structures) as an addition to the conventional oncologic therapy.

**Course of therapy and results:** Two standardized plant preparations based on lectin-sugar interactions were the patients given. The dose of the active sugar-binding mistletoe lectin (ML), applied subcutaneously by standardized mistletoe extract (ME) preparations, was between 0.5 and 1.0 ng/kg and the dose of arabinoxylan (given by standardized rice bran preparation, MGN-3/Biobran) was between 12 and 45mg/kg twice a week. In addition, wheat germ extract (WGE) standardized for 2, 6-dimethoxy-p-benzoquinone (50-80 mg/kg Avemar four times a week) was also given which can sensitize tumor cells against natural immune effector cells. Case reports gave an account of complete or nearly complete remissions in patients with sarcoma or with hepatic metastases treated with these standardized plant immunomodulators with and without conventional oncologic therapy.

**Conclusion:** Standardized plant extracts (such as ME/ML, MGN-3 and WGE) seem to be potent candidates to be regarded as a supportive therapy of metastatic tumors.

**Keywords:** Tumor; Immune dysfunction; Plant immunomodulatory; Viscum album lectin; Rice brain preparation; Wheat germ extract

## Introduction

### Immunological background

In tumor patients the prognostic significance of natural immune functions was often established. It is now generally recognized that immunocompetent cells of the innate immune system are committed in two separate directions: (1) M1 macrophages and CD1a+ dentritic cells (DC1) generating IL-12 and other pro-inflammatory cytokines activating cytotoxic effector cells such as natural killer (NK) and natural killer T (NKT) cells, potent inhibitors of tumor growth; (2) prototypic M2 macrophages generating IL-4 and IL-10, which facilitate the generation of Th2 cells while inhibiting Th1 cells. In patients with malignant tumors both branches of innate immunity are often affected. The basic function of macrophages of the M2 type is to induce inflammation and promote cell proliferation by producing growth factors and through initiation of the arginase pathway, neoangiogenesis and tissue repair [3]. In the presence of malignancy, a higher than normal proportion of macrophages belongs to this prototypic M2 population and this appears to alter the balance of immune responses [5]. For example, in healthy individuals M2 monocytes were found to comprise only 10% of the total monocytic population, and in tumor patients this proportion was 40% higher [6].

Since many years, a beneficial influence of certain bacterial infections on the progress of tumor disease was often observed. Now, it is also clear that bacterial Pathogenic Associated Molecular Pattern (PAMP) molecules can stimulate the type 1 natural immune cells by binding the Pattern Recognition Receptors (PRR) on their membrane. However, in spite of the fact that the effects of a great number of bacterial preparations on tumor disease were investigated, there are not in clinical use. They have toxic side effects and in case of endotoxin a tolerance was also observed. Therefore the hypothesis is interesting that plants may also contain PAMP like molecules without toxic side effects.

### Immunomodulatory effect of mistletoe lectin (ML)

The effect of ML given subcutaneously by standardized mistletoe extracts (ME) based on lectin –carbohydrate interaction on cell membrane of several immunocompetent cells of the innate immune system [7-10]. ML can selectively bind type-1 phagocytic cells and activates the "cascade"of cellular responses in innate immune, including granulocytes, macrophages, dentritic cells and natural killer (NK) cells. There is evidence accumulating that ML may also act as PAMP ligands and their binding to PRR on phagocytes shows some similarity with interactions between Toll-like receptors and PAMP ligands of microorganisms. Preclinical investigations in the tumor models (using nude mice xenotransplanted with human leiomyosarcoma and IL-12 deficient C57BL6 mice) show that without immunological reactions ML induce less anti-tumor efficacy [11]. ML, functioning as ligands for pattern recognition receptors of the natural immune system, is docked to ganglioside molecules (CD75) of monocytes and granulocytes, thereby stimulating the natural anti-tumor mechanisms. Through this interaction, ML is capable of partially restoring the immune imbalance in tumor patients [11-12].

### Immunomodulatory effect of arabinoxylan concentrate

Similar to mistletoe lectin, modified arabinoxylan preparation obtained from rice bran (MGN-3/BioBranR) was also found to stimulate type-1 cells in the innate immune system and Arabinoxylan isolated cautiously from rice bran may also exhibit (similar to mistletoe lectin) PAMP-like properties. Arabinoxylan given by MGN-3/BioBranR increased NK cell activity both in vivo and in vitro [13] and enhanced phagocytic function of macrophages [14]. Given as combined therapy, mistletoe lectin and arabinoxylan appear to have an additive effect (unpublished data).

### The effect of wheat germ extract

Wheat Germ Extract (WGE/AvemarR) containing 2, 6-dimethoxy-p-benzoquinone in 0.4 mg/g concentration as dry preparation [15]. Both in vitro and in vivo studies confirmed a significant antimetastatic effect by WGE [16-18]. The combination of WGE with NK stimulatory substances, such as ML in standardized mistletoe extracts and arabinoxylan in MGN3/BioBran is promising since WGE induces a down regulation in expression of major histocompatibility complex (MHC) class I proteins [19] and thus may have an additive effect to those of other immunomodulators. As known, the down regulation of MHC class I proteins reduce the effect of killing inhibitor receptors (KIR) resulting in enhanced killing of tumor targets by NK cells.

## Material and methods

### Standardized plant extracts

The application schema of standardized plant extracts used in treatment of patients is summarized in Table 1.

*Iscador*[R] is a fermented aqueous mistletoe plant extract manufactured and supplied by Weleda AG (CH-4144 Arlesheim, Switzerland). The active (sugar-binding) lectin content of commercially available mistletoe extracts (Iscador M spec 5 mg) was measured in the research laboratory of Pharmacochemical Department of Medical University Pécs.

The determination of sugar binding Mistletoe Lectins (MLs) level in ME was carried out by an optimized ELLA technique as published previously [13]. Standardized ME exhibited a bell-shaped dose-response relationship and 0.5-1.0 ng/kg lectin doses were found to be most effective as it was always assessed previously using healthy volunteers. Since two and three therapy-free days were found to be necessary for an immunologically optimal effect, the subcutaneous ME injections were regularly given twice a week.

| | Monday | Tuesday | Wednesday | Thursday | Friday | Saturday | Sunday |
|---|---|---|---|---|---|---|---|
| ML in standardized ME | 0.5-1.0 ng / kg s. c. | | | 0.5-1.0 ng / kg s. c. | | | |
| MGN-3 standardized for Arabinoxylan | 12-45 mg / kg per oral | | | 12-45 mg / kg per oral | | | |
| WGE standardized for 2,6 dimethoxy p-benzoquinon | 50-80 mg/kg per oral | 50-80 mg/kg per oral | | 50-80 mg/kg per oral | 50-80 mg/kg per oral | | |

**Table 1:** A schematic illustration of a proposed application of standardized plant extracts used as additive immunomodulatory treatment of patients with malignant tumors

The second immunomodulatory drug used in the combinative treatment of the presented patients is BioBran/MGN-3 which is manufactured and supplied by Daiwa Pharmaceutical Co, Ltd, Tokyo, Japan. BioBran/MGN-3 is composed of denaturated hemicellulose, which is obtained by rice bran hemicellulose reacting with multiple carbohydrate-hydrolyzing enzymes from shiitake mushrooms. BioBran/MGN-3 is standardized for its main chemical component: arabinoxylan with a xylose (in its main chain) and with an arabinose polymer (in its side chain). To the presented patients BioBran/MGN-3 was given per oral in doses between 12 and 45mg/kg twice a week parallel to the optimized, lectin-oriented ME therapy.

WGE (trade name AvemarR) is a complex of multiple, biologically active molecules obtained from fermented wheat-germ extract. Its biological effects are related to 2-methoxy-p-benzoquinone (2-MBQ) and 2, 6-dimethoxy-p-benzoquinone (2, 6-DMBQ) in the form of glucoside. During the fermentation the quinones are released by the glucosidase enzyme of the yeast fungus. The 1045 mg tablets are manufactured and supplied by Biopharma Kft, Kunfehértó, Hungary. WGE is standardized for its 2, 6-DMBQ content (0.4 mg/g concentration on dry matter basis). In presented cases WGE was given per oral in doses between 50 and 80 mg/kg/die four times a week (on the day of immunotherapy and 24h thereafter).

## Patients

### Ethics committee:

Ethics committee proposed to observe and publish case reports of own patients treated by standardized plant extracts. These and previous case reports may stimulate an interest for other research groups according to the opinion of the ethics committee. All patients have given an informed consent to process and publish their dates. They were informed that plant extracts can be regarded as a complementary therapy and it cannot substitute for conventional oncologic treatments. The patients were regularly controlled in various oncologic centers and parallel they were also treated with plant immunomodulators and monitored in private praxis (in Switzerland and Hungary).

### Eligibility criteria of patients with malignant tumors:

**Inclusion criteria:** 1. histological defined malignant tumor; 2. patients did not require nursing; 3. at begin of observation they did not receive morphine derivates; 4. measurable tumor parameters by CT scans or sonography.

**Exclusion criteria:** 1. no histological data; 2. Karnofsky index is less than 60; 3. undesired side effects (such as allergy).

## Results and Discussion

Previous clinical observations were published in case reports [20-23] and we present them only in a short form and discuss together with new clinical data.

### Clinical results with sarcoma patients published previously

As reported previously [20], six sarcoma patients show astonishing remission under optimized lectin-oriented doses of ME, partly in addition to other oncotherapies. A patient with lung metastases of liposarcoma was regularly given mistletoe therapy without other treatments. His clinical progress reveals that the optimized mistletoe dose alone was able to result in remission of metastases. Without lectin-oriented dose of ME the metastases of the lung recurred while as under a strict lectin oriented dose regression took place. Until today the patient has survived for 21 years with excellent quality of life. In another liposarcoma patient with inoperable metastases of peritoneum and of the lymph glands simultaneous chemotherapy and lectin-oriented ME-therapy brought about partial remission, solely under ME-therapy the remission has persisted for three years. As mentioned, preclinical data in the tumor model with xenotransplanted sarcoma [11] suggest that lectin-oriented ME therapy is capable of enhancing the efficacy of certain oncotherapies. Two patients with lung and peritoneal metastases of uterus stroma sarcoma were given lectin-oriented ME therapy in addition to hormone therapy (gonadotropin-releasing hormone analogue) or chemotherapy (epirubicin). In spite of the fact that the efficacy of hormone therapy on the recurrent low-grade stroma sarcoma is controversial its combination with ML resulted in a partial remission. In the second stroma sarcoma patient a complete remission already occurred after two chemotherapy cycles so that the planned sixth cycle could be abandoned. Two patients suffering from angiosarcoma were on the lectin-oriented ME therapy following operation. Both patients showed a complete remission and they have remained without relapse for three and four years now.

### Clinical results with hepatic metastases published previously

As in another case reports were published [21], using standardized plant extracts (see table 1) the clinical progress of seven patients showed a complete or nearly complete remission of hepatic metastases. These results are therefore surprising since as it well known, that after a chemotherapy hepatic tumors rarely disappear completely and the duration of responses is short. Hepatic resection in many cases also results in no long-term benefit. In one case the complete remission of hepatic metastasis was reached by immunomodulator alone [22]. In a 72-year-old patient, tumor extirpation of a malignant melanoma (IA SSM Clark level II, pT1 N0 M0, Breslow 0.375 mm) from the right upper arm was carried out in 1992, and because of a second nodular melanoma (IIA, pT3 pN0 pM0) on the right shoulder a second surgery was performed in 1999. In August 2001 three axillary lymph nodes (right) were removed. At the same time in segments 4/5 a solitary hepatic metastasis was detected. From October 2001 the patient was given lectin-standardized ME therapy. In June 2002 a complete remission of liver metastasis was established. Until 2014 no recurrence of the liver metastasis and normal liver functions were regularly observed. The quality of life of patient has been excellent. The multiple liver metastases of two breast cancer patients showed a complete and a partial remission after a combined therapy of hormones (anti-estrogens: Femara as well as Letrosol) and immunomodulators during the observation period of 11 and 10 months. As it is well known, anti-estrogens are able to inhibit the proliferation of mammary cancer cells and therefore it can be speculated that the effect of anti-tumor immune cells on tumor progression is enhanced by this hormone therapy.

Similarly to anti-estrogens, cytostatic drugs with antiproliferative effects seem to be helpful for anti-tumor immunological mechanisms. Because the now 50-year-old patient had ductal mammary carcinoma [T2 N1 (3/17) Mx], a tumorectomy in January 2010, and subsequently a hormone treatment (Femara) and chemotherapy (six cycles epirubicin and docetaxel) were carried out. In April 2011 multiple hepatic metastases were detected in PET/CT. In December 2011 seven liver metastases were removed by surgery. Six weeks later a considerable progression of hepatic metastases was established in PET/CT. Because of the bad liver functions and bad quality of life only a mono-chemotherapy with reduced dose (2500 later 1500 mg Xeloda /day) was given. In the same time an immunomodulatory treatment with lectin-standardized ME, MGN-3/Biobran and WGE was started. In April 2012 a considerable remission of the hepatic metastases (only three small metastases) were detected in CT. The liver functions and tumor markers have been normalized. In August 2012 a nearly complete remission of the hepatic metastases could be established. (The metastases were not measurable in CT). So far the quality of life has been excellent; the patient has been able to work 100% during an observation period of 11 months. These observations suggest the hypothesis that under certain circumstances these immunomodulatory treatments combined with low doses of chemotherapy may be more effective than their combination with high doses of cytostatic drugs.

Two case reports were also represented on patients whose hepatic metastases were removed by surgery [22]. These case reports supported the hypothesis that preoperative and postoperative treatments with these standardized immunomodulators may improve the prognosis of patients following a liver metastasis operation.

## Two new case reports presented now in figure 1 and 2

In a now 70 year old patient (Figure 1) an adenocarcinoma of stomach with coeliac lymph node metastases (T3N1Mx) was in November 2010 established by gastroscopy, biopsy and computed tomography (CT) scan. From December 2011 until May 2012 six cycles Epirubicin (79 mg/m$^2$), Cisplatin (76 mg/ m$^2$) and Xeloda (1000 mg/ m$^2$) were given. After three cycles the question arose as to whether her gastric tumor is responsive to this chemotherapy or not. Therefore in February 2012 a CT scan investigation was carried out and no change was established. The next three cycles of the same chemotherapy were combined with standardized plant immunomodulators and thereafter in May 2012 CT scan investigation showed a nearly complete remission. In Juni 2012 was the rest of tumor chirurgical removed. Until April 2014 the patient received only immunomodulators without an oncologic treatment and CT scan investigations did not show any relapse of her diseases. Her body weight increased by more than 10 kg and her quality of life is excellent.

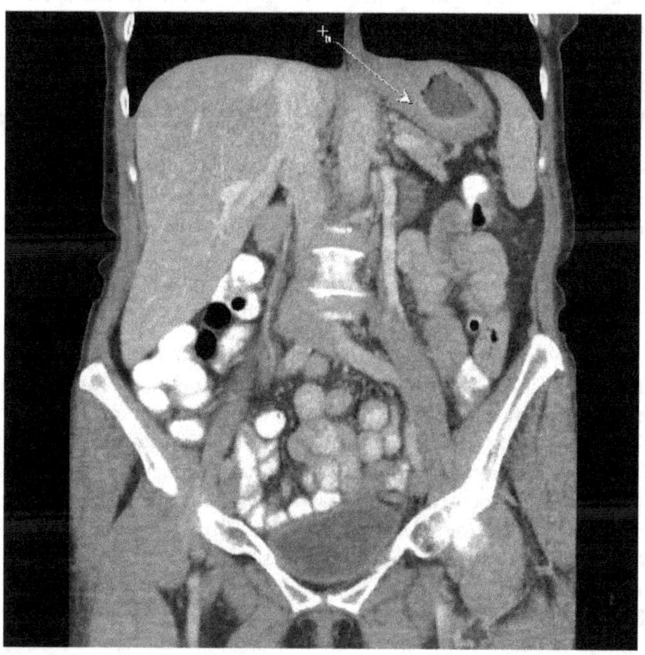

**Figure 1a:** Computed tomography (CT) scans of stomach cancer in a 70-year-old patient. She has received three cycles Epirubicin, Cisplatin and Xeloda and no change was established.

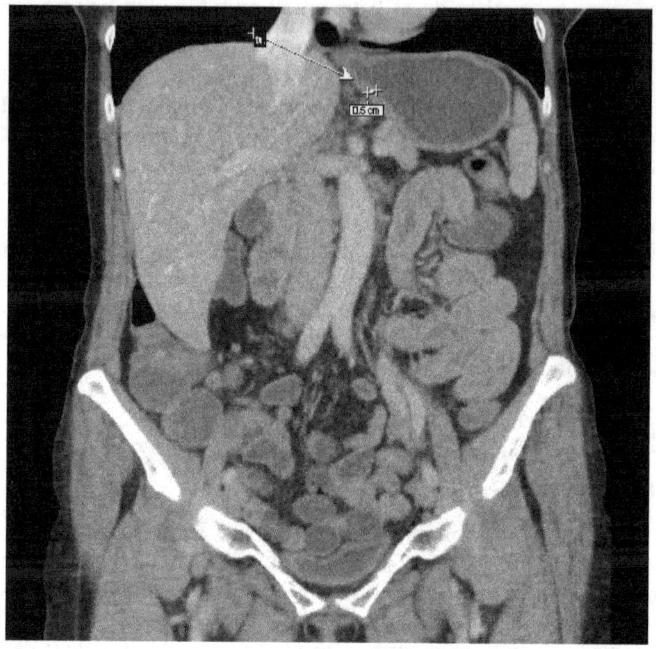


**Figure 1b: Figure 1:** The next three cycles chemotherapy were given in the same doses but combined with ME/ML, BioBran and WGE and after three months nearly complete remission was observed.

Another 65 years old patient (presented in figure 2) had a ductal mammary carcinoma [T2 N1 (2/14) M0], a tumorectomy was carried out in May 2003, and subsequently six cycles chemotherapy and irradiation (50GY) were adjuvant given. In June 2011 a lung metastasis was established in right segment 6 (S6) by PET/CT scan which was in July 2011 chirurgical removed by tumorectomy. In September 2012 a recidivation of lung metastasis in S6 was established by PET/CT scan. From Oktober 2012 low dose of Xeloda (2500mg/die) was applied and after four cycles the question arose as to whether her lung metastasis is responsive to this chemotherapy. Therefore a CT scan investigation was carried out in March 2013 which did not found any change. From March 2013 the same doses of Xeloda were combined with standardized plant immunomodulators and after the next four cycles in July 2013 a complete remission was established by PET/CT scan. The chemotherapy was stopped and only the immunomodulatory treatment was followed. The last PET/CT control in November 2013 did not find any relapse of her disease and her quality of life is excellent.

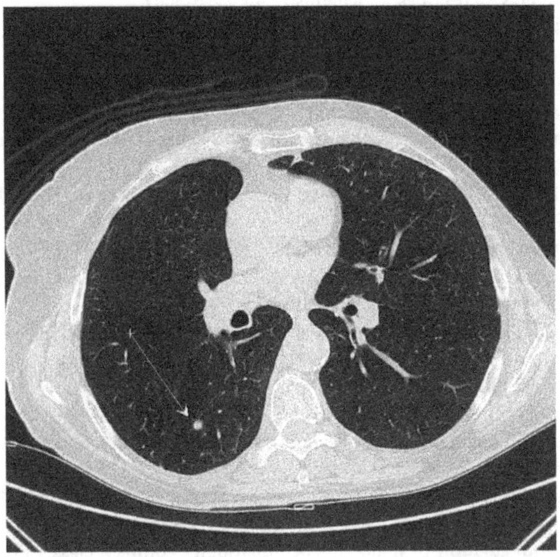

**Figure 2a:** Computed Tomography (CT) scans of lung metastasis of breast cancer in a 63-year-old patient. She has received five cycles Xeloda mono-chemotherapy and no change was established.

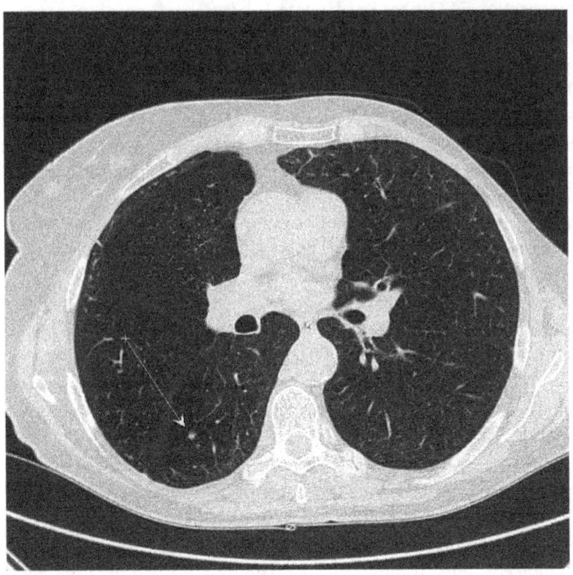

**Figure 2b:** The next four cycles of chemotherapy were given in the same doses but combined with ME/ML, BioBran and WGE. After four months nearly complete remission was observed, and the surgical operation was not necessary.

In the last two cases (illustrated on figure 1 and 2) the possibility cannot be ruled out that the remissions may be due to the time elapsed. Still, taking the previous clinical data into consideration these cases may also support the hypothesis that a combination of immune therapy with cytostatic drugs may be of additional benefit compared to a monotherapy with either substance. In addition, in second case report it is very improbable that low doses of Xeloda alone can induce a complete remission of lung metastasis suggesting a hypothesis that under certain circumstances these immunomodulatory treatments combined with low doses of chemotherapy may be more effective than their combination with high doses of cytostatic drugs.

## Standardizes plant immunomodulators, such as ME/ML, MGN-3/BioBran and WGE have no toxic side effects

Standardized plant extracts described above have a great advantage; they don't cause any side effects. In terms of safety and toxicity of ME, available studies indicate that mistletoe therapy is well tolerated, and serious adverse events were not reported [23]. MGN-3/BioBran has also been judged to be a highly safe food supplement as it was verified by conducting acute oral toxicity, mutagenicity, subacute toxicity, and antigenicity studies [24]. WGE has been put on the market as a non-toxic dietary supplement. Toxicological studies with high doses of WGE (3g/kg) did not show any deviation from the controls [19].

## Improvement of quality of life in tumor patients after an immunomodulatory treatment

Behavioral co-morbidities in cancer patients were often found to be associated with decreased activity of cellular innate immune responses and with an elevated activity of regulatory T cells [25]. The most often observed behavioral alterations of patients with cancer include fatigue, depression, pains and cognitive dysfunction [26]. Consequently, the influence of an immunomodulatory treatment on the cancer-related reduction of quality of life (QoL) attracts growing interest.

In a previous study [27] QoL was investigated in tumor patients who were treated with standardized plant immunomodulators. To monitor their QoL during this period, SF-36 questionnaires were regularly filled out at four months intervals. The score values of SF-36 questionnaires were regularly compared with untreated match pair control persons. The score values were evaluated 0, 4, 8, 1 2, 16, 20 and 24 months after the start of the observation period. Significant elevated differences in score values between patients and match pair control persons were found after 12, 16, 20 and 24 months. Particularly the tumor-related fatigue syndrome and pains were beneficially influenced. Consequently, it is suggested that the standardized plant immunomodulators can be helpful in the improvement of QoL of tumor patients.

## The role of external factors in clinical progress of tumor patients treated with standardized plant immunomodulators

Since an equilibrium disturbance in psychic situation and the tumor-induced immunological dysfunctions appear to be strongly associated with each other, the role of placebo effects may be also involved in the improvement of patients treated with standardized plant immunomodulators. Since the most frequent behavioral alterations of patients with cancer such as fatigue and depression can show an upturn during the immunomodulatory treatment, the patients are beginning to think more positively which can be helpful in the conventional oncologic therapy.

## Conclusion

Standardized plant extracts with PAMP-like activity may open new perspectives for oncologic therapy improving the tumor - related dysfunctions in innate immune system which can enhance the effectiveness of oncologic treatments and improve the quality of life. In order to further substantiate these claims, more rigorous research is urgently needed.

## Disclosure statement

The authors declare that there is no competing or other conflicting interest in relation to this paper. The sponsor had no influence on the design or conduct of the clinical reports, interpretation of data or approval of the manuscript.

## References


1. Nagtegaal ID, Marijnen CAM, Kranenbarg EK, Mulder-Stapel A, Hermans J, et al. (2001) Local and distant recurrences in rectal cancer patients are predicted by the nonspecific immune response; specific immune response has only a systemic effect. A histopathological and immunohistochemical study. BMC Cancer 1: 7-16.
2. Ostrand-Rosenberg S, Sinha P (2009) Myeloid-derived suppressor cells: linking inflammation and cancer. J Immunol 182: 4499-4506.
3. Mantovani A, (2007) Inflammation and cancer: the macrophage connection. Medicina (Buenos Aires), 67 (Suppl II): 32-34.
4. Terabe M, Berzofsky JA (2008) The role of NKT cells in tumor immunity. Adv Cancer Res 101: 277-348.
5. Baskic D, Acimovic L, Samardzic G, Vujanovic NL, Arsenijevic NN (2001) Blood monocytes and tumor-associated macrophages in human cancer: differences in activation levels. Neoplasma 48: 169-174.
6. Sánchez-Torres C, García-Romo GS, Cornejo-Cortés MA, Rivas-Carvalho A, Sánchez-Schmitz G (2001) CD16+ and CD16- human blood monocyte subsets differentiate in vitro to dendritic cells with different abilities to stimulate CD4+ T cells. Int Immunol 13: 1571-81.
7. Hajto T, Hostanska K, Gabius HJ (1989) Modulatory potency of the beta-galactoside-specific lectin from mistletoe extract (Iscador) on the host defense system in vivo in rabbits and patients. Cancer Res 49: 4803-4808.
8. Hostanska K, Hajto T, Spagnoli G.C, Saller R, 1996-97. A plant lectin, Viscum album agglutinin-I (VAA-I), stimulates cellular parameters of natural immunity in vivo and induces cytokine gene expression and apoptosis in cultures of peripheral blood mononuclear cells in vitro. Nat Immun 15: 196-201.
9. Hajto T, Hostanska K, Frei K, Rordorf K, Gabius HJ (1990) Increased secretion of tumor necrosis factor-alpha, interleukin-1 and interleukin-6 by human mononuclear cells exposed to beta-galactoside-specific mistletoe lectin. Cancer Res 50: 3322-3326.
10. Hajto T, Hostanska K, Weber K, Zinke H, Fischer J, et al. (1998) Effect of a recombinant lectin, Viscum album agglutinin on the secretion of interleukin-12 in cultured human peripheral blood mononuclear cells and on NK-cell-mediated cytotoxicity of rat splenocytes in vitro and in vivo. Nat Immun 16: 34-46.
11. Hajtó T, Fodor K, Perjési P, Németh P (2011) Difficulties and perspectives of immunomodulatory therapy with mistletoe lectins and standardized mistletoe extracts in evidence-based medicine. Evid Based Complement Alternat Med 2011: 298972.
12. Müthing J, Meisen I, Bulau P, Langer M, Witthohn K, et al. (2004) Mistletoe lectin I is a sialic acid-specific lectin with strict preference to gangliosides and glycoproteins with terminal Neu5Ac alpha 2-6Gal beta 1-4GlcNAc residues. Biochemistry 43: 2996-3007.
13. Ghoneum M (1998) Enhancement of human natural killer cell activity by modified arabinoxylan from rice bran (BioBrab/MGN-3). Int J Immunotherapy 14: 89-99.
14. Ghoneum M, Matsuura M (2004) Augmentation of macrophage phagocytosis by modified arabinoxylan rice bran (MGN-3/biobran). Int J Immunopathol Pharmacol 17: 283-292.
15. Hidvégi M, Rásó E, Tömösközi-Farkas R, Szende B, Paku S, et al. (1999) MSC, a new benzoquinone-containing natural product with antimetastatic effect. Cancer Biother Radiopharm 14: 277-289.
16. Szent-Györgyi A (1982) Biological oxidation and cancer. Int J Quant Chem Quant Biol Symp 9: 27-38.
17. Jakab F, Mayer A, Hoffmann A, Hidvégi M (2000) First clinical data of a natural immunomodulator in colorectal cancer. Hepatogastroenterology 47: 393-395.
18. Boros LG, Nichelatti M, Shoenfeld Y (2005) Fermented wheat germ extract (Avemar) in the treatment of cancer and autoimmune diseases. Ann N Y Acad Sci 1051: 529-542.
19. Fajka-Boja R, Hidvégi M, Shoenfeld Y, Ion G, Demydenko D, et al. (2002) Fermented wheat germ extract induces apoptosis and downregulation of major histocompatibility complex class I proteins in tumor T and B cell lines. Int J Onc, 20: 563-570.
20. Kirsch A, Hajto T (2011) Case reports of sarcoma patients with optimized lectin-oriented mistletoe extract therapy. J Altern Complement Med 17: 973-979.
21. Hajto T, Kirsch A (2013) Case reports of cancer patients with hepatic metastases treated by standardized plant immunomodulatory preparations. J Cancer Res Update 2: 1-9.
22. Kirsch A (2007) Successful treatment of metastatic malignant melanoma with Viscum album extract (Iscador M). J Altern Complement Med 13: 443-445.
23. Bock PR, Friedel WE, Hanisch J, Karasmann M, Schneider B, 2004. Efficacy abd safety of long-term complementary treatment with standardized European mistletoe extract (Viscum album L) in addition to the conventional adjuvant oncologic therapy in patients with primary non-metastasized mammary carcinoma. Results of a multi-center, comparative, epidemiological cohort study in Germany and Switzerland. Drug Res 54: 456-66.
24. Tsunekawa H (2004) Effect of long-term administration of immunomodulatory food on cancer patients completing conventional treatments. Clin Pharmacol Ther 14: 295-302.
25. Liu WM, Meyer B, Dalgleish AG (2009) How immunotherapy can enhance the response to other modalities and improve outcome and quality of life. J BUON 14 Suppl 1: S103-109.
26. Miller AH, Ancoli-Israel S, Bower JE, Capuron L, Irwin MR (2008) Neuroendocrine-immune mechanisms of behavioral comorbidities in patients with cancer. J Clin Oncol 26: 971-982.
27. Hajto T, Adámy A, Langmár Z, Kirsch A, Ábrahám L, et al. (2013) Enhanced effectiveness of conventional oncotherapy with plant immunomodulators: Overview of recent advances. Adv Med Plant Res 1: 56-65.

# Has Anyone so far Bridged the Gap between microRNA, Botanicals and Oropharyngeal Squamous Cell Carcinoma?

**Mohammed E Grawish[1*], Mathias Wagner[2], Benjamin Vicinus[3], Michael J Jack[4], Tereza Richards[5], Ahmed Ragheb Zaher[1] and Chen Xi[6]**

[1]*Department of Oral Biology, Mansoura University, Egypt*

[2]*Department of Pathology, Saar State University, Homburg Campus, Homburg Saar, Germany*

[3]*Department of General, Visceral, Vascular and Paediatric Surgery, Saar State University, Homburg Campus, Homburg Saar, Germany*

[4]*Competence Centre for Complementary Medicine and Naturopathy, Technical University Munich, Munich, Germany*

[5]*Medical Library, University of the West Indies, Mona Campus, Kingston, Jamaica, W.I.*

[6]*Department of Applied Biology and Chemical Technology, Hong Kong Polytechnic University, Hong Hom, Kowloon, Hong Kong*

*__Corresponding author__: Grawish ME, Georgetown University School of Medicine, USA, E-mail: Grawish2005@yahoo.com

**Abstract**

**Background/Context:** Current debate concerning properties of oropharyngeal squamous cell carcinoma (OSCC) is nothing new. More recent information can be found on functional aspects of microRNA (miRNA) in botanicals and mammals, suggesting that the aging process and cancer development are regulated by these molecules. Interestingly, some dietary supplements (especially botanicals) have been reported to have cancer chemopreventive and/or anti-cancer properties and are common ingredients in so-called "anti-aging" creams.

**Objective:** The present study was therefore conducted to determine the state-of-the-art on botanicals, OSCC, and their relationship to miRNA.

**Methods/Design:** PubMed and Google Scholar were interrogated for articles published in English between January 1, 2000 and December 31, 2010 that discuss botanicals and which could possibly be used in treating OSCC. Additional searches in Google, Google Scholar, PubMed and KoreaMed were conducted to detect possible associations between miRNAs and the aforementioned items.

**Results:** The current body of literature suggests that botanicals might deliver some of their properties via miRNAs. No report was found however that makes a direct connection to OSCC. It therefore has not been determined whether there is an association between botanicals, OSCC, and miRNA molecules that could possibly have "anti-aging" as well as cancer chemopreventive and/or anti-cancer properties.

**Conclusions:** Systematic studies are needed to determine whether it is miRNA that could dispense possible therapeutic properties of botanicals on OSCC.

**Keywords:** Botanicals; miRNA; Oropharyngeal Squamous cell carcinoma

## Introduction

MicroRNAs (miRNAs) are small post-transcriptional regulators found in animals and plants (Figure 1). Numerous miRNA sequences are evolutionarily conserved among plant species [1,2] as are their target sequences in the mRNAs [3]. This could possibly be due to the role of miRNAs in gene expression control. The average half-life of mammalian miRNAs has been calculated to be 119 hours which suggests that they are up to ten times more stable than mRNAs [4]. Among the differences between plant and animal miRNA biology are the processing, the position of target interaction and/or the degree of complementarity [5]. Health related functions may be mediated by miRNAs which regulate the expressome, metabolome or interactome [6] within plants (esp. botanicals) and/or molecules that modify the status of miRNAs within animals (esp. humans). Tanshinone IIA (Chemical Abstracts Service Registry Number, CAS *no*: 568-72-9) for instance, a constituent of the traditional Chinese medicine Dan shen (Salvia miltiorrhiza; National Center for Biotechnology Information, NCBI, Taxonomy Identifier: 226208) protects against **particular variants of** sudden cardiac death via repression of miRNA-1 which targets the inwardly rectifying potassium channel subunit Kir2.1 (Universal Protein Resource, UniProt, Identifier: **Q64273)** [7].

Oropharyngeal squamous cell carcinoma (OSCC, figure 2) has been defined as cancer of the anatomical regions that are covered by the classificators C00-C10 [8,9]. It is among the most common cancers worldwide, and continues to represent a public health problem [10]. Despite advances in therapy, cure rates and survival remain poor [11]. OSCC often appears to be preventable and is likely to be related to behavioral and lifestyle factors. Prevention of OSCC therefore remains the goal to reduce the incidence of this disease [12,13].

Anticancerous effects such as growth inhibition of OSCC cell lines can be mediated by miRNAs [14]. It is however noteworthy that some miRNAs can also promote cancer by supporting cell growth or metastasis [15], a phenomenon outside the scope of the present study.

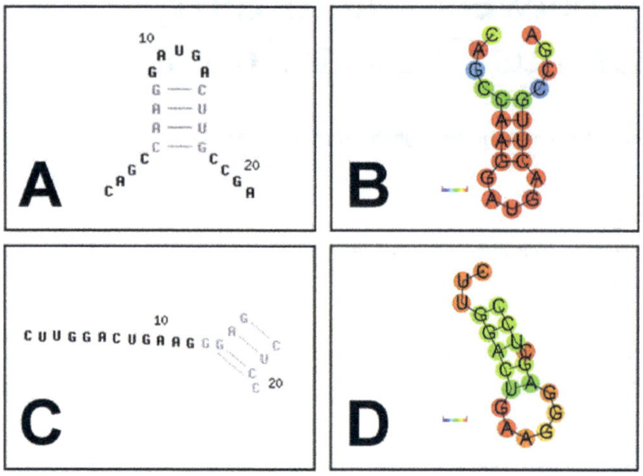

**Figure 1:** Graphic image representation of miRNA. Exemplarily selected results of single sequence RNA secondary structure prediction experiments for two miRNA species of *Solanum lycopersicum*, sly-miR169c [157] and sly-miR319 [160]. Two different computer programs, CONTRAfold (version: 2.02) [164] and RNAfold (Vienna RNA package version 2.0.0) [165, 166], were used to allow for visual comparison of geometries. [A] A secondary structure suggested for sly-miR169c based on conditional log-linear models (CLLM; CONTRAfold); [B] Coherence was found for the predicted minimum free energy structures and base pair probabilities for sly-miR169c (RNAfold); [C] A CLLM-based secondary structure suggested for sly-miR319 (CONTRAfold); [D] The secondary structure predicted for sly-miR319 based on minimum free energy structures and base pair probabilities (RNAfold) is not coherent, warranting further research

The use of dietary supplements, especially botanicals, or parts of them such as extracts or seeds as medicines predates recorded history and may be seen to represent an antecedent to modern medicine [16]. Technological advancement has facilitated the delivery of breakthrough bioactive compounds of botanicals with potency more or less comparable to those of conventional drugs [17]. Also their low cost, (per) oral bioavailability, and assumed low-risk profile at pharmacologically relevant concentrations have tremendous appeal. As a result of this assumed safety a considerable number of women for example use herbal remedies during pregnancy [18]. Phytochemicals have been evaluated for cancer chemoprevention and anti-cancer activities, increasingly throughout the course of the past decade [19-22]. Interestingly, some of these botanicals are among the top 10 ingredients in 2010 "anti-aging" creams [23]. This and previous reports [24-28] are suggesting that cancer chemopreventive agents and/or anti-aging drugs could have something in common. What they have in common could be effects mediated by miRNA as these molecules play a role in controlling the aging process [29] and cancer development [30]. It may therefore be hypothesized that botanicals could execute the aforementioned cancer chemopreventive and/or anti-cancer effects via miRNAs. The present study was conducted to determine whether miRNAs are currently seen as a link between botanicals and issues related to solid malignant tumors as exemplified by OSCC.

Google [31,32], PubMed [33], Google Scholar [34] and KoreaMed [35] were interrogated to identify scientific literature of relevance to this topic/area of research. This paper examines what these search engines present when interrogated for articles describing the possible role of miRNA in association with botanicals that have been applied in the context of chemoprevention of OSCC. Information on the role of botanicals in chemoprevention of OSCC published between January 1st, 2000, to December 3rd, 2010, is followed by a summary on miRNAs.

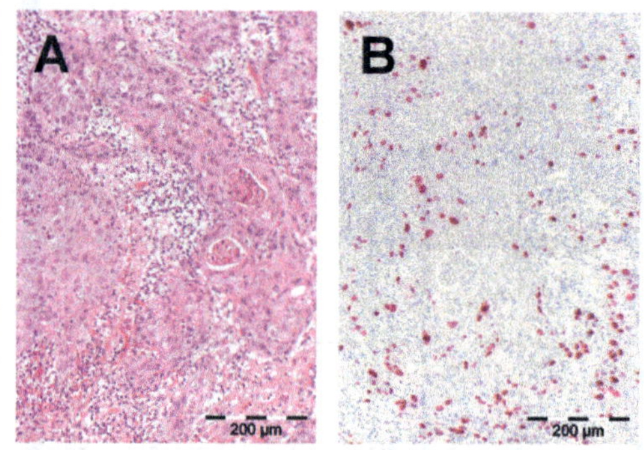

Figure 2: Microscopic image representation of the tumor. Oropharyngeal squamous cell carcinoma as exemplified by a pT1 G2 [9] lesion removed from the mouth floor (C04) of a 52 year old Caucasian male. [A] The histoarchitectonic pattern (Hematoxylin and Eosin, H&E, stain); [B] Late G1, S, M and G2 cell cycle phase (bright red signal), tumor cell nuclei, immunohistochemically contaminated with monoclonal mouse anti-human antibodies to the Ki67 antigen (clone: Mib1; Dako Deutschland GmbH, Hamburg, Germany; dilution: 1:100; BenchMark Series immunostainer, ultraView Universal Alkaline Phosphatase Red Detection Kit 760-501; Ventana Medical Systems, Inc., Tucson, AZ, USA)

## Leaves of the trees and shrubs

### Olive tree leaves

Olive tree (*Olea europaea* L; NCBI Taxonomy ID: 4146) leaves are well known as a traditional anti-diabetic and anti-hypertensive herbal drug [36]. Extracts rich in oleuropein (CAS *no*: 32619-42-4, 3 mg/kg body weight; bw) inhibited carcinogenesis in the oropharynx of *Rattus norvegicus* (NCBI Taxonomy *ID:* 10116), type Fischer (F344), after inductive treatment with 4-Nitroquinoline 1-oxide (4-NQO) (*CAS no*: 56-57-5) [37].

### Neem tree leaves, flowers and fruits

Neem (*Azadirachta indica*; NCBI Taxonomy ID: 124943) is a versatile tree of family Meliaceae (NCBI Taxonomy ID: 43707), the antiproliferative activity of neem tree flowers against some cancer cell lines was established [38]. Ethanolic neem leaf extract (200 mg/kg bw) and neem leaf fractions (1, 10, 100 mg/kg bw, in a dose dependent manner, ddm) have been reported to inhibit the development of OSCC in the buccal pouch of hamsters (NCBI Taxonomy ID: 10036) after application of 7,12-Dimethylbenz(a)anthracene (DMBA) (CAS no: 57-97-6) [39,40]. Apoptosis induction in neem treated hamsters was mediated by the expression of Bim (UniProt: Not Available), Bcl-2 (UniProt: Q687E0), caspase 3 (UniProt: Q60431), and caspase 8

(UniProt: Not Available) [41]. The neem fruit limonoids azadirachtin (CAS no: 11141-17-6; 10, 100 μg/kg bw) and neem flower nimbolide (CAS no: 25990-37-8; 10, 100 μg/kg bw) appeared to block cell proliferative activity and induce apoptosis. Comparatively, nimbolide is a more potent antioxidant and cancer chemopreventive agent [42, 43].

### Green, black and yerba mate shrub tea leaves

Tea, from the plant *Camellia sinensis L.* (NCBI Taxonomy ID: 4442), is one of the most common beverages and is generally consumed in its green, black, or oolong form. The main tea extract components are tea polyphenols and tea polysaccharides [44]. Green tea extract (GTE, 0.6% solution in tap water) and curcumin (CAS no: 458-37-7; 10 μmol) [45] had anticancerogenic effects by apoptosis induction, and the inhibition of cell proliferation and angiogenesis. It was proposed that green tea polyphenols (CAS no: 84650-60-2; 200 mg /kg bw/day) may act as a detoxifying agent, altering the expression of glycoconjugates and immunological markers [46], modulating lipid peroxidation and enhancing antioxidant ability [47] in an OSCC model. The recent effect was also associated with black tea polyphenols (BTP, CAS no: 84650-60-2; 0.05% Polyphenon) [47].

Epigallocatechin-3-gallate (CAS no: 989-51-5; 0 to 60 μM or 5, 10, 20, 50 μM, ddm) of green tea decreased the expression of matrix metalloproteinase (MMP) 2 (UniProt: **P08253**) and 9 (UniProt: **P14780**), urokinase plasminogen activator (UPA; UniProt: **P00749**) and inhibited the invasion and migration of carcinoma HSC-2 cells and normal HGF-2 fibroblasts cells [48-50]. A phase II randomized, placebo-controlled trial of GTE (500, 750, or 1,000 mg/m$^2$, ddm) concluded that GTE may suppress oropharyngeal premalignant changes, in part by reducing angiogenic stimulation [51].

Black tea was confirmed to have a beneficial effect on oropharyngeal leukoplakia (OLP) [52]. The BTP (30 to 40 mg/kg bw) exerted its preventive effects by inhibiting cell proliferation, modulating the oxidant-antioxidant status as well as markers of cell proliferation, cell survival, tumor infiltration, angiogenesis, apoptosis and xenobiotic-metabolizing enzymes [53-55]. The dietary administration of solitary or combined bovine lactoferrin (UniProt: **Q6LBN7**; 0.2%) and/or BTP (0.05% Polyphenon-B) has been reported to reduce tumor incidence in the hamster buccal pouch (HBP) [56]. Yerba mate tea (236 to 490 mg equiv of chlorogenic/g of dry leaves) is rich in phenolic constituents and can inhibit OSCC proliferation, topoisomerase 1 (UniProt: **P11387**), **topoisomerase** 2 (UniProt: **P11388**) [57].

### Seaside clerodendron shrub leaves

Seaside Clerodendron (*Clerodendrum inerme*; NCBI Taxonomy ID: 49994) is an evergreen sprawling shrub 1-1.8 m tall, containing two sterol constituents [58]. It was found that peroral administration of Clerodendron inerme aqueous leaf extract (500 mg/kg bw) reduced the incidence and size of DMBA-induced OSCC in the HBP [59].

## Roots, rhizomes and barks of shrubs herbaceous and trees

### Ashwaghanda shrub roots

Ashwaghanda (*Withania somnifera*; NCBI Taxonomy ID: 126910) root extracts are commonly used in Indian traditional Ayurveda as a general tonic for overall health and remedy for a variety of ailments [60]. Withaferin-A (CAS no: 5119-48-2; 20 mg/kg bw), a steroidal lactone isolated from *Withania somnifera*, appeared to prevent alterations of both p53 (UniProt: **Q00366**) and Bcl-2 and decreases micronucleus formation in the bone marrow once administered to DMBA-painted hamsters [61,62]. Withaferin-A prevented tumor formation and helped maintain erythrocyte integrity during DMBA induction of OSCC [63].

### Curcumin and ginger herbaceous plant rhizomes

Curcumin (diferuloylmethane), a polyphenol from the plant *Curcuma longa* (NCBI Taxonomy ID: 136217), traditionally called turmeric is used for cancer chemoprevention and treatment [64]. Meanwhile, ginger (*Zingiber officinale*; NCBI Taxonomy ID: 94328) is one of the plants family members that includes cardamom (NCBI Taxonomy ID: 105181) and turmeric [65]. Curcumin (0.1, 1.0, 10.0 μM, ddm) was considerably more potent than genistein (CAS no: 446-72-0) isoflavone and quercetin (CAS no: 117-39-5) flavonoid, but cisplatin (ATC/DDD: L01XA01; a platinum-based chemotherapy drug; CAS no: 15663-27-1) was fivefold more potent than curcumin in inhibition of growth and DNA synthesis in a cell line (SCC-25) in vitro [66]. In metabolism studies, curcumin (1, 5, 10, 25, and 50 μM, ddm) inhibited P-450 1A1 (UniProt: **P04798**)-mediated by benzo(a)pyrene diol (CAS no: 51689-89-5) bioactivation in both OSCC lines and intact oropharyngeal mucosa [67]. Curcumin (0.1 μM to 1mM) could also induce reactive oxygen species generation and early apoptotic changes in human gingival fibroblasts and human submandibular gland carcinoma cells [68]. It was reported that peroral administration of curcumin (80 mg/kg bw) and piperine (CAS no: 94-62-2; 50 mg/kg bw) to DMBA-painted hamsters helped prevent the formation of OSCC [69].

Moreover, dietary turmeric (1%) augmented apoptosis and decreased cell proliferation in DMBA-treated animals, reflected by decreased tumor burden, multiplicity and enhanced latency period [70]. In highly invasive human YD-10B OSCC cell lines, curcumin inhibited cell proliferation and motility through decreased expression of MMP2 and 9, UPA and UPA receptor (UniProt: Q03405) [71].

Ginger (400 mg powder added to labarotory chow) might have a preventive effect on oropharyngeal carcinogenesis through induction of apoptosis and suppression of tumor growth and proliferation [72].

### Portia tree barks

Portia tree or *Thespesia populnea* Soland ex Correa (NCBI Taxonomy ID: 3638; Family: Malvaceae; NCBI Taxonomy ID: 3629) is a large tropical tree found in coastal forests and India [73]. Ethanolic extract of *Thespesia populnea* bark (300 mg/kg bw) has been reported to execute cancer preventive effects in HBP contaminated with DMBA [74].

## Fruits and their seeds

### Black raspberries

Black raspberries (*Rubus occidentalis*; NCBI Taxonomy ID: 75079) contain many compounds with both in vitro and in vivo preventive properties [75]. The lyophilized black raspberries (5% and 10%) had a preventive activity and inhibited the tumor formation in the oral cavity [76]. Black raspberries inhibitory effects on growth of dysplastic human cells from the oropharynx were attributed to certain components that target specific signaling pathways regulating the progression of cell cycle [77]. Ethanolic extract (10, 50, 100 µg/ ml, ddm) of freeze-dried black raspberries was a promising agent for prevention of oropharyngeal epithelial dysplasia [75]. Application of black raspberry bioadhesive gel (10% w/w gel or 0.5 g of 10% gel) containing anthocyanins (CAS no: 15067-77-7) represented a promising strategy for human OSCC chemoprevention by modulation of gene expression and reduction of cyclooxygenase-2 (UniProt: Q9NNY7) protein [78,79].

### Cranberry and grape seeds

Cranberries (*Vaccinium macrocarpon*; NCBI Taxonomy ID: 13750) are a group of **evergreen** dwarf **shrubs** often used by pregnant or breastfeeding women as a preventive agent against urinary tract infections [80]. Grapes (*Vitis vinifera*; NCBI Taxonomy ID: 29760) are considered the world's largest fruit crops, with an approximate annual production of 58 million metric tons [81]. Grape seeds are rich sources of monomeric phenolic compounds, such as catechins (CAS no: 7295-85-4), epicatechin (CAS no: 490-46-0) and epicatechin-3-O-gallate (CAS no: 1257-08-5) and dimeric, trimeric and tetrameric procyanidins (CAS no: 4852-22-6) acting as antimutagenic and antiviral agents [82]. Grape seed proanthocyanidins (CAS no: 84929-27-1) differ from cranberry proanthocyanidins in that they are more likely to contain galloylated flavan-3-ols, and the monomers are primarily B linked [83]. Extracts of grape seed were more cytotoxic than grape peel extracts and 70% methanol extracts of grape seed selectively killed two human oropharyngeal tumor cell lines [84]. Cranberry and grape seed extracts (both 10 to 80 µg/ ml, ddm) inhibited the proliferation of OSCC cell lines (CAL27 and SCC25) in a dose-dependent manner [85].

### Tomato and its orange colored lycopene

Tomato is an edible fruit of the plant *Solanum lycopersicum* (NCBI Taxonomy ID: 4081) [86]. Combined administration of tomato (0.25 mg lycopene/ml; CAS no: 502-65-8;) and garlic (NCBI Taxonomy ID: 4682; 12.5 mg/ ml) inhibited the development of OSCC in the HBP by downregulation of Bcl-2 and upregulation of Bax (UniProt: Not Available), Bim, P53 and the caspases 3 and 8 [87]. They modulated xenobiotic-metabolizing enzymes mitigating the mutagenic and carcinogenic effects of DMBA [88]. Lycopene (a red carotene found in tomatoes; 2.5 mg/kg, bw) might exert its preventive effects by modulating lipid peroxidation and enhancing the activities of the enzymes in the glutathione redox cycle as it reduced glutathione (GSH; CAS no: 70-18-8), glutathione peroxidase (GPx; UniProt: P86215), glutathione S-transferase (GST; UniProt: P30116) and glutathione reductase (UniProt: Not Available) as biomarkers of cancer chemoprevention [89]. Lycopene (3 and 7 mol/L) inhibited proliferation and enhanced gap-junction communication of KB-1 tumor cells from the human oropharynx [90]. The observed effect of lycopene (4 or 8 mg/day) suggested that it can be effectively and safely used for the management of OLP [91]. Tomato paste containing weight lycopene (5 mg/kg bw reduced the incidence of OSCC in the HBP [92].

## Flavors and Spices

### Garlic and its water soluble extract S-allylcysteine

Garlic (*Allium sativum L.* fam. Allioideae; Taxonomy ID: 40553) is one of the most commonly used spices and herbal remedies. Alliinase (UniProt: D2CXF2), alliin (sulfur-containing compounds, CAS no: 556-27-4), and allicin (compounds produced enzymatically from alliin, CAS no: 539-86-6) are the main constituents of garlic [93]. Administration of S-allylcysteine (CAS no: 21593-77-1; 200 mg/kg bw) or aqueous garlic extract (250 mg/kg bw) suppressed DMBA-induced oropharyngeal carcinogenesis as revealed by the absence of neoplasms, induction of transglutaminase (UniProt: Not Available) and inhibition of Bcl-2 expression and restored retinoic acid receptor-beta mRNA (UniProt: Q8VHB7) expression to normal [94-97]. S-allylcysteine (0, 2, 5 10, 20 mM, ddm) effectively inhibited the proliferation, up-regulated the expression of E-cadherin (UniProt: Q9UII7) molecule and stabilized the E-cadherin/beta-catenin (UniProt: P35222) adherent junction complex in human OSCC cell lines [98]. Altered cytokeratin expression and enhanced quantities of circulatory antioxidants were suggested to be associated with garlic-mediated cancer chemoprevention (250 mg/kg bw) of experimental OSCC in the HBP [99,100].

In 4NQO-induced rat tongue carcinogenesis, garlic (25 mg/ml) might execute its preventive effects by modulating lipid peroxidation and enhancing the levels of GSH, GPx (UniProt: P04041) and GST (UniProt: Q6LDP3) [101].

### Pepper and its ingredients (piperine and capsaicin)

Piperine (CAS no: 94-62-2) extracted from *Piper longum* (long pepper; NCBI Taxonomy ID: 49511) and *Piper nigrum* (black pepper; NCBI Taxonomy ID: 13216) is an active alkaloid, consumed by a large number of individuals worldwide [102]. Piperine (50 mg/kg bw) had been suggested to execute a chemopreventive effect on DMBA-mediated induction of OSCC in the HBP [103]. The modifying effects of dietary capsaicin (CAS no: 404-86-4; ATC/DDD: N01BX04; active component of chili peppers; NCBI *Taxonomy ID:* 4073; 500 ppm, w/w) and rotenone (CAS no: 83-79-4; 500 ppm) on initiation or promotion phase of 4-NQO-induced rat tongue carcinogenesis reduced the frequency of OSCC [104].

### Plants used in Traditional Chinese Medicine

Levamisole (CAS no: 14769-73-4; ATC/DDD: P02CE01; antihelminthic drug) and/or Chinese medicinal herbs (root of *Astragalus*, NCBI Taxonomy ID: 20400; 12 g/day; fruit of *Ligustrum*, NCBI Taxonomy ID: 104487; 9 g/day; and fruit of *Ziziphi jujuba*; NCBI Taxonomy ID: 157914; 9 g/day) can modulate the level of the serum SCC associated antigen. For OLP patients, the combination therapy was superior to the single therapy of levamisole or of Chinese medicinal herbs [105]. Chinese herbal extracts of *Drynaria bonii* (NCBI Taxonomy ID: 272673), *Angelica sinensis* (NCBI Taxonomy ID: 165353) and *Cornus officinalis Sieb* (NCBI Taxonomy ID: 16906) were investigated for their antitumor potential on human OSCC cell lines (HSC-2 and NA) and the data demonstrated several unique antitumor properties of *Drynaria bonii* [106].

Ching waysan (0, 10, 25, 50, 75 and 100 µl/ ml, ddm; table 1) induced apoptosis via a Bax (UniProt: Q07812)-dependent pathway in human OSCC cell lines (OC2 and TSCCa) [107]. Shenyang (1,026 mg or 256.5 mg/100 g bw) had immune modulatory effects in rattus norvegicus, Sprague-Dawley type, with 4-NQO-induced OSCC [108]. Zeng sheng ping (6 g/kg bw/day by gavage) has been reported to prevent OSCC in humans with OLP as well as in animal models [109].

*Herba erigerontis* (NCBI Taxonomy ID: 124940) appeared to hamper the possible progression of OLP to tumor [110]. Also, Xian huayin (1.7 ml or 11.4 ml/kg bw/day) from China may exhibit a reversal effect on DMBA-induced premalignant lesions in the HBP [111]. The extract of the rhizome of *Coptidium* (NCBI Taxonomy ID: 568508, 13.5% w/w) induced cytochrome-c (UniProt: P99999) dependent apoptosis in immortalized and malignant human oropharyngeal keratinocytes via the mitochondrial signaling pathway [112].

Verticinone (CAS no: 18059-10-4; different concentrations for different cell lines), an alkaloid from *Fritillaria ussuriensis* (NCBI Taxonomy ID: 152096) induced apoptosis through a caspase pathway mediated by mitochondrial damage in immortalized keratinocytes and OSCC cell lines [113]. Rhein (CAS no: 478-43-3) is a anthraquinone (CAS no: 84-65-1) compound from *Rheum palmatum* (NCBI Taxonomy ID: 137221; 0, 25, 50, 100 μM) having inhibitory effects on OSCC as do emodin (CAS no: 518-82-1; 0, 20, 30, 40 μM) and aloe-emodin (CAS no: 481-72-1; 2.5, 5, 10, 20, 40 μM or 0, 25, 50, 100 μM) [114,115]. Shikonin (CAS no: 517-89-5; 0, 10, 20, 30, 40 μM, ddm), a naphthoquinone (CAS no: 130-15-4) pigment, seemed to alter growth and induce apoptosis in the human OSCC cell line Tca-8113 [116].

## Algae and their Extracts

### Spirulina platensis

Spirulina (NCBI Taxonomy ID: 1154) is a blue-green filamentous alga (NCBI Taxonomy ID; 1117) [117]. *Spirulina platensis* (*Arthrospira platensis*; NCBI Taxonomy ID: 118562; 10 mg/day) inhibited dysplastic changes occurring in the HBP mucosa and had a long-term cancer regression role on DMBA-induced OSCC [118,119].

## Miscellaneous Compounds

### Ferulic acid

Ferulic acid (hydroxycinnamic acid, CAS no: 1135-24-6), is found in the brans of grasses such as wheat (Triticum aestivum; NCBI Taxonomy ID: 4565), rice (Oryza sativa; NCBI Taxonomy ID: 4530), and oats (*Avena*; NCBI Taxonomy ID: 4496) [120]. It (40 mg/kg bw) has been said to reduce tumor incidence and size in DMBA-painted animals by exhibiting antilipidperoxidative effects as well as its ability to modulate the status of carcinogen detoxifying agents [121].

### Carnosic acid

Carnosic acid (CAS no: 3650-09-7; 10 mg/kg bw/day) from rosemary (*Rosmarinus officinalis;* NCBI Taxonomy ID: 39367) has been suggested to chemoprevent against DMBA-induced OSCC possibly due to likely carcinogen detoxification and antilipidperoxidative properties [122].

### Berberine

Berberine (CAS no: 2086-83-1), an isoquinoline (CAS no: 119-65-3) alkaloid present in roots, rhizome and stembark of a number of traditional medicinal plants such as *Berberis aquifolium* (NCBI Taxonomy ID: 203270), *Berberis vulgaris* (NCBI Taxonomy ID: 258209), *Berberis aristata* (NCBI Taxonomy ID: 659592) and *Tinospora cordifolia* (NCBI Taxonomy ID: 285590)[123]. The tumor size in xenograft mice treated with berberine (10 mg/kg bw) was smaller than that in the non-treated control group [124]. Prolonged exposure of human HSC-3 OSCC cell lines to berberine (0, 5, 10, 25, 50, 75 μM) increased apoptosis through reduced levels of MMP (UniProt: P03956), release of cytochrome c and activation of caspase 3 (UniProt: P42574) [125]. Moreover, berberine (0, 62.5, 100 μM) was found to down-regulate u-PA, MMP2 and MMP9 expression in SCC-4 cells through the focal adhesion kinase 1 (UniProt: Q05397), inhibitor of nuclear factor (NF) kappa B and NF kappa B mediated pathways and berberine inhibited the invasive capacity of malignant cells [126].

## A Few Notes on Dosages

Additional searches were conducted to compare the dosages previously discussed in cell line and animal models with those suggested for humans. The following databases have been interrogated: About Herbs, a web site provided by the Memorial Sloan Kettering Cancer Center (MSKCC Integrative Medicine Service) [127], Herbs at a Glance, and the Complementary and Alternative Medicine (CAM) subset of PubMed both of which have been established by the National Center for Complementary and Alternative Medicine (NCCAM) [128].

This part of the study revealed that the current body of literature contains only few peer reviewed articles on effective clinical dosages in humans specified by good scientific practice experimental design. At least in parts this may be attributable to the fact that botanicals come in a variety of dosage forms such as teas, creams, gels, capsules or tablets, and/or that they can be formulated for various types of drug delivery supporting extended, sustained or other modes of drug release. Different dosages can therefore be readily extracted from the body of literature (table 1). Comparative studies are warranted to learn more about dose-response relationships in this context.

| Botanical | Cell Lines | Animal model | Clinical Trial |
|---|---|---|---|
| Tea | Epigallocatechin-3-gallate: 0-60 μM [49]<br>Epigallocatechin-3-gallate: 5-50 μM [50] | Green Tea Extract: 0.6% in tap water [45]<br>Polyphenols: 200 mg/kg bw [46]<br>Polyphenon: 0.05% [47, 56]<br>Black Tea Polyphenon: 30-40 mg/kg bw [54]<br>Yerba Mate Tea: 236-490 mg [57] | Green Tea Extract: 500, 750, 1000 mg/m$^2$ [51]<br>§Catechin: 250 mg/day [167] |

| Curcumin | Curcumin: 0.1, 1.0 or 10.0 µM [66]; 1, 5, 10, 25, and 50 µM [67]; 0.1 µM to 1mM [68] | Curcumin: 80 mg/kg bw [69]<br>Turmeric: 1% [70] | §Curcumin: 8 g/day [168]; 3.6 g/day [169]; 1-4 g/day [170] |
|---|---|---|---|
| Black Raspberries | Ethanolic extract: 10, 50 or 100 µg/ml [75] | Lyophylized: 5% or 10% [76]<br>Bioadhesive Gel: 1g of 5% gel [78] | Bioadhesive Gel: 0.5g of 10% gel [79] |
| Tomato/<br>Lycopene | Lycopene: 3 and 7 mol/L [90] | Lycopene: 0.25 mg/ml [87]; 2.5 mg/kg bw [89]; 5 mg/kg bw [92] | Lycopene: 4 or 8 mg/day [91]<br>§Lycopene: 15 mg/day [171]; 4-30 mg/day [172] |
| Garlic | S-allylcysteine: 0, 2, 5 10, 20 mM [98] | S-allylcyteine: 200 mg/kg bw [94]; 250 mg/kg bw [96-100]; 25 mg/ml [101] | §Garlic: ~3.5 g/weak (range 0 to >28.8 g/weak) [173] |

**Table 1:** Dosage Variations. Differences in dosage and pharmaceutical formulation as exemplified above contribute to making systematic and reliable comparative evaluation a considerable challenge. The superscripted section sign ("§") marks entries on lesions other than OSCC

## MicroRNA

Medicinal plants may exert the carcinogenic potential by modulating carcinogen detoxification, inhibiting lipid peroxidation, or by improving in vivo antioxidants defense mechanism [90]. Only a few of the described botanicals exhibit articles which describe a role of miRNAs in the corresponding plants. Interrogating PubMed on July 2$^{nd}$ 2011 for entries containing for example the search terms "Salvia miltiorrhiza" and "miRNA" produced only a single hit, a publication mentioning the application of real-time reverse transcription polymerase chain reaction to determine the level of miRNA-1[7]. Entering "Salvia miltiorrhiza" and "miRNA" yielded no findings.

In *Camellia sinensis* there are around 13 conserved miRNAs which belong to 9 miRNA families [129]. Computational homology search in expressed sequencing tags revealed four candidate miRNAs from four miRNA families together with their target [130].

Computational predictions of *Vitis vinifera* genome identified 5.778 putative miRNAs [131]. High-throughput sequencing in *Vitis vinifera* tagged 24 conserved miRNA families, 26 non-conserved miRNA families and 21 grapevine-specific miRNAs [132]. Several grape genes contain putative binding sites of miRNAs [133]. Differential miRNA patterns in tissue development and fruit maturation indicate a function of miRNAs in these processes [134].

In *Solanum lycopersicum* 78 highly conserved mature miRNAs were found by a miRNA detecting microarray [135] and miRNAs play a role in the symbiosis with arbuscular mycorrhizal [136] and draught response (miRNA-169c) [137]. The miRNAs-159[138], 164 [139] and 319 [140] are involved in mechanisms like stamen regulatory network or leaf and flower development of *Solanum lycopersicum.*

In tomato plants the miRNA network is also associated with viral infection and is involved in: host defense response [141], altered host miRNA expression [142] and thereby miRNA mediated gene expression [143].

In safflower at least 236 miRNAs were identified which show different expression patterns in different tissues [144].

High throughput sequencing of wheat small RNAs revealed 58 miRNAs of 43 families from which 4 new miRNAs seem to be specific for monocots [145]. In the Triticeae 28 miRNA precursors were identified together with 337 target sequences in genes [146].

Approximately 40 potential miRNA genes were found in *Oryza sativa* [147]. Altered miRNA expression in rice was found as a result of heavy metal stress [148] and other biotic and abiotic stress factors [149]. Rice miRNAs control transcription factors which are involved in development and genes that regulate physiological processes [150].

Little is known about botanicals possibly inducing miRNAs in humans. Treatment of carcinoma cells with green tea polyphenons (polyphenon-60 or epigallocatechin gallate) leads to altered expression of miRNAs [151,152]. Epigallocatechin gallate changed miRNA expression in Hep G2 cells [153] and deregulated miRNA-21 and miRNA-330 in a mouse model of prostate carcinoma [154]. In a model of myocardial infarction miRNA-1 was downregulated by Tanshinone IIA a bioactive component of Salvia miltiorrhiza [7].

Curcumin up-regulated miRNA-15a and miRNA-16 in MCF-7 breast carcinoma cells and induced apoptosis of A549 human lung carcinoma cells by targeting miRNA-186*[155-157]. In pancreatic carcinoma cell lines miRNA-200 and miRNA-22 were up-regulated and miRNA-21 and miRNA-199* were down-regulated by curcumin (and its analogue CDF) [158,159]. Down-regulation of miRNA-21 by curcumin also inhibited invasion and metastasis in a chicken-embryo-metastasis model [160]. miRNA-146a and IRAK-2 were down-regulated by curcumin in stressed human astroglial cells in primary culture and a mouse model of Alzheimer's disease [161,162].

Extracts of Chinese herbal plant *Coptidis rhizoma* up-regulated miRNA-21 and miRNA-23a in human liver carcinoma cells (MHCC97-L) [163].

For the botanicals, ingredients, and properties that are not listed in this review, because there were no articles found which described the role of miRNAs in the plant or changes in human/animal miRNA expression upon treatment.

## Conclusion

Botanical and nutritional compounds have been used for the treatment of cancer throughout human history. So far little is known about the impact of miRNA on expression and function of botanicals. Nevertheless few studies indicate that miRNAs could mediate their health associated processes. Systematic studies are now warranted to determine their role in the chemoprevention of OSCC. To the knowledge of the authors no studies have so far directly bridged the gap between miRNA, botanicals, and the chemoprevention of OSCC. It remains therefore unclear if there is an association between botanicals, OSCC, and miRNA molecules that could possibly have "anti-aging" as well as cancer chemopreventive and/or anti-cancer properties.

## References


1. Axtell MJ, Bartel DP (2005) Antiquity of microRNAs and their targets in land plants. Plant Cell 17: 1658-1673.
2. Zhang B, Pan X, Cannon CH, Cobb GP, Anderson TA (2006) Conservation and divergence of plant microRNA genes. Plant J 46: 243-259.
3. Floyd SK, Bowman JL (2004) Gene regulation: ancient microRNA target sequences in plants. Nature 428: 485-486.
4. Gantier MP, McCoy CE, Rusinova I, Saulep D, Wang D, et.al (2011) Analysis of microRNA turnover in mammalian cells following Dicerl ablation. Nucleic Acids Res
5. Lelandais-Brière C, Sorin C, Declerck M, Benslimane A, Crespi M, et.al (2010) Small RNA diversity in plants and its impact in development. Curr Genomics 11: 14-23.
6. Bakry R, Rainer M, Huck CW, Bonn GK (2009) New stationary phases for enrichment and separation in the 'omics' era. Bioanalysis 1: 151-169.
7. Shan H, Li X, Pan Z, Zhang L, Cai B et al (2009) Tanshinone IIA protects against sudden cardiac death induced by lethal arrhythmias via repression of microRNA-1. Br J Pharmacol 158: 1227-1235.
8. Sankaranarayanan R, Dinshaw K, Nene BM, Ramadas K, Esmy PO, et al (2006) Cervical and oral cancer screening in India. J Med Screen 13: S 35-38.
9. Wittekind CH, Meyer HJ, Bootz F (2010) TNM-Klassifikation maligner Tumoren. 7th (edn) Springer-Verlag GmbH Berlin, Heidelberg, New York, London, Tokyo.
10. Warnakulasuriya S. (2010) Living with oral cancer: epidemiology with particular reference to prevalence and life-style changes that influence survival. Oral Oncol 46: 407-410.
11. Silverman S Jr, Kerr AR, Epstein JB (2010) Oral and pharyngeal cancer control and early detection. J Cancer Educ 25: 279-281.
12. Day TA, Davis BK, Gillespie MB, Joe JK, Kibbey M, et al (2003) Oral cancer treatment. Curr Treat Options Oncol 4 :27-41.
13. Saunders FR, Wallace HM (2010) On the natural chemoprevention of cancer. Plant Physiol Biochem 48: 621-626.
14. Shin KH, Bae SD, Hong HS, Kim RH, Kang MK, et.al (2011) miR-181a shows tumor suppressive effect against oral squamous cell carcinoma cells by downregulating K-ras. Biochem Biophys Res Commun 404: 896-902.
15. Yang CJ, Shen WG, Liu CJ, Chen YW, Lu HH, et al (2011) miR-221 and miR-222 expression increased the growth and tumorigenesis of oral carcinoma cells. J Oral Pathol Med 40: 560-566
16. Nobili S, Lippi D, Witort E, Donnini M, Bausi L, et al (2009) Natural compounds for cancer treatment and prevention. Pharmacol Res 59 : 365-378.
17. Rosenbloom RA, Chaudhary J, Castro-Eschenbach D (2011) Traditional botanical medicine: an introduction. Am J Ther 18 :158-161.
18. Low Dog T (2009) The use of botanicals during pregnancy and lactation. Altern Ther Health Med 15: 54-58.
19. Baskar AA, Ignacimuthu S, Paulraj GM, Al Numair KS (2010) Chemopreventive potential of beta-Sitosterol in experimental colon cancer model - an in vitro and In vivo study. BMC Complement Altern Med 10:24-34.
20. Gullett NP, Ruhul Amin AR, Bayraktar S, Pezzuto JM, Shin DM, et al (2010) Cancer prevention with natural compounds. Semin Oncol 37 : 258-281.
21. Khan N, Afaq F, Mukhtar H (2008) Cancer chemoprevention through dietary antioxidants: progress and promise. Antioxid Redox Signal 10 : 475-510.
22. Syed DN, Mukhtar H (2011) Botanicals for the prevention and treatment of cutaneous melanoma. Pigment Cell Melanoma Res 24 :688-702.
23. Cronin H, Draelos ZD (2010) Top 10 botanical ingredients in 2010 anti-ageing creams. J Cosmet Dermatol 9 : 218-225.
24. Donate LE, Blasco MA (2011) Telomeres in cancer and ageing. Philos Trans R Soc Lond B Biol Sci 366: 76-84.
25. Herranz D, Muñoz-Martin M, Cañamero M, Mulero F, Martinez-Pastor B, et al (2010) Sirt1 improves healthy ageing and protects from metabolic syndrome-associated cancer. Nat Commun 1:3.
26. Kiyono T (2007) Molecular mechanisms of cellular senescence and immortalization of human cells. Expert Opin Ther Targets 11 : 1623-1637.
27. Longo VD, Lieber MR, Vijg J (2008) Turning anti-ageing genes against cancer. Nat Rev Mol Cell Biol 9 : 903-910.
28. Svendsen L, Rattan SI, Clark BF (1994) Testing garlic for possible anti-ageing effects on long-term growth characteristics, morphology and macromolecular synthesis of human fibroblasts in culture. J Ethnopharmacol 43 : 125-133.
29. Noren Hooten N, Abdelmohsen K, Gorospe M, Ejiogu N, Zonderman AB, et al (2010) MicroRNA expression patterns reveal differential expression of target genes with age. PLoS One 5: e 10724.
30. Song FJ, Chen KX (2011) Single-nucleotide polymorphisms among microRNA: big effects on cancer. Chin J Cancer 30 :381-391.
31. Kingsley K, Galbraith GM, Herring M, Stowers E, Stewart T, et al (2011) Why not just Google it? An assessment of information literacy skills in a biomedical science curriculum. BMC Med Educ 11:17.
32. Giglia E (2008) To Google or not to Google, this is the question. Eur J Phys Rehabil Med 44 :221-230.
33. Roberts RJ (2001) PubMed Central: The GenBank of the published literature. Proc Natl Acad Sci USA 98 : 381-382.
34. Walters WH Google scholar search performance: comparative recall and precision. Portal Libr Acad 9 : 5-24.
35. Kim SY, Hahm CK, Bae CW, Cho HM (2008) Duplicate Publications in Korean medical journals indexed in KoreaMed. J Korean Med Sc 23 : 131-133.
36. Sato H, Genet C, Strehle A, Thomas C, Lobstein A, et al (2007) Anti-hyperglycemic activity of a TGR5 agonist isolated from Olea europaea. Biochem Biophys Res Commun 362 : 793-798.
37. Grawish ME, Zyada MM, Zaher AR (2010) Inhibition of 4-NQO-induced F433 rat tongue carcinogenesis by oleuropein-rich extract. Med Oncol 28: 1163-1168
38. Roy MK, Kobori M, Takenaka M, Nakahara K, Shinmoto H, et al (2007) Antiproliferative effect on human cancer cell lines after treatment with nimbolide extracted from an edible part of the neem tree (azadirachta indica). Phytother Res 21 : 245-250.
39. Subapriya R, Bhuvaneswari V, Ramesh V, Nagini S. (2005) Ethanolic leaf extract of neem (Azadirachta indica) inhibits buccal pouch carcinogenesis in hamsters. Cell Biochem Funct 23 : 229-238.
40. Manikandan P, Letchoumy PV, Gopalakrishnan M, Nagini S (2008) Evaluation of Azadirachta indica leaf fractions for in vitro antioxidant potential and in vivo modulation of biomarkers of chemoprevention in the hamster buccal pouch carcinogenesis model. Food Chem Toxicol 46 : 2332-2343.
41. Subapriya R, Bhuvaneswari V, Nagini S (2005) Ethanolic neem (Azadirachta indica) leaf extract induces apoptosis in the hamster buccal pouch carcinogenesis model by modulation of Bcl-2, Bim, caspase 8 and caspase 3. Asian Pac J Cancer Prev. 6 : 515-520.
42. Harish Kumar G, Vidya Priyadarsini R, Vinothini G, Vidjaya Letchoumy P, Nagini S (2010) The neem limonoids azadirachtin and nimbolide inhibit cell proliferation and induce apoptosis in an animal model of oral oncogenesis. Invest New Drugs 28 : 392-401.
43. Priyadarsini RV, Manikandan P, Kumar GH, Nagini S (2009) The neem limonoids azadirachtin and nimbolide inhibit hamster cheek pouch carcinogenesis by modulating xenobiotic-metabolizing enzymes, DNA damage, antioxidants, invasion and angiogenesis. Free Radic Res 43 : 492-504.

44. Monobe M, Ema K, Tokuda Y, Maeda-Yamamoto M (2010) Enhancement of the phagocytic activity of macrophage-like cells with a crude polysaccharide derived from green tea (Camellia sinensis) extract. Biosci Biotechnol Biochem 74 :1306-1308.

45. Li N, Chen X, Liao J, Yang G, Wang S, et al (2002) Inhibition of 7,12-dimethylbenz[a]anthracene (DMBA)-induced oral carcinogenesis in hamsters by tea and curcumin. Carcinogenesis 23 : 1307-1313.

46. Srinivasan P, Suchalatha S, Babu PV, Devi RS, Narayan S, et al (2008) Chemopreventive and therapeutic modulation of green tea polyphenols on drug metabolizing enzymes in 4-nitroquinoline 1-oxide induced oral cancer. Chem Biol Interact 172 : 224-234.

47. Chandra Mohan KV, Hara Y, Abraham SK, Nagini S (2005) Comparative evaluation of the chemopreventive efficacy of green and black tea polyphenols in the hamster buccal pouch carcinogenesis model. Clin Biochem 38 : 879-886.

48. Babich H, Krupka ME, Nissim HA, Zuckerbraun HL (2005) Differential in vitro cytotoxicity of (-)-epicatechin gallate (ECG) to cancer and normal cells from the human oral cavity. Toxicol In vitro 19 : 231-242.

49. Ho YC, Yang SF, Peng CY, Chou MY, Chang YC (2007) Epigallocatechin-3-gallate inhibits the invasion of human oral cancer cells and decreases the productions of matrix metalloproteinases and urokinase-plasminogen activator. J Oral Pathol Med 36 : 588-593.

50. Kato K, Long NK, Makita H, Toida M, Yamashita T, et al (2008) Effects of green tea polyphenol on methylation status of RECK gene and cancer cell invasion in oral squamous cell carcinoma cells. Br J Cancer 99 : 647-654.

51. Tsao AS, Liu D, Martin J, Tang XM, Lee JJ, et al (2009) Phase II randomized, placebo-controlled trial of green tea extract in patients with high-risk oral premalignant lesions. Cancer Prev Res (Phila) 2 : 931-941.

52. Halder A, Raychowdhury R, Ghosh A, De M (2005) Black tea (Camellia sinensis) as a chemopreventive agent in oral precancerous lesions. J Environ Pathol Toxicol Oncol. 24 :141-144.

53. Letchoumy PV, Chandra Mohan KV, Kumaraguruparan R, Hara Y, Nagini S (2006) Black tea polyphenols protect against 7,12-dimethylbenz[a]anthracene-induced hamster buccal pouch carcinogenesis. Oncol Res 16 : 167-178.

54. Letchoumy PV, Mohan KV, Prathiba D, Hara Y, Nagini S (2007) Comparative evaluation of antiproliferative, antiangiogenic and apoptosis inducing potential of black tea polyphenols in the hamster buccal pouch carcinogenesis model. J Carcinog 6:19.

55. Vidjaya Letchoumy P, Chandra Mohan KV, Stegeman JJ, Gelboin HV, Hara Y, et al (2008) Pretreatment with black tea polyphenols modulates xenobiotic-metabolizing enzymes in an experimental oral carcinogenesis model. Oncol Res 17 : 75-85.

56. Chandra Mohan KV, Devaraj H, Prathiba D, Hara Y, Nagini S (2006) Antiproliferative and apoptosis inducing effect of lactoferrin and black tea polyphenol combination on hamster buccal pouch carcinogenesis. Biochim Biophys Acta 1760 : 1536-1544.

57. Gonzalez de Mejia E, Song YS, Ramirez-Mares MV, Kobayashi H (2005) Effect of yerba mate (ilex paraguariensis) tea on topoisomerase inhibition and oral carcinoma cell proliferation. J Agric Food Chem 53 : 1966-1973.

58. Pandey R, Verma RK, Singh SC, Gupta MM (2003) 4alpha-methyl-24beta-ethyl-5alpha-cholesta-14,25-dien-3beta-ol and 24beta-ethylcholesta-5, 9(11), 22E-trien-3beta-ol, sterols from clerodendrum inerme. Phytochemistry 63: 415-420.

59. Manoharan S, Kavitha K, Senthil N, Renju GL (2006) Evaluation of anticarcinogenic effects of clerodendron inerme on 7,12-dimethylbenz(a) anthracene-induced hamster buccal pouch carcinogenesis. Singapore Med J 47:1038-1043.

60. Kataria H, Shah N, Kaul SC, Wadhwa R, Kaur G (2011) Water extract of ashwagandha leaves limits proliferation and migration, and induces differentiation in glioma cells. Evid Based Complement Alternat Med 267614

61. Bargagna-Mohan P, Hamza A, Kim YE, Khuan Abby Ho Y, Mor-Vaknin N, et al (2007) The tumor inhibitor and antiangiogenic agent withaferin A targets the intermediate filament protein vimentin. Chem Biol 14 : 623-634.

62. Panjamurthy K, Manoharan S, Balakrishnan S, Suresh K, Nirmal MR, et al (2008) Protective effect of withaferin-A on micronucleus frequency and detoxication agents during experimental oral carcinogenesis. Afr J Tradit Complement Altern Med 6 :1-8.

63. Manoharan S, Panjamurthy K, Pugalendi P, Balakrishnan S, Rajalingam K, et al (2008) Protective role of withaferin-A on red blood cell integrity during 7,12-dimethylbenz[a]anthracene induced oral carcinogenesis. Afr J Tradit Complement Altern Med 6 :94-102.

64. Aggarwal BB, Kumar A, Bharti AC (2003) Anticancer potential of curcumin: preclinical and clinical studies. Anticancer Res 23 :363-398.

65. White B (2007) Ginger: an overview. Am Fam Physician 75 : 1689-1691.

66. Elattar TM, Virji AS (2000) The inhibitory effect of curcumin, genistein, quercetin and cisplatin on the growth of oral cancer cells in vitro. Anticancer Res 20 : 1733-1738.

67. Rinaldi AL, Morse MA, Fields HW, Rothas DA, Pei P, et al (2002) Curcumin activates the aryl hydrocarbon receptor yet significantly inhibits (-)-benzo(a)pyrene-7R-trans-7,8-dihydrodiol bioactivation in oral squamous cell carcinoma cells and oral mucosa. Cancer Res 62 : 5451-5456.

68. Atsumi T, Tonosaki K, Fujisawa S (2006) Induction of early apoptosis and ROS-generation activity in human gingival fibroblasts (HGF) and human submandibular gland carcinoma (HSG) cells treated with curcumin. Arch Oral Biol 51:913-921.

69. Manoharan S, Balakrishnan S, Menon VP, Alias LM, Reena AR (2009) Chemopreventive efficacy of curcumin and piperine during 7,12-dimethylbenz[a]anthracene-induced hamster buccal pouch carcinogenesis. Singapore Med J 50:139-146.

70. Garg R, Ingle A, Maru G (2008) Dietary turmeric modulates DMBA-induced p21ras, MAP kinases and AP-1/NF kappa B pathway to alter cellular responses during hamster buccal pouch carcinogenesis. Toxicol Appl Pharmacol 232 : 428-439.

71. Shin HK, Kim J, Lee EJ, Kim SH (2010) Inhibitory effect of curcumin on motility of human oral squamous carcinoma YD-10B cells via suppression of ERK and NF-kappaB activations. Phytother Res 24 : 577-582.

72. Khater DS (2010) The influence of ginger as a chemopreventive agent on proliferation and apoptosis in chemically induced oral carcinogenesis. Nature and Science 8 : 44-51.

73. Ilavarasan R, Vasudevan M, Anbazhagan S, Venkataraman S (2003) Antioxidant activity of thespesia populnea bark extracts against carbon tetrachloride-induced liver injury in rats. J Ethnopharmacol 87:227-230.

74. Dhanarasu S, Al-hazimi AM, Sethuraman P, Selvam M (2010) Chemopreventive and antilipidperoxidative potential of thespesia populnea (L.) on experimental buccal pouch carcinogenesis. Ibnosina J Med BS. 2 :269-277.

75. Rodrigo KA, Rawal Y, Renner RJ, Schwartz SJ, Tian Q, et al (2006) Suppression of the tumorigenic phenotype in human oral squamous cell carcinoma cells by an ethanol extract derived from freeze-dried black raspberries. Nutr Cancer 54 : 58-68.

76. Casto BC, Kresty LA, Kraly CL, Pearl DK, Knobloch TJ, et al (2002) Chemoprevention of oral cancer by black raspberries. Anticancer Res 22 : 4005-4015.

77. Han C, Ding H, Casto B, Stoner GD, D'Ambrosio SM (2005) Inhibition of the growth of premalignant and malignant human oral cell lines by extracts and components of black raspberries. Nutr Cancer 51 :207-217.

78. Mallery SR, Stoner GD, Larsen PE, Fields HW, Rodrigo KA, et al (2007) Formulation and in vitro and in-vivo evaluation of a mucoadhesive gel containing freeze dried black raspberries: implications for oral cancer chemoprevention. Pharm Res 24 : 728-737.

79. Mallery SR, Zwick JC, Pei P, Tong M, Larsen PE , et al (2008) Topical application of a bioadhesive black raspberry gel modulates gene expression and reduces cyclooxygenase 2 protein in human premalignant oral lesions. Cancer Res 68 :4945-4957.

80. Dugoua JJ, Seely D, Perri D, Mills E, Koren G (2008) Safety and efficacy of cranberry (vaccinium macrocarpon) during pregnancy and lactation. Can J Clin Pharmacol 15: e 80-86.
81. Li MH, Jang JH, Sun B, Surh YJ (2004) Protective effects of oligomers of grape seed polyphenols against beta-amyloid-induced oxidative cell death. Ann N Y Acad Sci 1030 :317-329.
82. Stanković M, Tesević V, Vajs V, Todorović N, Milosavljević S, et al (2008) Antioxidant properties of grape seed extract on human lymphocyte oxidative defence. Planta Med 74 :730-735.
83. Hayasaka Y, Waters EJ, Cheynier V, Herderich MJ, Vidal S (2003) Characterization of proanthocyanidins in grape seeds using electrospray mass spectrometry. Rapid Commun Mass Spectrom 17:9-16.
84. Shirataki Y, Kawase M, Saito S, Kurihara T, Tanaka W, et al (2000) Selective cytotoxic activity of grape peel and seed extracts against oral tumor cell lines. Anticancer Res 20:423-426.
85. Chatelain K, Phippen S, McCabe J, Teeters CA, O'Malley S, et al (2008) Cranberry and grape seed extracts inhibit the proliferative phenotype of oral squamous cell carcinomas. Evid Based Complement Alternat Med
86. Luengwilai K, Fiehn OE, Beckles DM (2010) Comparison of leaf and fruit metabolism in two tomato (solanum lycopersicum L.) genotypes varying in total soluble solids. J Agric Food Chem 58:11790-11800.
87. Bhuvaneswari V, Rao KS, Nagini S (2004) Altered expression of anti and proapoptotic proteins during chemoprevention of hamster buccal pouch carcinogenesis by tomato and garlic combination. Clin Chim Acta 350:65-72.
88. Bhuvaneswari V, Abraham SK, Nagini S (2005) Combinatorial antigenotoxic and anticarcinogenic effects of tomato and garlic through modulation of xenobiotic-metabolizing enzymes during hamster buccal pouch carcinogenesis. Nutrition 21:726-731.
89. Bhuvaneswari V, Velmurugan B, Balasenthil S, Ramachandran CR, Nagini S (2001) Chemopreventive efficacy of lycopene on 7,12-dimethylbenz[a]anthracene-induced hamster buccal pouch carcinogenesis. Fitoterapia 72:865-874.
90. Livny O, Kaplan I, Reifen R, Polak-Charcon S, Madar Z, et al (2002) Lycopene inhibits proliferation and enhances gap-junction communication of KB-1 human oral tumor cells. J Nutr 132:3754-3759.
91. Singh M, Krishanappa R, Bagewadi A, Keluskar V (2004) Efficacy of oral lycopene in the treatment of oral leukoplakia. Oral Oncol 40:591-596.
92. Bhuvaneswari V, Velmurugan B, Nagini S (2004) Dose-response effect of tomato paste on 7,12-dimethylbenz[a]anthracene-induced hamster buccal pouch carcinogenesis. J Exp Clin Cancer Res 23:241-249.
93. Aviello G, Abenavoli L, Borrelli F, Capasso R, Izzo AA, et al (2009) Garlic: empiricism or science? Nat Prod Commun 4:1785-1796.
94. Balasenthil S, Nagini S (2000) Inhibition of 7,12-dimethylbenz[a]anthracene-induced hamster buccal pouch carcinogenesis by S-allylcysteine. Oral Oncol 36:382-386.
95. Balasenthil S, Ramachandran CR, Nagini S (2001) S-allylcysteine, a garlic constituent, inhibits 7,12-dimethylbenz[a]anthracene-induced hamster buccal pouch carcinogenesis. Nutr Cancer 40:165-172.
96. Balasenthil S, Rao KS, Nagini S (2002) Garlic induces apoptosis during 7,12-dimethylbenz[a]anthracene-induced hamster buccal pouch carcinogenesis. Oral Oncol 38:431-436.
97. Balasenthil S, Rao KS, Nagini S (2003) Retinoic acid receptor-beta mRNA expression during chemoprevention of hamster cheek pouch carcinogenesis by garlic. Asia Pac J Clin Nutr 12:215-218.
98. Tang FY, Chiang EP, Chung JG, Lee HZ, Hsu CY (2009) S-allylcysteine modulates the expression of E-cadherin and inhibits the malignant progression of human oral cancer. J Nutr Biochem 20:1013-1020.
99. Balasenthil S, Rao KS, Nagini S (2002) Altered cytokeratin expression during chemoprevention of experimental hamster buccal pouch carcinogenesis by garlic. J Oral Pathol Med 31:142-146.
100. Balasenthil S, Arivazhagan S, Nagini S (2000) Garlic enhances circulatory antioxidants during 7, 12-dimethylbenz[a]anthracene-induced hamster buccal pouch carcinogenesis. J Ethnopharmacol 72:429-433.
101. Balasenthil S, Ramachandran CR, Nagini S (2001) Prevention of 4-nitroquinoline 1-oxide-induced rat tongue carcinogenesis by garlic. Fitoterapia 72:524-531.
102. Koul IB, Kapil A (1993) Evaluation of the liver protective potential of piperine, an active principle of black and long peppers. Planta Med. 59:413-417.
103. Krishnakumar N, Manoharan S, Palaniappan PR, Venkatachalam P, Manohar MG (2009) Chemopreventive efficacy of piperine in 7,12-dimethyl benz [a] anthracene (DMBA)-induced hamster buccal pouch carcinogenesis: an FT-IR study. Food Chem Toxicol 47:2813-2820.
104. Tanaka T, Kohno H, Sakata K, Yamada Y, Hirose Y, et al (2002) Modifying effects of dietary capsaicin and rotenone on 4-nitroquinoline 1-oxide-induced rat tongue carcinogenesis. Carcinogenesis 23:1361-1367.
105. Sun A, Chiang CP (2001) Levamisole and/or Chinese medicinal herbs can modulate the serum level of squamous cell carcinoma associated antigen in patients with erosive oral lichen planus. J Oral Pathol Med 30:542-548.
106. Chu Q, Satoh K, Kanamoto T, et al (2009) Antitumor potential of three herbal extracts against human oral squamous cell lines. Anticancer Res. 29:3211-3219.
107. Liao PH, Chen SL, Shih HC, Chou MY (2005) Induction of apoptosis in human oral cancer cell lines, OC2 and TSCCa, by Ching waysan. Am J Chin Med 33:21-27.
108. Jiang C, Ye D, Qiu W, Zhang X, Zhang Z, et al (2007) Response of lymphocyte subsets and cytokines to shenyang prescription in Sprague-Dawley rats with tongue squamous cell carcinomas induced by 4NQO. BMC Cancer 7:40.
109. Sun Z, Guan X, Li N, Liu X, Chen X (2010) Chemoprevention of oral cancer in animal models, and effect on leukoplakias in human patients with Zeng sheng ping, a mixture of medicinal herbs. Oral Oncol 46:105-110.
110. Zhou Z, Zhang S, Hua L, Zhong W, Jin Z (2000) Leukoplakia and angiopoiesis resistance of Herba Erigerontis. Chin J Dent Res 3:56-62.
111. Xu YZ, Qiu YL, An ZG, Yang FY (2010) Role of the Chinese herbal medicine Xian huayin on the reversal of premalignant mucosal lesions in the golden hamster buccal pouch. Int J Oral Sci 2:53-58.
112. Lee HJ, Son DH, Lee SK, Lee J, Jun CD, et al (2006) Extract of Coptidis rhizoma induces cytochrome-c dependent apoptosis in immortalized and malignant human oral keratinocytes. Phytother Res 20:773-779.
113. Yun YG, Jeon BH, Lee JH, Lee SK, Lee HJ, et al (2008) Verticinone induces cell cycle arrest and apoptosis in immortalized and malignant human oral keratinocytes. Phytother Res 22:416-423.
114. Xiao B, Guo J, Liu D, Zhang S (2007) Aloe-emodin induces in vitro G2/M arrest and alkaline phosphatase activation in human oral cancer KB cells. Oral Oncol 43:905-910.
115. Chen YY, Chiang SY, Lin JG, Ma YS, Liao CL, et al (2010) Emodin, aloe-emodin and rhein inhibit migration and invasion in human tongue cancer SCC-4 cells through the inhibition of gene expression of matrix metalloproteinase-9. Int J Oncol. 36:1113-1120.
116. Min R, Tong J, Wenjun Y, Wenhu D, Xiaojian Z, et al (2008) Growth inhibition and induction of apoptosis in human oral squamous cell carcinoma Tca-8113 cell lines by Shikonin was partly through the inactivation of NF-kappa B pathway. Phytother Res 22:407-415.
117. Hayashi T, Hayashi K, Maeda M, Kojima I (1996) Calcium spirulan, an inhibitor of enveloped virus replication, from a blue-green alga spirulina platensis. J Nat Prod 59:83-87.
118. Grawish ME (2008) Effects of Spirulina platensis extract on Syrian hamster cheek pouch mucosa painted with 7,12-dimethylbenz[a]anthracene. Oral Oncol 44:956-962.
119. Grawish ME, Zaher AR, Gaafar AI, Nasif WA (2010) Long-term effect of Spirulina platensis extract on DMBA-induced hamster buccal pouch carcinogenesis (immunohistochemical study). Med Oncol 27:20-28.
120. Mathew S, Abraham TE (2004) Ferulic acid: an antioxidant found naturally in plant cell walls and feruloyl esterases involved in its release and their applications. Crit Rev Biotechnol 24:59-83.

121. Balakrishnan S, Menon VP, Manoharan S (2008) Ferulic acid inhibits 7,12-dimethylbenz[a]anthracene-induced hamster buccal pouch carcinogenesis. J Med Food 11:693-700.

122. Manoharan S, Vasanthaselvan M, Silvan S, Baskaran N, Kumar Singh A, et al (2010) Carnosic acid: a potent chemopreventive agent against oral carcinogenesis. Chem Biol Interact 188:616-622.

123. Craig WJ (1999) Health-promoting properties of common herbs. Am J Clin Nutr 70:491-499.

124. Ho YT, Yang JS, Lu CC, Chiang JH, Li TC, et al (2009) Berberine inhibits human tongue squamous carcinoma cancer tumor growth in a murine xenograft model. Phytomedicine 16:887-890.

125. Lin CC, Yang JS, Chen JT, Fan S, Yu FS, et al (2007) Berberine induces apoptosis in human HSC-3 oral cancer cells via simultaneous activation of the death receptor-mediated and mitochondrial pathway. Anticancer Res 27:3371-3378.

126. Ho YT, Yang JS, Li TC, Lin JJ, Lin JG, et al (2009) Berberine suppresses in vitro migration and invasion of human SCC-4 tongue squamous cancer cells through the inhibitions of FAK, IKK, NF kappa B, u-PA and MMP-2 and -9. Cancer Lett 279:155-162.

127. Cassileth BR, Heitzer M, Wesa K (2009) The public health impact of herbs and nutritional supplements. Pharm Biol 47:761-767.

128. Marcus DM, Grollman AP (2006) Science and government. Review for NCCAM is overdue. Science 313:301-302.

129. Das A, Mondal TK (2010) Computational identification of conserved microRNAs and their targets in tea (camellia sinensis). Am J Plant Sci. 1:77-86.

130. Prabu GR, Mandal AK (2010) Computational identification of miRNAs and their target genes from expressed sequence tags of tea (Camellia sinensis). Genomics Proteomics Bioinformatics 8:113-121.

131. Lazzari B, Caprera A, Cestaro A, Merelli I, Del Corvo M, et al (2009) Ontology-oriented retrieval of putative microRNAs in Vitis vinifera via GrapeMiRNA: a web database of de novo predicted grape microRNAs. BMC Plant Biol 9:82.

132. Pantaleo V, Szittya G, Moxon S, Miozzi L, Moulton V, et al (2010) Identification of grapevine microRNAs and their targets using high-throughput sequencing and degradome analysis. Plant J 62:960-976.

133. Faccioli P, Stanca AM, Morcia C, Alberici R, Terzi V (2010) Identification of a set of widely expressed genes in grape (Vitis vinifera L.) and its functional characterisation: a multi-evidence based study. Vitis 49:175-179.

134. Mica E, Piccolo V, Delledonne M, Ferrarini A, Pezzotti M, et al (2010) Correction: High throughput approaches reveal splicing of primary microRNA transcripts and tissue specific expression of mature microRNAs in vitis vinifera. BMC Genomics 11:109.

135. Zhang J, Zeng R, Chen J, Liu X, Liao Q (2008) Identification of conserved microRNAs and their targets from Solanum lycopersicum Mill. Gene 423:1-7.

136. Gu M, Xu K, Chen A, Zhu Y, Tang G, et al (2010) Expression analysis suggests potential roles of microRNAs for phosphate and arbuscular mycorrhizal signalling in solanum lycopersicum. Physiol Plant 138:226-237.

137. Zhang X, Zou Z, Gong P, Zhang J, Ziaf K, et al (2011) Over-expression of microRNA169 confers enhanced drought tolerance to tomato. Biotechnol Lett 33:403-409.

138. Buxdorf K, Hendelman A, Stav R, Lapidot M, Ori N, et al (2010) Identification and characterization of a novel miR159 target not related to MYB in tomato. Planta 232:1009-1022.

139. Berger Y, Harpaz-Saad S, Brand A, Melnik H, Sirding N, et al (2009) The NAC-domain transcription factor GOBLET specifies leaflet boundaries in compound tomato leaves. Development 136:823-832.

140. Ori N, Cohen AR, Etzioni A, Brand A, Yanai O, et al (2007) Regulation of LANCEOLATE by miR319 is required for compound-leaf development in tomato. Nat Genet 39:787-91.

141. Naqvi AR, Choudhury NR, Mukherjee SK, Haq QM (2011) In silico analysis reveals that several tomato microRNA/microRNA ? sequences exhibit propensity to bind to tomato leaf curl virus (ToLCV) associated genomes and most of their encoded open reading frames (ORFs). Plant Physiol Biochem 49:13-17.

142. Naqvi AR, Haq QM, Mukherjee SK (2010) MicroRNA profiling of tomato leaf curl New Delhi virus (tolcndv) infected tomato leaves indicates that deregulation of mir159/319 and mir172 might be linked with leaf curl disease. Virol J 7:281.

143. Cillo F, Mascia T, Pasciuto MM, Gallitelli D (2009) Differential effects of mild and severe Cucumber mosaic virus strains in the perturbation of microRNA-regulated gene expression in tomato map to the 3' sequence of RNA 2. Mol Plant Microbe Interact 22:1239-1249.

144. Li H, Dong Y, Sun Y, Zhu E, Yang J, et al (2011) Investigations of the microRNAs in safflower seed, leaf and petal by high-throughput sequencing. Planta 233:611-619.

145. Yao Y, Guo G, Ni Z, Sunkar R, Du J, et al (2007) Cloning and characterization of microRNAs from wheat (Triticum aestivum L.). Genome Biol 8:R96.

146. Dryanova A, Zakharov A, Gulick PJ (2008) Data mining for miRNAs and their targets in the Triticeae. Genome 51:433-443.

147. Li Y, Li W, Jin YX (2005) Computational identification of novel family members of microRNA genes in Arabidopsis thaliana and Oryza sativa. Acta Biochim Biophys Sin (Shanghai) 37:75-87.

148. Huang SQ, Peng J, Qiu CX, Yang ZM (2009) Heavy metal-regulated new microRNAs from rice. J Inorg Biochem 103:282-287.

149. Sanan-Mishra N, Kumar V, Sopory SK, Mukherjee SK (2009) Cloning and validation of novel miRNA from basmati rice indicates cross talk between abiotic and biotic stresses. Mol Genet Genomics 282:463-474.

150. Wu L, Zhang Q, Zhou H, Ni F, Wu X, et al (2009) Rice MicroRNA effector complexes and targets. Plant Cell 21:3421-3435.

151. Fix LN, Shah M, Efferth T, Farwell MA, Zhang B (2010) MicroRNA expression profile of MCF-7 human breast cancer cells and the effect of green tea polyphenon-60. Cancer Genomics Proteomics 7:261-277.

152. Tsang WP, Kwok TT (2010) Epigallocatechin gallate up-regulation of miR-16 and induction of apoptosis in human cancer cells. J Nutr Biochem 21:140-146.

153. Ahn JI, Jeong MJ, Shin HJ, Kim HS, Chung HJ, et al (2010) Changes of miRNA and mRNA expression in HepG2 cells treated by epigallocatechin gallate. Mol Cell Toxicol 6:169-177.

154. Siddiqui IA, Asim M, Hafeez BB, Adhami VM, Tarapore RS, et al (2011) Green tea polyphenol EGCG blunts androgen receptor function in prostate cancer. FASEB J 25:1198-1207.

155. Zhang J, Du Y, Wu C, Ren X, Ti X, et al (2010) Curcumin promotes apoptosis in human lung adenocarcinoma cells through miR-186* signaling pathway. Oncol Rep 24:1217-1223.

156. Zhang J, Zhang T, Ti X, et al (2010) Curcumin promotes apoptosis in A549/DDP multidrug-resistant human lung adenocarcinoma cells through an miRNA signaling pathway. Biochem Biophys Res Commun 399:1-6.

157. Yang J, Cao Y, Sun J, Zhang Y (2010) Curcumin reduces the expression of Bcl-2 by upregulating miR-15a and miR-16 in MCF-7 cells. Med Oncol 27:1114-1118.

158. Ali S, Ahmad A, Banerjee S, Padhye S, Dominiak K, et al (2010) Gemcitabine sensitivity can be induced in pancreatic cancer cells through modulation of miR-200 and miR-21 expression by curcumin or its analogue CDF. Cancer Res 70:3606-3617.

159. Sun M, Estrov Z, Ji Y, Coombes KR, Harris DH, et al (2008) Curcumin (diferuloylmethane) alters the expression profiles of microRNAs in human pancreatic cancer cells. Mol Cancer Ther 7:464-473.

160. Mudduluru G, George-William JN, Muppala S, Asangani IA, Kumarswamy R, et al (2011) Curcumin regulates miR-21 expression and inhibits invasion and metastasis in colorectal cancer. Biosci Rep 31:185-197.

161. Cui JG, Li YY, Zhao Y, Bhattacharjee S, Lukiw WJ (2010) Differential regulation of interleukin-1 receptor-associated kinase-1 (IRAK-1) and

IRAK-2 by microRNA-146a and NF kappa B in stressed human astroglial cells and in Alzheimer disease. J Biol Chem 285:38951-38960.

162. Li YY, Cui JG, Hill JM, Bhattacharjee S, Zhao Y, et al (2011) Increased expression of miRNA-146a in Alzheimer's disease transgenic mouse models. Neurosci Lett 487:94-98.

163. Zhu M, Wang N, Tsao SW, Yuen MF, Feng Y, et al (2011) Up-regulation of microRNAs, miR21 and miR23a in human liver cancer cells treated with Coptidis rhizome aqueous extract. Exp Ther Med 2: 27-32.

164. Do CB, Foo CS, Batzoglou S (2008) A max-margin model for efficient simultaneous alignment and folding of RNA sequences. Bioinformatics 24:168-176.

165. Gruber AR, Lorenz R, Bernhart SH, Neuböck R, Hofacker IL (2008) The Vienna RNA Websuite. Nucleic Acids Res 36: W 70-74.

166. Hofacker IL, Stadler PF (2006) Memory efficient folding algorithms for circular RNA secondary structures. Bioinformatics 22:1172-1176.

167. Boehm K, Borrelli F, Ernst E, Habacher G, Hung SK, et al (2009) Green tea (Camellia sinensis) for the prevention of cancer. Cochrane Database Syst Rev CD005004.

168. Dhillon N, Aggarwal BB, Newman RA, Wolff RA, Kunnumakkara AB, et al (2008) Phase II trial of curcumin in patients with advanced pancreatic cancer. Clin Cancer Res. 14:4491-4499.

169. Sharma RA, Euden SA, Platton SL, Cooke DN, Shafayat A, et al (2004) Phase I clinical trial of oral curcumin: biomarkers of systemic activity and compliance. Clin Cancer Res 10:6847-6854.

170. Williamson EM (2002) Major Herbs of Ayurveda. (1st edn) Churchill Livingstone Oxford UK

171. Schwarz S, Obermüller-Jevic UC, Hellmis E, Koch W, Jacobi G, et al (2008) Lycopene inhibits disease progression in patients with benign prostate hyperplasia. J Nutr 138:49-53.

172. Van Patten CL, de Boer JG, Tomlinson Guns ES (2008) Diet and dietary supplement intervention trials for the prevention of prostate cancer recurrence: a review of the randomized controlled trial evidence. J Urol 180:2314-2321.

173. Fleischauer AT, Poole C, Arab L (2000) Garlic consumption and cancer prevention: meta-analyses of colorectal and stomach cancers. Am J Clin Nutr 72:1047-1052.

7

# Treating Cancer with Snake Venom and Serum

**Federica Facchin[1,6], Margherita Ciano[1,2], Silvia Canaider[1,6], Fernando Ferretti[3], Anna Ferretti[3], Gianluigi Veronesi[3], Stefano Iotti[4,6]* and Pierluigi Lenzi[3,5,6]**

[1]*Department of Experimental, Diagnostic and Specialty Medicine (DIMES), University of Bologna, Italy*
[2]*Section of Molecular Medicine, National Heart and Lung Institute, Imperial College London, UK*
[3]*Institute Of Human Physiology, University Of Bologna, Italy*
[4]*Professor of Biochemistry, Department of Pharmacy and Biotechnology, University of Bologna, Italy*
[5]*Former professor of Physiology, Faculty of Medicine, University of Bologna, Italy*
[6]*National Institute of Biostructures and Biosystems, Rome, Italy*

**Abstract**

**Introduction:** A new anti-cancer immunological approach devised and experimented for years by Dr. Fernando Ferretti, is presented. Cobra Venom Factor is incubated with filtered Naja Naja Kaouthia serum and the mix obtained is injected subcutaneously. Due to the close functional similarity between Cobra Venom Factor and human Complement C3b, as well as the likely similarity between their inhibitors, the induced antibodies are hypothesized to cross react with Complement inhibitors and help restore the immune anti-cancer mechanisms.

**Methods and results of mix component analysis:** The electrophoretic analysis of Cobra Venom Factor, Naja serum and the therapeutic mix was performed and it showed that complex interactions occur between Cobra Venom Factor and serum, leading to the formation of new molecules in the mix.

**Case report:** We describe 8 cases of cancer treated with the present approach. Following immunogen injections, the patients generally experienced a transient increase in pain in the regions of primary and secondary cancer lesions, then the pain reduced and they felt better that before the injection. Overall, the effects observed ranged from complete healing to an increase of life duration beyond medical expectancy, together with a state of general well-being, decrease or disappearance of pain, new energy, a new positive sense of life.

**Discussion:** This therapy is aimed at balancing the various molecular components of the immune system, so as to restore its natural antitumor activity. A specific link is suggested between mix immunogens and the malignancy process.

**Keywords:** Cancer; Complement inhibitors; Immunological therapy; CVF; NNK; SDS-PAGE

## Introduction

New anti-cancer strategies are worth considering as conventional therapies are not always successful and the cancer death toll is still awfully high. Besides surgery, chemotherapy and radiotherapy, new hopes are oriented to the immune system potentialities [1,2]. It is now recognized that the immune system has the ability to identify and eliminate nascent tumor cells with no toxicity to normal tissue, together with long-term memory that can prevent cancer recurrence [3]. If some tumor cells escape detection, cancer may develop and such tumor cells, by the effect of the selective pressure exerted by the immune system, become progressively less immunogenic, so that tumor tolerance grows up [4]. New immune-based therapies are directed to break tumor tolerance and reactivate anti-tumor immunity to induce effective anti-tumor responses [5]. In this paper we present a new anti-cancer immunological therapy, studied and applied for years by Dr. Fernando Ferretti, aimed at restoring the proper functioning of the natural anti-cancer immune mechanisms, in particular the activity of the Complement System, which are likely impaired in cancer patients. This therapy is protected by US patent [6]. The Complement System plays a key role against invading bacteria by the Membrane Attack Complex forming pores and lysing the bacteria. Moreover, as a mediator between the innate and adaptive immune response, the complement system can directly neutralize viruses and modulate pathogen elimination [7]. Complement components may however be pathogenic in chronic diseases as atherosclerosis. For what concerns cancer, the relationship between complement and tumor cells is complex. On the one hand, the activated complement proteins through different mechanisms may lead to complement-mediated destruction of tumor cells. However tumor cells have natural mechanisms of self-protection against the complement system, as membrane and soluble complement inhibitors released by tumor cells interfere with the activation of the complement cascade. On the other hand, complement proteins may also favor tumor growth and immunosuppression [7]. The C3 molecule is a key component of complement, as it is involved in classical, lectin and alternative pathways. The alternative pathway not only serves as an individual activation pathway, but also provides an amplification loop of the classical and lectin pathways. The alternative pathway is continuously low level activated by the hydrolysis of C3 to $C3(H_2O)$ ("tick-over") and an initial C3 convertase $C3(H_2O)Bb$ is formed in the presence of Factor B and Factor D. The C3 convertases from all pathways cleave C3 in the anaphylatoxin C3a and the opsonin C3b and a final C3 convertase (C3bBb), if not prevented by inhibitors, is formed and cleaves more C3 [8]. Years ago Dr. Fernando Ferretti hypothesized that transformed cells secrete a molecule closely related to complement C3b, capable of reacting with Factor B and forming a C3/C5 convertase. This would activate the alternative pathway and

***Corresponding author:** Stefano Iotti, Department of Pharmacy and Biotechnology, University of Bologna, Italy, E-mail: stefano.iotti@unibo.it lead to the lysis of the transformed cells through the lytic cascade and/or the cell mediated cytotoxicity. This hypothesized molecule, named by Dr. Ferretti as RUHC3bL from "Relatively un-modulated human C3b like" [6], is supposed not to be regulated by fluid-phase and membrane-bound complement regulatory proteins and then to have long lasting action. Once secreted, two possible outcomes could result: either adequate complement activation occurs and the transformed cells are eliminated, or too much inhibitor are present and inadequate complement activation gives rise to inflammation but not cell elimination, so that a tumor may develop. Interestingly, complement inhibitors have been found on nearly all developed tumors and cancer cell lines that have been examined, while some studies indicate that complement-inhibitory proteins are up-regulated on tumor cells [9]. In most patients, chronic inflammation and immune suppression are the dominant effects in the tumor microenvironment [10]. The basic idea of Dr. Ferretti was to stimulate the production of antibodies against the inhibitors hindering complement activation. He exploited the close functional similarity between Cobra Venom Factor (CVF) and human C3b. In fact, CVF reacts with human Factor B and forms a C3/C5 convertase, (CVF)Bb, which is not regulated by complement regulatory proteins and has long lasting action [11], as it is supposed to be for the hypothesized RUHC3bL molecule. Basing on the well-known resistance of snakes to their own venom, due among others to venom inhibitors present in their serum [12], Dr. Ferretti hypothesized that by incubating CVF with Naja serum, a mix would be obtained containing complexes of CVF or CVF fragments with inhibitors. These inhibitors are likely related to human C3b or RUHC3bL inhibitors, but are definitely non-self. Injecting this mix in cancer patients, the non-self-epitopes would stimulate the formation of antibodies hypothetically cross-reacting with human C3b and RUHC3bL inhibitors, thus enhancing complement activation and complement mediated attack against transformed cells. In this paper a sample of the clinical results obtained over the years by Dr. Ferretti's therapy, together with a preliminary analysis of the therapeutic mix and its components are presented. We underline that the present study is aimed at evaluating whether the serum-CVF interaction produce adducts that could be compatible with Dr. Ferretti hypothesis. Of course, to obtain a conclusive confirm to this hypothesis further and more detailed studies are needed.

## Case History

### Patient characteristics and diagnosis

Patients having received cancer diagnosis were considered. Two of the oldest cases, relative to the years 1965-1970, together with two more recent cases, are presented below. The oldest cases concern skin cancers, documented by their images. For the more recent cases, clinical information is available, documented by clinical reports. Four more cases are presented in supplementary information. The cases here reported are just a sample of the many cases treated over the years by Dr. Ferretti. Many of the patients treated by Dr. Ferretti had been abandoned by the medical establishment as the conventional therapy was no more effective. In other cases, the therapy was applied in parallel with standard treatments, outside the control of the official medical team. For patients abandoned by the medical establishment, only the direct observation by Dr. Ferretti, the patients themselves and their relative could account for the effects of the immunological therapy. For patients in follow-up, the effects of the immunological therapy could be inferred from the clinical information provided by the official medical team. In all cases the immunological therapy was applied on request and informed consent of the patient.

## Methods and Intervention

### Immunological therapy

Dr. Ferretti's immunological therapy is based on injecting in cancer patients a mix obtained by incubating CVF with Naja Naja Kaouthia (NNK) serum. The mix is prepared according to the procedure presented below. Doses and incubation times, as well as serum filter cut-off, were slightly modified over the years, aiming at optimizing the outcome. Pre-clinical toxicity of a mixture of whole NNK serum and its crude venom was evaluated in 1973 at the Institute of Pharmacology of the Bologna University. Acute and chronic toxicity in rats, embryo-toxicity in rabbits and direct active anaphylaxis in the guinea pig were tested. At doses comparable with the therapeutic ones, no toxicity, either acute or chronic, was found in the mix analyzed. Dr. Ferretti started experimenting his immunological therapy on mice in the '60$^{th}$ and the results obtained encouraged him to treat cancer patients. The cases here reported represent only a small sample of the many cases treated by Dr. Ferretti, who worked in the silence for more than 30 years to develop his therapeutic mix, engaging all his intellectual and economical resources, as he always applied his therapy for free in all the patients treated. Dr. Ferretti's therapy and mix are protected by US patent [6].

### Treatment

Typically, a 500 µL dose of the mix was injected subcutaneously at intervals ranging from 5 to 30 days, depending on patient reactions. The duration of treatment ranged from many months to years, as during the treatment the patients enjoyed a better quality of life. Some patients wanted to continue the therapy even if they felt healed.

### Composition of the therapeutic mix

Two different mixes utilized over the years were considered, with serum 10 kDa and 50 kDa filter cut off (here named S10 and S50, respectively). The mixes were obtained according to the following procedure:

NNK serum and CVF were obtained from ACZON (BOLOGNA, ITALY). 2 ml of NNK serum were diluted with 38 ml of sterile distilled water and kept shaking for 20 minutes. The serum was filtered by centrifugal filter devices, with 10 or 50 kDa cut off (AMICOM ULTRA-15 10K and 50K, MILLIPORE, IRELAND). The diluted serum was placed at the top of the filter and centrifuged (5800 rpm×60 minutes×4°C). Filtrates were separately collected for 10 kDa and 50 kDa filter cut-off. 200 µg of CVF were mixed with filtrates, oscillated for 2 hours at 26°C and aliquoted.

The mix was concentrated to 7 ml (SAVANT concentrator)-The mix was filtrated through MILLEX Syringe Filter Unit 0.45 µm (MILLIPORE, IRELAND) this mix yielded an overall volume of 7200 µl. This mix was added with the following:- 3000 µL of Aluminum Hydroxide 3%, colloidal aluminum for subcutaneous vaccines approved by the Italian health authorities)

110 µL of Tyrosine 400 µM solution. It is an adjuvant normally used in vaccines [13] (SIGMA, ST. LOUIS, MO)-110 µL of THIMEROSAL (10 µg/µl) (SIGMA, ST. LOUIS, MO).This amount lead to a final THIMEROSAL concentration of 1:10000. It is germicide, utilized for subcutaneous vaccines and once allowed by the Italian health authorities.The final volume of the above components was 10420 µl. The unit dosage is 500 µl. The mix obtained is thus equivalent to about 20 doses, every single dose containing 10 µg CVF+10 µL of 10 kDa or

50 kDa cut-off filtered serum+other accessory adjuvants added (here named S10V and S50V, respectively).

## Native PAGE, SDS-PAGE and 2D-PAGE: CVF, serum and therapeutic mix protein analysis

Protein content of each sample was determined with a BCA protein assay kit (PIERCE, PIERCE BIOTECHNOLOGY, and ROCKFORD, IL, USA) and NANODROP technologies (NANODROP ND 1000 v.3.8.1, WILMINGTON, DELAWARE, USA) were used for the quantification. The protein content of each sample was analyzed in both native and denaturing conditions. Preliminary tests were performed to find the correct protein balance to get a good visualization. For the Native-PAGE, samples were diluted 1:4 with Native loading buffer (62.5 mM Tris-HCl pH 6.8, 40% Glycerol w/v, 0.01% BPB) then shaken for 10 minutes. The electrophoresis was performed using gradient gels (4–20% precast polyacrylamide gel, BIO-RAD, MILANO, ITALY) with native buffer (25 mM Tris, 192 mM Glycine pH 8.3) at 4°C to avoid denaturation due to high temperature.For the SDS-PAGE, samples were diluted 1:4 with denaturing loading buffer (1 M Tris base, pH 6.8, 8% SDS, 20% Glycerol, 0.24% BPB, 4% beta-mercaptoethanol) and boiled for 10 minutes. SDS-PAGE was performed using a standard method on a vertical slab gel. Proteins were analyzed on 4-20% precast gel or 6% or 12% or 15% homemade polyacrylamide gels and the electrophoresis was performed with Glycine buffer (25 mM Tris, 192 mM glycine, 0.1% SDS, pH 8.3) at room temperature.

To investigate the potential interaction between CVF and S10 proteins a two-dimensional polyacrylamide gel electrophoresis (2D-PAGE) was performed. Native PAGE as above was used for one-step isolation of protein complexes. The whole lane or the bands of interest were cut out, treated with 10% SDS for 15 minutes and placed on top of a 10% or 12% or 15% polyacrylamide gel and subjected to Glycine/SDS–PAGE [14].

After all the electrophoresis, the protein bands were visualized by staining with bio-safe COOMASSIE (BIO-RAD) or with silver stain using a mass spectrometry compatible protocol (161-0449 SILVER STAIN PLUS, BIO-RAD). PRECISION PLUS PROTEIN DUAL XTRA standards (BIO-RAD) were used as a molecular weight marker. The bands produced in the electropherogram were scored, and their molecular weights were compared with the standard protein marker.

## Results of Mix Component Analysis

Native-PAGE (Native Polyacrylamide Gel Electrophoresis) of CVF showed three bands. Besides the expected 150 kDa band [11], two more bands of about 70 and 75 kDa appeared (Figure 1A). When CVF was analyzed with two-dimensional electrophoresis system (2D-PAGE), the three bands were confirmed in denaturing condition, indicating that no interactions were present in native CVF (Figure 1B). The SDS (Sodium Dodecyl Sulfate) - PAGE of CVF showed many bands (Figure 1C), including the three expected products (69, 45 and 29 kDa, [11]).

In both native-PAGE S10 and S50, a 70 kDa band appeared (Figure 2A). To better visualize protein bands in SDS-PAGE of S10 and S50, several experiments were performed with different polyacrylamide gel concentrations (4-20%, 6%, 12%, 15%). In all experiments, a 70 kDa band was visualized (Figure 2B), while in some experiments up to three bands were present (approximately 70, 65 and 50 kDa, Figure 2C).

Two therapeutic mixes (CVF added to S10 or S50, here named S10V and S50V, respectively) were analyzed. Native-PAGE of S10V showed at least three bands corresponding to those of native CVF (150,

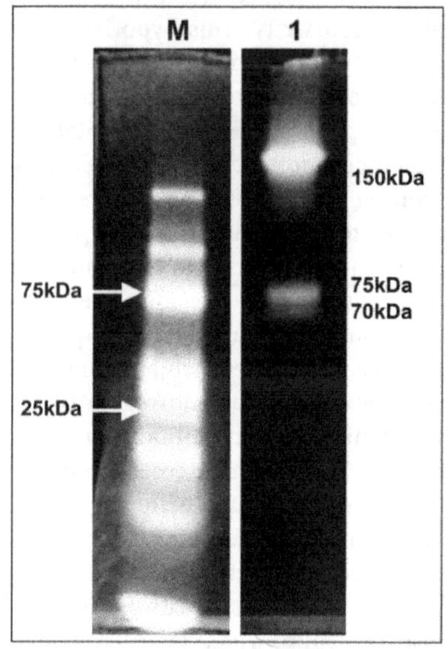


**Figure 1a**: CVF protein analysis. (A), Representative gel of 4-20% Native PAGE of CVF. Lane M, 5 µl Precision Plus Protein Dual Xtra standards marker. Lane 1, 15 µg CVF sample.

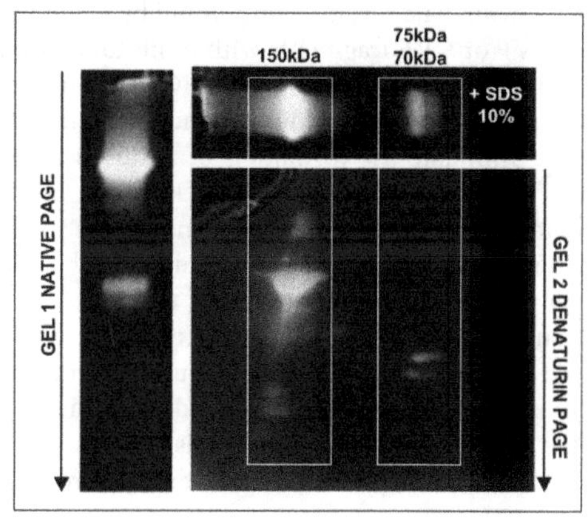


**Figure 1b:** 2D-PAGE of CVF. Gel 1 (left), CVF 4-20% Native PAGE. Gel 2 (right), CVF 12% denaturing PAGE.

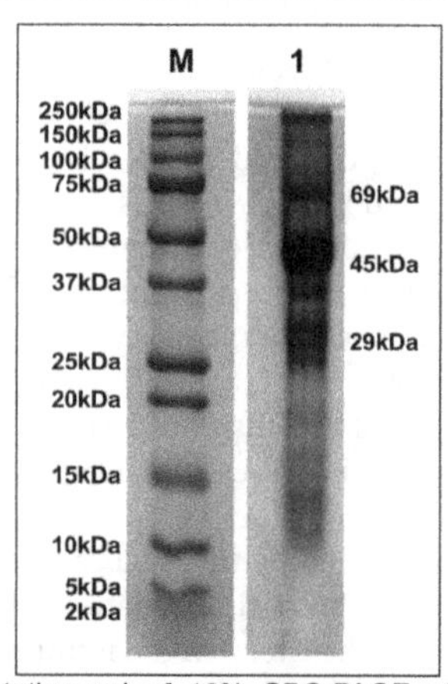


**Figure 1c:** Representative gel of 12% SDS-PAGE of CVF. Lane M, 5 µl Precision Plus Protein Dual Xtra standards marker. Lane 1, 15 µg CVF sample (arrows indicate expected size bands: 69, 45 and 29 kDa). The gels in Figure 1 resulted from three independent experiments. Gel staining was made with bio-safe comassie.

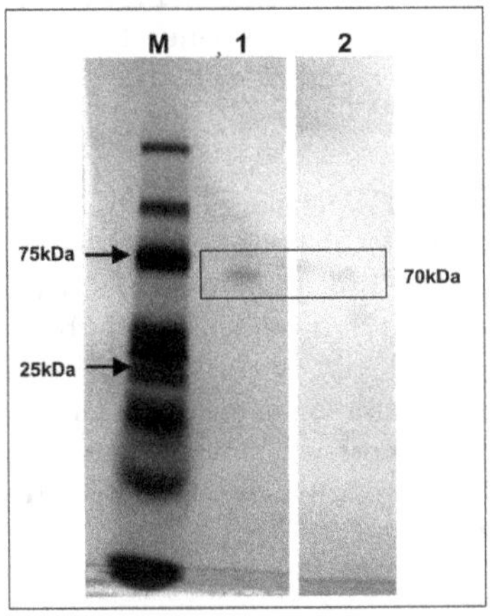


**Figure 2a:** S10 and S50 protein analysis. (A) Representative gel of 4-20% Native PAGE of S10 and S50. Lane M, 5 μl Precision Plus Protein Dual Xtra standards marker. Lane 1, 60 μg S10 sample. Lane 2, 95 μg S50 sample. Gel staining by bio-safe comassie

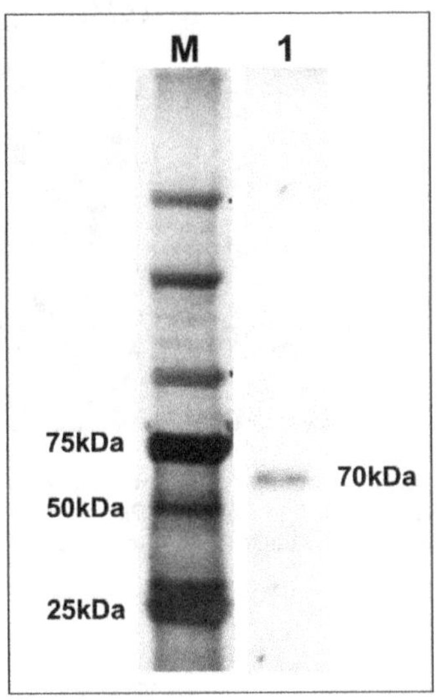


**Figure 2b:** Representative gel of S10 6% SDS-PAGE of S10. Lane M, 5 μl Precision Plus Protein Dual Xtra standards marker. Lane 1, 36 μg S10 sample. Gel staining by bio-safe comassie.

75 and 70 kDa approximately) or native S10 (70 kDa). Native-PAGE of S50V showed at least two bands (approximately 70 and 75 kDa) corresponding to those of native CVF and/or of native S50, together with another band (higher than 150 kDa), possibly representing the product of protein interaction (Figure 3A). All the bands obtained from S10V in native conditions (some of which detected also in S50V), were analyzed with 2D-PAGE (data not shown). The bands suspected to be the product of protein interaction (>150 kDa) were analyzed at least three times in denaturing-condition electrophoresis and they revealed a single spot. After denaturation, the bands corresponding to native CVF revealed only one spot on the gel, in accordance with the previous CVF behavior (Figure 1B). SDS-PAGE of S10V showed many bands with molecular weight in the range 200 to 4 kDa approximately (Figure 3B), while SDS-PAGE of S50V showed at least three bands (Figure 3C).

Both in S10V and S50V (Figure 3B and 3C) two bands (70 and 45/50 kDa approximately) could be assigned to S10 or S50 respectively and the 69 kDa band to CVF, while in S10V bands with molecular weight lower than about 50 kDa could be assigned to CVF (in particular 29 kDa band).

On the contrary, some SDS-PAGE CVF bands were not present in S10V or S50V and in the SDS-PAGE of S10V some bands were not easily assigned to CVF or S10, thus showing that molecular changes occurred in the therapeutic mix. Moreover, the CVF fragments appreciable in S10Vwere no more visible in S50V, demonstrating that proteolytic enzymes with molecular weight >10 KDa are present in serum,

The analysis of S10V showed the same band pattern before and after freezing (-20°C). This has been verified with both native (Figure 4A) and SDS-PAGE (Figure 4B). The same evidence appeared for S50V (data not shown).

## Treatment Outcome

### Case AB

The first case treated by Dr. Ferretti was the patient AB, affected

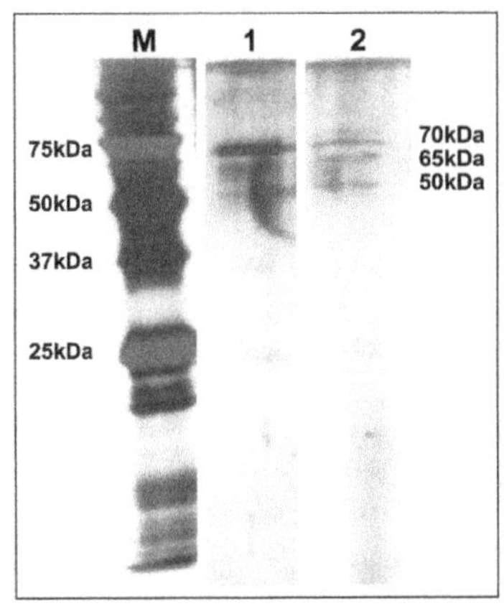


**Figure 2c:** Representative gel of 12% SDS-PAGE of S10 and S50. Lane M, 5 μl Precision Plus Protein Dual Xtra standards marker. Lane 1, 36 μg S10 sample. Lane 2, 57 μg S50 sample. Gel staining by silver. The gels in Figure 2 resulted from three independent experiments.

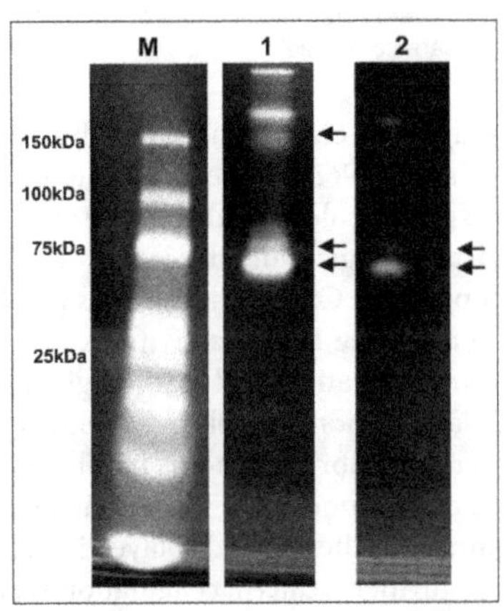


**Figure 3a:** S10V and S50V protein analysis. (A), Representative gel of 4-20% Native PAGE of S10V and S50V. Lane M, 5 μl Precision Plus Protein Dual Xtra standards marker. Lane 1, 100 μg S10V sample. Lane 2, 100 μg S50V sample. The arrows indicate the bands assigned to CVF and/or S10 and S50 (see text).

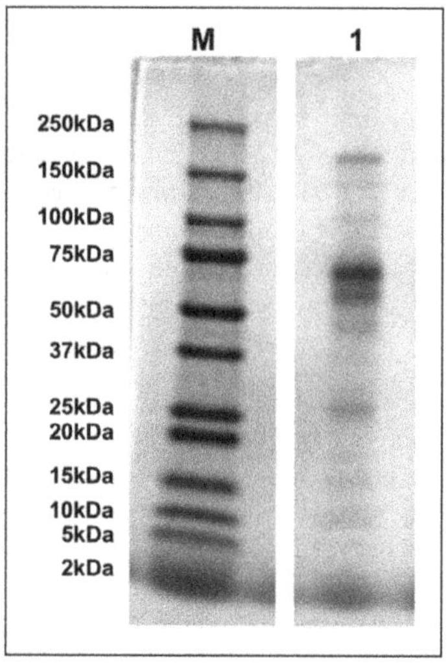


**Figure 3b:** Representative gel of 4-20% SDS-PAGE of S10V. Lane M, 5µl Precision Plus Protein Dual Xtra standards marker. Lane 1, 56 µg S10V sample.

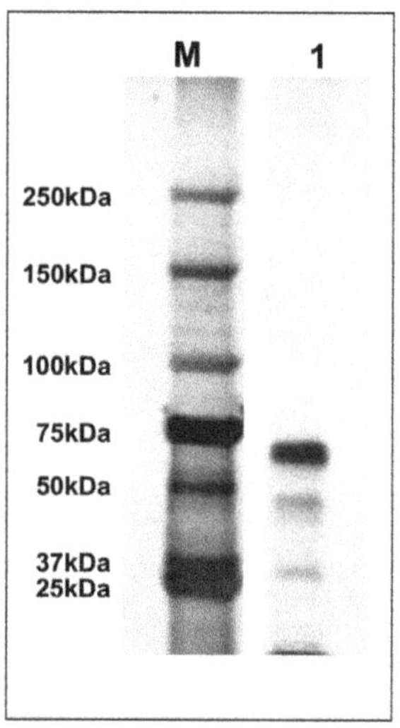


**Figure 3c:** Representative gel of 6% SDS-PAGE of S50V. Lane M, 5 µl Precision Plus Protein Dual Xtra standards marker. Lane 1, 56 µg S50V sample. All gels were stained with bio-safe comassie.

by a devastating squamous-cell carcinoma, with poor prognosis in the short term (Figure 5A), in 1965. The neoplastic lesion was characterized by irregular edges and colors and these traits recalled chronic inflammation and pathologic wound healing. This suggested to Dr. Ferretti that in neoplasms a C3-like protein was present, characterized by poor regulation and long lasting activity. A lesser duration would occur in chronic inflammation and pathologic wound healing. In Figure 5B the neoplastic lesion is displayed 60 days after the beginning of therapy. It appears that fibrinolysis was highly reduced, coagulation was getting normal and wound edges were drying up. The situation 90 days after the beginning of therapy is displayed in Figure 5C. It appears that fibrinolysis was further reduced, coagulation was effective, wound edges were dried and more regular. Eventually, cancer regressed, the edges healed and became dry and new epithelium developed. Pain ceased completely (painkillers passed from 8 to 1 per day at bedtime), as well as paresthesias, local circulatory alterations and hyperthermia. The elderly patient resumed feeding and led a worth living life for 6 years, until he fell and fractured his femur. He died a few months later due to complications from pneumonia caused by immobilization.

## Case PB

The patient PB had a hyper-fibrinolytic basal cell carcinoma in the back in 1969. In Figure 6A the neoplastic lesion before the beginning of the therapy is shown. In Figures 6B-6D the same neoplastic lesion is displayed 60, 90 and 120 days after the beginning of therapy, respectively. Eventually, the basal cell carcinoma regressed with dry scarring and re-epithelialization of the edges. Pain completely stopped, as well as regional parenthesis and alterations in macro- and micro-circulation. Local hyperthermia ceased as well. The patient was still alive and in good health in 2005.

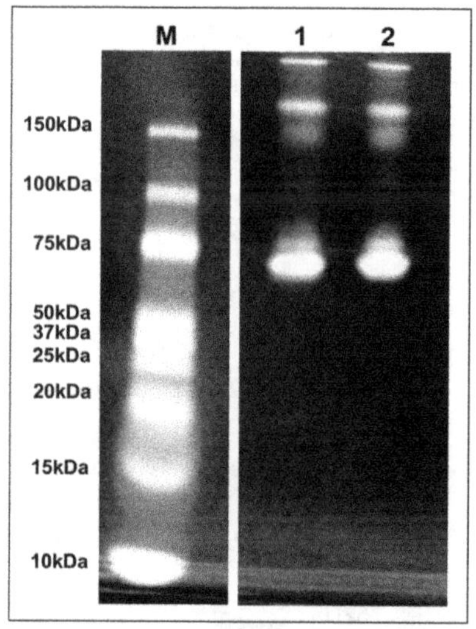


**Figure 4a**: Analysis of S10V before and after freezing. (A) Representative gel of 4-20% Native PAGE. Lane M, 5 µl Precision Plus Protein Dual Xtra standards marker. Lane 1, 100 µg S10V. Lane 2, 100 µg S10V (three times frozen and defrozen sample).

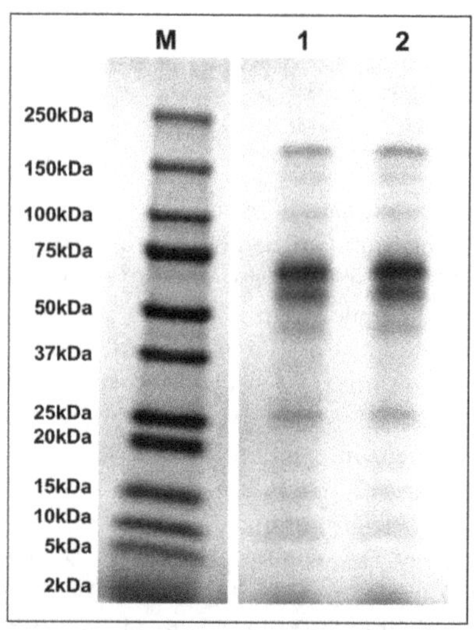


**Figure 4b**: Representative gel of 4-20% SDS-PAGE of S10V. Lane M, 5µl Precision Plus Protein Dual Xtra standards marker. Lane 1, 56 µg S10V. Lane 2, 56 µg. S10V (after three times freezing and defreezing processes). Gels were stained by bio-safe comassie.

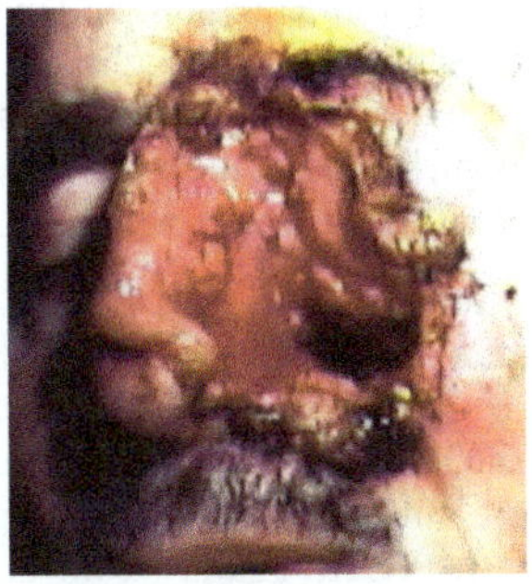

**Figure 5a:** Squamous-cell carcinoma in the left side of the face. (A) Before the beginning of the immunological therapy. An overall irregularity is apparent in edges and colors, with traits recalling chronic inflammation and pathological wound healing.

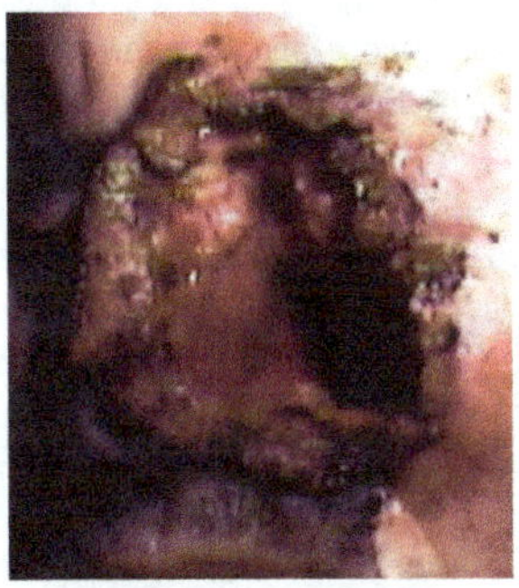

**Figure 5b:** 60 days after the beginning of therapy. Fibrinolysis was markedly reduced, clotting was getting normal and the edges of the neoplastic lesion were drying up.

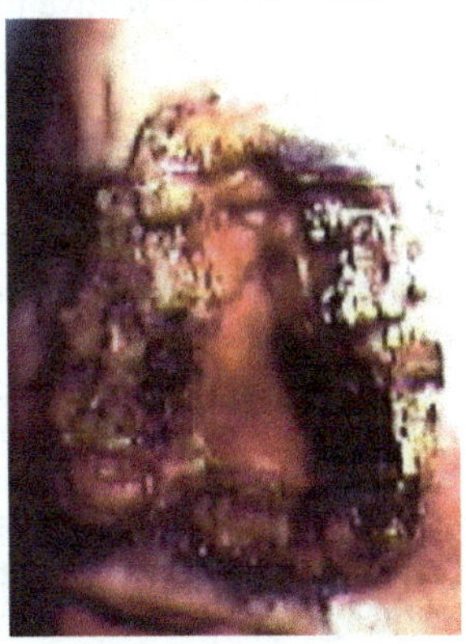

**Figure 5c:** 90 days after the beginning of therapy. Fibrinolysis was further decreased, clotting was effective, the edges of the neoplastic lesion were dry, less indented and more regular.

## Case GG

GG was born in 1947. At the beginning of 1998, a swelling appeared in the medial part of the left thigh, near the groin, without pain or obstacles to walking. On June 26, the MRI performed on his left thigh led to the diagnosis of "solid neoplasm of about 9 cm, suggestive of mixoid liposarcoma". On June 30, the CT scan of lower limbs, abdomen and chest, confirmed the previous data and, though not showing clear signs of secondary lesions, showed the presence of simildense tissue between pericardium and the aortic arch, as well as the enlargement of the left seminal vesicle. On July 7, on the basis of a biopsy specimen, the first histopathological diagnosis of "undifferentiated neoplasm, characterized by round cells with vacuoles and morphological features consistent with a round cell liposarcoma" was issued. From July 22 to late August 1998, antero-posterior tele-cobalt radiotherapy was applied in the left thigh, but on August 25 the CT scan showed that the known lesion was still present. On September 2, surgery was performed at Rizzoli hospital in Bologna and the histological examination of the surgical specimens supported the diagnosis of infiltrating pleomorphic liposarcoma, with large necrotic regions and reactive lymph adenitis. On September 16 the patient was discharged from the hospital with a drainage that leaked about 400 mL/day. Chemotherapy was prescribed (Zimat 500, Cytotec, Calciparin, Contramal, Ferrograd). On October 2, an opening 4 cm long formed at the surgical edge, with a marked loss

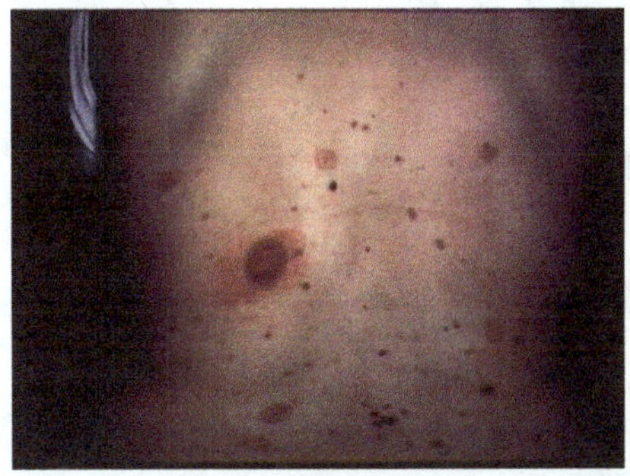

**Figure 6a:** Basal cell carcinoma. (A) before the beginning of the immunological therapy.

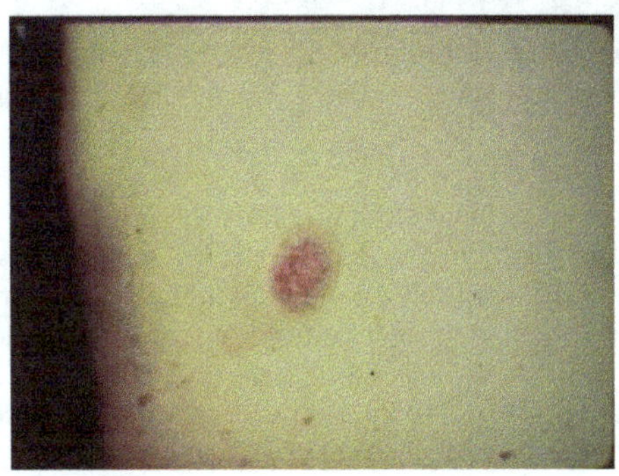

**Figure 6b:** The neoplastic lesion 60, 90 and 120 days after the beginning of therapy, respectively. The basal cell carcinoma regressed with dry scarring and re-epithelialization of the edges.

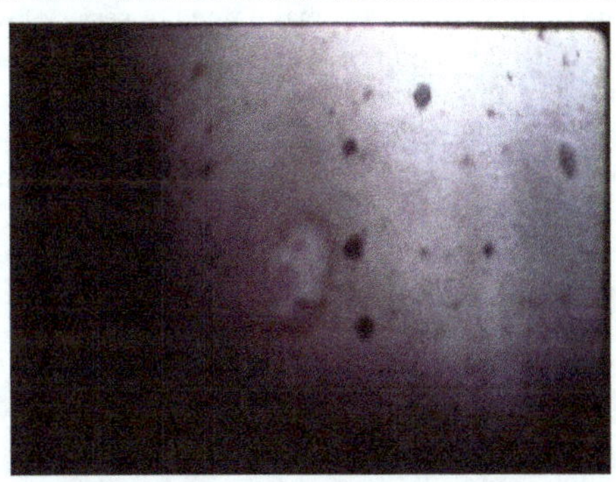

**Figure 6c:** The neoplastic lesion 60, 90 and 120 days after the beginning of therapy, respectively. The basal cell carcinoma regressed with dry scarring and re-epithelialization of the edges.

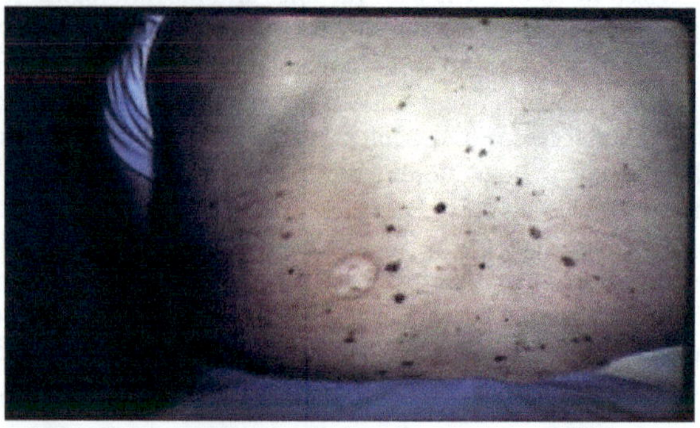

**Figure 6d:** The neoplastic lesion 60, 90 and 120 days after the beginning of therapy, respectively. The basal cell carcinoma regressed with dry scarring and re-epithelialization of the edges.

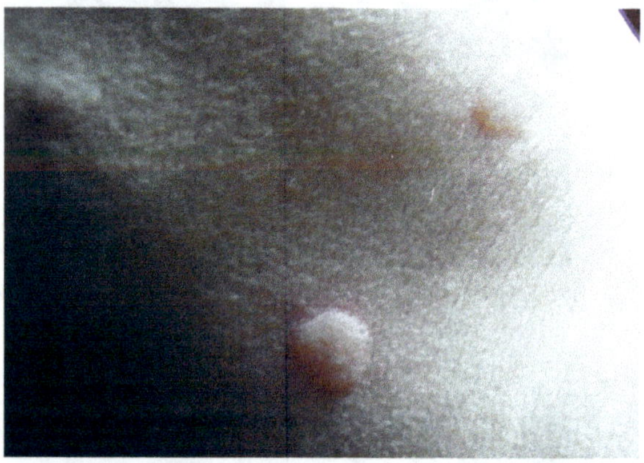

**Figure 7:** Example of blisters in sites of past immunogen injections in the left arm.

of blood serum. This opening was repeatedly sutured, but the loss and the smell continued. On October 26, the CT scan of chest, abdomen and legs showed a large volume of liquid in the place where the tumor mass had been removed. After clinical examination, Tiklid, Persantin and Trental were prescribed. Overall, the patient was getting clinically worse. According to his family, the patient decided to discontinue any cancer treatment.

**Beginning of immunological therapy:** As the patient was discharged from the hospital, at the suggestion of Dr. Ferretti, the cancer treatments previously prescribed were gradually removed. Only Multicentrum (1 tablet per day), Contramal (10 drops if necessary) and Cibalgina (if necessary) were maintained. A series of wet poultices (saline solution, 1 tablespoon of salt in 500 ml of water) were applied on the opening of the wound, to hold it open. On October 27, the first injection of Dr. Ferretti's immunogen was made and injections of immunogen were repeated at intervals ranging from a week to a month, depending on patient's reactivity. Following removal of chemotherapy and the beginning of Dr. Ferretti's therapy, the patient started feeling better and both serum leakage and the size of the opening in the thigh started reducing. After the second and third injection, made on November 11 and December 12, respectively, the size of opening, serum leakage and smell declined progressively. The thigh circumference also reduced, but in spite of these slight improvements the patient felt worse, with general fatigue, dissatisfaction with food, weight loss and psychological discomfort. The patient refused to take any kind of painkiller and occasionally felt pain in the site of surgical wound, as well as in two left thorax regions and in the left pelvic region, roughly corresponding to the sites were slight alterations were found in previous CT. On palpation, a massive enlargement could be felt in the left pelvic region, with thickening of the vas deferens, where the patient felt sharp stitches alternating with tingling.

About two weeks after the onset of these painful sensations, in urine, faeces and sweat a smell of dead rat could be perceived and Dr. Ferretti informed the patient that his therapeutic strategy contemplated this apparent worsening before the beneficial effects would appear. The patient did not believe this explanation; he became very depressed and refused to meet Dr. Ferretti again. However, on January 29 and February 13 the patient voluntarily received the fourth and fifth injections of immunogen. The following period was characterized by increased painful sensations in the locations above reported. Brief episodes of dead rat smell in urine, faeces and sweat also occurred. The emotional discomfort improved and periods of relief ensued. The thigh circumference also decreased and the functional capacity of the leg slowly recovered. On February 29, the patient received the sixth application and the painful sensations became rarer, with no bad smell. The patient began to drive a modified car and received further immunogenic injections on March 25 and 31, April 7 and 21 and May 2, respectively. Similar episodes of pain and mood swings between depression and well-being continued, but with a definitely lower intensity and the patient were able to sleep without any drug. On June 5, the patient received the twelfth application and a clear improvement was evident. On June 22 the thirteenth application was made and the patient for the first time reported feeling healed. He could walk without a cane. Electromyography was performed, which showed a neurological impairment due to surgery. In August 1999, the patient began physical therapy. The injections of immunogen continued until April 2000. From 2000 until 2006, the patient received an injection of immunogen every 4 months for preventive purposes. During this period further analysis were performed and no clinical signs of relapse were apparent. GG died on 2011 by other pathology.

## Case BS

BS was born in 1984. On November 16, 2005, BS underwent thyroidectomy. The diagnosis was papillary carcinoma 3.7×7 cm wide, also involving perithyroid tissues, with surgical margins infiltrated by neoplastic cells and multiple lymph node metastases. In December 2005, she received ablative metabolic radiotherapy (5550 MBq of 131 iodine), after which areas of radioalogen uptake were still present in the anterior region of the neck and in both lung fields. On January 2006, a CT-scan without contrast medium did not show densitometric changes in the thorax. In April 2006, chest and bone scan, as well as abdominal ultrasounds, were negative, however under Levothyroxine therapy, detectable values of thyroglobulin (TG, 20 ng/ml) were suggestive of biochemical relapse. In June 2006 the patient underwent the second metabolic treatment (same parameters as the first one). After the metabolic therapy, total body scan displayed "two areas of moderate uptake in the anterior region of the neck and a widespread activity in both lung fields, significantly reduced with respect to the previous control". Due to detectable values of TG (12 ng/ml) during a TSH suppressing therapy, on July 2007 another treatment of metabolic radiotherapy was applied (3700 MBq of 131 Iodine, after Thyrogen administration). TSH and TG values were 145 and 27 ng/ml, respectively. The PET scan (370 MBq, 18F-FDG) did not display areas of radioisotope pathological accumulation suggesting lesions with high metabolic activity.

**Beginning of immunological therapy:** The immunological therapy started on March 2008 paralleling the standard follow-up therapy and is still continuing. On February 2008, just a month before the start of therapy, plasma TG concentration was 11 ng/ml. On March 2008, TG concentration by needle aspiration cytology from right lymph node III-IV level was 2.0 ng/ml. The cytologic diagnosis was consistent with reactive lymph node. Plasma TG concentration in successive measurements from 2008 to 2009 ranged between 7.10 and 10.9 ng/ml.

On February 2009 a PET scan with 370 MBq of 18 F-FDG did not show areas of increased metabolism related with certainty to neoplastic type lesions. A hypermetabolic lymph node was however observed in the right armpit. On April 2009 a total body bone scan with 99 Tc-MDP 740 MBq did not show areas of pathological accumulation of the tracer related to bone lesions. The full abdomen echography as well as the high-resolution CT (HRCT) showed no alterations worth noting. However, according to laboratory tests performed on June 2009, reactive lymph nodes were still present in the right supraclavicular region. Plasma TG concentration in successive measurements from 2009 to 2010 ranged between 2.20 and 3.40 ng/ml.

The full abdomen echography as well as the chest high-resolution CT, performed on March 2010 showed no pathological changes worth noting. On June 2010, a biopsy was performed at the mediastinal VII level. The diagnosis was "reactive lymph nodes. No evidence of neoplasia ".

On December 2010, on the specific question of metastases of papillary thyroid cancer, a lymph node biopsy was performed. The report was A) reactive lymph nodes, no evidence of neoplasia, B) thymic tissue unaffected.

After the beginning of the immunological therapy, the patient experienced an increase in appetite, joy of life and energy. This allowed her to resume the work of nursery school teacher, work she still retains.

**Overall treatment outcome:** In some cases, such as AB and PB, healing took place as a result of immunological therapy alone. In other cases, such as GG, healing occurred as a result of immunological treatment applied following conventional anti-cancer therapies, such as radiotherapy, surgery and chemotherapy. In the case BS and in the cases MV, KV and DC reported in supplementary information, healing took place as a result of the immunological therapy applied in parallel with conventional anti-cancer therapies. In the case SG, reported in the supplementary information, the immunological therapy was applied after all conventional therapies had been abandoned. Life duration increased beyond medical expectancy, associated with an acceptable life quality. Basing on the many cases treated over the years, the overall outcome of Dr. Ferretti's therapy may be depicted. In general, a substantial improvement in quality of life was observed. Starting from the 3rd-5th day after the immunogen injection, the patients felt a kind of pain awakening in the regions of neoplastic lesions. The pain lasted a few days, rarely requiring the administration of mild analgesics. Then it disappeared and the patients felt better than before the injection. Sometimes sparse itching blisters appeared in sites of past immunogen injections and in no other body sites. The blisters remained visible for 2-4 hours, then disappeared without leaving any visible sign (Figure 7). For what concerns the general effects of therapy, the marked pain decrease until total disappearance was accompanied by an increased desire to live. In some cases, the patient resumed the work activities previously interrupted because of the disease. Apparently, the therapy eliminated the systemic effects of cancer. Even in the presence of large and even increasing tumor masses, the patient maintained a state of well-being and absence of pain. An increased survival beyond the medical prognosis was also observed. Although theoretically possible, in thousands of injections, adverse reactions never occurred.

## Discussion

### CVF, serum and therapeutic mix

The band profile of native CVF appearing in Figure 1A showed a greater complexity than published [11]. The CVF analyzed was from the same stock as that utilized in the more recent cases. The low weight bands appearing in SDS-PAGE CVF (Figure 1C) may result from denaturation and reduction of the 70 and 75 kDa native bands.

In both Native-PAGE S10 and S50, a 70 kDa band is present (Figure 2A). According to the filter nominal cut-off values, the band weights in the filtrate should be lower than 10 or 50 kDa, respectively. However, manufacturer's specifications indicate that a minor percentage of higher weight proteins may pass through the filter [15,16]. More restrictive conditions could have been realized, but this protocol was maintained since it was the one used to prepare the therapeutic mix. Seemingly, only the most abundant proteins (70 kDa) showed up in the gel, but the presence of other less represented hight weight proteins cannot be excluded. Indeed, cut-off filter excludes high molecular weight serum proteins. However this was done on purpose by Dr. Ferretti to cut-off albumin and other high concentration proteins that could overstimulate the immune system with no relation to anti-cancer mechanisms. Moreover, as CVF inhibitors also include proteolytic enzymes, CVF fragments possibly complexed with serum low molecular weight proteins may appear in the mix. Thus the CVF-serum interaction is demonstrated by both low and high molecular weight adducts.

For what concerns high molecular weight bands (>150 Kda) in native S10V and S50V, they possibly represent the products of protein interaction (Figure 3C). Bands higher than 250 kDa (the upper weight limit of the molecular marker used) cannot be excluded (Figure 3A).

On the basis of the overall data above reported, it appears that a complex interaction occurred between CVF and filtered S10 and S50 serum. For what concerns S10V, the three bands detectable in native S10V (150, 75 and 70 kDa approximately) likely arose from the products assigned to CVF or S10 in SDS-PAGE of S10V. Native S10 and CVF could interact through both proteolysis and aggregation processes and products with molecular weight higher than the gel resolution could arise. These products could result in the bands that in SDS-PAGE conditions cannot be assigned to CVF or S10. Furthermore, the native products of S10V not easily assigned to native CVF or S10 likely arose from the interaction of CVF and S10 by S-S bonds.

Interestingly, in the SDS-PAGE condition, the products assignable to CVF were fewer and less abundant in S50V than in S10V. This different molecular rearrangement can be explained by the hypothesis that serum contained proteases with molecular weight higher than 10 kDa, together with protease inhibitors with molecular weight higher than 50 kDa. Therefore, while S10 contained few proteases and almost no inhibitors, S50 contained many proteases and few inhibitors. As a consequence, larger protein degradation occurred in S50V than in S10V.

The results concerning freezing (see Figures 4A and 4B) indicate that freezing may be a good preservation method for the therapeutic mix, allowing not adding Thimerosal, a germicide previously utilized, but no more allowed by the Italian health authorities.

### Immunological therapy

Dr. Ferretti's therapy is aimed at balancing the various molecular components of the immune system, so as to restore its natural antitumor activity. According to his hypothesis, this is obtained by stimulating the production of antibodies that neutralize the excess inhibitors, thus reactivating the lytic cascade and the cell-mediated toxicity. If the immune response elicited is not adequate to eliminate the transformed cells, a tumor develops. Even in this case the improvement of the immune function may be beneficial in slowing down tumor development and reducing its systemic effects. The beneficial effects of Dr. Ferretti's therapy might be explained by alternative hypotheses, such as unspecific effects of the immune reaction. For instance, diphtheria toxin (DT) showed anti-tumor activity in mice [17] and in humans [18]. Even a nontoxic mutant of DT exerted some degree of biological anti-tumor activity [19]. Intravesical induction and maintenance of Bacillus Calmette-Guerin has proven to reduce tumor recurrence and progression [20]. Concomitant active tuberculosis prolongs the patient survival in non-small cell lung cancer [21]. In mice, the anticancer effects of cyclophosphamide are in part immune mediated, as cyclophosphamide alters the composition of microbiota in the small intestine and induces the translocation of selected species of Gram-positive bacteria into secondary lymphoid organs, thus stimulating immune responses [22]. However, some data point to a specific immune mediated link between Dr. Ferretti's immunogen and malignancy processes. First, the injected immunogen initially increases pain in the neoplastic lesions and no elsewhere. Seemingly, the immunogen-induced antibodies cross-react with malignancy processes. Second, blisters form in sites of past immunogen injections. Likely, immunogen and/or cancer induced antibodies cross-react with the injected immunogen. Both events are compatible with a specific link between Dr. Ferretti's immunogen and malignancy processes. This link deserves further studies, as it could provide the basis of new therapeutic strategies. Most cancer vaccines contain antigens normally expressed by the host. This may lead the host to develop immunological tolerance [23]. In the present therapeutic mix the epitopes eliciting antibodies are definitely non-self and unlikely to induce immunological tolerance. Moreover, neither toxicity nor adverse effects were ever found in the many patients treated up to now. In addition, the hypothesized link between immunogen and malignancy may also provide a diagnostic tool, as the sites of unknown secondary lesions become apparent through the increased pain elicited by immunogen injections. Possibly, the therapy mainly affects the transformed cells peripheral to the tumor mass, preventing their aggression against normal cells. Even if tumor mass increases, the increase possibly occurs through the sole circulating nutrients, without affecting the normal peri-tumoral tissue. In general, besides a state of general well-being, decrease or disappearance of pain, new energy and a new positive sense of life, the patients also reported a better resistance to infectious diseases, which is consistent with the improvement of the immune function.

## Conclusion

Dr. Ferretti's therapy is aimed at balancing the various molecular components of the immune system, so as to restore its natural anti-tumor activity. This therapy likely acts on tumors through improving the immune function and therefore the general state of the patient and his quality of life, as consistently observed. A specific immune mediated link between Dr. Ferretti's immunogen and malignancy processes is suggested. This link could provide the basis of new therapeutic and diagnostic strategies.

## Future perspectives of Dr. Ferretti's immunotherapy

The important results obtained by Dr. Ferretti deserve further studies and researches. Dr. Ferretti's therapy and mix are protected by US patent [6], previously assigned to the Fernando and Anna Foundation, Chicago IL (US). The present assignee is the Fondazione Fernando e Anna Ferretti, a nonprofit institution according to the Italian law. This institution is willing to grant the use of the patent for scientific and commercial purposes.

## References


1. Vergati M, Intrivici C, Huen NY, Schlom J, Tsang KY (2010) Strategies for cancer vaccine development. J Biomed Biotechnol 596432.
2. Perez SA, von Hofe E, Kallinteris NL, Gritzapis AD, Peoples GE et al. (2010) A new era in anticancer peptide vaccines. Cancer 116: 2071-2080.
3. Finn OJ (2012) Immuno-oncology: understanding the function and dysfunction of the immune system in cancer. Ann Oncol 23: 6-9.
4. Quezada SA, Peggs KS (2013) Exploiting CTLA-4, PD-1 and PD-L1 to reactivate the host immune response against cancer. Br J Cancer 108: 1560-1565.
5. Topalian SL, Weiner GJ, Pardoll DM (2011) Cancer Immunotherapy Comes of Age. J Clin Oncol 29: 4828-4836.
6. Ferretti F, Ferretti A (2010) Compositions and methods for treating cancer. Patent No. US7,723,292 B2
7. Shishido SN, Varahan S, Yuan K, Li X, Fleming SD (2012) Humoral innate immune response and disease. Clin Immunol 144: 142-158.
8. Qu H, Ricklin D, Lambris JD (2009) Recent developments in low molecular weight complement inhibitors. Mol Immunol 47: 185-195.
9. Chen S, Caragine T, Cheung NK, Tomlinson S (2000) CD59 expressed on a tumor cell surface modulates decay-accelerating factor expression and enhances tumor growth in a rat model of human neuroblastoma. Cancer Res 60: 3013-3018.
10. Liu Y, Zeng G (2012) Cancer and Innate Immune System Interactions: Translational Potentials for Cancer Immunotherapy. J Immunother 35: 299–308.
11. Kock MA, Hew BE, Bammert H, Fritzinger DC, Vogel CW (2004) Structure and function of recombinant cobra venom factor. J Biol Chem 279: 30836-30843.
12. Hains PG, Broady KW (2000) Purification and inhibitory profile of phospholipase A2 inhibitors from Australian elapid sera. Biochem J 346: 139-146.
13. Baldrick P, Richardson D, Wheeler AW (2002) Review of L-tyrosine confirming its safe human use as an adjuvant. J Appl Toxicol 22: 333-344.
14. Rais I, Karas M, Schägger H (2004) Two-dimensional electrophoresis for the isolation of integral membrane proteins and mass spectrometric identification. Proteomics 4: 2567–2571.
15. http://www.millipore.com/userguides/tech1/centrifugal_ivd_userguide
16. http://www.millipore.com/publications.nsf/a73664f9f981af8c852569b9005b4eee/f01ae45d5551b0588525792200680bbb/$FILE/PB2778ENEU%20MM.pdf
17. Buzzi S, Maistrello I (1973) Inhibition of growth of Erlich tumors in Swiss mice by diphtheria toxin. Cancer Res 33: 2349-2353.
18. Buzzi S (1982) Diphtheria toxin treatment of human advanced cancer. Cancer Res 42: 2054-2058.
19. Buzzi S, Rubboli D, Buzzi G, Buzzi AM, Morisi C et al. (2004) CRM197 (nontoxic diphtheria toxin): effects on advanced cancer patients. Cancer Immunol Immunother 53: 1041-1048.
20. Ajili F, Darouiche A, Chebil M, Boubaker S (2013) The efficacy of intravesical

bacillus Calmette-Guerin in the treatment of patients with pT1 stage non-muscle-invasive bladder cancer. Ultrastruct Pathol 37: 278-283.

21. Kuo CH, Lo CY, Chung FT, Lee KY, Lin SM et al. (2012) Concomitant active tuberculosis prolongs survival in non-small cell lung cancer: a study in a tuberculosis-endemic country. PLoS One 7: e33226

22. Viaud S, Saccheri F, Mignot G, Yamazaki T, Daillère R, et al. (2013) The intestinal microbiota modulates the anticancer immune effects of cyclophosphamide. Science 342: 971-976.

23. Church SE, Jensen SM, Twitty CG, Bahjat K, Hu HM et al. (2011) Multiple Vaccinations: Friend or Foe. Cancer J 17: 379-396.

# Radioprotective Potential of Nigella Sativa Extract in Swiss Albino Mice Exposed to Whole Body γ-Radiation

**Ganesh Chandra Jagetia*** **and Ravikiran PB**

*Department of Zoology, Mizoram University, India*

***Corresponding author**: Ganesh Chandra Jagetia, Professor, Department of Zoology, Mizoram University, Aizawl - 796 004, India, E-mail: gc.jagetia@gmail.com

**Abstract**

The radioprotective activity of *Nigella sativa* extract (NSE) was ascertained by administering mice orally with 25, 50, 100, 150, 200, 400 or 500 mg/kg b. wt. of NSE, once daily for five consecutive days prior to 10 Gy γ-irradiation. One hour after the last administration of NSE on fifth day, the animals were whole body exposed to 10 Gy radiation. The exposure of animals to 10 Gy irradiation resulted in the death of all irradiated animals within 16 days post-irradiation, whereas administration of mice with different doses of NSE reduced the radiation-induced mortality and increased the animal survival significantly ($p<0.05$). The maximum number of survivors (60%) was observed in the group of animals treated with 150 mg/kg NSE. A further increase in the NSE dose up to 500 mg/kg did not significantly elevate the animal survival when compared to 150 mg/kg. Since maximum number of survivors was observed with 150 mg/kg of NSE, it was considered as an optimum dose for radioprotection and further experiments were performed using this dose. In another set of experiments the animals were administered with 150 mg/kg b. wt. of NSE orally once daily for five consecutive days before exposure to 7, 8, 9, 10 or 11 Gy γ-radiation, where the animals were monitored daily up to thirty days post-irradiation for the development of symptoms of radiation sickness and mortality. Treatment of mice with NSE before irradiation delayed the onset of mortality and reduced the symptoms of radiation sickness when compared with the double distilled water (DDW) treated irradiated controls. The $LD_{50/30}$ was found to be 8 Gy for DDW + irradiation group, whereas the NSE treatment increased $LD_{50/30}$ up to 9.6 Gy with a dose reduction factor (DRF) of 1.2. The in vitro studies in cell free system revealed that NSE inhibited the generation of various free radicals including 2,2-diphenyl-2-picryl hydrazyl (DPPH), 3-ethyl benzothiazoline-6-sulphonic acid ($ABTS^{\bullet+}$), hydroxyl ($OH^{\bullet}$) and superoxide ($O2^{\bullet-}$) in a concentration dependent manner. The radioprotective effect of NSE may be due to free radical scavenging and increased antioxidant status.

**Keywords:** Mice; Nigella sativa; Free radicals; Radiation; Survival

## Introduction

The discovery of ionizing radiations led to its widespread applications in various fields immediately. Ionizing radiations are regularly used in the diagnosis of various diseases, cancer treatment, nuclear power production, industry, research, weapon testing, nuclear warfare, and space explorations. These applications have led to increased exposure of humans to ionizing radiations advertently or inadvertently, which may result in the numerous deleterious health effects including cancer [1,2]. The longest sought and the most elusive goal in radiobiology research has been the development of potent multifunctional, multi target pharmacological agents, which are able to alleviate the ill effects of ionizing radiation on human health. It is fairly well established that the ionizing radiations interact with biological tissues mainly by indirect effect and induce cellular damage principally by the generation of free radicals in the cellular milieu [1]. These free radicals or reactive oxygen species (ROS) are generated by the interaction of ionizing radiations with aqueous milieu of cells that induce radiolysis of water [1]. The ROS thus generated are highly reactive and interact with molecular oxygen or various important biomolecules such as DNA, lipids, proteins and also with membranous structures of cells leading to oxidative stress, and subsequently disrupting the homeostasis between the pro-oxidants and antioxidants inside the microenvironment of the cell that causes damage to cell components [3].

With the realization of harmful effects of ionizing radiation, the need for the protection of mankind against the radiation induced deleterious effects was realized as early as 1949, when Patt and his co-workers tried cysteine, a sulphydryl group containing amino acid in rats to protect them against the deleterious effects of ionizing radiations and reported for the first time that cysteine protected the rats against the X-irradiation-induced sickness and mortality [4]. Thereafter several sulphydryl containing compounds were tried; however, practical applicability of the majority of these synthetic compounds remained limited owing to their high toxicity at their optimum protective dose [5]. One of the best known radioprotector so far, the amifostine has been tired in clinical condition however; its widespread application remained limited because of its systemic toxicities and exorbitant cost. Over the years, although considerable advancement has been made in the field of radioprotection by screening various types of pharmacological agents for their radioprotective ability, none of these agents were found to be clinically useful [6,7].

An ideal radioprotector is a pharmacological agent, which is non-toxic, economically cheaper, and orally administrable and acts by multiple mechanisms [7]. A non-toxic radioprotector could be useful in occupational settings including defense, airline, military, research, dentistry, radiotherapy, nuclear medicine and/or nuclear accidents. A chemical radioprotector will be very useful in situations, where radioactivity is released accidentally in the environment eg. Three Mile Island, Chernobyland Goiania, and Fukushima. It may be also useful during air and/or space travel to protect humans from the deleterious effects of radiation associated with solar flares [2,6-8]. With the recent developments and increased accessibility of terrorists to improvised nuclear devices, threat of such attacks seems to be also imminent. This indicates the need to devise countermeasures to combat such situations and reduce the causalities to as minimum as possible. This could be achieved using effective pharmacological agents to protect humans [7]. The dietary agents have received little attention for their radioprotective activities. The dietary agents, if found radioprotective will be advantageous, as they are in regular use, economically cheaper and widely acceptable to humans and also do not have known untoward side effects [9].

Kalonji, the seeds of *Nigella sativa Linn.* (family: *Ranunculaceae*) have been used as a spice, condiment and food additive. The ancient system of medicine, the Ayurveda, is a Sanskrit word which means Science of Life (Ayur=life and veda=knowledge) and is the oldest human healthcare system of medicine. Kalonji has been used as a curative remedy for several disorders in the Ayurvedic system of medicine. It is effective in alopecia, asthma, mad dog bites, respiratory diseases, paralysis, palsy, migraine, amnesia, palpitation and diabetes mellitus [10,11]. Experimentally, kalonji has been reported to be antiasthmatic [12], anticancerous [13,14], anti-inflammatory [15], lactogogue and vermifuge [16]. It has been reported to be cytotoxic to multidrug resistant cells *[17]. Nigella sativa* has been reported to reduce cisplatin induced toxicity in rats [14]. The principle component of *Nigella sativa*, the thymoquinone has been reported to be hepatoprotective [18]. Kalonji has also been reported to inhibit histamine release in mast cells [19]. However the radioprotective activity of kalonji has not been yet studied. Therefore, the aim of the present study was to investigate the radioprotective potential of kalonji (*Nigella sativa Linn.*) in mice exposed to different doses of γ-radiation in a preclinical setting.

## Materials and Methods

### Chemicals

2,2-diphenyl-2-picryl hydrazyl (DPPH), sodium nitroprusside, Greiss reagent, 2,2-azino-bis(3-ethyl benzothiazoline-6-sulphonic acid) diammonium salt (ABTS) glutathione, chloro-2,4-dinitrobenzene (CDNB), 5,5-dithiobis-2-nitrobenzoic acid (DTNB), trichloroacetic acid (TCA), thiobarbituric acid (TBA) and fetal calf serum (FCM) were purchased from Sigma Chemical Co. (St. Louis, MO, USA). The other chemicals such as absolute alcohol, dimethyl sulphoxide (DMSO), ethylene diamine tetraacetic acid (EDTA), sodium bicarbonate, sodium chloride, potassium hydrogen phosphate, disodium hydrogen phosphate, potassium chloride and hydrochloric acid were purchased from Merck India Ltd; Mumbai.

### Collection of Plant material and extraction

The dried seeds of kalonji, *Nigella sativa Linn.* (family: *Ranunculaceae*) were commercially procured, identified and authenticated by Dr. P. K. Rajgopal, Taxonomist, Department of Botany, Mahatma Gandhi Memorial College, Udupi, India. The powdered material of *Nigella sativa* (NS) was sequentially extracted in a Soxhlet apparatus using petroleum ether (60°C), chloroform and finally, the chloroform free marc was extracted in methanol. The methanol extract of NS was concentrated under reduced pressure and freeze dried. The dried methanol extract was stored at -70°C until use. Henceforth the *Nigella sativa* extract will be referred as NSE throughout the manuscript.

### Animals

The care of animals and handling were done according to the guidelines issued by the World Health Organization, Geneva, Switzerland and the INSA (Indian National Science Academy, New Delhi, India). Usually, six to eight weeks old Swiss albino mice weighing 22 to 24 g of either sex were selected from an inbred colony maintained under the controlled conditions of temperature (23 ± 2°C), humidity (50 ± 5%) and 12 h of light and dark cycle, respectively. The animals had free access to the sterile food and water, five animals were housed in a polypropylene cage containing sterile paddy husk (procured locally) as bedding throughout the experiment. The study was approved by the Institutional Animal Ethical Committee of Manipal University, Manipal, where the entire study was carried out.

### Mode of administration

The NSE was freshly dissolved in double distilled water (DDW) and administered orally using an oral gavage.

### Experimental design

The radioprotective activity of NSE was determined by performing the following experiments:-

### Maximum tolerated dose (MTD)

The acute toxicity of NSE was determined according to the method Prieur et al., [17] with minor modifications. Briefly, mice weighing 25-35 g were fasted for 18 h by withdrawing food and water. The fasted animals were divided into two groups of 10 each. Each group of animals was administered p.o. with a single dose of 500, 1000, 2000, 3000, and 5000 mg/kg b. wt. of NSE. The animals were provided with food and water immediately after the drug administration. The animals were monitored carefully and continuously for the first hour and thereafter for a period of 4 h at an interval of every 30 min and subsequent observations were made at 24, 48 and 72 h and until 14 days post- drug treatment. $LD_{50}$ was calculated using the probit analysis as described [18].

### Radioprotective effect

The radioprotective effect of NSE was determined by dividing the animals into the following groups:-

**DDW + irradiation**: The animals of this group were administered with 0.1 ml/kg b. wt. of double distilled water (DDW).

**NSE+irradiation:** This group of animals was administered with NSE orally for five consecutive days before radiation exposure.

### Irradiation

The prostate and immobilized animals, restrained in a specially designed well-ventilated acrylic box were wholebody exposed to γ-radiation from a $^{60}$Co gamma teletherapy source (Theratron, Atomic Energy Agency, Canada) at the Shirdi Sai Baba Cancer Hospital, Manipal, at a dose rate of 1.33 Gy/min in a field size of 25×25 cm$^2$ and at a distance (SSD) of 57.8 cm.

### Optimum dosing schedule

A separate experiment was performed to select the optimum NSE administration schedule. The animals were divided into two groups of 10 each, where grouping and other conditions were essentially similar to that described in experimental design section. The animals were administered with 150 mg/kg b. wt. of NSE p.o. once daily for one (one hour before irradiation), three, five or seven consecutive days before exposure to 10 Gy of γ-radiation. Ten animals were used for each schedule of administration and a total of 50 animals were used for the whole experiment.

### Administration route selection

Another experiment was conducted to select the best route of administration, where the animals were divided into two groups of 10 each. The grouping and other conditions were essentially similar to that described earlier. The most effective route of NSE administration was determined by administering mice with 150 mg/kg of NSE through different routes including intraperitoneal (i.p), intramuscular (i.m) or oral (p.o.) once daily for five consecutive days. One hour after the last administration on fifth day, the animals were exposed to 10 Gy of γ- radiation. Ten animals were used for each route of administration and a total of 30 animals were used for the whole experiment.

### Optimum dose selection

The optimum radioprotective dose of NSE was selected by conducting a separate experiment, where the animals were divided into two groups of 10 each as described above and administered with 0, 25, 50, 100, 150, 200, 300 or 500 mg/kg b. wt. of NSE orally once daily for five consecutive days. One hour after the last administration on day fifth, the animals were exposed to 10 Gy of γ-radiation [19].

### Radioprotective effect

An another experiment was conducted to determine the radioprotective activity of NSE where the animals were divided into two groups as described in section 2.5.2, except that the animals were administered with 150 mg/kg b. wt. of NSE for five consecutive days before exposure to 7, 8, 9, 10 or 11 Gy of γ-radiation. A total of 120 animals were used for this experiment.

The dose reduction factor (DRF) was calculated according to the methods as follows:

$$DRF = \frac{\text{LD50 of the NSE + irradiation group}}{\text{LD50 of the DDW + irradiation group}}$$

### Estimation of Free radical scavenging activity

The free radical scavenging ability of NSE was determined in cell free system in vitro for the following radical species:

### DPPH radical

The effect of NSE on the inhibition of DPPH radical was estimated according to the method of Mensor et al., where an antioxidant reacts with the stable DPPH radical and converts it into 1,1-diphenyl-2-picryl hydrazine. The ability to scavenge the stable DPPH radicals is measured as a decrease in the absorbance at 517 nm. Aliquots containing various concentrations of NSE (10-120 μg) in a final volume of 2 ml were mixed with 2 ml of 0.05 mM DPPH (in methanol). DPPH (2 ml) with an equal amount of PBS served as control. The reaction mixture was incubated at 37°C for 20 minutes and the optical density (OD) was measured at λ=517 nm using spectrophotometer. The DPPH radical scavenging activity was calculated as follows:-

$$\% \text{ Scavenging [DPPH]} = [(A0-A1) / A0]\times 100$$

Where A0 is the absorbance of the control and A1 is the absorbance in the presence of the samples and standard.

### Hydroxyl radical

Hydroxyl radical scavenging assay was performed by the oxidation of deoxyribose as described by Halliwell et al. [22]. The OH• were generated by Fenton reaction in Fe3+- EDTA-ascorbate-H2O2 system. The degradation of deoxyribose by OH• was estimated by measuring the thiobarbituric acid reactive substances (TBARS). Briefly, the reaction mixture contained ascorbic acid (50 mM), EDTA (2 mM), H2O2 (1.42 mM), deoxyribose (2.8 mM) and various concentrations of NSE in a final volume of 1.0 ml. The reaction mixture was incubated at 37°C for 30 minutes, followed by the addition of 1 ml of 5% trichloroacetic acid (TCA) and 1 ml of thiobarbituric acid (TBA), and heated in a water bath at 75°C for 30 minutes and cooled. The reaction mixture without NSE served as control. The absorbance was read at 534 nm using UV-VIS spectrophotometer (Shimadzu UV-260, Shimadzu Corp, Tokyo, Japan). Percent inhibition was calculated by the following equation:-

$$\% \text{ Inhibition} = [(A0-A1) / A0]x100$$

Where A0 is the absorbance of the control and A1 is the absorbance in the presence of the samples and standard.

### Superoxide radical

Superoxide scavenging activity of NSE was performed by the photooxidation of riboflavin according to the method of Hyland et al. [23]. The 3 ml of reaction mixture, contained 20 mM phosphate buffer, 100 mM EDTA-sodium cyanide, 2 mM of riboflavin, 75 μM nitrobluetetrazolium and various concentrations of NSE. The control consisted of reaction mixture without NSE. The test samples along with control were illuminated under incandescent light for 20 minutes and the absorbance was recorded at 513 nm. The percentage inhibition of superoxide anion generation was calculated using the following formula:-

$$\% \text{ Inhibition} = [(A0-A1) / A0]\times 100$$

Where A0 is the absorbance of the control and A1 is the absorbance in the presence of the samples and standard.

### ABTS radical

ABTS diammonium salt radical cation decolorisation test was performed using spectrophotometric method described by Miller et al. [24]. The ABTS reacts with potassium persulphate to produce the ABTS•+ radical cation, a blue green chromogen. In the presence of antioxidant, the colored radical is converted back to colorless ABTS. Various concentrations of NSE (10-120 μg) in a final volume of 1 ml of PBS were mixed with 1ml of ABTS working solution. ABTS working solution with equal volume of PBS served as control. The reaction mixture was incubated at room temperature (28°C) for 30 minutes and the absorbance was measured at 734 nm.

All the experiments were performed thrice and test of homogeneity was applied to find out variation among each experiment if any. The data of each experiment did not differ significantly from one another and hence, all the data have been combined and means calculated.

### Statistical analysis

All data are expressed as Mean ± SEM (Standard Error of Mean). The significance between different groups was determined by Mantel-Cox Log Rank test, except free radical estimations, where statistical significance was determined by the Students 't' test. A p value of $<0.05$ was considered as significant.

## Results

The results are expressed as mean ± SEM (Standard Error of the Mean) in Table 1 and Figures 1-7.

### Maximum tolerated dose (MTD)

Administration of 500 to 1000 mg/kg b. wt. NSE did not show any adverse clinical signs and symptoms of toxicity up to day 14 post-drug treatment. Similarly, the body weights also remained unaltered in the animals treated with NSE when compared with the DDW treated control group. A further increase in the NSE dose resulted in a corresponding decrease in the animal survival and an administration of 2000 mg/kg b. wt. NSE resulted in a 50% reduction in the animal survival [Figure 1]. When the NSE dose was increased up to 3000 mg/kg b. wt. the animal survival reduced up to 30% leading to a mortality of 70% and no animals survived when the NSE dose was further raised up to 5000 mg/kg b. wt. [Table 1]. The $LD_{50(14)}$ was determined by probit analysis as described by Litchfield and Wilcoxon was found to be 2000 mg/kg b. wt. NSE [Table 1 and Figure 1].

| NSE dose (mg/kg.b.wt.) | Mortality (%) | Corrected (%) | Probit values |
|---|---|---|---|
| 500 | 0 | 2.5 | 3.04 |
| 1000 | 00 | 2.5 | 3.04 |
| 2000 | 50 | 50 | 4.75 |
| 3000 | 70 | 70 | 5.52 |
| 5000 | 100 | 97.5 | 6.96 |
| LD50(14) value = 2000 mg/kg b.wt. | | | |

**Table 1**: Acute toxicity of oral administration of NSE in Swiss albino mice

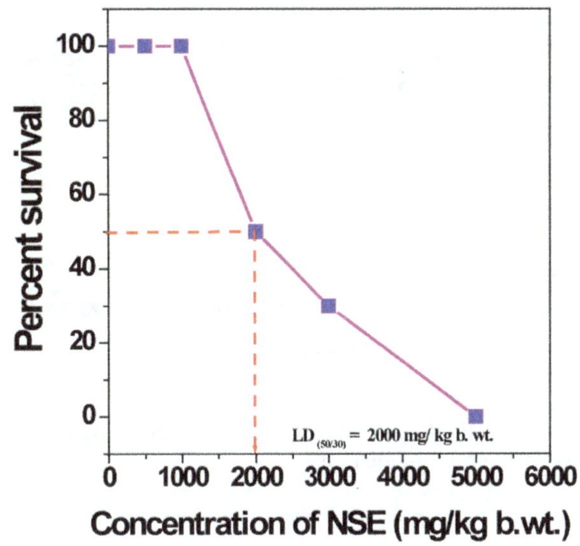


**Figure 1**: Acute toxicity of various doses of NSE after oral administration in Swiss albino mice. $LD_{50}(14)$ value=2000 mg/kg b. wt

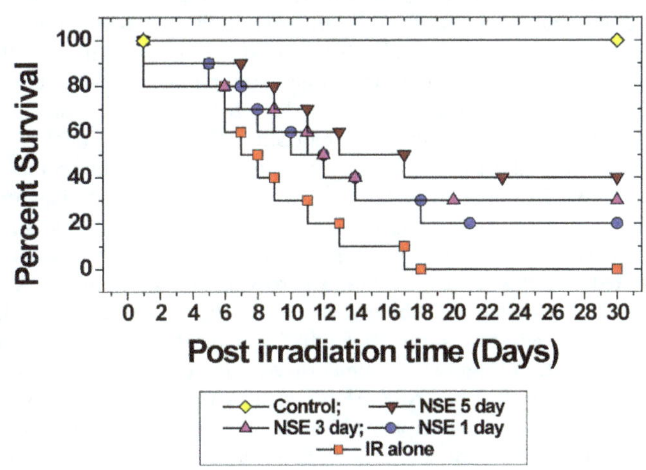


**Figure 2**: Effect of various dosing schedules of 150 mg/kg b. wt. NSE pre-treatment on the survival of mice exposed to 10 Gy of γ-radiation

### Optimum dosing schedule

The optimum dosing schedule was determined by orally administering the animals with 150 mg/kg NSE once daily for one, three, or five consecutive days before 10 Gy irradiation and monitoring the animals for 30 days post-irradiation. A greatest number of animals receiving the oral administration of 150 mg/kg NSE for five days survived at day 30 post-irradiation, when compared to other administration schedules i.e. 1, 3 and 5 days [Figure 2]. Therefore, administration of NSE once daily for five consecutive days before irradiation was considered the best and further studies were carried out using this regimen.

### Administration route

The administration of 150 mg/kg NSE, once daily, consecutively for five days by oral (po), intraperitoneal (ip) or intramuscular (im) route before irradiation to 10 Gy showed an increase in 30 day survival of mice. The analysis of thirty-day survival revealed that the optimum radioprotective activity was observed when the drug was administered through oral route rather than through ip or im route, where 40% animals survived after 30 days post irradiation than the other routes of administration [Figure 3].

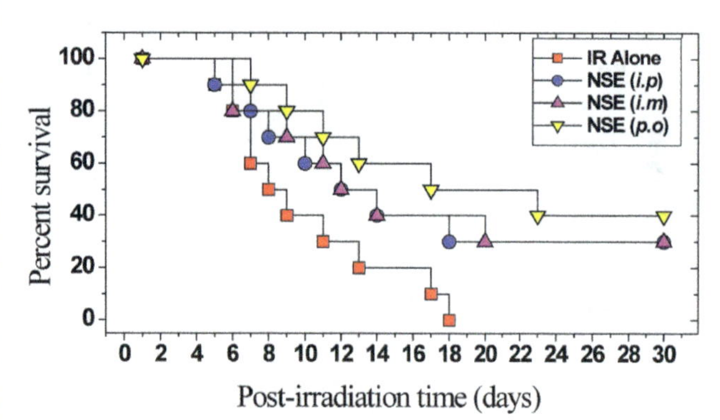


**Figure 3**: Effect of different routes of administration of 150 mg/kg b. wt. NSE on the Kaplan Meir's estimate of the survival of mice exposed to 10 Gy of γ-radiation

## Optimum dose

The optimum radioprotective dose was determined by injecting different doses of NSE before whole-body exposure to 10 Gy γ-radiation. Oral administration of 500 mg/kg of NSE (¼ of $LD_{50}$) alone for five consecutive days did not cause any drug induced mortality up to 30 days. Exposure of animals to 10 Gy γ-irradiation resulted in a decline in the animal survival and the first death was observed on day 3 and majority of the animals died by 16 days post-irradiation in the DDW +10 Gy irradiation group. Administration of mice with various doses of NSE for five consecutive days before 10 Gy irradiation reduced the radiation-induced mortality. The administration of animals with different doses of NSE before 10 Gy irradiation increased the survival in a dose dependent manner up to 150 mg/kg NSE, where 40% animals survived as against nil in the DDW+10 Gy irradiation group. The administration of 50, 100, 200 and 400 mg/kg NSE to mice resulted in a 30% animal survival, whereas treatment of animals with 25 and 500 mg/kg NSE before 10 Gy irradiation resulted in 20% survival as against no survivors for 10 Gy alone at the end of 30 days after irradiation [Figure 4]. Animal survival increased significantly ($p < 0.05$) for all doses of NSE treated groups when compared to the DDW-treated group, except for 25 and 500 mg/kg b. wt. NSE, where this increase was non-significant. Since a maximum survival was observed in the animals treated with 150 mg/kg of NSE before 10 Gy irradiation, it was considered as an optimum dose for radioprotection and further experiments were performed using this dose.

## Radiation Protection

The radioprotective activity of NSE was determined by administering animals with 150 mg/kg of NSE orally once daily for five consecutive days before whole-body exposure to 0-11 Gy of γ-radiation. Irradiation resulted in a dose-dependent decline in the animal survival, where the first mortality was observed on day 4 post-irradiation in the group of animals receiving 9 Gy irradiation and all animals succumbed to death even before the end of 30th day after exposure to 10 and 11 Gy radiation in the DDW + irradiation group [Figure 5]. As 50% of the animals died after 30 days in the group receiving 8 Gy irradiation. The $LD_{50/30}$ was found to be 8 Gy for DDW + irradiation group. Administration of 150 mg/kg NSE resulted in a significant elevation in the animal survival after irradiation to 10 and 11 Gy. Treatment of mice with 150 mg/kg NSE delayed the gastrointestinal deaths when compared to DDW + irradiation group, especially 9 Gy, where it was delayed by 5 days [Figure 6]. This increased the LD50/30 up to 9.6 Gy resulting in an increase in the LD50/30 by 1.6 Gy. The dose reduction factor (DRF) was found to be 1.2 [Figures 5 and 6].

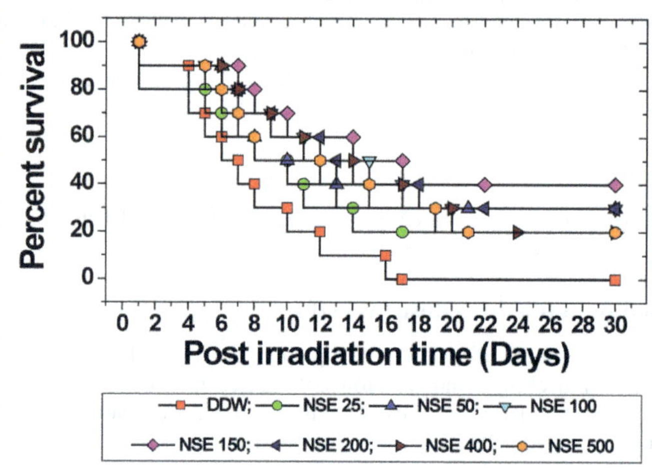


**Figure 4**: Kaplan Meir's estimate of the survival of mice treated with different doses of NSE p.o. before whole body exposure to 10 Gy γ-radiation

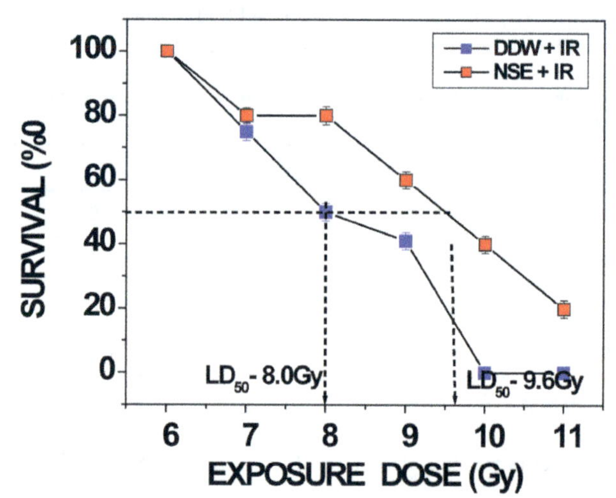


**Figure 5**: Radiation dose response curves for 30 day survival of mice after whole body γ-radiation with or without NSE (150 mg/kg b. wt.) before exposure to 7–11 Gy

## Free radical scavenging activity

### DPPH radical

Introduction of different concentration in vitro resulted in a concentration dependent inhibition of DPPH radicals and a maximum reduction of 74% in DPPH radicals was observed at a concentration of 200 μg/ml [Figure 7a].

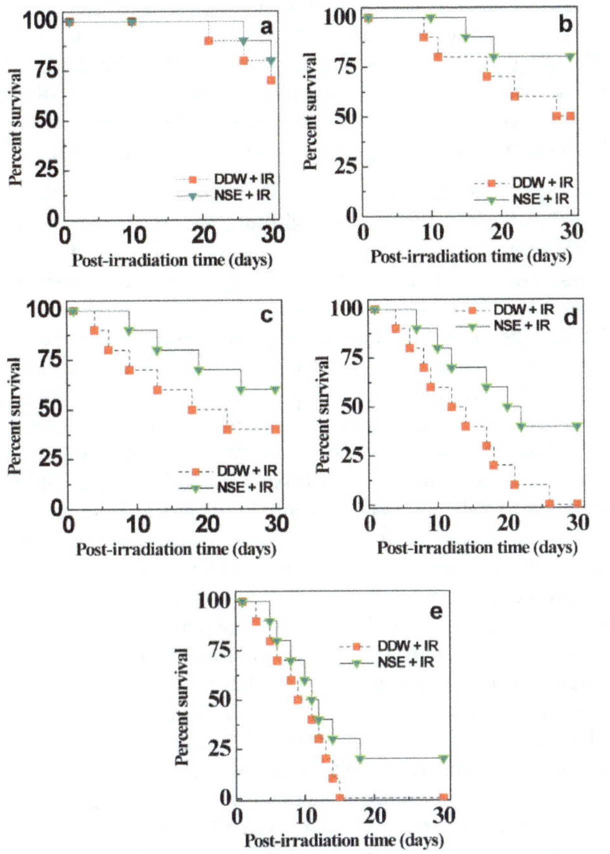


Figure 6: Kaplan-Meir's estimate of survival of mice treated with 150 mg/kg b. wt. of NSE before exposure to various doses of γ-radiation. a) 7, b) 8, c) 9, d) 10, e) 11 Gy radiation

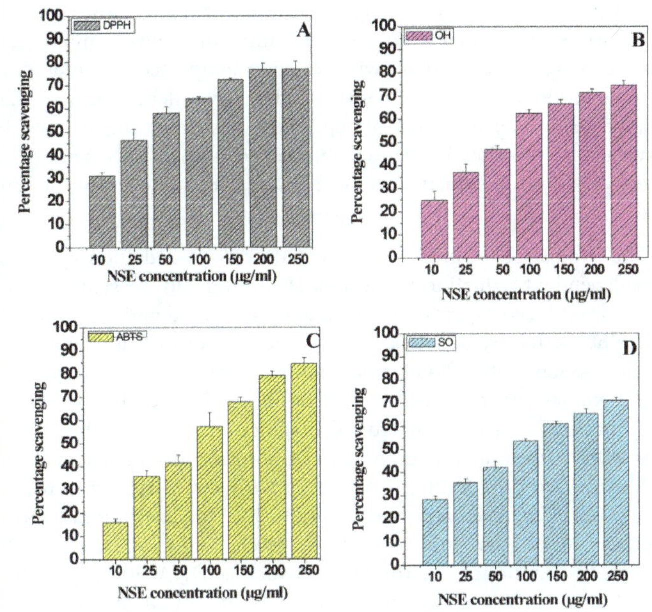


Figure 7: Effect of various concentrations of NSE on the scavenging of various free radicals generated in vitro. a) DPPH b) Hydroxyl c) $ABTS^{•+}$ d) Superoxide anion

## Hydroxyl radical

NSE treatment significantly ($p<0.05$) inhibited 2-deoxyribose degradation in a concentration dependent manner [Figure 7b] and a maximum inhibition was observed at a concentration of 200 μg/ml (75%) and a plateau thereafter [Figure 7b].

## Superoxide anion radical

The generation of superoxide radicals was inhibited by NSE in a concentration dependent manner and a greatest inhibition was observed for 200 μg/ml NSE where a 70% inhibition was reported for the superoxide radicals [Figure 7c]

## ABTS radical

The total antioxidant capacity of the NSE was estimated as the decolouration of ABTS•+, upon interaction with the NSE that suppressed the absorbance of the ABTS•+ radical and the results are expressed as percent inhibition of absorbance as shown in Figure 7d. The ABTS cation radical was inhibited in a concentration dependent manner by NSE and a maximum inhibition was observed for 250 μg/ml [Figure 7d].

## Discussion

Ionizing radiations induce a wide range of molecular damages, which subsequently lead to a spectrum of cellular responses causing cellular damage and cell death [1,25]. Numerous earlier studies on synthetic compounds have demonstrated their ability to protect against deleterious effects of ionizing radiation in various organisms. However, inherent toxicity of these agents at radioprotective concentrations precluded their clinical use [5], and more extensive pursuits for safe and efficacious radioprotectors have been underway since then. The increasing terror attacks and possibility of possession of improvised nuclear devices or dirty bomb in the hands of terrorist organization has reemphasized the need for an effective radioprotector, which is able to counter the deleterious effect of ionizing radiations. Several pharmacological agents have been screened for their radioprotective potential however; none meet the required properties that can be used as a countermeasure against the deleterious effects of ionizing radiations [2,7,26]. This implies that there is a continued need to search and screen newer pharmacological agents that are less toxic and highly effective as radioprotector/s. Therefore, the aim of the present study was to evaluate the radioprotective effect of *Nigella sativa* extract in mice exposed to different doses of γ-radiation.

The maximum tolerated dose of NSE was found to be 1000 mg, where no mortality was observed. With increasing dose the animals succumbed to death and 50% survival was recorded for 2000 mg/kg NSE. Most of the plant extracts have been reported to have higher toxic doses earlier [27-34]. Dichloromethane extract of guduchi was found to have LD50 of 1.2 g/kg b. wt. [35].

Administration of mice with different doses of NSE resulted in a dose dependent elevation in the animal survival after exposure to 10

Gy up to a dose of 150 mg/kg NSE, where a maximum number of survivors were observed. The administration of higher doses of NSE before irradiation actually reduced the animal survival. A similar effect has been reported earlier with other radioprotectors including phytoceuticals [4,7,26-34]. These studies have demonstrated that radioprotective agents have an optimum dose and the decline in survival after this dose is due to the induction of toxic effects at higher doses [4,26-34]. A similar effect of NSE is discernible in the present study.

The irradiation of mice to different doses of γ-radiation caused a dose dependent reduction in the animal survival and the symptoms of radiation-induced sickness like reduction in the food and water intake, irritability lethargy, diarrhea, weight loss, emaciation and epilation within 3–5 days after 10 Gy irradiation is in good agreement with the earlier studies, where a similar effect has been observed [26-34,36,37]. The intestinal and bone marrow damage reduced the survival up to 40% within 10 days and the remaining animals succumbed to death within next 20 days is in corroboration with earlier studies, where a similar effect has been reported [26-34,36,37]. The ionizing radiations interact at cellular and molecular levels inducing damage to biologically important macromolecules such as DNA, RNA, proteins, lipids and carbohydrates of various organs. Usually molecular damages are expressed early, whereas the cellular and tissue damages may be expressed over a period of time depending on the cellular kinetics and radiation tolerance of the tissues. It is well established that the dividing cells are highly sensitive to the effect of ionizing radiations and the effect of whole body irradiation is mainly experienced by germinal epithelium, the gastrointestinal epithelium and the bone marrow progenitor cells, which are under constant renewal at a rapid rate. Since the germinal epithelium does not play any active role in the life supporting functions of the exposed individual, damage to it is inconsequential as far as organismal survival is concerned. In contrast, the gastrointestinal epithelium and the bone marrow progenitor cells are vital for the sustenance of life, and any damage or destruction of these cells will be felt by the whole organism. This will impair the normal physiological processes drastically leading to the death of animals depending upon the severity of damage suffered by these tissues. Despite the fact that the gastrointestinal epithelium is less sensitive than the bone marrow progenitor cells, its cell transit time is quick, and hence the radiation-induced damage is expressed earlier in the gastrointestinal epithelium than the hemopoietic system [37]. This is the reason that gastrointestinal syndrome is expressed earlier in the irradiated organisms than the bone marrow syndrome. In mice death within 10 days post-irradiation is due to the damage inflicted by radiation to the gastrointestinal epithelium and remaining deaths due to irradiation within 11 to 30 days post-irradiation is mainly due to hemopoietic damage inflicted by radiation to the bone marrow cells [26-34,36,37].

The NSE treatment before exposure to different doses of γ-radiation increased the animal survival by 30, 20, 40 and 20% after exposure to 8, 9, 10 and 11 Gy γ-radiation, respectively. A similar increase in the animal survival has been reported earlier when the animals were pretreated with other botanical extracts including *Zinger officinale, Mentha arvensis, Aegle marmelos, Ageratum conzoides, Syzyzium cumini* and *Tinospora cordifolia* before exposure to various doses of ionizing radiations [27-30,38,39]. Likewise, several other chemicals have been shown to elevate the survival of the animals after exposure to lethal doses of radiation [4,40,41]. Similarly, delta-tocotrienol, a vitamin E analogue and a strong antioxidant has been found to protect mice exposed to 9.2 Gy of γ-radiation [42]. The dose reduction factor (DRF) is an indication of the extent of protection offered by any pharmacological agents. NSE treatment has elevated the LD50/30 up to 9.6 Gy resulting in an approximate increase of 1.6 Gy for NSE+ irradiation group as against the 8 Gy for DDW + irradiation group. The administration of NSE before irradiation resulted in a DRF of 1.2. Different agents have been reported to provide different DRF values and WR-2721 have been reported to give a DRF of 2.7 [7,43].

The exact mechanism of action of radioprotection by NSE is not known. However, it may have used multiple putative mechanisms to provide protection to the animals against the radiation-induced sickness and mortality. The ionizing radiations interact with biomolecules by inducing various free radicals, which subsequently inflict damage to cells, tissues and organisms as a whole depending on the dose of radiation. The radioprotective action of NSE may have been mediated through scavenging of the radiation-induced primary free radicals and subsequent prevention of other reactive oxygen species. This contention is supported by our observations that NSE inhibited the generation of hydroxyl, superoxide and DPPH free radicals in the cell-free system. Similarly, it has also inhibited ABTS free radicals in vitro. A similar effect has been reported previously in essential oils obtained from *N. sativa* [44,45]. The other plausible mechanism of radioprotection by NSE may be increase in glutathione, antioxidant enzymes including glutathione peroxidase, glutathione-S-transferase, catalase and superoxide dismutase. NSE has been reported to upregulate the messenger RNA (mRNA) levels of glutathione-S-transferase [46]. As it has reduced the generation of free radicals NSE may have reduced the radiation-induced lipid peroxidation thereby by protecting cell damage. The NSE has been reported to scavenge lipid peroxidation in brain homogenate in vitro [44]. Although no effort has been made to study the molecular mechanisms of radioprotection by NSE, there is no reason to believe that NSE would have not employed the molecular pathways to exert its protective effect. The ionizing radiation induces DNA double strand breaks, which subsequently induce transactivation of NF-κB and expression of COX-II in normal cells [47-49]. Therefore, blockage of transactivation of NF-κB and expression of COX-II may be one of the important molecular mechanisms of radioprotection by NSE [50]. Recently, Nfr2 gene has been identified to play an important role in antioxidant defense and ionizing radiation has been found to disrupt its activation [51]. The presence of NSE before irradiation may have inhibited this action of radiation against the Nfr2 gene keeping the antioxidant enzyme system in good shape leading to radioprotection [52].

The *Nigella sativa* seeds contain thymoquinone, *nigellidine,p-cymene (rho), carvacrol,* 4-terpineol, *t-anethole (tau)* and the sesquiterpene longifolene [53,54]. The observed radioprotective activity of NSE may be due to one of its components or as a concerted action of all these phytochemicals present in NSE.

In conclusion, administration of NSE protected mice against the radiation-induced sickness and mortality. The principle mechanism of radioprotection seems to be scavenging of various radiation-induced free radicals and increase in the activity of antioxidant enzymes. The molecular mechanisms that may have played important role in radioprotection by NSE include inhibition of radiation-induced transactivation of NF-κB, suppression of radiation-induced elevation in COX-II expression, inhibition of the radiation-induced decline in GST mRNA and Nfr2/HO gene, which is supported by various studies on the NSE. The radioprotective action of NSE may be mediated by the presence of various phytochemicals including thymoquinone, nigellidine,*p-cymene (rho)*, carvacrol, 4-terpineol, *t-anethole (tau)* and the sesquiterpene longifolene.

## Acknowledgements

We are thankful to Dr. M.S. Vidyasagar, Professor and Head, and Dr. J.G.R. Solomon, Department of Radiotherapy and Oncology, Kasturba Medical College Hospital, Manipal, for providing the necessary irradiation facilities and for dosimetric calculations, respectively. This work was carried out under a grant sanctioned to GCJ by the Council of Scientific and Industrial Research, Govt. of India, New Delhi.

## References

1. Hall EJ (2000) Acute Effects of Total-Body Irradiation. "In: Radiobiology for the Radiologist" Lippincott Williams & Wilkins, Philadelphia PA
2. Jagetia GC (2007) Radioprotection and radiosensitization by curcumin. Adv Exp Med Biol 595: 301-320.
3. O'Neill P, Fielden EM (1993) Primary radical process in DNA. Adv Radiat Biol 17: 53-120.
4. Patt HM, Tyree EB, Straube RL, Smith DE (1949) Cysteine protection against X-irradiation. Science 110: 213-214.
5. Sweeney TR (1979) A survey of compounds from the antiradiation drug development program of the U.S. Army Medical Research and development command. Government printing office, Washington DC publication 308-318.
6. Weiss JF, Landauer MR (2003) Protection against ionizing radiation by antioxidant nutrients and phytochemicals. Toxicology 89: 1-20.
7. Jagetia GC (2007) Radioprotective Potential of Plants and Herbs against the Effects of Ionizing Radiation. J Clin Biochem Nutr 40: 74-81.
8. Roberts L (1987) Radiation Accident Grips Goiania. Science 238: 1028-1031.
9. Jagetia GC, Venkatesha VA (2005) Effect of mangiferin on radiation-induced micronucleus formation in cultured human peripheral blood lymphocytes. Environ Mol Mutagen 46: 12-21.
10. Chopra RN, Nayar SL, Chopra IC (1956) Clossary of Indian Medicinal Plants. CSIR New Delhi India 175.
11. Warrier PK (1994) Indian Medicinal Plants : a compendium of 500 species Hyderabad Orient Longman 5: 245-247.
12. el-Tahir K, M Ashour, M Al-Harbi (1993) The cardiovascular actions of the volatile oil of the blackseed (Nigella sativa) in rats, elucidation of the mechanism of action. Gen. Pharmacol., 24: 1123-1131.
13. Salomi NJ, Nair SC, Jayawardhanan KK, Varghese CD, Panikkar KR (1992) Anti-tumor principles from Nigella sativa seeds. Cancer Lett 63: 41-46.
14. El Daly ES (1998) Protective effect of cysteine and vitamin E, Crocus sativus and Nigella sativa extracts on cisplatin-induced toxicity in rats. J Pharm Belg 53: 87-89
15. Houghton PJ, R Zarka, de las Heras B, JR Hoult (1995) Fixed oil of Nigella sativa and derived thymoquinone inhibit eicosanoid generation in leukocytes and membrane lipid peroxidation. Planta Med 61: 33-36.
16. Ipor IB, Oyen LPA, de Guzman CC, Siemonsma JS (1999) Nigella sativa Lin: Plant Resources of South-East Asia No. 13: Spices. Backhuys Publisher, Leiden, The Netherlands 148-151.
17. Worthen DR, Ghosheh OA, Crooks PA (1998) The in vitro anti-tumor activity of some crude and purified components of blackseed, Nigella sativa L Anticancer Res 18: 1527-1532.
18. Daba MH, MS Abdel-Rahman (1998) Hepatoprotective activity of thymoquinone in isolated rat hepatocytes. Toxicol Lett 95: 23-29.
19. Chakravarty N (1993) Inhibition of histamine release from mast cells by nigellone. Ann Allergy 70: 237-242.
20. Prieur DJ, Young DM, Davis RD, Cooney DA, Homan ER, et al. (1973) Procedures for preclinical toxicologic evaluation of cancer chemotherapeutic agents: protocols of the laboratory of toxicology. Cancer Chemother Rep 4: 1-28.
21. Mensor LL, Menezes FS, Leitao GG, Reis AS, dos Santos TC, et al. (2001) Screening of Brazilian plant extracts for antioxidant activity by the use of DPPH free radical method. Phytother Res 15: 127-130.
22. Halliwell B, Gutteridge JM, Aruoma OI (1987) The deoxyribose method: a simple "test-tube" assay for determination of rate constants for reactions of hydroxyl radicals. Anal Biochem 165: 215-219
23. Hyland K, Voisin E, Banoun H, Auclair C (1983) Superoxide dismutase assay using alkaline dimethylsulfoxide as superoxide anion-generating system. Anal Biochem 135: 280-287.
24. Miller NJ, Castelluccio C, Tijburg L, Rice-Evans C (1996) The antioxidant properties of theaflavins and their gallate esters--radical scavengers or metal chelators? FEBS Letters 392: 40-44.
25. Ryan JL (2012) Ionizing radiation: the good, the bad, and the ugly. J Invest Dermatol 132: 985-993.
26. Pandey BN, Kumar A, Tiwari P, Mishra KP (2010) Radiobiological basis in management of accidental radiation exposure Int J Radiat Biol 86: 613-35.
27. Jagetia GC, Baliga MS, Venkatesh P, Ulloor JN (2003) Influence of ginger rhizome (Zingiber officinale Rosc) on survival, glutathione and lipid peroxidation in mice after whole-body exposure to γ-radiation. Radiat Res 160: 584-592.
28. Jagetia GC, Shirwaikar A, Rao, SK, Bhilegaonkar PM, (2003) Evaluation of the radioprotective effect of Ageratum conyzoides Linn. extract in mice exposed to different doses of gamma radiation. J Pharm Pharmacol 8: 1151-1158.
29. Jagetia GC, Venkatesh P, Baliga MS (2004) Evaluation of the radioprotective effect of bael leaf (Aegle marmelos) extract in mice. Int J Radit Biol 4: 281-290.
30. Jagetia GC, Baliga MS, Venkatesh P (2005) Influence of seed extract of Syzygium cumini (Jamun) on mice exposed to different doses of γ-radiation. J Radiat Res 46: 59-65.
31. Jagetia GC, Baliga MS (2002) Cystone, an ayurvedic herbal drug imparts protection to the mice against the lethal effects of γ - radiation: a preliminary study. Nahrung/Food 5: 332- 336.
32. Jagetia GC, Baliga MS (2003) Treatment of mice with a herbal preparation mentat protects against radiation-induced mortality. Phytother Res 8: 876-881.
33. Jagetia GC, Baliga MS (2004) Polyherbal extract of septilin protects mice against whole body lethal dose of gamma radiation. Phytother Res 18: 619-623.
34. Jagetia GC, Baliga MS (2004) Evaluation of the radioprotective action of geriforte in mice exposed to different doses of gamma-radiation. Am J Chinese Med 4: 551-567.
35. Jagetia GC, Nayak V, Vidhyasagar MS (2002) Enhancement of radiation effect by guduchi (Tinospora cordifolia) in HeLa cells. Pharmaceutical Biology 40: 179-188.
36. Jagetia GC, Ganapathi NG, Venkatesh P, Rao N, Baliga MS (2006)Evaluation of the radioprotective effect of Liv 52 in mice. Environmental and Molecular Mutagenesis 47: 490-502.
37. Bond VP, Fliedner T, Archambeau JO (1965) Mammalian Radiation Lethality. Academic Press New York USA
38. Tayagi S, Singh L, Devi MM, Goel HC, Rizvi MA (2009) Augmentation of Antioxidant Defense System by Tinospora cordifolia: Implications in Radiation Protection. J Complement Integrat Med 6: 36.
39. Jagetia GC, Baliga MS (2002) Influence of the leaf extract of Mentha arvensis Linn. (mint) on the survival of mice exposed to different doses of gamma radiation. Strahlenther Onkol 178: 91-98.
40. Ghosh SP, Perkins MW, Hieber K, Kulkarni S, Kao TC (2009) Radiation protection by a new chemical entity, Ex-Rad: efficacy and mechanisms. Radiat Res 171: 173-179
41. Kuntić VS, Stanković MB, Vujić ZB, Brborić JS, Uskoković-Marković SM (2013) Radioprotectors - the evergreen topic. Chem Biodivers 10: 1791-1803.

42. Singh VK, Wise SY, Scott JR, Romaine PL, Newman VL, et al (2014) Radioprotective efficacy of delta-tocotrienol, a vitamin E isoform, is mediated through granulocyte colony-stimulating factor. Life Sci 98: 113–122.
43. Yuhas JM, Storer JB (1969) Chemoprotection against three modes of radiation death in the mouse. Int J Radiat Biol Relat Stud Phys Chem Med 15: 233-237.
44. Burits M, Bucar F (2000) Antioxidant activity of Nigella sativa essential oil. Phytotherapy Research 14: 323–328.
45. Abdel-Wahhab MA, Aly SE (2005) Antioxidant property of Nigella sativa (black cumin) and Syzygium aromaticum (clove) in rats during aflatoxicosis. Journal of Applied Toxicology. 25: 218-223.
46. El-Sayed WM (2011) Upregulation of Chemoprotective Enzymes and Glutathione by Nigella sativa(Black Seed) and Thymoquinone in CCl4-Intoxicated Rats. Int J Toxicol 30: 707-714.
47. Meng A, Yu T, Chen G, Brown SA, Wang Y, et al (2003) Cellular origin of ionizing radiation-induced NF-kappaB activation in vivo and role of NF-kappaB in ionizingradiation-induced lymphocyte apoptosis. Int J Radiat Biol 79: 849-861.
48. Dong XR, Luo M, Fan L, Zhang T, Liu L (2010) Corilagin inhibits the double strand break-triggered NF-kappaB pathway in irradiated microglial cells. Int J Mol Med 25: 531-536.
49. Moore ED, Kooshki M, Metheny-Barlow LJ, Gallagher PE, Robbins ME (2013) Angiotensin-(1-7) prevents radiation-induced inflammation in rat primary astrocytes through regulation of MAP kinase signaling. Free Radic Biol Med 65: 1060-1068.
50. Kundu JK, Liu L, Shin JW, Surh YJ (2013) Thymoquinone inhibits phorbol ester-induced activation of NF-κB and expression of COX-2, and induces expression of cytoprotective enzymes in mouse skin in vivo. Biochem Biophys Res Commun 438: 721-727.
51. Kim SB, Pandita RK, Eskiocak U, Ly P, Kaisani A, et al (2012) Targeting of Nrf2 induces DNA damage signaling and protects colonic epithelial cells from ionizing radiation. Proc Natl Acad Sci USA 109: 2949-2955
52. Ulu R, Doğukan A, Tuzcu M, Gürel A, Muqbil I, et al (2013) Modulation of Nrf2/HO-1 by Thymoquinone During Cisplatin-Induced Nephrotoxicity. Turk Neph Dial Transpl 22: 182-187
53. Ali BH, Blunden G (2003) Pharmacological and toxicological properties of Nigella sativa. Phytotherapy Research 17: 299–305.
54. Ali Z, Ferreira D, Carvalho P, Avery MA, Khan IA (2008) Nigellidine-4-O-sulfite, the first sulfated indazole-type alkaloid from the seeds of Nigella sativa. J Nat Prod 71: 1111–1112.

# The Non-Electromagnetic Action of Photons on Biological Systems: Spin Supercurrent

**Liudmila B Boldyreva***

*The State University of Management, Moscow, Russia*

***Corresponding author:** Liudmila B Boldyreva PhD in Engineering, Associate Professor, The State University of Management, Moscow, Russia, E-mail: boldyrev-m@yandex.ru

**Abstract**

The paper aims at showing that there is a physical process that might account for the non-electromagnetic action of photons on biological systems.

An analogy is shown between the effects of low-intensity electromagnetic radiation and the effects of biologically active substances in ultra-low doses on biological systems and also the features of quantum correlation of photons. The analogy may be due to the same physical mechanism underlying the phenomena. It is of importance that quantum correlations of photons are effected by non-electromagnetic forces.

A comparison is drawn between the features of quantum correlations in such quantum macrosystem as superfluid $^3$He-B and the experimentally established properties of quantum correlations of photons.

It is shown that quantum correlations (and, consequently, the effects of low-intensity electromagnetic radiation on biological systems) may be due to spin supercurrents, whose properties are like those of spin supercurrents emerging between spin structures in superfluid $^3$He-B, the spin supercurrents being of non-electromagnetic nature.

It is shown that the non-electromagnetic action of photons on a biological system may be performed by spin supercurrents emerging between the spin structures produced by the photons and biological system in the physical vacuum. The spin supercurrent speed may exceed that of light, because the spin supercurrent is not accompanied by the birth of a mass, as it is in the motion of a body (the relativistic increase in mass) or in the motion of photon (the kinetic mass of photon), and therefore has no inertial properties.

**Keywords:** Ultra-low doses; Non-electromagnetic action of photon; Low-intensity electromagnetic radiation; Quantum correlations; Spin supercurrent; Superfluid physical vacuum

## Abbreviations

BS: Biological System; HPD: Homogeneously Precessing Domain.

## Introduction

There is a number of phenomena that are indicative, expressly or by implication, of non-electromagnetic action of light on bodies, including biological systems. Let us discuss such phenomena.

### The action of low-intensity electromagnetic radiation on a biological system (BS)

Electromagnetic radiation is referred to as a low-intensity radiation if its flux density is less than 1 $\mu W/cm^2$ [1,2].

Figure 1 shows the difference Y between the normalized blood clotting time for test group rats (exposed to an alternating electromagnetic field) and that for control group rats (not exposed to the alternating electromagnetic field) against the amplitude of magnetic field strength *H*. The frequency *f* of the electromagnetic field is 5 Hz. Helmholtz coils were used to produce the field [3].

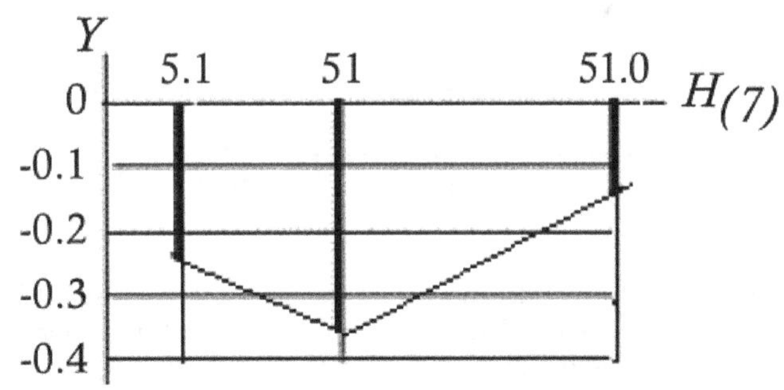


**Figure 1:** The difference *Y* between the normalized blood clotting time for test group rats and that for control group rats (not exposed to the alternating electromagnetic field) against the amplitude of magnetic field strength *H*. The frequency *f* of the field is 5 Hz.

Figure 2 shows the results of the experiment where test group rats were exposed to a low-frequency alternating electromagnetic field, in particular the difference *A* between the normalized erythrocyte count in the blood of test group rats and that of control group rats (not exposed to the alternating magnetic field) against the amplitude of magnetic field strength *H*. The frequency *f* of the magnetic field is 10 Hz [3].

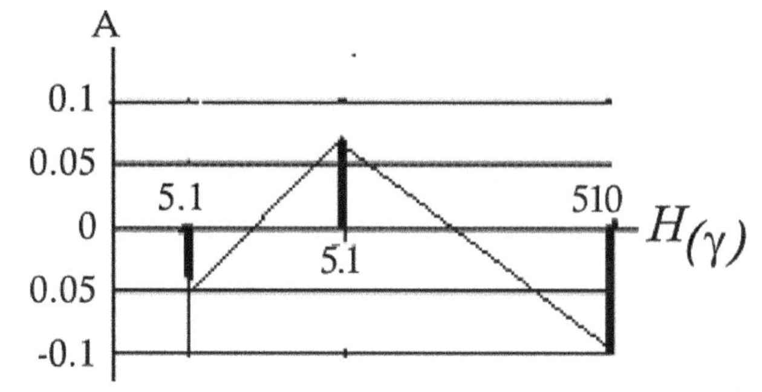


**Figure 2**: The difference *A* between the normalized erythrocyte count in the blood of test group rats and that in the blood of control group rats (not exposed to the alternating magnetic field) against the amplitude of magnetic field strength *H*. The frequency *f* of the field is 10 Hz

One more phenomenon characteristic of the action of ultra-low doses of irradiation is the type of dependence of human mortality (caused by leukemia) on the equivalent dose *d* of irradiation (including the Υ-radiation of cesium-137) (Figure 3). The curve is based on the data collected under E. Burlakova's guidance [2,4]. As the death rate *K* the ratio of the number of deaths per 100000 person-years to the number of deaths caused by the equivalent dose of about 23 mSv is used.

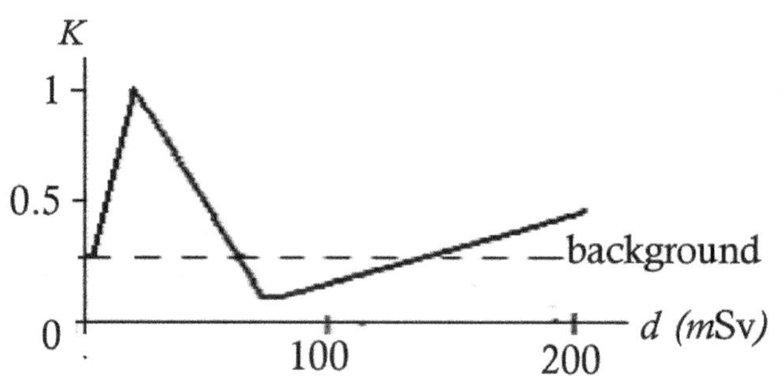


**Figure 3**: The type of dependence of human mortality (caused by leukemia) on the equivalent dose *d* (including the Υ-radiation of cesium-137). *K* is the ratio of the number of deaths per 100000 person-years caused by arbitrary value of equivalent dose *d* to the number of deaths caused by the equivalent dose of about 23 mSv

As is shown by the above data, in the action of low-intensity electromagnetic radiation on BS the "dose-effect" (or "dose-response") dependence is non-monotonic. In some cases, the same effects are produced by low-doses differing in 5 to 8 orders of magnitude. There are also cases (an example is shown in Figure 2) where a change in the "sign" of the effect is observed in the dose dependence. Let us compare the above cases of "dose-effect" dependence with similar cases of dependence in the action of biologically active substances in ultra-low doses on BS.

Figure 4 shows the type of variation of the content of protein p53 with mice of F1 line as a function of dose *D* of the injected antioxidant phenosan [5,6]. The value *D*= $10^{14}$ mole/kg corresponds to an ultra-low dose.

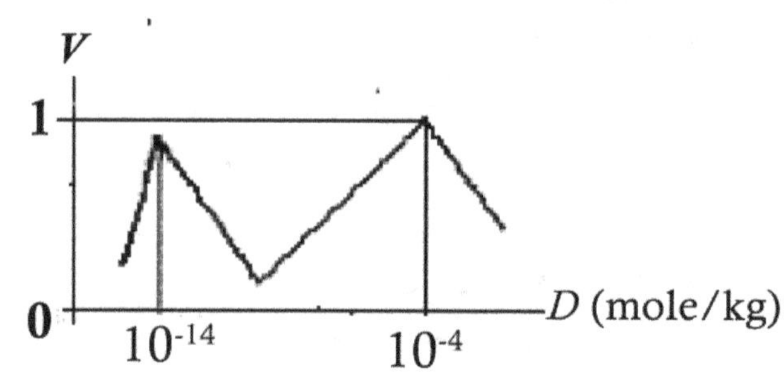


**Figure 4**: The type of dependence of the content of protein p53 with mice of F1 line as a function of dose *D* of the injected antioxidant phenosan

Figure 5 shows the dependence of normalized toxicity rate T/T' (T=T' at d=9 nm)of silver nanoparticles (AgNP) in experiments with *E.coli* [7] on the nanoparticle size d. The conclusion was made that AgNP interaction with bacteria [8,9] cannot be reduced to the action of $Ag^+$ ions in equivalent concentrations. Therefore there are grounds to assume that the biological action of silver NPs can be effected through the mechanism different from that of $Ag^+$ ions (that is, it is not due to electric forces).

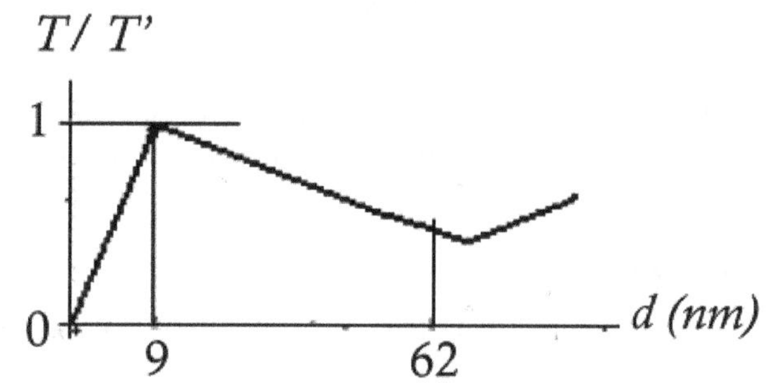


**Figure 5**: The type of dependence of normalized toxicity rate T/T' (T=T'at d=9nm) on the nanoparticle size *d*.

The non-monotonic "dose-effect" dependence (shown in Figures 1-5) is not the only similarity between the features of the effects of low-intensity electromagnetic radiation on BS and the effects of biologically active substances in ultra-low doses on BS. There are other analogies [1,10-13]: a change in sensitivity (generally, an increase) of the BS with respect to a subsequent exposure to ultra-low dose; dependence of the "sign" of the effect (inhibition or stimulation) on the initial state of the BS being treated; disappearance of side effects with a decreased dose (while retaining its activity). The analogies suggest that the effects of low-intensity electromagnetic radiation on BS and those of biologically active substances in ultra-low doses on BS may be due to the same physical mechanism. Since the action of biologically active substances in ultra-low doses on BS is performed by non-electric and non-magnetic forces, the action of low-intensity electromagnetic radiation on BS is likely to be of non-electromagnetic nature too.

The main difficulty in determining the physical mechanism accounting for the effects of ultra-low doses is the low concentration of the substance introduced. The ultra-low doses are taken to be those with concentrations of $10^{13}$M or lower [1]. Note that introduction of a substance in doses of $10^{12}$-$10^{13}$M into an organism will result in about 10 down to 1 molecules of the substance to be contained in a cell. That is, at concentrations of less than $10^{13}$M there will be, from the point of view of classical physics, no molecules of the substance in a cell. This accounts for the difficulty of explaining the effects on the basis of modern physics, in particular, on the basis of the laws of statistical physics.

## Quantum correlations of photons

The phenomenon of quantum correlation can be explained by the following example. Let two photons *a* and *b* at the output of a beam splitter, which are described by the same wave function (that is, they have the same frequency and phase), move in different directions and interact with different BS. Photon *a* is directed, depending on the position (1 or 2) of switch *P*, either towards BS $A_1$ or BS $A_2$; photon *b* is directed towards BS *B*. Since in quantum mechanics any interaction results in a reduction of wave function, two different interactions of photon *a* with BS may result in two different states of photon *b*, that is, the properties of photon *b* will depend on which BS photon *a* interacts with. Thus the biological systems irradiated by the photons emitted by the same source appear to be connected with each other by quantum correlations of the photons.

The following properties of quantum correlations were determined in the experiments. Quantum correlations take place:

1) For quantum entities having either zero rest mass (e.g. photon) or nonzero rest mass [14].

2) Independent of the distance between the detectors; this was established over distances of the order of 10 km [15].

3) Not only in the process of simultaneous detection of both photons, but also in the case of different times of traveling of the photons from their sources to the detectors. That is quantum correlation takes place between the photon interacting with a detector and the photon which has not yet reached its detector and is found in the physical vacuum [16].

4) Quantum correlations have a non-electromagnetic nature.

There are experimental data [17] that quantum correlations may take place between the photons that have the same frequency, but have been emitted by different sources.

Note that the effects of ultra-low doses on BS and quantum correlations have some similar features:

1. They take place for quantum entities having either zero rest mass (e.g. photon) or nonzero rest mass;

2. They are caused not by electric or magnetic forces;

3. They do not present a cooperative effect, that is, they take place between single quantum entities (between two photons in Figure 6), not between ensembles of quantum entities.

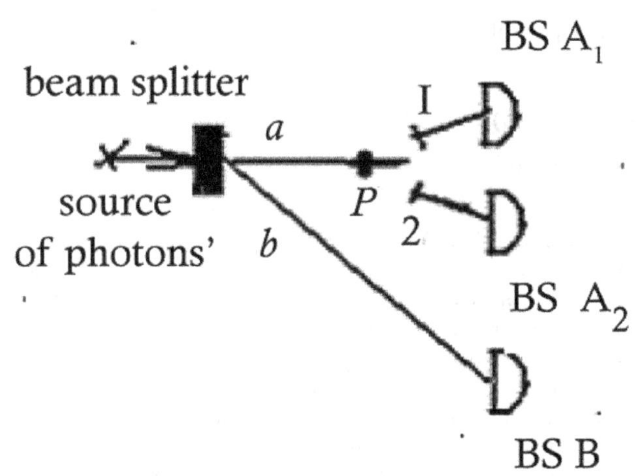


**Figure 6**: Photon *a* arrives at either BS $A_1$ or BS $A_2$ depending on the position of switch P (1 or 2), photon *b* arrives at BS B.

Both phenomena, the quantum correlation and the action of ultra-low doses (including the action of low-intensity electromagnetic radiation) on BS, may be assumed to be caused by the same physical mechanism.

Theoretically, quantum correlations occur instantaneously, and the only explanation based on the classical cause-and-effect relationship might be the introduction of unknown "superluminal" (non-electromagnetic) forces between quantum entities. The only obstruction to "legalization" of such forces is the relativity postulate according to which the speed of transmission of energy (signal) cannot exceed the speed of light [16].

*Note.* There is the Copenhagen interpretation of quantum correlations, but it does not consider in principle the processes taking places between the quantum entities in the physical vacuum. At the same time the above third property of quantum correlations suggests that quantum correlations take place specifically in the physical vacuum.

Using as an example the quantum correlations in such quantum macrosystem as superfluid $^3$He-B it is shown in this paper that there is a physical process responsible for quantum correlations, namely, spin supercurrent. Thus the non-electromagnetic action of photons on BS may be effected by spin supercurrents arising in the physical vacuum. The spin supercurrent speed may exceed the speed of light, because spin supercurrent is not accompanied by the birth of a mass, as it is in the motion of a body (the relativistic increase in mass) or in the motion of photon (the kinetic mass of photon), and therefore has no inertial properties.

# Materials and Methods

### The properties of quantum correlations in superfluid $^3$He-B

The superfluid $^3$He-B consists of atoms having spin. One of the properties of superfluid $^3$He–B is that areas with coherently precessing spins of $^3$He atoms, the so-called homogeneously precessing domains (HPDs), may exist there. Examples of HPDs are given in Figure 7;

these HPDs are characterized by spin $S$ and by respective precession angles $\alpha_1$ and $\alpha_2$, nutation angles $\beta_1$ and $\beta_2$, precession frequencies $\omega_1$ and $\omega_2$, and energies $U_1$ and $U_2$, the energies being dependent on the characteristics of the respective spin structures:

$$U_1 = f(S, \omega_1, \beta_1), \quad (1)$$

$$U_2 = f(S, \omega_2, \beta_2). \quad (2)$$

Since superfluid $^3$He-B is a quantum system, the HPDs produced in it are quantum entities too. The precession and nutation angles determine the spin part of the order parameter for superfluid $^3$He–B and there are processes that tend to make equal the respective characteristics of the spin part of the order parameter throughout the whole volume of the superfluid. Such processes in superfluid $^3$He–B are spin supercurrents [18-20], that is, quantum correlations are effected in this quantum system by spin supercurrents. The value of spin supercurrent $J$ between two HPDs is proportional to differences in their precession angles and nutation angles ($\alpha_1$ - $\alpha_2$ and $\beta_1$ - $\beta_2$ in Figure 7).

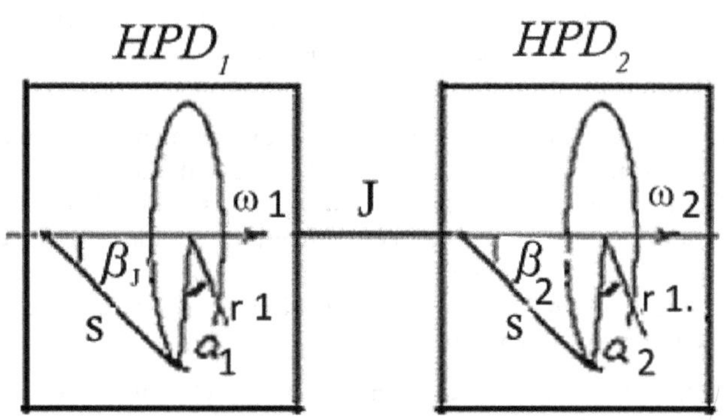


**Figure 7:** Spin structures $HPD_1$ and $HPD_2$ : $\omega_1$ and $\omega_2$ are precession frequencies, $\alpha_1$ and $\alpha_2$ are precession angles, $\beta_1$ and $\beta_2$ are nutation angles, S is spin; r.l. is the reference line, J is spin supercurrent

There exists such a phenomenon in $^3$He–B as phase slippage. At a certain difference in precession angles, $\Delta\alpha_c$, for two HPDs there takes place a precession phase slippage, or phase drop, by $2\pi n$ (n=1, 2...). The critical spin supercurrent $J_c$ corresponds to $\Delta\alpha_c$ [19]. Figures 8a and 8b show examples of the character of dependence of normalized spin supercurrent $J/J_c$ between two HPDs with respective precession frequencies $\omega_1$ and $\omega_2$ ($\omega_1 \neq \omega_2$) on the hypothetical difference in the precession angles, $\Delta\varphi$, which is defined as $\Delta\varphi = (\omega_1-\omega_2)t$, t being time. Up to the value of $\Delta\varphi$ equal to $\Delta\alpha_c$, the hypothetical difference is equal to the precession angles difference determining the spin supercurrent, $\Delta\alpha$, that is, $\Delta\varphi = \Delta\alpha$. On the curves the line 1-1 corresponds to the change in the supercurrent in the process of phase slippage, the $2\pi$ phase slip taking place. In Figure 8a we have $\Delta\alpha_c = \pi$. In Figure 8b $\Delta\alpha_c \approx 3\pi$ [18].

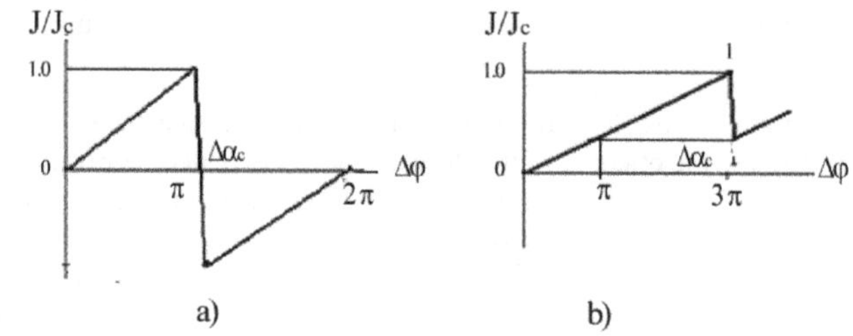


**Figure 8:** Versions of dependency of the normalized spin supercurrent $J/J_c$ on the hypothetical difference in the phases of precession, $\Delta\varphi$. Up to point $\Delta\varphi = \Delta\alpha_c$, $\Delta\varphi = \Delta\alpha$.The phase slippage is shown by line 1-1. The $2\pi$ phase slippage is taking place. Version a) $\Delta\alpha_c = \pi$; version b) $\Delta\alpha_c \approx 3\pi$

Generally, the determination of time dependency of the magnitude of the spin supercurrent between two regions with precessing spins is a difficult problem, because the speed of transmission of information of the existence of a gradient of the order parameter is, in theory, infinite, and the speed of the spin supercurrent is finite [19]. Besides, a possibility of phase slippage should be taken into account. One of the conditions for the respective precession and nutation angles of interacting HPDs to become equal is the following:

$$\Delta\omega \to 0, \quad (3)$$

where $\Delta\omega$ is the difference between the precession frequencies of interacting HPDs.

## Results

Comparison of the properties of quantum correlations and those of spin supercurrents in superfluid $^3$He-B

According to postulates of quantum mechanics, quantum entities (including photons) produce virtual particles in the physical vacuum. The spin of those particles is the same as for the real particles. Hence it follows that 1) the virtual particle spin has no definite direction, and by the magnitude of spin the magnitude of its projection onto a preferential direction is meant; this can be interpreted as a precession of the spin about the preferential direction; 2) spin correlations can take place.

Thus the spin structures produced by the biologically active substances, photons and the target biological systems as consisting of quantum entities are characterized by respective frequencies of precession, precession angles and nutation angles, the total spin $S_s$ and energy $U_s$

$$U_s = S_s \omega_s, \quad (4)$$

where $\omega_s$ is the frequency of precession of spin in the structure consisting of virtual particles. Spin correlations may take place between these spin structures.

In this section it will be shown that under the assumption that the properties of these spin correlations are analogous to those of spin supercurrents in superfluid $^3$He-B, the properties of quantum correlations mentioned in Introduction can be explained on the basis of the properties of spin supercurrents between spin structures in superfluid $^3$He-B.

*Correlations take place between quantum entities with zero or non-zero rest mass.*

Spin supercurrents may emerge in superfluid $^3$He-B between any structures having spin. Consequently, quantum correlations may take place between any quantum entities producing spin structures with total nonzero spin in the physical vacuum. No matter by which type of quantum entities the spin structures have been produced: with zero or non-zero rest mass.

Note. Quantum correlations may not take place between quantum entities producing spin structures with total zero spin in the physical vacuum. For example, according to [21], there will be no quantum correlations in superconductors between Cooper pairs of electrons with s-pairing.

*Correlations take place independent of the distance between the detectors.*

Spin supercurrents in superfluid $^3$He-B may emerge between any spin structures, independent of the distance between them.

*Correlations take place between quantum entities not only at the moment of simultaneous registration of the entities.*

Spin supercurrent arises between spin structures in superfluid $^3$He-B instantly, in theory, after the emergence of differences in the precession angles or/and nutation angles of the structures, whether the difference is a result of an external action on one of the structures or on both ones simultaneously.

*The quantum correlations may take place between photons of the same frequency, emitted by different sources.*

The virtual particles produced by photons in the physical vacuum are converted into real particles (electron-positron pairs, proton-antiproton pairs), if the energy of the photon equals the total energy of the pair of real particles produced. This means that the energy of a pair of virtual particles, that is, the energy of the spin structure produced by the photon in the physical vacuum $(Us)_{ph}$ is equal to the energy of photon, Uph:

$$(Us)_{ph} = U_{ph}. \quad (5)$$

For the total spin of the pair of virtual particles produced by the photon, $(Ss)_{ph}$, we have:

$$(Ss)_{ph} = \hbar. \quad (6)$$

Taking Eq. (4) into account and comparing the well-known relation between energy Uph and photon frequency ωph, Uph = hωph with Eqs. (5) and (6), we obtain that the precession frequency in the spin structure produced by a photon in the physical vacuum $(\omega s)_{ph}$ is equal to the photon frequency.

$$(\omega s)_{ph} = \omega_{ph}. \quad (7)$$

According to Eq. (3), the efficacy of spin supercurrents in superfluid 3He-B is maximum if the interacting spin structures have equal precession frequencies. But according to (7) the frequency of precession in the spin structure produced by the photon in the physical vacuum is equal to the photon frequency. Thus, the main condition for the photons to be quantum-correlated, i.e. the equality of the photon frequency, is transformed into the condition of the equality of the precession frequencies in the spin structures created by the photons in the physical vacuum

*Quantum correlations are effected by a process propagating at a superluminal speed.*

The question arises whether the speed of spin supercurrent can exceed the speed of light in vacuum, c, which is a speed limit not only for light but for moving bodies with nonzero rest mass?

To answer the question let us discuss the phenomenon which is characteristic of both light and moving particles: the increase in mass. This quantity for the photon is equal to $\hbar\omega_{ph}/c2$ (c is the speed of light). With due account of (7), it may be assumed that the formation of the mass is associated with the spin precession frequency in the spin structure produced by the photon in the physical vacuum. According to postulates of quantum mechanics any quantum entities produce virtual particles in the physical vacuum; consequently any body as consisting of quantum entities produces a spin structure in the physical vacuum. It is shown in [21] that the additional mass of any moving body (the so-called relativistic increase in mass), Δm, is related to the precession frequency $\omega_m$ of the spin structure produced by the body by the following equation: $\Delta m = \hbar\omega_m/c^2$. Thus any moving object that produces a spin structure in the physical vacuum possesses inertial properties, and its speed, at least relative to the gravitational field (since the formation of mass is due to a process in the gravitational field), cannot exceed the speed of light in vacuum.

The spin supercurrent arises between spin structures, but it does not produce the latter. Therefore, *spin supercurrent is not accompanied by the birth of a mass and thus does not possess any inertial properties. So its speed may be greater than the speed of light in vacuum.* A change in the characteristics of interacting spin structures results, according to equations (1)-(2), in a change of energy of the structures. *Consequently, the spin supercurrent transports energy between spin structures, but there is no mass associated with the energy, that is, the equation which relates energy E to mass m ($E=mc^2$) is not valid in this case.*

Thus the properties of quantum correlations mentioned in Introduction can be explained by the action of spin supercurrents emerging between the spin structures created by quantum entities in the physical vacuum [22]. The properties of spin supercurrent are similar to those of spin supercurrent emerging between spin structures in superfluid $^3$He-B.

## Discussion

I. In [21] it is shown that the spin precession frequency in the spin structure created by a biological system in the physical vacuum is determined by the energy of the biological system and may coincide with one of the frequencies of the intrinsic electromagnetic radiation of the system. In this case condition (3) – the condition of the effective action of light on the biological system – is transformed into the requirement of equality of the frequency of the irradiating light and the frequency of the intrinsic electromagnetic radiation of the biological object being irradiated. This can elucidate the long-lived principle of treatment of various diseases: "Like cures like." Here are some well-known recommendations based on that principle: erysipelatous inflammation having red color is treated by application of red cloth; choledochitis by yellow cloth.

II. According to the properties of spin supercurrent, for the action of ultra-low doses on a biological system by spin supercurrents to be effective the condition (3) has to be met. Therefore, taking into account (7), the following conclusion can be drawn: *the action of a biologically active substance in ultra-low dose on a biological system can be replaced by the action of light whose frequency is equal to the spin precession frequency in the spin structure created by the biologically active substance in the physical vacuum.* It agrees with Paracelsus' views on treatment of diseases. The outstanding medieval physician and philosopher thought that light emitted by celestial bodies can cure certain diseases: for example, the disease whose symptoms are like those of anaemia should be cured by radiation of Mars. Note that in the modern medicine anaemia is treated by iron-containing preparations; and Mars is characterized by the presence of iron oxide on its surface, which accounts for the color of the planet: "red planet".

The converse is valid as well: *the therapeutic action of electromagnetic radiation on a biological system can be replaced by the action of a biologically active substance provided the spin precession frequency in the spin structure created by the substance in the physical vacuum is equal to the frequency of electromagnetic radiation.* There are a number of experiments where the properties of water were affected by low-intensity electromagnetic radiation [1] and then this water exerted the same therapeutic effect as the low-intensity electromagnetic radiation.

III. There is much evidence that in the periods of enhanced solar activity outbreaks of diseases (typhus, cholera, etc.) occurred most frequently [23]. Quite possible that epidemics burst out when in the spectrum of solar radiation there were frequencies equal to the spin precession frequencies in the spin structures created by bacterial agents of corresponding diseases in the physical vacuum.

IV. Assuming that the non-electromagnetic action of photons on a biological system is due to spin supercurrents, similar to those which emerge between spin structures in superfluid $^3$He-B, we endow the physical vacuum with the properties of superfluid $^3$He-B.

The validity of ascribing the properties of superfluid $^3$He-B to the physical vacuum is substantiated in a number of works. For example, in [24] a possibility of laboratory simulation of cosmic string formation in the early Universe using superfluid $^3$He was shown; in [25-27] there were revealed analogies between some properties of superfluid $^3$He-B and gravitational properties of space. It was proved in [21,28] that if the physical vacuum had the properties of superfluid $^3$He-B, the waves described by Maxwell's equations could propagate through the vacuum. The spin supercurrents similar to those which emerge between spin structures in superfluid $^3$He-B may underlie the effects of cavity structures on biological systems [29].

## Conclusion

It is shown in the paper that light may exert a non-electromagnetic action on biological systems through spin supercurrents similar to those which emerge between the spin structures in superfluid $^3$He-B.

The spin supercurrent speed may exceed the speed of light, because the spin supercurrent is not accompanied by the birth of mass, as it is in the motion of a body ("relativistic" increase in mass) or in the case of photon (kinetic mass of photon), and consequently does not possess any inertial properties.

## References

1. Burlakova EB, Konradov AA, Maltseva EL (2008) The effects of ultra-low doses of biologically active substances and low-intensity physical factors. Proceedings of the IV International Symposium on Action Mechanisms of Ultra-low Doses Moscow the Russian Academy of Sciences: In Russian 123-149.
2. Burlakova EB, Goloshchapov AN, Zhizhina GP, Konradov AA (1999) New aspects of the mechanisms of effects of low-intensity irradiation in small doses. Radiation Biology. Radioecology 39: 26-33.
3. Makeev VB, Temuryanz NA (1982) The study of frequency dependence of biological efficacy of magnetic field in the micropulsation range of geomagnetic field (0.01-100 Hz). Problemy kosmicheskoi biologii (Problems of Space Biology) : In Russian 43: 116-128
4. Nussbaum R, Kőhnlein W (1994) Inconsistencies and open questions regarding low-dose health effects of ionizing radiation. Environ Health Perspect 102: 657-667.
5. Mil' EM, Myshlyakova OV, Burlakova EB (2005) Behavior of the p53 Protein under the Action of Weak Physical and Chemical Factors (Ionizing Radiation and Antioxidant). Biophysics 50: 69-73.
6. Mil' EM, Albantova AA, Burlakova EB (2008) Ultra-low doses of phenosan cause activation of p53 protein and bcl-2 with mice F1(CBAxC57B1) and AKR. Proceedings of the IV International Symposium on Action Mechanisms of Ultra-low Doses Moscow the Russian Academy of Sciences: In Russian 71-72
7. Lok CN, Ho CM, Chen R, He QY, Yu WY et al. (2007) Silver nanoparticles: partial oxidation and antibacterial activities. J Biol Inorg Chem 12: 527-534.
8. Egorova EM (2010) "Biological effects of silver nanoparticles," In: Audrey E. Welles, editor. Silver Nanoparticles: Properties, Characterization and Applications. Chapter 5. Nova Science Publishers, Inc : 221-258.
9. Neal AL (2008) What can be inferred from bacterium-nanoparticle interactions about the potential consequences of environmental exposure to nanoparticles? Ecotoxicology 17: 362-371.
10. Boldyreva LB (2013) The Physical Aspect of Action of Biologically Active Substances in Ultra-Low Doses and Low-Intensity Physical Factors on Biological Objects: Spin Supercurrents. Alternative and Integrative Medicine 1000110(2): 6.
11. Boldyreva LB (2011) An analogy between effects of ultra low doses of biologically active substances on biological objects and properties of spin supercurrents in superfluid 3He-B. Homeopathy 100, issue 3: 187-193.
12. Boldyreva LB, Boldyreva EM (2012) The Model of Superfluid Physical Vacuum as a Basis for Explanation of Efficacy of Highly Diluted Homeopathic Remedies. Journal of Homeopathy & Ayurvedic Medicine
13. Boldyreva LB (2014) The Physical Aspect of the Effects of Metal Nanoparticles on Biological Systems. Spin Supercurrents. Nanomaterials and Nanosciences 2(1):6
14. Lamehi–Rachti M, Mittig W (1976) Quantum mechanics and hidden variables: A test of Bell's inequality by the measurement of the spin correlation in low-energy proton-proton scattering. Physical Review D 14: 2543-2555.
15. Tittel W, Brendel J, Gisin B, Herzog T, Zbinden H et al (1998) Experimental demonstration of quantum-correlations over more than 10 kilometers. Physical Review A 57: 3229.
16. Belinskii AV (2003) Quantum nonlocality and the absence of a priori values for measurable quantities in experiments with photons. Physics Uspekhi 46: 877–881.
17. Klyshko DN (1994) Quantum optics: quantum, classical, and metaphysical aspect. Physics Uspekhi 37: 1097–1122.
18. Borovic-Romanov AS, Bunkov YuM, Dmitriev VV, Mukharskii YuM, Sergatskov DA (1989) Investigation of Spin Supercurrents in 3He-B. Physical Review Letters 62, No. 14: 1631.
19. Bunkov YuM (2009) Spin Superfluidity and Coherent Spin Precession. Journal of Physics: Condensed Matter 16: 164201.
20. Dmitriev VV, Fomin IA (2009) Homogeneously precessing domain in 3He-B: formation and properties. Journal of Physics: Condensed Matter 16: 164202.
21. Boldyreva LB (2012) What does this give to physics: attributing the properties of superfluid 3He-B to physical vacuum? URSS. Moscow.

22. Boldyreva LB (2014) Quantum correlations — Spin supercurrents. International Journal of Quantum Information 12(1): 14500.
23. Wolfgang Lillge (2001) Vernadsky's Method-Biophysics and the Life Process. 21st Century Science & Technology Magazine.
24. Bauerle C, Bunkov YuM, Fisher SN, Godfrin H, Pickett GR (1996) Laboratory simulation of cosmic string formation in the early Universe using superfluid 3He. Nature 382: 332.
25. Ruutu VMH, Eltsov VB, Gill AJ, Kibble TWB, Krusius M, et. al (1996) Vortex formation in neutron-irradiated superfluid 3He as an analog of cosmological defect formation. Nature 382: 334.
26. Winkelmann CB Elbs J, Bunkov YM, Godfrin H (2006, May) Probing "cosmological" defects in superfluid 3He-B with a vibrating-wire resonator. Physical Review Letters 96(20): 205301.
27. Volovic GE (2003) The Universe in a Helium Droplet. Clar Press Oxford.
28. Boldyreva LB, Sotina NB (1992) Superfliud Vacuum with Intrinsic Degrees of Freedom. Physics Essays 5: 510-513.
29. Boldyreva LB (2013) The cavity structure effect in medicine: the physical aspect. Forschende Komplementärmedizin/Research in Complementary Medicine 20: 322-326.

# Minimum Inhibitory and Bactericidal Concentrations (MIC and MBC) of Honey and Bee Propolis against Multi-Drug Resistant (MDR) Staphylococcus sp. Isolated from Bovine Clinical Mastitis

**Aamer AA**[1*], **Abdul-Hafeez MM**[2] **and Sayed SM**[2]

[1]*Department of Animal Medicine, Faculty of Veterinary Medicine, Assiut University, Assiut, Egypt*

[2]*Animal Health Research Institute, Assiut Lab, Assiut, Egypt*

[*]**Corresponding author**: Aamer AA, Department of Animal Medicine, Faculty of Veterinary Medicine, Assiut University, Assiut, Egypt, E-mail: aamer_ahmad@ymail.com

**Abstract**

With the emergence of antibiotic-resistant *Staph. sp.,* search for antimicrobial agents other than antibiotic is of great concern. The study aimed to determine both MIC and MBC of different honey samples against these strains. The study was conducted with 64 different *Staph sp.* isolated from bovine mastitis and tested *in vitro* against 11 antimicrobial agents. The most MDR strains (19) were tested *in vitro* against six honey batches; marjoram, cotton, two fennel samples and two different trefoil samples as well as against 10% propolis-fennel honey mixture. Both MIC and MBC of the tested honey samples against every tested strain were determined. Propolis-fennel honey mixture showed the lowest both MIC AND MBC values against all *Staph sp.* all over the study with highly significant differences, while against different *Staph sp.,* also it had the lowest MIC and MBC values against *S. intermedius* followed by *S. aureus*. The study revealed that among the different *Staph. sp., S. aureus* was the most sensitive species to the honey antimicrobial action with highly significant differences. The study concluded that all tested *Staph. sp.* –despite of being MDR- were sensitive to the antimicrobial activity of all tested honeys where *S. aureus* was the most sensitive one, while adding 10% propolis powder would maximize its antimicrobial activity significantly.

**Keywords:** MIC; MBC; Apitherapy; Antimicrobial; Staphylococcus; Mastitis

## Introduction

As the traditional knowledge about the use of natural products or substances should be scientifically investigated [1] and the antimicrobial application requires safe preparations, knowledge of the composition of antibacterial factors and standardized antibacterial activity [2], the *in vitro* study of honey therapeutic action is of great necessity for its applicability. Honey possesses therapeutic potential and its antimicrobial activity is widely documented as a large number of *in vitro* studies of MIC and MBC confirmed its broad-pectrum antimicrobial properties either in solo use [3-6] or in combination with other agents as royal jelly [7], bee propolis [8], ginger starch [9], garlic extract [1] or rifampicin [10] even on MDR such as *S. aureus* methicillin resistant (MRSA) [11] or vancomycin-resistant enterococci (VRE) [12]. Propolis extract also proved to possess antimicrobial activity [13-17] Moreover, subinhibitory concentration of honey in combination with oxacillin restored oxacillin susceptibility to MRSA [11]. The present work aimed to investigate the *in vitro* MICs and MBCs of different honey batches and propolis powder against different MDR *Staph. spp.* isolated from bovine clinical mastitis.

## Material and Methods

### Bacterial isolation

Out of 101 milk samples from clinical mastitic cows through a previous work for the same author [18], 64 *Staph. sp.* strains were recovered and be the baseline of the present study where the most MDR strains (no 19) as *Staph aureus* (6), *Staph intermedius* (3), *Staph saprophyticus* and *Staph epidermedis* (5 for each)were tested against all honey patches.

### Antimicrobial sensitivity testing

All these 64 isolated *Staph. sp.* strains were tested against 11 antimicrobial agents [Oxacillin (OX) 1 µg, Ampicilin (AM) 10 µg, Cefotaxime (CTX) 30 µg, Doxycycline (DO) 30 µg, Enrofloxacin (ENR) 5 µg, Gentamicin (CN) 10 µg, Lincomycin (L) 2 µg, Oxytetracycline (T) 30 µg, Penicillin (P) 10 µ, Trimethoprim – Sulflamethaxzole (SXT) 25 µg and Cloxacillin (CX) 10 µg][*] to determine the MDR strains using disc diffusion sensitivity method according to Kirby-Bauer as described in the guidelines of the National Committee for Laboratory Standards (NCCLS) [19]. For Oxacillin inhibition zones around the disc were measured after 24 and 48 h using the following breakpoints: susceptible (S) ≥ 18 mm; resistance (R) ≤ 17 mm [20].

### Honey batches

Six row full strength different unprocessed honey batches were used in the study; A (marjoram), B (cotton), C (fennel-1)[**], D (fennel-2)[**], E (trefoil-1)[**] and F (trefoil-2)[**] as well as G (10% propolis- Fennel honey mixture) as 10% w/v bee propolis powder[***] in fennel honey. To study the synergistic action and to detect the sole antimicrobial action of propolis, 50 mg propolis powder (the added amount in propolis honey mixture) was tested plain for its MIC and MBC against all tested strains.

## Determination of MIC

Three to six strains of the most MDR strains from each species were chosen for the *in vitro* MIC and MBC study. Honey batches were investigated for their MIC and MBC against the chosen isolated *Staph. sp.* strains where 1 ml of the tested honey was used in bifold dilution method [21] with series of 6 tubes containing 1 ml of Mueller Hinton broth (Accumix - Verna, India) to achieve final dilutions of 50, 25, 12.5, 6.25, 3.12 and 1.62% v/v. Standard bacterial inoculums ($5\times10^5$) of the chosen isolated *Staph. spp.* were inoculated into all 6 dilutions post thorough honey mix. The inoculated tubes were overnight incubated at 37°C. The highest dilution of the tested honey to inhibit growth (no turbidity in the tube) was considered as the MIC value of this honey batch against the tested bacterial species.

## Determination of MBC

From all tubes showed no visible signs of growth/turbidity (MIC and higher dilutions), loopfuls were inoculated onto sterile Mueller Hinton agar (Accumix - Verna, India) plates by streak plate method. The plates were then overnight incubated at 37°C. The least concentration that did not show any growth of tested organisms was considered as the MBC value of the tested honey against the tested bacterial species.

## Statistical analysis

Mean values, standard deviation (SD) and ANOVA analysis were adopted by means of PASW V.18 (2010, spss Inc, Chicago, Illinois, USA). Results were considered statistically significant when P>0.05 and highly significant when P>0.01.

*Antibiotic sensitivity discs were purchased from Bioanalyse - Turkey.

**Fennel or Trefoil 1 and 2: honey batches were collected from two different pasture locations.

***Chinese bee propolis provided kindly from Plant Protection Research Institute (PPRI)- Assiut unit.

## Results

The present study was conducted with 64 *Staph. sp.* strains isolated from bovine mastitis, where the most MDR strains which showed MDR pattern > 6 antimicrobials were chosen and be prepared for MIC and MBC study as shown in Table 1. Against *Staph. sp.*, all tested strains - which showed at least 6 MDR pattern - were sensitive to all tested honey batches with MICs ranged from 20.83% (trefoil-2) up to 33.33% (fennel-2) (Figure 1) and MBCs from 37.92% (cotton) up to 45.83 % v/v (for both fennel-1 and trefoil-1) (Figure 2). However, 10% propolis fennel honey mixture showed the most favorable results as the lowest both MIC and MBC (13.96% and 28.26 % v/v respectively) with highly significant differences p>0.01 (Figures 1 and 2).

Propolis powder alone gave no any bacterial inhibition. *S. aureus* showed the lowest MIC (13.3%) and MBC (27.1%) v/v with highly significant differences P>0.01 (Figures 3 and 4) among all tested *Staph. sp.* By the statistical analysis for the antibacterial activity of different honey batches against different *Staph. sp.*, it was found that propolis honey mixture had the lowest MIC value against both coagulase positive *Staph. sp.* (*S. intermedius and S. aureus*) all over the present study as 6.2% and 7.25% v/v respectively with highly significant differences P>0.01 (Figure 5), while MBC values were 12.5 and 14.58% respectively (Figure 6).

| Isolates | Antimicrobial testing | | Honey tested strains | |
|---|---|---|---|---|
| | MDR | | | |
| | No. | ≥5 antimicrobials | No. | MDR pattern |
| *S. aureus* | 35 | 30 | 6 | 9 antimicrobials |
| *S. intermedius* | 9 | 5 | 3 | (6-7) antimicrobials |
| *S. saprophyticus* | 11 | 8 | 5 | (7-9) antimicrobials |
| *S. epidermidis* | 9 | 8 | 5 | 8 antimicrobials |
| Total | 64 | 51 | 19 | |

**Table 1:** *Staph. sp.* isolated from bovine clinical mastitis and MDR pattern of the honey tested strains.

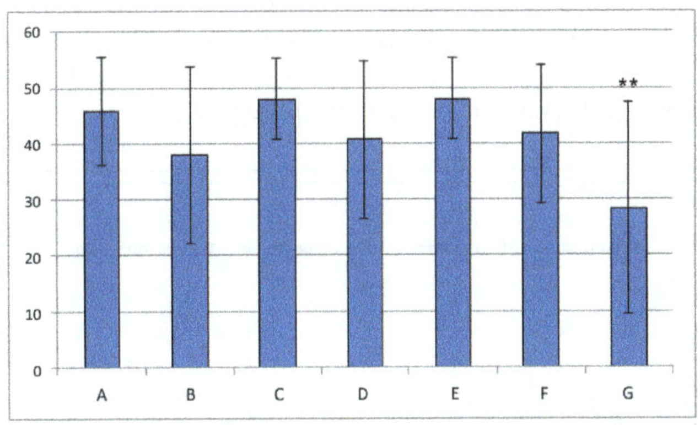


**Figure 1:** MIC values of different honey batches against *Staph. Sp.*

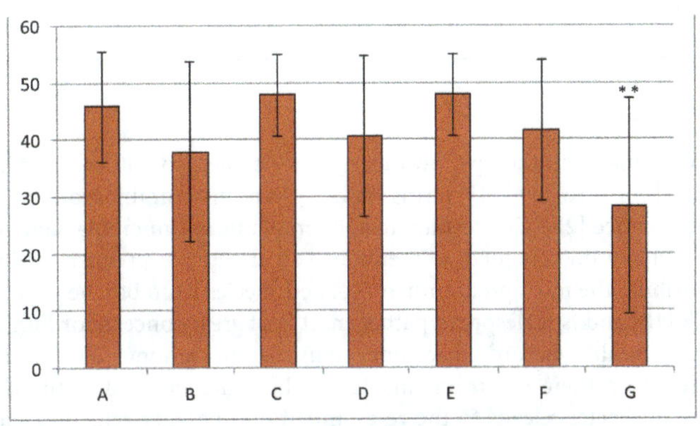


**Figure 2:** MBC values of different honey batches against *Staph. Sp.*

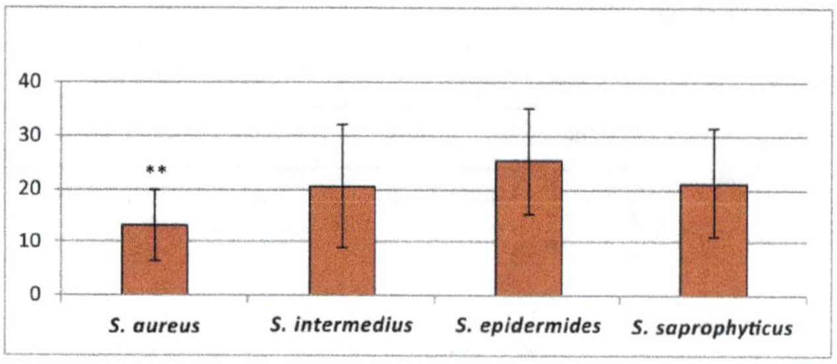


**Figure 3**: MIC values of honey against different *Staph. Sp.*

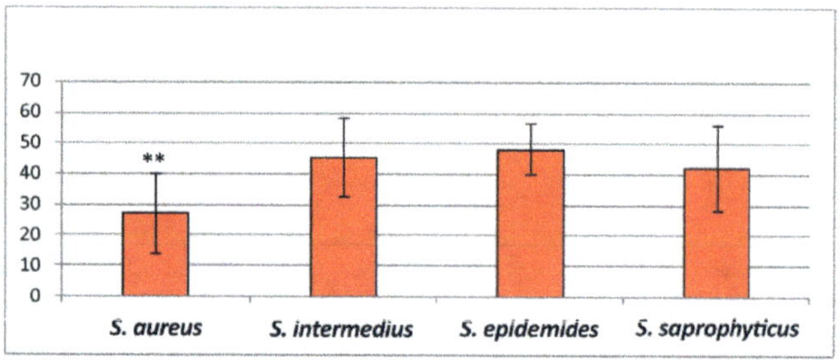


**Figure 4**: MBC values of honey against different *Staph. Sp*

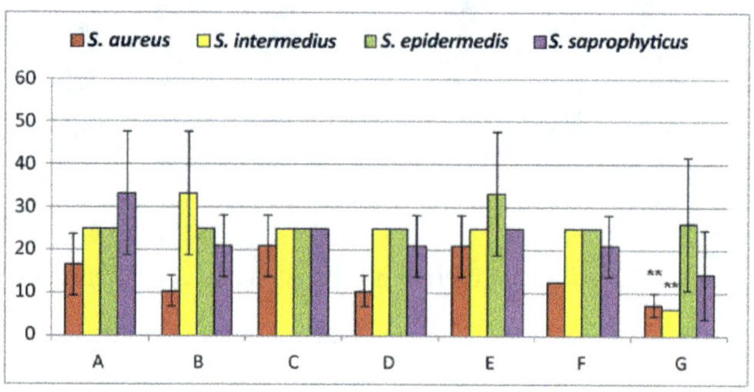


**Figure 5**: MIC values of different honey batches against different *Staph. Sp.*

## Discussion

Veterinary apitherapy nowadays is documented either in dairy [22,23] or broiler [24] farms rather than in immunomodulation performance [25]. Concerning to apitherapeutic antimicrobial activity, it is widely documented as mentioned in the above premise. MRSA contribute the most predominant isolated species from bovine mastitis milk [18] and is widespread pathogen. It is of great concern for human public health hazard threatens transmission among dairy farm workers or their environments [26]. The emergence of antibiotic-resistant bacteria leads to the re-examination of earlier remedies such as honey [7] or propolis [27]. The antibacterial potency differences among different studied honey samples could be attributed to the natural variations in floral sources of nectar and the different geographical locations since honey micro components possess physicochemical and phytochemical characteristics resulting in its potency that differs associated with botanical and geographical origins [28].

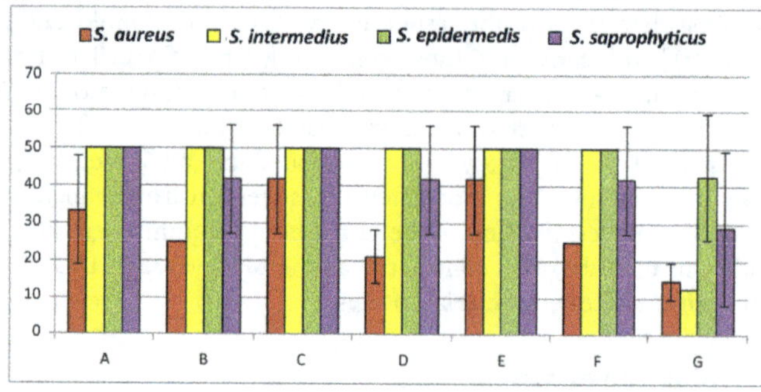


**Figure 6**: MBC values of different honey batches against different *Staph. Sp*

Different honey samples of different botanical or geographical origins; Egyptian honey had MIC and MBC values as 12.5 and 50% v/v [29], Malysian honey as 5% and 6.25% w/v [6], UK Manuka honey had MIC as 6% w/v [11] and Ethiopian honey as 6.25% w/v [3]. Honey antimicrobial action involves several mechanisms but mainly the presence of bacteriostatic and bactericidal action is due to production of hydrogen peroxide [30]. H2O2 alone may not be sufficient to the full activity [31], since it is in conjunction with other unknown honey components produce bacterial cytotoxic effects and DNA degradation. The concentration of polyphenols and H2O2 in different honeys may be of critical importance for bacterial cell survival [32]. Another mechanism of honey antimicrobial activity may be due to its lysosomal contents [33] or micro components as polyphenols, phenolic acids and flavonoids [34] or due to increase in cytokine release [35]. On the other hand, the mechanism of propolis antimicrobial activity is more complex and might be attributed to the synergistic activity between its various potent biological ingredients [8] that more than 300 compounds mainly phenolics and flavonoids [36]. It was found that propolis affects bacterial cytoplasmic membrane, and it inhibits motility, enzyme activity, cell division, and protein synthesis through inhibition of RNA-polymerase which can explain partially the synergism of propolis with drugs [37]. Moreover, galagin and caffeic acid derived[38] Since the synergistic action might be detected when the MIC of the combination of both studied antimicrobial agents is lower than the MIC of each alone [8], the present study was designed to test the added propolis powder (50 mg) alone where did not inhibit the tested *Staph. sp.* The present study chose Egyptian fennel honey for propolis mixture as our previous studies [25,29] recommendations. Although fennel showed low results for both MIC and MBC through the present study, its antimicrobial action was maximized giving highly significant difference (P>0.01) when propolis be added 10% w/v. The synergy of honey antimicrobial activity when be added to another antimicrobial was fully studied [1,7-10] and for propolis, the added flavonoids and phenolic acids - have antibacterial, antifungal and antiviral properties [39]- might maximize the action of these micro components present in honey resulting in synergy of its antimicrobial action. Fortunately, *S. aureus* (either MRSA or methicillin sensitive) which is the most predominant and virulent pathogen was the most sensitive *Staph. sp.* to honey antimicrobial action with highly significant. It is documented and proved that S.

aureus was the most sensitive species to the antimicrobial activity of honey among all tested bacterial species studied [1,2,40].

## Conclusion

It was concluded that all tested MDR *Staph. sp.* were sensitive to the antimicrobial activity all tested honey samples, where S. aureus was the most sensitive one among the four tested *Staph. sp.* It was concluded that adding 10% w/v propolis powder to the chosen honey patch would maximize its antimicrobial activity with highly significant difference. The promising results encourage the utilization of propolis extract in combination with the chosen honey patch for treatment of subclinical bovine mastitis to achieve the synergistic antimicrobial action.

## References


1. Andualem B (2013) Combined antibacterial activity of stingless bee (Apis mellipodae) honey and garlic (Allium sativum) extracts against standard and clinical pathogenic bacteria. Asian Pac J Trop Biomed 3: 725-731.
2. Kwakman PH1, Te Velde AA, de Boer L, Vandenbroucke-Grauls CM, Zaat SA (2011) Two major medicinal honeys have different mechanisms of bactericidal activity. PLoS One 6: e17709.
3. Ewnetu Y, Lemma W1, Birhane N (2013) Antibacterial effects of Apis mellifera and stingless bees honeys on susceptible and resistant strains of Escherichia coli, Staphylococcus aureus and Klebsiella pneumoniae in Gondar, Northwest Ethiopia. BMC Complement Altern Med 13: 269.
4. Hammond EN, Donkor ES (2013) Antibacterial effect of Manuka honey on Clostridium difficile. BMC Res Notes 6: 188.
5. Kronda JM1, Cooper RA, Maddocks SE (2013) Manuka honey inhibits siderophore production in Pseudomonas aeruginosa. J Appl Microbiol 115: 86-90.
6. Zainol MI1, Mohd Yusoff K, Mohd Yusof MY (2013) Antibacterial activity of selected Malaysian honey. BMC Complement Altern Med 13: 129.
7. Boukraa L1, Benbarek H, Moussa A (2008) Synergistic action of starch and honey against Candida albicans in correlation with diastase number. Braz J Microbiol 39: 40-43.
8. Al-Waili N, Al-Ghamdi A, Ansari M, Salom YK (2012) Synergistic Effects of Honey and Propolis toward Drug Multi-Resistant Staphylococcus aureus, Escherichia coli and Candida albicans isolates in single and polymicrobial cultures. Int J Med Sci 9: 793-800
9. Moussa A1, Noureddine D, Hammoudi SM, Saad A, Bourabeh A, et al. (2012) Additive potential of ginger starch on antifungal potency of honey against Candida albicans. Asian Pac J Trop Biomed 2: 253-255.
10. Muller P, Alber D G, Turnbull L, Schlothauer R C, Carter D A et al (2013) Synergism between Medihoney and rifampicin against methicillin-resistant Staphylococcus aureus (MRSA). PLOSO ne 8: e57679
11. Jenkins R1, Cooper R (2012) Improving antibiotic activity against wound pathogens with manuka honey in vitro. PLoS One 7: e45600.
12. Mavric E1, Wittmann S, Barth G, Henle T (2008) Identification and quantification of methylglyoxal as the dominant antibacterial constituent of Manuka (Leptospermum scoparium) honeys from New Zealand. Mol Nutr Food Res 52: 483-489.
13. Monzote L1, Cuesta-Rubio O, Campo Fernandez M, Márquez Hernandez I, Fraga J, et al. (2012) In vitro antimicrobial assessment of Cuban propolis extracts. Mem Inst Oswaldo Cruz 107: 978-984.
14. Liberio SA1, Pereira AL, Dutra RP, Reis AS, Araújo MJ, et al. (2011) Antimicrobial activity against oral pathogens and immunomodulatory effects and toxicity of geopropolis produced by the stingless bee Melipona fasciculata Smith. BMC Complement Altern Med 11: 108.
15. Possamai MM1, Honorio-França AC, Reinaque AP, França EL, Souto PC (2013) Brazilian propolis: a natural product that improved the fungicidal activity by blood phagocytes. Biomed Res Int 2013: 541018.
16. Skaba D1, Morawiec T, Tanasiewicz M, Mertas A, Bobela E, et al. (2013) Influence of the toothpaste with brazilian ethanol extract propolis on the oral cavity health. Evid Based Complement Alternat Med 2013: 215391.
17. Wojtyczka RD1, Dziedzic A, Idzik D, KÄ™pa M, Kubina R, et al. (2013) Susceptibility of Staphylococcus aureus clinical isolates to propolis extract alone or in combination with antimicrobial drugs. Molecules 18: 9623-9640.
18. Sayed SM (2014) Bacteriological study on staphylococcal bovine clinical mastitis with reference to methicillin-resistant Staph. aureus (MRSA). Assiut Vet Med J 60: 38-46
19. NCCLS (2000) Performance Standards for Antimicrobial Disk Susceptibility Test. Approved Standard M2 - A7, M100 - S10. PA: National Committee for Laboratory Standards
20. Bogado I, Sutich E, Krapp A, Marchiaro P, Marzi M (2001) Methicillin resistance study in clinical isolates of coagulase-negative staphylococci and determination of their susceptibility to alternative antimicrobial agents. J of applied Microbiology 91: 344-350
21. Quinn PJ, Carter ME, Markey B, Carter GR (2004) Bacteriology: Clinical veterinary microbiology. (6th edn) Mosby Edinburgh London New York Oxord Philadelphia St Louis Sydney Toronto
22. Abdul Hafeez MM, Ali MM, Abdel-Rahman MF, Nahed–Wahba M (2005) Antibacterial activity of honey for treatment of subclinical mastitis: 2- Intramammary infusion as a tool to manage non responding antibiotic cases. 8th Scientific Congress of Cattle disease Egypt 146-149
23. Nahed M Wahba, Niveen A El Nisr, Sayed MS, Abdallah MR, et al (2011) Intramammary honey infusion: A new trend in the management of bovine subclinical mastitis. J of Anim and Vet Advances 10: 2740–2744
24. Attia YA, Abd Al-Hamid AE, Ibrahim MS, Al-Harthi M A, Bovera F, et al (2014) Productive performance, biochemical and hematological traits of broiler chickens supplemented with propolis, bee pollen, and mannan oligosaccharides continuously or intermittently. Livestock science journal.
25. Sayed SM1, Abou El-Ella GA, Wahba NM, El Nisr NA, Raddad K, et al. (2009) Immune defense of rats immunized with fennel honey, propolis, and bee venom against induced staphylococcal infection. J Med Food 12: 569-575.
26. Lim SK1, Nam HM, Jang GC, Lee HS, Jung SC, et al. (2013) Transmission and persistence of methicillin-resistant Staphylococcus aureus in milk, environment, and workers in dairy cattle farms. Foodborne Pathog Dis 10: 731-736.
27. da Cunha MG1, Franchin M, de Carvalho Galvão LC, de Ruiz AL, de Carvalho JE, et al. (2013) Antimicrobial and antiproliferative activities of stingless bee Melipona scutellaris geopropolis. BMC Complement Altern Med 13: 23.
28. Alzahrani HA1, Alsabehi R, Boukraâ L, Abdellah F, Bellik Y, et al. (2012) Antibacterial and antioxidant potency of floral honeys from different botanical and geographical origins. Molecules 17: 10540-10549.
29. Ali MWN, Abdel-Rahman M, Abdel-Hafeez MM (2005) Antibacterial activity of honey for treatment of subclinical bovine Mastitis: 1- In vitro study of bacterial inhibits and chemical bioassay of some different honeys. 8th Sci cong Egyptian society for cattle diseases Assiut Egypt 139-146.
30. Feás X1, Iglesias A, Rodrigues S, Estevinho LM (2013) Effect of Erica sp. honey against microorganisms of clinical importance: study of the factors underlying this biological activity. Molecules 18: 4233-4246.
31. Chen C1, Campbell LT, Blair SE, Carter DA (2012) The effect of standard heat and filtration processing procedures on antimicrobial activity and hydrogen peroxide levels in honey. Front Microbiol 3: 265.
32. Brudzynski K1, Lannigan R (2012) Mechanism of Honey Bacteriostatic Action Against MRSA and VRE Involves Hydroxyl Radicals Generated from Honey's Hydrogen Peroxide. Front Microbiol 3: 36.
33. León-Ruiz V1, González-Porto AV, Al-Habsi N, Vera S, San Andrés MP, et al. (2013) Antioxidant, antibacterial and ACE-inhibitory activity of four monofloral honeys in relation to their chemical composition. Food Funct 4: 1617-1624.

34. Al-Hindi RR1, Bin-Masalam MS, El-Shahawi MS (2011) Antioxidant and antibacterial characteristics of phenolic extracts of locally produced honey in Saudi Arabia. Int J Food Sci Nutr 62: 513-517.
35. Aparna S1, Srirangarajan S, Malgi V, Setlur KP, Shashidhar R, et al. (2012) A comparative evaluation of the antibacterial efficacy of honey in vitro and antiplaque efficacy in a 4-day plaque regrowth model in vivo: preliminary results. J Periodontol 83: 1116-1121.
36. Khalil ML (2006) Biological activity of bee propolis in health and disease. Asian Pac J Cancer Prev 7: 22-31.
37. Mirzoeva OK1, Grishanin RN, Calder PC (1997) Antimicrobial action of propolis and some of its components: the effects on growth, membrane potential and motility of bacteria. Microbiol Res 152: 239-246.
38. Koo H1, Rosalen PL, Cury JA, Park YK, Bowen WH (2002) Effects of compounds found in propolis on Streptococcus mutans growth and on glucosyltransferase activity. Antimicrob Agents Chemother 46: 1302-1309.
39. MediÄ‡-SariÄ‡ M1, Rastija V, BojiÄ‡ M, Males Z (2009) From functional food to medicinal product: systematic approach in analysis of polyphenolics from propolis and wine. Nutr J 8: 33.
40. Sherlock O, Dolan A, Athman R, Power A, Gethin G et al (2010) Comparison of the antimicrobial activity of Ulmo honey from Chile and Manuka honey against methicillin-resistant Staphylococcus aureus, Escherichia coli and Pseudomonas aeruginosa. BMC Complementary and Alternative Medicine 10:47

11

# Anti-Inflammatory and Pro-apoptotic Effects of Curcumin and Resveratrol on the Human Lung Fibroblast Cell Line MRC-5

**Burkhard Kloesch[1*], Elisabeth Dietersdorfer[1], Silvia Loebsch[1] and Guenter Steiner[1,2]**

[1]*Ludwig Boltzmann Institute for Rheumatology and Balneology, Cluster Rheumatology, Balneology and Rehabilitation, Vienna, Austria*

[2]*Division of Rheumatology, Department of Internal Medicine III, Medical University Vienna, Austria*

***Corresponding author:** Burkhard Kloesch, Ludwig Boltzmann Institute for Rheumatology and Balneology Kurbadstrasse 14 1100 Vienna, Austria, E-mail: burkhard.kloesch@gmx.at

**Abstract**

**Background:** The naturally occuring polyphenols curcumin and resveratrol are considered to be powerful antioxidants and anti-inflammatory compounds and both inhibit the proliferation of different types of cancer cells. In the present study, we investigated possible anti-inflammatory and pro-apoptotic effects of curcumin and resveratrol on the human lung fibroblast cell line MRC-5.

**Methods:** MRC-5 cells were stimulated for 6 h with interleukin (IL)-1β or phorbol 12- myristate 13-acetate (PMA) in the absence or presence of different concentrations of curcumin or resveratrol. The release of interleukin (IL)-6 was quantified by enzyme-linked immunosorbent assay (ELISA). The modulation in phosphorylation of the transcription factor nuclear factor-kappa B (NF-κB) and mitogen-activated protein kinases (MAPKs) such as $p^{38}$ and ERK1/2 were analyzed by Western blot. Cytotoxic and pro-apoptotic effects of curcumin and resveratrol were monitored by the measurement of lactate dehydrogenase (LDH) activity and by Annexin-V/7-AAD staining.

**Results:** Both curcumin and resveratrol effectively attenuated IL-1β and PMA-induced IL-6 expression in MRC-5 cells. Furthermore, curcumin treatment induced apoptosis via caspase-3 signaling and caused endoplasmic reticulum (ER) stress. Salubrinal, an inhibitor of serine/threonine phosphatase PP1, and antioxidants such as N-acetyl-cysteine (NAC), reduced glutathione (GSH) and sodium hydrogen sulfide (NaHS) diminished the cytotoxic effects of curcumin on MRC-5 cells. In contrast to curcumin, resveratrol had no negative effects on cell viability.

**Keywords:** MRC-5 cells; Curcumin; Resveratrol; IL-6; Apoptosis.

## Introduction

Curcumin (diferuloylmethane) is a yellow pigment found in the rhizome of turmeric (*Curcuma longa L., Zingiberaceae*) with a wide range of pharmacological activities [1,2]. Antioxidant, anti-carcinogenic, anti-inflammatory and pro-apoptotic effects of this compound have been assessed in various *in vitro* and *in vivo* systems [3]. Numerous studies have demonstrated its role in suppressing expression of the cell cycle protein cyclin D1 and transcription factors that are implicated in carcinogens is such as nuclear factor kappa-B (NF-κB) and activator protein-1 (AP-1). Furthermore, curcumin induced programmed cell death (apoptosis) in tumor cells by activating caspases and down-regulating Bcl-2 family proteins [4,5]. Recent reports have also demonstrated that curcumin inhibits proteosomal activity [6], triggers accumulation of cytosolic $Ca^{2+}$ [7], and disrupts protein disulfide bond formation [8], all of which initiate ER stress response.

Resveratrol (*trans*-3,4,9,5-trihydroxystilbene) is a natural phytoalexin found in large quantities in grapes and other food products [9,10]. Resveratrol was found to have a potent anti-carcinogenic activity in several animal models of cancer [9]. The anti-carcinogenic properties of resveratrol are closely associated with its antioxidant activity and the ability to inhibit cyclooxygenase-2 (COX-2), hydroperoxidase, protein kinase C (PKC), Bcl-2 phosphorylation, Akt, NF-κB, matrix metalloprotease-9 (MMP-9), and programmed cell death [11-14].

In the present study, we investigated possible anti-inflammatory and pro-apoptotic properties of curcumin and resveratrol in the human lung fibroblast cell line MRC-5. Data demonstrate that both curcumin and resveratrol effectively blocked interleukin (IL)-1β and phorbol 12-myristate 13-acetate (PMA)-induced interleukin (IL)-6 expression in MRC-5 cells. Furthermore, curcumin suppressed activation of NF-κB and inhibited degradation of IκBα, respectively. Beside its potent anti-inflammatory properties, curcumin, at high concentrations, had pronounced cytotoxic effects on MRC-5 cells, induced apoptosis and triggered ER stress response via activation of caspase-3 and phosphorylation of translation initiation factor 2 (eIF-2α). In strong contrast to curcumin, resveratrol did not negatively influence cell viability.

## Materials and Methods

### Reagents

Unless stated otherwise, all reagents were from Sigma Aldrich (Vienna, Austria) and C Roth (Karlsruhe, Germany). IL-1β was purchased from ProSpecTany Technogene (Tel Aviv, Israel). Antibodies for p38 MAPK and ERK1/2, NF-κB, IκBα, caspase-3/-7/-9, and eIF-2α were from Cell Signaling (New England Biolabs, Frankfurt am Main, Germany).

### Cell culture and experimental methods

The human lung fibroblast cell line MRC-5 was kindly provided by B Lohberger (Department of Orthopaedics, Medical University of Graz, Austria). Cells were cultivated in Dulbecco's modified Eagle's medium (DMEM) supplemented with 10% heat-inactivated foetal bovine serum (FBS), 50 IU/ml penicillin, 50 µg/ml streptomycin, and 2 mmol/l-L-glutamine in a humidified incubator with 5% $CO_2$ and 95% air. Stock solutions of curcumin and resveratrol were prepared with ethanol (96% v/v) and diluted properly into medium. To induce IL-6 expression, MRC-5 cells were stimulated for 6 h either with IL-1β (10 ng/ml) or PMA (100 ng/ml). All experiments were performed in duplicates and were repeated twice.

### Lactatdehydrogenase (LDH) assay

MRC-5 cells were seeded in 12-well cell culture plates (2 x 105/well) and cultured overnight in DMEM plus 10% (v/v) FBS. The next day, culture medium was changed and replaced by DMEM containing 1% FBS (v/v) lacking phenol red. Curcumin and resveratrol were added and cells were incubated for another 6 h. LDH activity in cell culture supernatants was determined with a commercially available kit (Roche, Vienna, Austria).

### Annexin-V/7-AAD-assay

MRC-5 cells were cultured overnight in 6-well cell culture plates (6 x 105/well) in DMEM supplemented with 10% (v/v) FBS. The next day, culture medium was changed and curcumin or resveratrol were added to the desired concentrations and cells were incubated for another 6 h. Then, cells were trypsinized and labeled with the Muse$^{TM}$ Annexin-V & Dead Cell reagent (Merck-Millipore, Germany). Detection of living cells, cells in the early or late apoptotic stage and dead cells was performed with the Muse$^{TM}$ Cell Analyzer (Merck-Millipore, Germany).

### Cytokine measurement

Ready-to-go enzyme-linked immunosorbent assay (ELISA) kit from ebioscience (Vienna, Austria) was used to quantify IL-6 levels in cell culture supernatants.

### Gel electrophoresis and Western blot analysis

SDS-PAGE and Western blots were performed by standard methods. Briefly, at the end of the experiment, cells were washed twice with PBS ($p^H$ 7.4) and lysed with SDS-loading buffer. Cell lysates were boiled for 5 min at 95°C and treated with a short pulse of ultrasound (10 sec) to minimize viscosity. Equal amounts were then loaded onto SDS gels. Proteins were separated on 12% polyacrylamide mini gels, blotted by semi-dry electrotransfer to nitrocellulose membranes and probed with specific antibodies. Proteins were visualized using Roti-Lumin (Roth, Karlsruhe, Germany) and the GeneGnome chemiluminescence detection device (Syngene, Cambridge, UK).

### Statistical analysis

Statistical analysis was performed using GraphPad Prism version 5.04. Data were expressed as means ± SEM. Differences between three or more groups were calculated by 1 and 2-way ANOVA, respectively. A probability level of 0.05 was used to define significance.

## Results

### Curcumin and resveratrol attenuate IL-1β and PMA-induced IL-6 expression

To evaluate possible anti-inflammatory properties of curcumin and resveratrol, MRC-5 cells were stimulated for 6 h with IL-1β or PMA in the absence or presence of increasing concentrations of curcumin or resveratrol (12.5–100 µM). As shown in Figure 1A, IL-1β induced IL-6 expression in MRC-5 cells to a high extent (~8 ng/ml). IL-6 production induced by PMA was much less pronounced, approximately 20-fold lower (Figure 1B). Data show that relatively low concentrations of curcumin (12.5 µM) almost completely blocked IL-6 expression, regardless of whether IL-1β or PMA was used for stimulation (Figure 1A and 1B). The inhibitory effect of curcumin on IL-6 expression was much higher compared to that of the same concentration of resveratrol (95 versus 15% inhibition at 12.5 µM; Figure 1A). In fact, 100 µM resveratrol was required to obtain the same degree of suppression of IL-6 production as observed with 12.5 µM curcumin. The half maximal inhibitory concentration ($IC_{50}$) of curcumin on IL-6 expression was estimated by a dose-response curve; $IC_{50} \sim 5$ µM (Figure 1C). Next, we investigated whether curcumin may amplify the inhibitory effects of resveratrol on IL-6 expression. MRC-5 cells were stimulated for 6 h with IL-1β in the absence or presence of resveratrol or resveratrol plus curcumin. As shown in Figure 1D, 50 µM resveratrol reduced IL-6 expression at about 60%, whereas resveratrol in combination with 5 µM curcumin blocked IL-6 release almost completely (~95%) indicating that resveratrol and curcumin have additive effects.

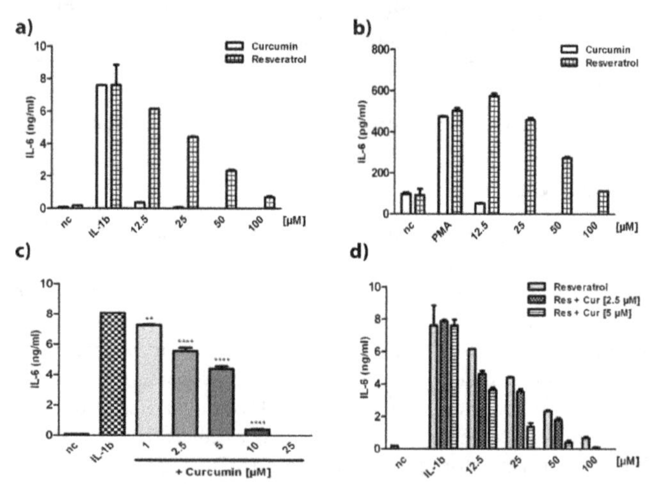


**Figure 1:** Curcumin and resveratrol diminish IL-1β and PMA-induced IL-6 expression in MRC-5 cells. Cells were stimulated for 6 h with IL-1β or PMA in the absence or presence of indicated concentrations of curcumin or resveratrol (A, B). (C) Dose-response curve of curcumin. MRC-5 cells were stimulated for 6 h with IL-1β in the absence or presence of indicated concentrations of curcumin. (D) MRC-5 cells were stimulated for 6 h with IL-1β in the absence or presence of resveratrol or resveratrol plus curcumin. IL-6 levels in cell culture supernatants were quantified by ELISA. Data from 2 independent experiments are presented as mean ± SEM (**p<0.01; ****p<0.0001).

## Curcumin blocks activation of NF-κB

Next, we tried to identify potential signaling pathways (NF-κB, etc.) affected by curcumin and resveratrol. MRC-5 cells were pre-incubated for 30 min with curcumin or resveratrol (12.5–100 μM) before being stimulated for 20 min with IL-1β. Activation of NF-κB (phosphorylation of the $p^{65}$ subunit at serine 536) and degradation of IκBα, respectively, were analyzed by Western blot. As shown in Figure 2A, NF-κB was rapidly phosphorylated after the addition of IL-1β. Interestingly, phosphorylation of NF-κB and degradation of IκBα were blocked only at 100 μM curcumin, lower concentrations (12.5–50 μM), however, were inefficient (Figure 2A). In comparison to curcumin, resveratrol completely failed to inhibit NF-κB activation (Figure 2B).

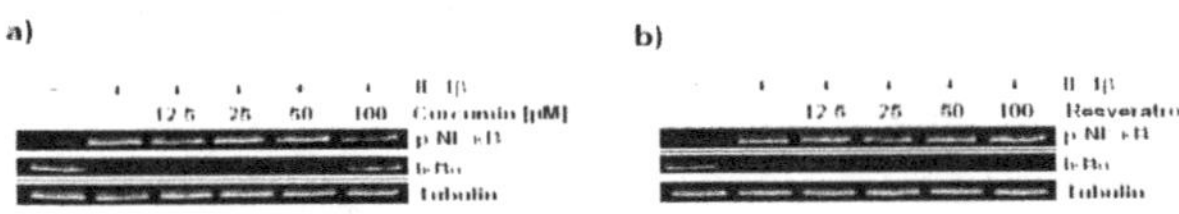


**Figure 2**: Curcumin inhibits phosphorylation of NF-κB$p^{65}$ in IL-1β-stimulated MRC-5 cells. Cells were pre-incubated for 30 min with indicated concentrations of curcumin or resveratrol before being stimulated for 20 min with IL-1β. Total cell proteins were subjected to SDS-PAGE electrophoresis and blotted onto nitrocellulose membranes. Phospho-NF-κB (p-NF-κB) and IκBα were detected with specific antibodies; (A) Cells were stimulated with IL-1β -/+ curcumin; (B) Cells were stimulated with IL-1β -/+ resveratrol.

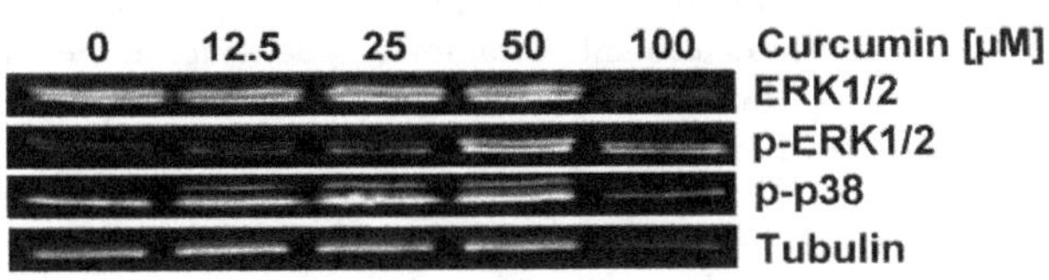


**Figure 3**: Curcumin induces phosphorylation of ERK1/2. MRC-5 cells were treated for 60 min with indicated concentrations of curcumin or resveratrol. Total cell proteins were subjected to SDS-PAGE electrophoresis and blotted onto nitrocellulose membranes. Phospho-ERK1/2 (p-ERK1/2) and phospho-$p^{38}$ MAPK (p-$p^{38}$) were detected with specific antibodies against Thr202/Tyr204 (p-ERK1/2) and Thr180/Tyr182 (p-$p^{38}$); (A), Curcumin-treated cells; (B), Resveratrol-treated cells.

## Curcumin activates extracellular signal-regulated kinase (ERK)-1/2

Besides NF-κB, mitogen-activated protein kinases (MAPKs) play a central role in proliferation, gene expression, differentiation, cell survival, and apoptosis. Therefore, we investigated the effects of curcumin and resveratrol on MAPK activation ($p^{38}$ MAPK and ERK1/2) in MRC-5 cells. Cells were treated for 60 min with different concentrations of curcumin or resveratrol (12.5–100 μM) and phosphorylation of $p^{38}$ MAPK and ERK1/2 was analyzed by Western blot. As shown in Figure 3, phosphorylation of ERK1/2 was induced at 50 μM curcumin, whereas lower concentrations did not affect ERK1/2. Notably, treatment of MRC-5 cells with 100 μM curcumin led to a dramatic decrease of total protein content (Figure 3) indicating that curcumin at high concentrations had cytotoxic effects. In contrast to ERK1/2, $p^{38}$ MAPK was only slightly affected (Figure 3).

## Curcumin induces cell death through apoptosis

To analyze cytotoxic and pro-apoptotic effects of curcumin and resveratrol, we measured lactate dehydrogenase (LDH) activity in cell culture supernatants and performed Annexin-V/7-AAD staining of curcumin and resveratrol-treated cells. Treatment of MRC-5 cells with 25 μM curcumin led to a significant increase in LDH activity (Figure 4A) whereas resveratrol, however, did not. Next, we asked whether cell death observed in curcumin-treated cells was due to apoptosis. MRC-5 cells were incubated for 6 h with increasing concentrations of curcumin (12.5–100 μM) and apoptotic activity was analyzed by Annexin-V/7-AAD staining. Data show that treatment with 12.5 μM curcumin had no significant effect on cell viability (Figure 4B). At 25 μM curcumin, about 40% of the total cell population was in the early apoptotic stage, at 50 μM, already 80%. At 100 μM curcumin, 90% of the cells were in the late apoptotic/dead stage (Figure 4B). In contrast, treatment of MRC-5 cells with resveratrol (up to 24 h) did not negatively affect cell viability (data not shown). In addition, we investigated whether apoptosis was induced via the caspase signaling pathway. As shown in Figure 4C, degradation of pro-caspase-3 was evident 1 h post-treatment. Interestingly, a decrease of pro-caspase-7/-9 could not be detected (Figure 4C). Confirming the data shown in Figure 3, a dramatic decline in total protein content was observed at 100 μM curcumin (Figure 4C) suggesting that curcumin at high concentrations led to irreversible cell damage. In cells treated with resveratrol, however, caspases were not activated (Figure 4E).

## Curcumin induces endoplasmic reticulum (ER) stress

Phosphorylation of the alpha subunit of the eukaryotic initiation factor-2 (eIF-2α) is a well-documented mechanism of down-regulating protein synthesis triggered by agents that induce apoptosis, ER stress and protein misfolding. To clarify whether curcumin may also induce ER stress in MRC-5 cells, cells were left untreated or were exposed for 30 min to curcumin (6.25–100 μM). As shown in Figure 5A, treatment of cells with 100 μM curcumin resulted in marked phosphorylation of eIF-2α. Salubrinal (Sal) as an inhibitor of serine/threonine phosphatase PP1 blocks eIF-2α dephosphorylation. When MRC-5 cells were treated for 6 h with 25 μM curcumin in the presence of Sal (50 μM), the survival rate significantly increased (> 40%) (Figure 5B and 5C). At higher concentrations of curcumin, however, Sal failed to maintain cell viability (Figure 5A). Interestingly, the caspase inhibitor Q-VD-OPh did not reduce curcumin-induced cell death (Figure 5B).

## Antioxidants and the MEK1/2 inhibitor U0126 prevent curcumin-induced cell death

Antioxidants such as N-acetylcysteine (NAC), reduced glutathione (GSH) and sodium hydrogen sulfide (NaHS) are substances with known cytoprotective properties and potent scavengers of reactive oxygen species (ROS). To study whether curcumin-induced cytotoxicity might be diminished by these substances, MRC-5 cells were loaded for 1 h with NAC, GSH (each 1 mM) or NaHS (0.1 mM) before being treated for 6 h with curcumin (25 μM). In comparison to curcumin-treated cells, NAC reduced LDH activity by about 80%, GSH and NaHS by about 50–60%, suggesting that antioxidants had strong beneficial effects on cell viability (Figure 6). The MEK1/2 inhibitor U0126, which blocks activation of ERK1/2, also reduced curcumin-induced cell death (~ 50%) (Figure 6).

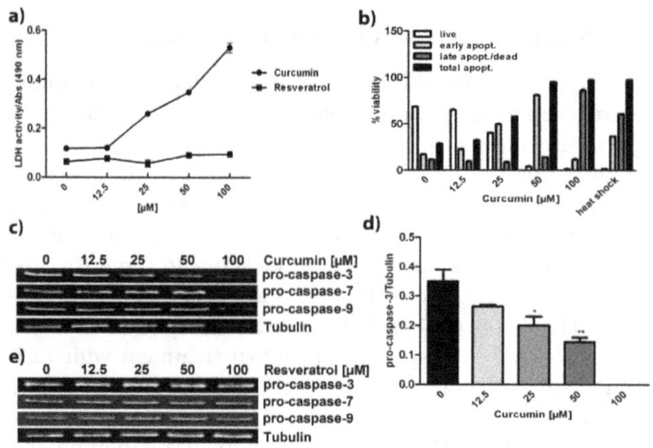


**Figure 4:** Cytotoxic and pro-apoptotic effects of curcumin and resveratrol on MRC-5 cells.(A) Cells were treated for 6 h with indicated concentrations of curcumin or resveratrol and LDH activity was then measured in cell culture supernatants. (B) MRC-5 cells were treated for 6 h with indicated concentrations of curcumin and cells were stained with Annexin-V/7-AAD to differentiate between cells being alive or in the early or late apoptotic stage. (C, E) MRC-5 cells were treated for 1 h with indicated concentrations of curcumin or resveratrol and activation of caspase-3/-7/-9 was analyzed by Western blot. (D) Levels of pro-caspase-3 in curcumin-treated cells were semi-quantitatively determined by densitometry. Data are representative of 2 experiments ($^{*}p<0.05$; $^{**}p<0.01$).

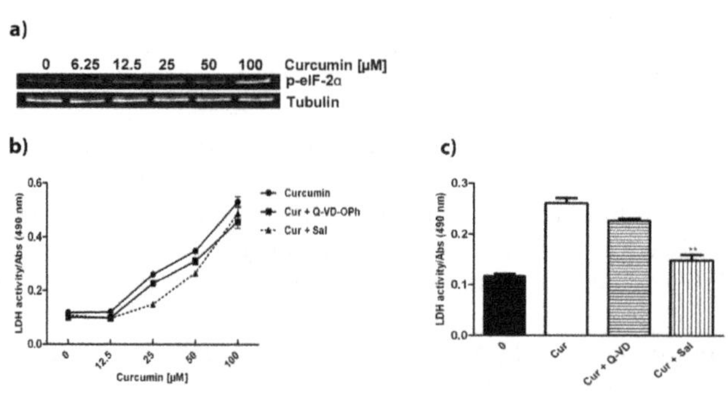


**Figure 5:** Curcumin induces ER stress in MRC-5 cells. Cells were treated for 30 min with indicated concentrations of curcumin. Total cell proteins were subjected to SDS-PAGE and blotted onto nitrocellulose membranes. (A) Phospho-eIF-2α (p-eIF-2α) was detected with a specific antibody against ser51. (B, C) Cells were treated for 6 h with indicated concentrations of curcumin in the absence or presence of Salubrinal (50 µM) or Q-VD-OPh (25 µM) and LDH activity was then monitored in cell culture supernatants.

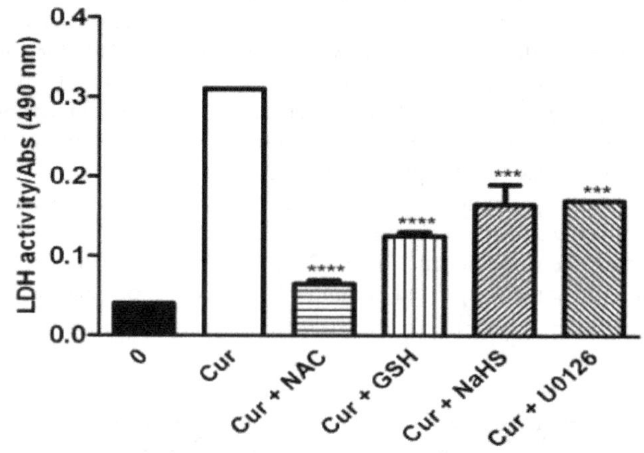


**Figure 6:** NAC, GSH, NaHS and U0126 reduce the cytotoxic effects of curcumin in MRC-5 cells. Cells were loaded for 1 h with NAC, GSH (each 1 mM), NaHS (0.1 mM) or U0126 (10 µM) and were then incubated with 25 µM curcumin for another 6 h. LDH activity was measured in cell culture supernatants. Data from 2 independent experiments are presented as mean ± SEM ($^{***}p<0.001$; $^{****}p<0.0001$).

## Discussion

Our data demonstrate that the phytochemicals curcumin and resveratrol had pronounced anti-inflammatory activities in the human lung fibroblast cell line MRC-5. Both compounds diminished IL-1β and PMA-induced IL-6 gene expression in a concentration-dependent manner. In the NF-κB signaling cascade, NF-κB once activated immediately initiates the transcription of IL-6 mRNA and many other pro-inflammatory genes (TNF-α, IL8, COX-2, etc.). Our data show that curcumin at 12.5 µM almost completely blocked IL-6 expression in MRC-5 cells. In strong contrast, Western blot analysis revealed that curcumin suppressed phosphorylation of NF-κB only at a concentration of 100 µM. It has been shown that besides the phosphorylation of the NF-κB subunit $p^{65}$ (RelA) at serine 276/536, acetylation at lysine 218, 221, and 310 differentially regulates the DNA binding activity of RelA along with its assembly with IκBα, and transcriptional activity [15]. The acetyltransferases p300 and CBP appear to play a major role in the *in vivo* acetylation of RelA [16]. Balasubramanyam et al. has been reported that curcumin repressed acetylation of histone/nonhistone proteins and histone acetyltransferase-dependent chromatin transcription [17]. Therefore, we suggest that the inhibitory effects of curcumin on IL-6 expression may be due to its ability to prevent acetylation of RelA but in further experiments we will clarify this hypothesis. In contrast to curcumin, the inhibitory effect of resveratrol on IL-6 expression was significantly lower (~10 fold less). Western blot data demonstrate that resveratrol blocked neither RelA phosphorylation nor degradation of IκBα. Recently, it has been reported that activation of Sirtuin1 (Sirt1) by resveratrol inhibited TNF-α-induced inflammation in mouse embryonic fibroblasts [18]. Sirt1, a mammalian homolog of Sir2, is a $NAD^{+}$ -dependent class III histone deacetylase. Sirt1 is involved in a variety of physiological and pathophysiological processes, such as cell growth, inflammation and modulation of cancer cell metabolism

[19,20]. Knockout of Sirt1 led to an increase in cytokine expression, whereas Sirt1 activation inhibited production of TNF-α, monocyte chemoattractant protein 1 (MCP-1) and IL-8 [21]. Suppression of pro-inflammatory cytokines production by Sirt1 is highly related to its negative regulation of NF-κB activity via the deacetylation of the RelA subunit at lysine 310 [22]. Based on these findings we conclude that curcumin and resveratrol are both anti-inflammatory compounds but may act by different molecular mechanisms. On the one hand, curcumin may prevent acetylation of RelA at lysine 310 thereby blocking acetyltransferase p300 and CBP, while resveratrol, on the other hand, may induce deacetylation of RelA by activation of Sirt1.

Caspases play a key role in programmed cell death mediated by various apoptotic stimuli [23]. Curcumin was found to act as an antioxidant at low dose, whereas at higher concentrations its prooxidant properties prevailed, a virtue that may be of importance in cell apoptosis [24]. We demonstrated that curcumin, even at relatively low concentrations (25 μM) had negative effects on cell viability. This finding stays in contrast to the results of another group which has been demonstrated that NIH3T3 mouse fibroblasts and HEK-293 cells were largely resistant to curcumin treatment and displayed minimal cell death toxicity at 100 μM suggesting different sensitivities of distinct cell types to curcumin [25]. Additionally, our data show that curcumin induced cell death through apoptosis via activation of caspase-3. Apoptosis is often associated with the induction of endoplasmic reticulum (ER) stress [26]. Phosphorylation of the alpha unit of the eukaryotic initiation factor-2 (eIF-2α) is a marker for ER stress [27]. Our findings demonstrate that curcumin besides its capability to induce apoptosis also induced phosphorylation of eIF-2α. Inhibition of dephosphorylation eIF-2α by Salubrinal significantly protected cells from curcumin-induced cell damage. Furthermore, antioxidants such as NAC, GSH and NaHS also increased the survival rate of curcumin-treated cells. It has recently been shown that in the leukemic monocyte cell line THP-1, curcumin-induced apoptosis was induced via phosphorylation of ERK1/2 [28]. We showed that in MRC-5 cells, phosphorylation of ERK1/2 was induced at 50 μM curcumin, a concentration which definitely led to programmed cell death. Therefore, we suggest that the underlying mechanisms for the initiation of apoptosis in THP-1 and MRC-5 cells might be similar. In contrast to curcumin, resveratrol had no negative influence on cell viability and did not induce apoptosis.

## Conclusion

Recently, we reported about the anti-inflammatory and pro-apoptotic effects of curcumin on human synovial fibroblasts derived from rheumatoid arthritis patients [29,30]. In the present study, we investigated the effects of curcumin and resveratrol on the human lung fibroblast cell line MRC-5 and data demonstrated that the effects of curcumin were very similar. In accordance with our results, Smith et al. reported that curcumin inhibited fibrosis-related effects in idiopathic pulmonary fibrosis (IPF), a progressive and fatal lung disease for which not therapy has been identified. Curcumin reduced lung fibroblast cell proliferation and inhibited collagen secretion by IPF fibroblasts [31]. The potential use of curcumin and resveratrol as a therapeutic option is very limited through its low bioavailability. Therefore, in cooperation with the Department of Nanobiotechnology (University of Natural Resources and Life Sciences, Vienna, Austria) we plan to evaluate the effects of so called "CurcuEmulsomes" in our *in vitro* assays. CurcuEmulsomes are spherical solid nanoparticles and increase the bioavailability of curcumin by up to 10.000 fold as recently reported [31,32]. CurcuEmulsomes might be a valuable tool to study the beneficial effects of curcumin in various therapeutic applications *in vivo.*

## References


1. Aggarwal BB, Kumar A, Bharti AC (2003) Anticancer potential of curcumin: preclinical and clinical studies. Anticancer Res 23: 363-398.
2. Ammon HP, Wahl MA (1991) Pharmacology of Curcuma longa. Planta Med 57: 1-7.
3. Park C, Moon DO, Choi IW, Choi BT, Nam TJ, et al. (2007) Curcumin induces apoptosis and inhibits prostaglandin E(2) production in synovial fibroblasts of patients with rheumatoid arthritis. Int J Mol Med 20: 365-372.
4. Bush JA, Cheung KJ Jr, Li G (2001) Curcumin induces apoptosis in human melanoma cells through a Fas receptor/caspase-8 pathway independent of p53. Exp Cell Res 271: 305-314.
5. Shishodia S, Chaturvedi MM, Aggarwal BB (2007) Role of curcumin in cancer therapy. Curr Probl Cancer 31: 243-305.
6. Jana NR, Dikshit P, Goswami A, Nukina N (2004) Inhibition of proteasomal function by curcumin induces apoptosis through mitochondrial pathway. J Biol Chem 279: 11680-11685.
7. Logan-Smith MJ, East JM, Lee AG (2002) Evidence for a global inhibitor-induced conformation change on the Ca(2+)-ATPase of sarcoplasmic reticulum from paired inhibitor studies. Biochemistry 41: 2869-2875.
8. Pae HO, Jeong SO, Jeong GS, Kim KM, Kim HS, et al. (2007) Curcumin induces pro-apoptotic endoplasmic reticulum stress in human leukemia HL-60 cells. Biochem Biophys Res Commun 353: 1040-1045.
9. Jang M, Cai L, Udeani GO, Slowing KV, Thomas CF, et al. (1997) Cancer chemopreventive activity of resveratrol, a natural product derived from grapes. Science (Wash DC) 275: 218-220.
10. Soleas GJ, Diamandis EP, Goldberg DM (1997) Wine as a biological fluid: history, production, and role in disease prevention. J Clin Lab Anal 11: 287-313.
11. Banerjee S, Bueso-Ramos C, Aggarwal BB (2002) Suppression of 7,12-dimethylbenz(a)anthracene-induced mammary carcinogenesis in rats by resveratrol: role of nuclear factor-kappaB, cyclooxygenase 2, and matrix metalloprotease 9. Cancer Res 62: 4945-4954.
12. Baur JA, Sinclair DA (2006) Therapeutic potential of resveratrol: the in vivo evidence. Nat Rev Drug Discov 5: 493-506.
13. Bhat KPL, Kosmeder JW 2nd, Pezzuto JM (2001) Biological effects of resveratrol. Antioxid Redox Signal 3: 1041-1064.
14. Dorrie J, Gerauer H, Wachter Y, Zunino SJ (2001) Resveratrol induces extensive apoptosis by depolarizing mitochondrial membranes and activating caspase-9 in acute lymphoblastic leukemia cells. Cancer Res 61: 4731-4739.
15. Chen LF, Williams SA, Mu Y, Nakano H, Duerr JM, et al. (2005) NF-kappaB RelA phosphorylation regulates RelA acetylation. Mol Cell Biol 25: 7966-7975.
16. Chen LF, Mu Y, Greene WC (2002) Acetylation of RelA at discrete sites regulates distinct nuclear functions of NF-kappaB. EMBO J 21: 6539-6548.
17. Balasubramanyam K, Varier RA, Altaf M, Swaminathan V, Siddappa NB, et al. (2004) Curcumin, a novel p300/CREB-binding protein-specific inhibitor of acetyltransferase, represses the acetylation of histone/ nonhistone proteins and histone acetyltransferase-dependent chromatin transcription. J Biol Chem 279: 51163-51171.
18. Zhu X, Liu Q, Wang M, Liang M, Yang X, et al. (2011) Activation of Sirt1 by resveratrol inhibits TNF-Î± induced inflammation in fibroblasts. PLoS One 6: e27081.
19. Howitz KT, Bitterman KJ, Cohen HY, Lamming DW, Lavu S, et al. (2003) Small molecule activators of sirtuins extend Saccharomyces cerevisiae lifespan. Nature 425: 191-196.

20. Kojima K, Ohhashi R, Fujita Y, Hamada N, Akao Y, et al. (2008) A role for SIRT1 in cell growth and chemoresistance in prostate cancer PC3 and DU145 cells. Biochem Biophys Res Commun 373: 423-428.
21. Yang SR, Wright J, Bauter M, Seweryniak K, Kode A, et al. (2007) Sirtuin regulates cigarette smoke-induced proinflammatory mediator release via RelA/p65 NF-kappaB in macrophages in vitro and in rat lungs in vivo: implications for chronic inflammation and aging. Am J Physiol Lung Cell Mol Physiol 292: L567-576.
22. Yeung F, Hoberg JE, Ramsey CS, Keller MD, Jones DR, et al. (2004) Modulation of NF-kappaB-dependent transcription and cell survival by the SIRT1 deacetylase. EMBO J 23: 2369-2380.
23. Philchenkov A, Zavelevich M, Kroczak TJ, Los M (2004) Caspases and cancer: mechanisms of inactivation and new treatment modalities. Exp Oncol 26: 82-97.
24. Schröder M, Kaufman RJ (2005) ER stress and the unfolded protein response. Mutat Res 569: 29-63.
25. Manson MM (2005) Inhibition of survival signalling by dietary polyphenols and indole-3-carbinol. Eur J Cancer 41: 1842-1853.
26. Bakhshi J, Weinstein L, Poksay KS, Nishinaga B, Bredesen DE, et al. (2008) Coupling endoplasmic reticulum stress to the cell death program in mouse melanoma cells: effect of curcumin. Apoptosis 13: 904-914.
27. Harding HP, Calfon M, Urano F, Novoa I, Ron D (2002) Transcriptional and translational control in the Mammalian unfolded protein response. Annu Rev Cell Dev Biol 18: 575-599.
28. Boyce M, Bryant KF, Jousse C, Long K, Harding HP, et al. (2005) A selective inhibitor of eIF2alpha dephosphorylation protects cells from ER stress. Science 307: 935-939.
29. Yang CW, Chang CL, Lee HC, Chi CW, Pan JP, et al. (2012) Curcumin induces the apoptosis of human monocytic leukemia THP-1 cells via the activation of JNK/ERK pathways. BMC Complement Altern Med 12: 22.
30. Kloesch B, Becker T, Dietersdorfer E, Kiener H, Steiner G (2013) Anti-inflammatory and apoptotic effects of the polyphenol curcumin on human fibroblast-like synoviocytes. Int Immunopharmacol 15: 400-405.
31. Smith MR, Gangireddy SR, Narala VR, Hogaboam CM, Standiford TJ, et al. (2010) Curcumin inhibits fibrosis-related effects in IPF fibroblasts and in mice following bleomycin-induced lung injury. Am J Physiol Lung Cell Mol Physiol 298: L616-625.
32. Ucisik MH, Küpcü S, Schuster B, Sleytr UB (2013) Characterization of CurcuEmulsomes: nanoformulation for enhanced solubility and delivery of curcumin. J Nanobiotechnology 11: 37.

# 12

# Phytochemical Isoliquiritigenin Inhibits Angiogenesis *Ex Vivo* and Corneal Neovascularization in Mice

**Lingling Yang[1], Wenxiao He[1], Huihua Qu[2], Changkai Jia[1], Yao Wang[1], Yiqiang Wang[1,3*] and Dongmin Liu[2*]**

[1]*Shandong Provincial Key Lab of Ophthalmology, Shandong Eye Institute, Shandong Academy of Medical Sciences, Qingdao, China*

[2]*Department of Human Nutrition, Foods and Exercise, Virginia Tech, Blacksburg, USA*

[3]*University Research Center, Beijing University of Traditional Chinese Medicine, Beijing, China*

[*]**Corresponding author**: Dongmin Liu, Department of Human Nutrition, Foods and Exercise, Virginia Tech, USA, Email: doliu@vt.edu

**Abstract**

Neovascularization is often involved in many diseases and there is no effective treatment for this pathological process. In searching for potential therapies for neovascularization, we screened nineteen pre-selected small molecules isolated from herbal extracts for their possible anti-angiogenic effect *in vitro* and *in vivo*. We found that isoliquiritigenin, a chalconoid compound isolated from Chinese herb medicine licorice, potently inhibited vascular endothelial cell (EC) proliferation, migration, tube -like structure formation *ex vivo*. Western blot analysis shows that exposure of ECs to isoliquiritigenin inhibited extracellular signal-regulated kinase 1/2 (ERK1/2) phosphorylation. In Matrigel plug assay, isoliquiritigenin effectively blocked fibroblast growth factor-induced in vivo angiogenesis in mice. Consistently, topical application of isoliquiritigenin significantly inhibited chemical injury-induced corneal neovascularization in mice. Collectively, these results suggest that isoliquiritigenin may be a low-cost and effective natural agent to treat angiogenesis-dependent diseases.

**Keywords:** Isoliquiritigenin; Vascular endothelial cell; Proliferation; Migration; Angiogenesis; Neovascularization

## Introduction

Angiogenesis is a complex phenomenon long known to be under the tight control by a large panel of cytokines, cells, hormones, etc. [1]. While angiogenesis might occur under both physiological and pathological conditions, neovascularization is often referred to the development of new blood vessels in tissues that are normally not or less vascularized. Except for situations where neovascularization helps to heal and reconstitute the structure of injured tissues, all other instances of neovascularization are associated with the dysfunction of the affected tissues or with the expansion of undesirable tissues (e.g. tumor) [2]. The cornea is normally avascular. Under pathological conditions however, blood vessels from the limbal vascular plexus could invade the cornea, leading to its pathological vascularization that can cause visual impairment and blindness [3,4]. Previous studies showed that corneal neovascularization can be triggered by various factors, including infection [5], trauma [6] and inflammation [7]. While several strategies have been tested for their anti-neovascularization efficacy, such as multiple anti-angiogenic gene therapy [8], recombinant anti-angiogenic factor therapy [9], and anti-inflammation therapy with monoclonal antibody against pro-inflammatory molecules [10], these approaches are not very effective in the treatment of corneal neovascularization [11].

Natural products (e.g. medicinal herbs) have been proposed as alternative resources for anti-angiogenic agents [8,12]. Indeed, traditional Chinese Medicine practitioners have been prescribing herbal medicines to treat various diseases that are associated with neovascularization, although not all of herbal therapies are based on evidence from the results of modern biomedical studies [13]. In addition, the components that are responsible for the anti-angiogenic action of these herb medicines are largely unknown. In the present study, we first screened 19 small molecules isolated from presumably angiogenesis-modulating herbs for their potential to modulate endothelial cell (EC) behavior ex vitro. We then studied the anti-angiogenic effect of the identified compound in vivo and further determined the mechanism underlying this action. We found that isoliquiritigenin, a chalconoid compound isolated from Licorice Roots, is a potent agent for the treatment of pathological neovascularization.

## Materials and Methods

### Herbal isolates

All compounds were isolated and provided by the National Pharmaceutical Engineering Center for Chinese Herbal Medicine in Jiangxi Herbfine Hi-tech Co., Ltd, Nanchang, Jiangxi, China. The purity of all compounds is >98% as determined by high performance liquid chromatography. The compounds were dissolved, either in PBS or dimethyl sulfoxide (DMSO), according to the manufacturer's instructions.

### Cell proliferation assay

Primary human umbilical vein endothelial cells (HUVECs) were used for the proliferation analyses. Cell proliferation was measured using the coloregenic Cell Counting Kit-8 (CCK, Dojindo laboratories, Kumamoto, Japan) as previously described [14]. In brief, HUVECs were grown to about 30% confluence followed by the addition of the individual compounds or vehicle at a single concentration of 40 μM. After 48 h of incubation, CCK-8 solution was added and the cells were incubated for additional 4 h. The absorbance at 450 nm was measured using a microplate reader (Molecular Devices, Sunnyvale, CA, USA).

### Cell migration assay

Migration of HUVECs was evaluated by using a monolayer wound healing and the Transwell migration assays. For the wound healing assay, cells were plated on 24-well culture plates and allowed to grow to confluence. A scratch was made with a micropipette tip and the cultures were rinsed to remove detached cells. Cells were then cultured in medium with or without various concentrations of tanshinone IIA or isoliquiritigenin. On the outer surface of the culture wells facing the scratches, ink lines were made perpendicular to the inside scratch and the width of the scratches at the crossing site were photographed before and after the 24 h of incubation. The cell migration rates were calculated as previously described [15].

For Transwell migration assay, HUVECs were placed in the upper compartment of Transwell Boyden chambers with fibronectin-coated polycarbonate filters (8-μm pore size, Corning Inc., Acton, MA) at 1×105 cells/well in 0.2 mL medium containing 1% serum. The lower chamber contained 0.7 mL of complete medium supplemented with increasing concentrations of isoliquiritigenin (0, 25, 50, or 100 μM). After 6 h of incubation at 37°C, cells remaining on the upper surface of filter were removed using a cotton swab. The cells that had transmigrated to the lower surface of the membranes were stained with 0.1% crystal violet and counted under microscope.

### In vitro angiogenesis assay

Thirty μL of Matrigel™ Matrix (BD Bioscience, San Jose, CA) was dispensed in 96-well plates and allowed to polymerize for 1 h at 37°C. HUVECs were labeled with Vybrant Dil cell-labeling solution (Invitrogen, Carlsbad, CA, USA) and seeded at a density of 1.5×104 cells/well in medium containing various concentrations of isoliquiritigenin (0, 6.25, 12.5, 25, 50 or 100 μM). Cells were then incubated at 37°C. 6 h later, random fields were photographed using an Eclipse TE2000-U microscope (Nikon, Japan) with a 594 nm filter.

### Western blot analysis

Protein extracts from treated and untreated HUVECs were resolved on 10% SDS-PAGE gel and then transferred to nitrocellulose membranes. The membranes were probed with antibody against phosphorylated extracellular signal-regulated kinase 1/2 (ERK1/2; Santa Cruz Biotechnology, Santa Cruz, CA) according to the manufacturer's instructions and the immunoreactive proteins were detected by chemilluminescence. The membranes were then stripped and re-probed with ERK 1/2 antibody (Santa Cruz).

### In vivo Matrigel plug angiogenesis assay

C57BL/6 mice (6-10 weeks old) were used for in vivo assays of angiogenesis. Mice were purchased from the Laboratory Animal Center of the Academy of Military Medical Sciences (Beijing, China) and all experimental procedures were carried out in accordance with the guidelines of the Association for Research in Vision and Ophthalmology Statement for the Use of Animals in Ophthalmic and Vision Research. To assess the effect of isoliquiritigenin on angiogenesis *in vivo*, 300 μl of Matrigel (BD Bioscience, San Jose, CA, USA) containing 60 ng of fibroblast growth factor (R&D System, Minneapolis, MN, USA) and 3U of heparin (B.Braun Melsungen AG, Melsungen, Germany), with or without 100 μM of isoliquiritigenin, were injected subcutaneously into the abdominal wall of mice (n=4 mice/group). Ten days after implantation, mice were euthanized and the Matrigel plugs were removed and photographed. Hemoglobin contents in the plugs were measured as described by others [16] with modification. Briefly, the implants were snap frozen, lyophilized overnight, and weighted. The dried Matrigel was re-suspended in 0.4 mL of 0.1% Triton X-100 for 1 h, disrupted by vigorous pipetting, and then centrifuged at 14,000×g for 15 min to remove any particulate debris. Absorbance of hemoglobin in the supernatants was read at 405 nm with a microplate reader, and its concentration was calculated according to the standard curve obtained with pure hemoglobin.

### Corneal neovascularization studies

Under general anesthesia with intraperitoneal injection of ketamine and chloropromazine (50 mg/kg and 5 mg/kg, respectively), *corneal neovascularization in mice were* generated by application of a 2 mm sized filter soaked with 2 μL of 1 N NaOH to the central cornea for 40 sec followed by immediate rinsing with normal saline for 40 sec, a widely used mouse model for pathological corneal neovascularization. Isoliquiritigenin or resveratrol (100 μM in saline eye drops) was applied topically (5 μL) to the burned eyes 4 times daily for 7 consecutive days. Control eyes were similarly burnt but treated with saline only. At day 7, eyes were photographed under a slit lamp. All mice were killed and their corneas were collected and subjected to conventional histology with hematoxylin-eosin (H&E) staining and immunohistochemistry as detailed below.

### Histology and immunohistochemistry

Eyeballs were either fixed with formalin or snap-frozen in Optimal Cutting Temperature (OCT) compound (Sakura Finetechnical, Tokyo, Japan). Formalin-fixed tissues were stained with H&E. For immunofluorescence staining, cryosections (6 μm) were prepared from OCT-embedded eyeballs and were fixed in ice-cold acetone for 10 min. The sections were blocked with 10% normal goat serum for 15 min and then stained with PE-conjugated anti-CD31 monoclonal antibody (1:100, BD Biosciences, San Jose, CA, USA) overnight at 4°C. After counterstaining with DAPI, the stained sections were viewed under an Eclipse TE2000-U microscope (Nikon, Japan). Negative controls were stained in parallel by omitting primary antibody.

### Reverse-transcription quantitative real-time PCR analysis

Total RNA from mouse corneas was extracted using a NucleoSpin RNAII kit (Macherey-Nagel, Düren, Germany) and reverse transcribed using a PrimeScript RT Reagent Kit (Takara, BIO INC., Shiga, Japan) following the manufacturer's protoocls. Quantitative PCR analysis of vascular endothelial growth factor (VEGF), basic fibroblast growth factor (bFGF), and transforming growth factor-β1 (TGF- β1) was performed in an ABI 7500 Detection System (Applied Biosystems, Foster City, CA, USA) using TaqMan Mastermix (Tiangen Biotech, Beijing China). RPL5 gene was used as internal control. Reactions were carried out with an initial 10-min incubation at 95°C followed by 45 cycles at 95°C for 15 sec and then at 60°C for 1 min. The raw data were analyzed using SDS 7500 software (Applied Biosystems) and Ct values for each gene in each sample were determined. The relative amount of each target gene mRNA to RPL5 was calculated as the 2− ΔCt (where ΔCt = Ct − CtRPL5) and expressed as folds of control. The primers used in quantitative real-time RT-PCR were listed below (Table 1):

| Gene Symbol (Accession Number) | Primer sequences F: forward; R:reverse | Amplicon (bp) |
|---|---|---|
| VEGF (NM_009505) | F- GCTACTGCCGTCCGATTGAG<br>R- CACACAGGACGGCTTGAAGA | 86 bp |
| bFGF2 (NM_008006) | F- AGAGCGACCCACACGTCAA<br>R- AAGGTACCGGTTGGCACACA | 86 bp |
| TGFβ1 (NM_011577) | F- ACGGAATACAGGGCTTTCGA<br>R- GCTGATCCCGTTGATTTCCA | 86 bp |
| RPL5 (NM_016980) | F- GGAAGCACATCATGGGTCAGA<br>R- TACGCATCTTCATCTTCCTCCATT | 70 bp |

**Table 1:** Sequences of primers used for RT-qPCR assay.

## Statistical analysis

Data from in vitro experiments were derived from at least three independent experiments with duplicated determination each. Variation within treatments is expressed as the standard error (SE) of the mean (SEM) for in vitro assays and SE for in vivo studies. All data were subjected to a one-way ANOVA using the SigmaPlot software and treatment differences were subjected to Tukey's multiple comparison tests, where P<0.05 was considered significant.

# Results

## Effects of herb-derived small molecules on EC proliferation

For this study, 19 pure compounds were carefully selected based on the following reasons. First, the herbs from which these molecules were isolated have been used in complex recipes of traditional Chinese Medicine for treating various angiogenesis-related diseases; and second, these selected chemicals had been thought to be bioactive components responsible for some biological effects of corresponding herb(s). These 19 molecules are arteannuinum succinate, baicalein, berberine hydrochloride, ginkgolide B, ginsenoside Rg3, hydroxycamptothecin, isoliquiritigenin, L-epicatechin, ligustrazine hydrochloride, notoginsenoside R1, procyanidin B2, protocatechuic aldehyde, puerarin, quercetin, resveratrol, salvianic acid A sodium, silybin, tanshinone IIA, and wogonin. Beside we first tested their effects on the proliferation of primary human umbilical vascular ECs (HUVECs). In that regard, cells were cultured in the medium with the presence of vehicle or 40 μM various isolated compounds for 24 h. The results showed that baicalein, tanshinone II A, resveratrol, ginsenoside Rg3, arteannuinum succinate, berberine hydrochloride, isoliquiritigenin, and 10-hydroxy camptothecin inhibited cell proliferation, whereas ligustrazine hydrochloride, pueraria, notoginsenoside R1, epicatechin, and silybin stimulated cell proliferation as compared to the control (Figure 1). The order of potency for the inhibition of EC proliferation at this concentration is tanshinone IIA≈isoliquiritigenin>arteannuinumsuccinate≈berberinehydrochloride>hydroxycamptothecin>ginsenoside Rg3>resveratrol≈Baicalein, with tanshinone IIA and isoliquiritigenin blocking cell proliferation by 97.0% and 93.7%, respectively. We further tested does-dependent effects of tanshinone IIA and isoliquiritigenin on EC proliferation. Both tanshinone IIA (Figure 2A) and isoliquiritigenin (Figure 2B) dose-dependently inhibited EC proliferation. Tanshinone IIA as low as 5 μM significantly inhibited EC proliferation with 10 μM and 20 μM concentrations blocking cell proliferation by 64% and 94%, respectively, whereas isoliquiritigenin at ≤10 μM concentrations was ineffective with 10 μM reducing proliferation by 42%, suggesting that low-dose tanshinone IIA is more potent than isoliquiritigenin in inhibiting EC proliferation. To confirm that the effect of Tanshinone IIA and isoliquiritigenin in our experiments was on cell proliferation, rather than due to induction of cell death, we assessed if tanshinone IIA and isoliquiritigenin induce apoptosis of HUVECs. In that regard, cells were treated with various doses of tanshinone IIA or isoliquiritigenin for 24 h. The results showed that tanshinone IIA or isoliquiritigenin ISL at ≤80 μM had no effect on cell apoptosis (data not shown). Since the long-term purpose of this study is to identify herb-derived small molecules that will be potentially used in managing human neovascularization diseases, we focused following studies on these two most potent compounds that inhibited HUVEC proliferation.

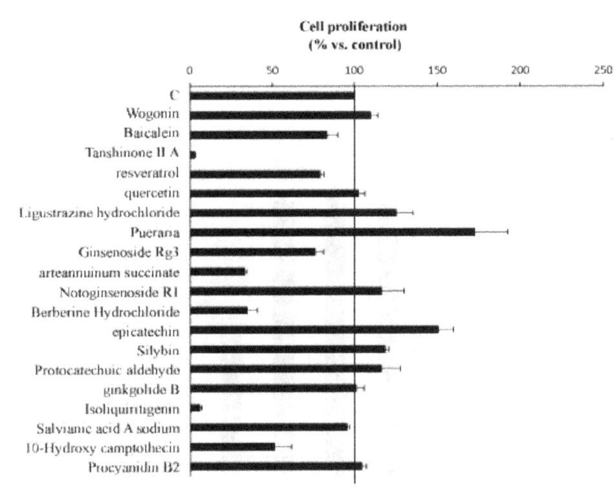


**Figure 1:** The effect of herb-derived compounds on EC proliferation. HUVECs were incubated with vehicle or 40 μM individual compounds. After 48 h of incubation, cell proliferation was measured as described in Methods. Data are expressed as mean ± SEM of three separate experiments with quadruplicate determinations each. *P<0.05 vs vehicle alone-treated cells.

## Effects of tanshinone IIA and isoliquiritigenin on EC migration

The chemotactic migration of ECs is one of the critical steps in the process of angiogenesis. We therefore examined whether tanshinone IIA and isoliquiritigenin can further inhibit migration of HUVECs. We first performed the monolayer wound healing assay to evaluate whether these compounds affect EC migration. The results showed that both tanshinone IIA and isoliquiritigenin dose-dependently inhibited cell migration from the edge of the wound into the open area, but isoliquiritigenin is more potent than Tanshinone IIA in inhibiting the migration of HUVECs (Figure 3A and 3B). Next, we performed transwell assays by using modified Boyden chambers to further evaluate whether isoliquiritigenin affects cell migration in HUVECs. As shown in Figure 3C, isoliquiritigenin significantly reduced the number of migrated cells through the membrane barrier of the transwell.

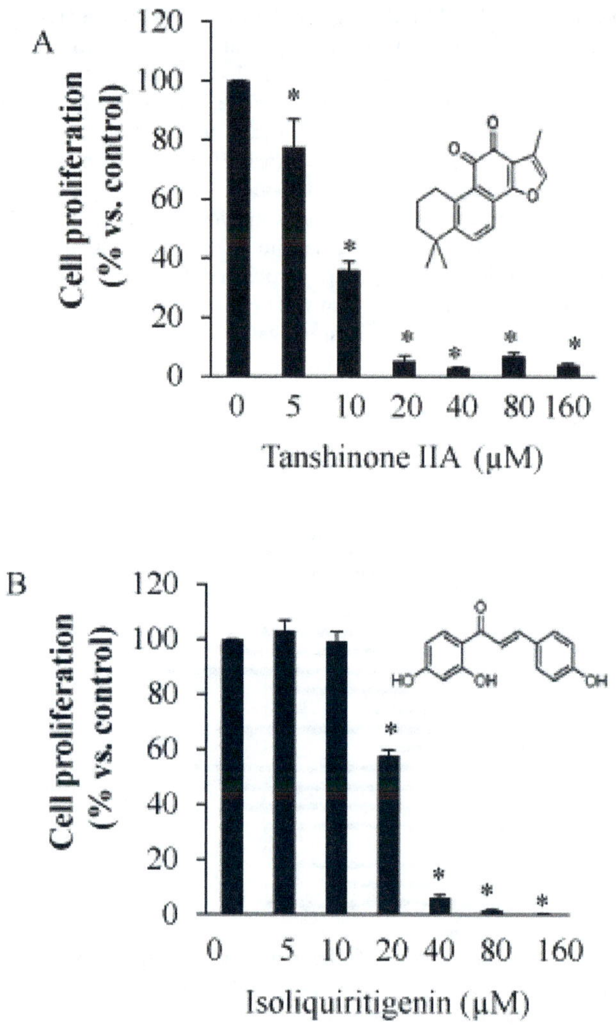


**Figure 2:** Does-dependent effects of Tanshinone IIA and isoliquiritigenin on EC proliferation. HUVECs were incubated with vehicle or various concentrations of Tanshinone IIA (A) or isoliquiritigenin (B) After 48 h of incubation, cell proliferation was measured as described in Methods. Data are expressed as mean ± SEM of three separate experiments with quadruplicate determinations each. *P<0.05 vs vehicle alone-treated cells.

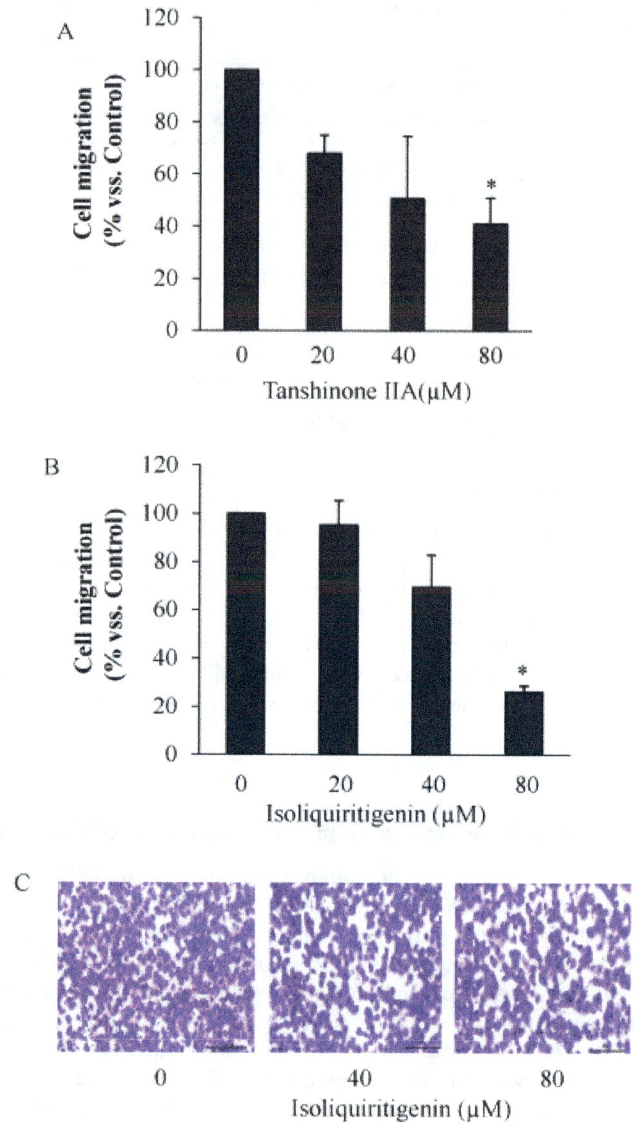


**Figure 3:** The effects of Tanshinone IIA and isoliquiritigenin on migration of HUVECs. Cell cultures were "wounded" and incubated in medium with or without various concentrations of Tanshinone IIA (A) or isoliquiritigenin (B) for 24 h. The distance between the two wound edges was measured before and after treatment and are expressed as a percentage of the control. Representative photographs are shown of cells immediately after wound induction or after 24 h incubations with or without compounds from three independent experiments. Cell migration was determined by modified Boyden chamber assay in the presence of isoliquiritigenin or vehicle (C), as described in Methods. Data are expressed as mean ± SEM of three separate experiments with quadruplicate determinations each. Inserts in bar graphs are chemical structures. * p<0.05 vs. control.

## Isoliquiritigenin abolishes in vitro angiogenesis

Angiogenesis is a complex process involving EC proliferation, migration, and the formation of vascular tube structures. Next, we evaluated if isoliquiritigenin affects EC tube structure formation, a widely used in vitro model of angiogenesis. In that regard, cells were plated onto Matrigel, followed by incubation with or without isoliquiritigenin. As shown in Figure 4, ECs developed tube/cord-like networks after 6 h of incubation. However, exposure of cells to isoliquiritigenin substantially ablated tube-like structure formation.

## Isoliquiritigenin may inhibit angiogenesis through suppression of ERK1/2 activity

It is well recognized that the ERK 1/2 signaling pathway plays an important role in cell proliferation and growth. Next, we investigated the possible pathways involved in the modulation of angiogenesis by comparing the total and activated ERK1/2 levels in isoliquiritigenin-treated and untreated HUVECs. The results from Western blot analysis showed that isoliquiritigenin induced a dose-dependent inhibition of the phosphorylation of ERK1/2, a magnitude similar to its effect on cell proliferation and migration (Figure 5). However, isoliquiritigenin had no effect on total ERK protein expression in the cells.

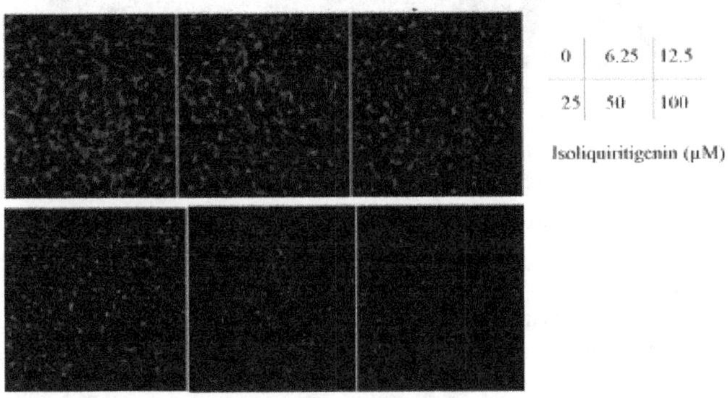


**Figure 4:** Isoliquiritigenin inhibits tube-like structure formation by HUVECs. Cells were fluorescently labeled as described in "Methods" and seeded onto Matrigel in the presence or absence of various concentrations of isoliquiritigenin for 6 h. A set of representative photographs from three independent experiments with similar results is shown.

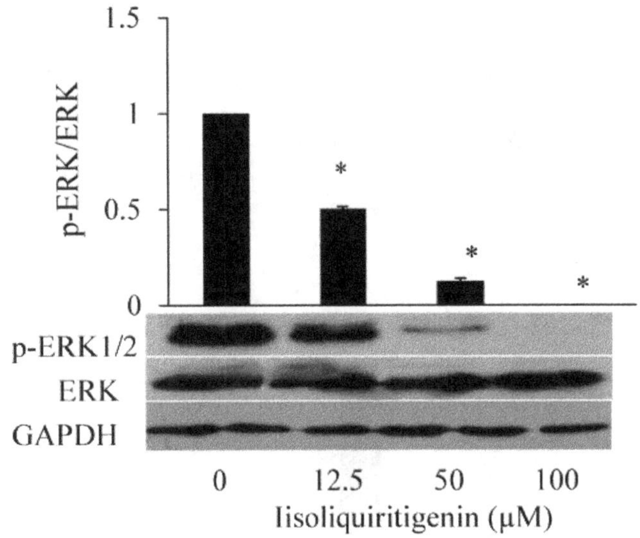


**Figure 5:** Isoliquiritigenin inhibits ERK1/2 phosphorylation in HUVEs. HUVECs were incubated with vehicle or various concentrations of isoliquiritigenin for 48 h. Western analysis was performed to detect phosphorylated ERK1/2 (p-ERK1/2), which was normalized to total ERK 1/2 from the same sample. Mean±SE of normalized densitometry measurements from three separate experiments, along with representative blots, are shown.

## Isoliquiritigenin suppresses vasculogenesis and corneal neovascularization

To confirm the anti-angiogenic activity of isoliquiritigenin in vivo, we first used the mouse Matrigel plug model of angiogenesis. Resveratrol was chosen as the positive control because it is often used as an anti-angiogenic agent to treat various angiogenesis-related diseases [17-19]. As shown in Figure 6A, significant blood vessel formation was observed in Matrigel plugs supplemented with fibroblast growth factor (FGF) as compared to the plugs harvested from the control mice. However, microvessel formation induced by FGF was profoundly reduced in the presence of 100 μM isoliquiritigenin, as demonstrated by relatively pale color of isoliquiritigenin-supplemented plugs compared to that of vehicle-treated plugs, which was more effective than that of resveratrol treatment (Figure 6A). Consistently, isoliquiritigenin potently reduced the hemoglobin content of the plugs (Figure 6B), further confirming that isoliquiritigenin is a potent inhibitor of growth factor-induced angiogenesis *in vivo.*

To further test the therapeutic potential of isoliquiritigenin in treating corneal neovascularization, we generated a mouse model of corneal neovascularization by alkali burning of the mouse cornea, which causes injury to the corneal surface and subsequent neovascularization, a well-established model for the study of corneal neovascularization. As shown in Figure 7A, topical application of isoliquiritigenin (100 μM in eye drops) to the corneas injured by chemical burn greatly inhibited the development of corneal neovascularization, an effect that was more potent than that of resveratrol. Analysis of sections from H&E (Figure 7B) and immunohistochemistry staining (Figure 7C) further showed that isoliquiritigenin greatly decreased the numbers of blood/lymphatic vessels in the corneas, which was also more effective than that of resveratrol.

## Isoliquiritigenin has no effect on the gene expression of angiogenic factors in cornea

It is recognized that overexpression of several growth factors in the cornea, including vascular endothelial growth factor (VEGF), basic fibroblast growth factor (bFGF) and transforming growth factor beta1 (TGFβ1), plays pivotal roles in promoting angiogenesis and corneal neovascularization [3,20-22], we then performed RT-PCR to determine whether isoliquiritigenin suppresses neovascularization through suppressing the production of angiogenic factors. The results show that chemical burn drastically increased gene expression of VEGF, bFGF, and TGFβ1 by 11.8, 142.9 and 3.2 fold, respectively, in the neovascularized corneas from mice. However, neither isoliquiritigenin nor resveratrol significantly affected chemical injury-induced up regulation of these angiogenic factors (data not shown).

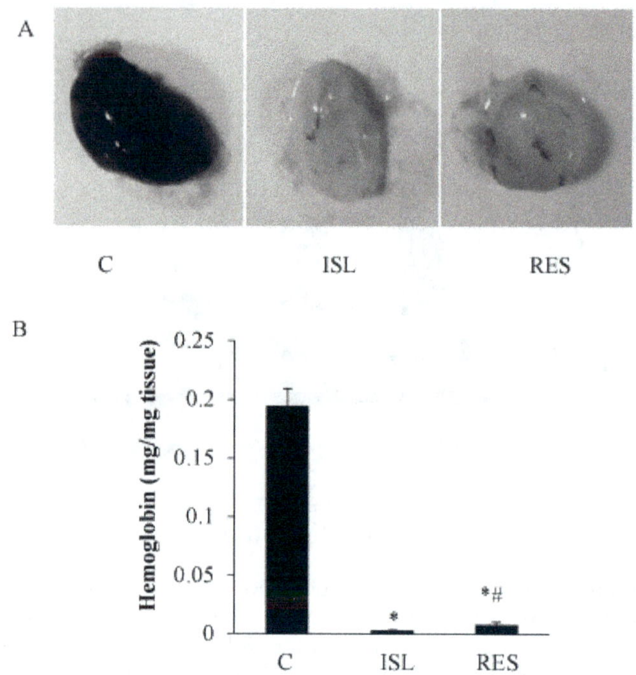


**Figure 6:** Isoliquiritigenin inhibits angiogenesis in vivo. Matrigels in the presence of basic fibroblast growth factor (bFGF) and heparin with or without 100 μM isoliquiritigenin (ISL) or resveratrol (RES) were injected subcutaneously into the abdominal wall of mice. (A) Representative photographs of Matrigel plugs at 10 d after implantation are shown (n=4 mice/group). (B) Hemoglobin levels in the Matrigel plugs were quantified and are expressed as mean ± SE. *, $p<0.05$ vs. bFGF alone-treated group.

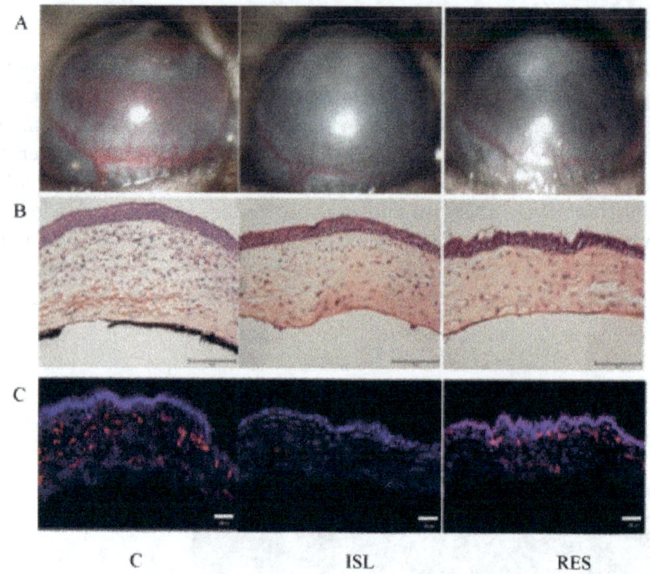


**Figure 7:** Isoliquiritigenin inhibits corneal neovascularization. Corneal neovascularization in mice was induced as described in the "Methods". Isoliquiritigenin (ISL) or resveratrol (RES) in 100 μM solution was then applied topically (5 μL) to the eyes 4 times daily for 7 consecutive days. Control eyes were treated with vehicle only. (A) Neovascularization was examined by slit lamp and representative photographs of cornea at day 7 after induction of corneal neovascularization (n=4 mice/group) are shown. (B) H&E staining of corneal sections. Corneal neovascularization assessed by CD31 staining. As demonstrated, the area of neovascularized cornea dramatically increased in the control groups but was significantly reduced in mice treated with isoliquiritigenin.

## Discussion

Angiogenesis is a complex process with EC cell proliferation, migration, and tubulogenesis playing an essential role in ultimate new blood vessel formation [15] Corneal angiogenesis causes vascularization of avascular cornea that can lead to the decline of vision and even blindness. The pathogenesis of corneal neovascularization is still not fully understood, but it is stimulated by various growth factors, notably VEGF and bFGF that are secreted in response to hypoxia, chemical burn, chronic inflammation, infection, and trauma [22]. Isoliquiritigenin is a naturally occurring flavonoid that reportedly has an array of biological activities, such as vasorelaxation [23], anti-platelet aggregation [24], anti-inflammation [25], and anti-cancer [26]. While studies examining the effects of this compound on vascular ECs are limited, a recent study showed that isoliquiritigenin suppressed growth factor-stimulated proliferation of ECs [27]. In the present study, we identify that isoliquiritigenin potently inhibits EC proliferation, migration, and the formation of tube-like structure *ex vivo*. Consistently, we demonstrate that this compound is a strong inhibitor of angiogenesis and corneal neovascularization induced by growth factor and chemical injury in vivo. These data suggest that isoliquiritigenin may have great therapeutic for ocular neovascularization and other disorders associated with angiogenesis.

The exact mechanism for isoliquiritigenin to inhibit corneal neovascularization is presently unclear. It is well recognized that the ERK1/2 signaling pathway in vascular ECs plays an important role in cell proliferation. migration, and angiogenesis [28,29]. ERK1/2 are activated in response to a large array of extracellular stimuli, including growth factors [29-31]. In the present study, we show that isoliquiritigenin greatly suppressed ERK1/2 activation, suggesting that its inhibitory action on angiogenesis may be primarily mediated via inhibiting the ERK1/2 signaling pathway. Interestingly, isoliquiritigenin treatment had no effect on ERK1/2 protein expression, suggesting that isoliquiritigenin ablates ERK1/2 activity via a non-genomic mechanism. ERK1/2 is directly activated by MEK, which is activated by its upstream kinase, Raf-1 [32]. However, how isoliquiritigenin interacts with the ERK 1/2 pathway remains to be elucidated.

Accumulating evidence show that several growth factors, particularly VEGF and bFGF, play a critical role in corneal angiogenesis [3,20,21]. Indeed, studies showed that these angiogenic factors are over-expressed and increasingly secreted from neovascularized cornea [6]. Accordingly, corneal neovascularization can be reduced by anti-VEGF or anti-bFGF treatment [22,33]. In the present study, our data show that the expression of these angiogenic factors in neovascularized mouse cornea was greatly increased. However, treatment with isoliquiritigenin had no significant effect on these molecules, suggesting that the anti-angiogenesis action of isoliquiritigenin is not mediated through suppressing the expression of VEGF and bFGF in the cornea.

Tanshinone IIA, isolated from the root of Salvia miltiorrhiza, is widely used in the prescriptions for treating vascular diseases. While the scientific evidence supporting its beneficial effect on vasculature in humans is not well established, some studies showed that tanshinone IIA protects against vascular inflammation and promotes vasodilatation [34-36]. In addition, tanshinone IIA has been shown to inhibit proliferation and migration of cancer cells [37-39]. In the present study, we demonstrate that tanshinone IIA is a potent agent inhibiting EC proliferation and does-dependently inhibits cell migration, but it is less potent than isoliquiritigenin in inhibiting EC migration, which is essential to angiogenesis. Given this result, we then solely focused on further characterizing the anti-angiogenic action of isoliquiritigenin. However, there is possibility that tanshinone IIA is still a potent anti-angiogenesis agent in vivo, as it may be able to suppress angiogenesis by inhibiting migration of smooth muscle cells, as reported [40].

In summary, by screening herb-derived small molecules, we identified that isoliquiritigenin is a potent inhibitor of angiogenesis and corneal neovascularization in vivo. These effects are ascribed at least in part to the inhibition of proliferation, migration, and tubulogenesis of ECs. These data suggest that isoliquiritigenin may have great therapeutic potential as a low-cost natural compound for neovascularization-associated corneal disorders or other diseases. However, the detailed anti-angiogenic mechanisms of isoliquiritigenin remain to be determined.

## References


1. Iruela-Arispe ML, Dvorak HF (1997) Angiogenesis: a dynamic balance of stimulators and inhibitors. Thromb Haemost 78: 672-677.
2. Isner JM, Asahara T (1999) Angiogenesis and vasculogenesis as therapeutic strategies for postnatal neovascularization. J Clin Invest 103: 1231-1236.
3. Suryawanshi A, Veiga-Parga T, Reddy PB, Rajasagi NK, Rouse BT (2012) IL-17A differentially regulates corneal vascular endothelial growth factor (VEGF)-A and soluble VEGF receptor 1 expression and promotes corneal angiogenesis after herpes simplex virus infection. J Immunol 188: 3434-3446
4. Maruyama K, Ii M, Cursiefen C, Jackson DG, Keino H, et al. (2005) Inflammation-induced lymphangiogenesis in the cornea arises from CD11b-positive macrophages. J Clin Invest 115: 2363-2372.
5. Xue ML, Thakur A , Willcox M (2002) Macrophage inflammatory protein-2 and vascular endothelial growth factor regulate corneal neovascularization induced by infection with Pseudomonas aeruginosa in mice. Immunol Cell Biol 80: 323-327
6. Amano S, Rohan R, Kuroki M, Tolentino M, Adamis AP (1998) Requirement for vascular endothelial growth factor in wound- and inflammation-related corneal neovascularization. Invest Ophthalmol Vis Sci 39: 18-22
7. Sivak JM, Ostriker AC, Woolfenden A, Demirs J, Cepeda R, et al. (2011) Pharmacologic uncoupling of angiogenesis and inflammation during initiation of pathological corneal neovascularization. J Biol Chem 286: 44965-44975.
8. Chen P, Yin H, Wang Y, Mi J, He W, et al. (2010) Multi-gene targeted antiangiogenic therapies for experimental corneal neovascularization. Mol Vis 16: 310-319.
9. Wang Y, Yin H, Chen P, Xie L, Wang Y (2011) Inhibitory effect of canstatin in alkali burn-induced corneal neovascularization. Ophthalmic Res 46: 66-72.
10. Li C, Zhang F, Wang Y (2010) S100A proteins in the pathogenesis of experimental corneal neovascularization. Mol Vis 16: 2225-2235.
11. Maddula S, Davis DK, Maddula S, Burrow MK, Ambati BK (2011) Horizons in therapy for corneal angiogenesis. Ophthalmology 118: 591-599.
12. Koltermann A, Liebl J, Fürst R, Ammer H, Vollmar AM, et al. (2009) Ginkgo biloba extract EGb 761 exerts anti-angiogenic effects via activation of tyrosine phosphatases. J Cell Mol Med 13: 2122-2130.
13. Fan TP, Yeh JC, Leung KW, Yue PY, Wong RN (2006) Angiogenesis: from plants to blood vessels. Trends Pharmacol Sci 27: 297-309.
14. Ishiyama M, Tominaga H, Shiga M, Sasamoto K, Ohkura Y, et al. (1996) A combined assay of cell viability and in vitro cytotoxicity with a highly water-soluble tetrazolium salt, neutral red and crystal violet. Biol Pharm Bull 19: 1518-1520.
15. Liu D, Iruthayanathan M, Homan LL, Wang Y, Yang L, et al. (2008) Dehydroepiandrosterone stimulates endothelial proliferation and angiogenesis through extracellular signal-regulated kinase 1/2-mediated mechanisms. Endocrinology 149: 889-898.
16. McMahon GA, Petitclerc E, Stefansson S, Smith E, Wong MK, et al. (2001) Plasminogen activator inhibitor-1 regulates tumor growth and angiogenesis. J Biol Chem 276: 33964-33968.
17. Khan AA, Dace DS, Ryazanov AG, Kelly J, Apte RS (2010) Resveratrol regulates pathologic angiogenesis by a eukaryotic elongation factor-2 kinase-regulated pathway. Am J Pathol 177: 481-492.
18. Bråkenhielm E, Cao R, Cao Y (2001) Suppression of angiogenesis, tumor growth, and wound healing by resveratrol, a natural compound in red wine and grapes. FASEB J 15: 1798-1800.
19. Athar M, Back JH, Kopelovich L, Bickers DR, Kim AL (2009) Multiple molecular targets of resveratrol: Anti-carcinogenic mechanisms. Arch Biochem Biophys 486: 95-102.
20. Oliveira HB, Sakimoto T, Javier JA, Azar DT, Wiegand SJ, et al. (2010) VEGF Trap(R1R2) suppresses experimental corneal angiogenesis. Eur J Ophthalmol 20: 48-54.
21. Ghanem RC, Han KY, Rojas J, Ozturk O, Kim DJ, et al. (2011) Semaphorin 7A promotes angiogenesis in an experimental corneal neovascularization model. Curr Eye Res 36: 989-996.
22. Shakiba Y, Mansouri K, Arshadi D, Rezaei N (2009) Corneal neovascularization: molecular events and therapeutic options. Recent Pat Inflamm Allergy Drug Discov 3: 221-231.
23. Liu B, Yang J, Wen Q, Li Y (2008) Isoliquiritigenin, a flavonoid from licorice, relaxes guinea-pig tracheal smooth muscle in vitro and in vivo: role of cGMP/PKG pathway. Eur J Pharmacol 587: 257-266.
24. Tawata M, Aida K, Noguchi T, Ozaki Y, Kume S, et al. (1992) Anti-platelet action of isoliquiritigenin, an aldose reductase inhibitor in licorice. Eur J Pharmacol 212: 87-92.
25. Kumar S, Sharma A, Madan B, Singhal V, Ghosh B (2007) Isoliquiritigenin inhibits IkappaB kinase activity and ROS generation to block TNF-alpha induced expression of cell adhesion molecules on human endothelial cells. Biochem Pharmacol 73: 1602-1612
26. Wang KL, Hsia SM, Chan CJ, Chang FY, Huang CY, et al. (2013) Inhibitory effects of isoliquiritigenin on the migration and invasion of human breast cancer cells. Expert Opin Ther Targets 17: 337-349.
27. Cao L, Liu H, Lam DS, Yam GH, Pang CP (2010) In vitro screening for angiostatic potential of herbal chemicals. Invest Ophthalmol Vis Sci 51: 6658-6664.
28. Wu L, Mayo L, Dunbar J, Kessler K, Baerwald M, et al. (2000) Utilization of distinct signaling pathways by receptors for vascular endothelial cell growth factor and other mitogens in the induction of endothelial cell proliferation. Journal of Biological Chemistry 275: 5096-5103
29. Pedram A, Razandi M, Levin ER (1998) Extracellular signal-regulated protein kinase/Jun kinase cross-talk underlies vascular endothelial cell growth factor-induced endothelial cell proliferation. Journal of Biological Chemistry 273: 26722-26728

30. Razandi M, Pedram A, Park ST, Levin ER (2003) Proximal events in signaling by plasma membrane estrogen receptors. J Biol Chem 278: 2701-2712.
31. Jo H, Sipos K, Go Y, Law R, Rong J, et al. (1997) Differential effect of shear stress on extracellular signal-regulated kinase and N-terminal Jun kinase in endothelial cells. Gi2- and Gbeta/gamma-dependent signaling pathways. J Biol Chem 272: 1395-1401
32. Simoncini T, Mannella P, Fornari L, Varone G, Caruso A, et al. (2003) Dehydroepiandrosterone modulates endothelial nitric oxide synthesis via direct genomic and nongenomic mechanisms. Endocrinology 144: 3449-3455.
33. Chang JH, Garg NK, Lunde E, Han KY, Jain S, et al. (2012) Corneal neovascularization: an anti-VEGF therapy review. Surv Ophthalmol 57: 415-429.
34. Xu W, Yang J, Wu LM (2009) Cardioprotective effects of tanshinone IIA on myocardial ischemia injury in rats. Pharmazie 64: 332-336.
35. Fan GW, Gao XM, Wang H, Zhu Y, Zhang J, et al. (2009) The anti-inflammatory activities of Tanshinone IIA, an active component of TCM, are mediated by estrogen receptor activation and inhibition of iNOS. J Steroid Biochem Mol Biol 113: 275-280.
36. Yin X, Yin Y, Cao FL, Chen YF, Peng Y, et al. (2012) Tanshinone IIA attenuates the inflammatory response and apoptosis after traumatic injury of the spinal cord in adult rats. PLoS One 7: e38381.
37. Wang X, Wei Y, Yuan S, Liu G, Lu Y, et al. (2005) Potential anticancer activity of tanshinone IIA against human breast cancer. Int J Cancer 116: 799-807.
38. Won SH, Lee HJ, Jeong SJ, Lee HJ, Lee EO, et al. (2010) Tanshinone IIA induces mitochondria dependent apoptosis in prostate cancer cells in association with an inhibition of phosphoinositide 3-kinase/AKT pathway. Biol Pharm Bull 33: 1828-1834.
39. Tang C, Xue HL, Huang HB, Wang XG (2010) Tanshinone IIA inhibits constitutive STAT3 activation, suppresses proliferation, and induces apoptosis in rat C6 glioma cells. Neurosci Lett 470: 126-129.
40. Jin UH, Suh SJ, Chang HW, Son JK, Lee SH, et al. (2008) Tanshinone IIA from Salvia miltiorrhiza BUNGE inhibits human aortic smooth muscle cell migration and MMP-9 activity through AKT signaling pathway. J Cell Biochem 104: 15-26

# 13

# Neuropsychiatric Effects of *Nigella sativa* (Black Seed)

**Mohammad Akram Randhawa**[1*] **and Shehab Ahmed Alenazi**[2]

[1]*Department of Pharmacology, College of Medicine, Northern Border University, Arar, Saudi Arabia*

[2]*Department of Pediatrics, College of Medicine, Northern Border University, Arar, Saudi Arabia*

[*]**Corresponding author:** Mohammad Akram Randhawa, Professor, Department of Pharmacology, College of Medicine, Northern Border University, P.O. Box 1321, Arar 91431, Saudi Arabia, E-mail: mrakramsa@yahoo.co.uk

**Abstract**

*Nigella sativa* (*N. sativa*) seed, commonly known as 'Black Seed' in English and 'Al-Habba Al-Sauda' in Arabic, had been frequently used as a folk medicine for a large number of diseases since ancient times. *N. sativa* seed, its oil, various extracts and active components are reported to possess very useful pharmacological effects to include: immune stimulation, anti-inflammatory, antioxidant, anticancer, hypoglycemic, antihypertensive, anti-asthmatic, antimicrobial and anti-parasitic, etc. Some authors have reviewed these pharmacological activities in general but their neuropsychiatric effects are not separately and adequately described. The literature search has revealed a lot of publications pertaining to the actions of *N. sativa* in neurological and psychiatric problems, e.g., the control of pain, epilepsy, Parkinsonism, anxiety and drug dependence, as well as improvement of learning and memory, alertness, elevation of mood and feeling of good health, etc. Besides, because of its antioxidant, anti-inflammatory and other useful actions, was shown to provide neuro-protection from spinal cord injury and prevent damage to brain cells from various nerve toxins in experimental animal models. Moreover, black seed showed promising prophylactic and therapeutic effects on murine toxoplasmosis and demonstrated excellent antimalarial activity against various Plasmodium species in in vivo experiments, including *Plasmodium falciparum* strains notorious for causing cerebral malaria. The present article is intended to briefly review the valuable efforts of scientists to investigate the pharmacological activities and therapeutic potential of this precious natural herb pertaining to the neuropsychiatric diseases. It is hoped that the present manuscript would be of particular interest to the neurologists and psychiatrists, and the information provided would also benefit general physicians, medical students and the community.

**Keywords:** *Nigella sativa*; Black seed oil; Extracts; Active components; Neurological and psychiatric problems

## Introduction

*Nigella sativa* (*N. sativa*) is a small annual flowering plant, about 20-30 cm tall, commonly grown in Middle East, Middle Asia and North Africa. It has finely divided green leaves and beautiful, delicate, pale blue and white flowers. The inflated capsule of its ripe fruit is comprised of 3-7 united follicles, each containing numerous oval shaped black tiny seeds, about 1mm in diameter. *N. sativa* belongs to the botanical family of Ranunculaceae and its seeds are named as 'Black Seed' or 'Black Cumin' in English, 'Habba Al-Sauda' or 'Habba Al-Barakah' in Arabic, 'Kalonji' in Urdu, 'Siyah Daneh' in Persian and 'Corek Out' in Turkish language. The scientific name is a derivative of Latin 'niger' meaning 'black' [1].

*N. sativa* seed and its oil have been found in several sites from ancient Egypt, including Tutankhamun's tomb (1350 BD). Items entombed with a pharaoh were carefully selected to assist in the life hereafter [2]. *N. sativa* was included in the list, perhaps, because of its healing effect in many ailments. Interestingly, the cause of death for the boy king of ancient Egypt, who died at the age of 19 years only, has been suggested to be linked to cerebral malaria and temporal lobe epilepsy [3-5]; and recently some studies have reported the beneficial effects of *N. sativa* in malaria as well as epilepsy in *in vivo* experimental models [6,7]. *N. sativa* seed was a traditional condiment of the Old World and since classical times has been extensively used to flavor food [2]. Moreover, black seed and its oil have been employed for the treatment of a variety of conditions in the ancient systems of medicine: Unani, Ayurveda, Chinese and Arabic Medicines [8]. Ibne-Sina in his famous book 'Al-Qanoon fi el-Tibb' or 'The Canon of Medicine' has mentioned many medicinal uses of *N. sativa* including treatment of fever, common cold, headache, asthma, rheumatic diseases, 'Sartan' (cancer), scorpion and spider stings and bites of snake, cat and dog. Moreover, it is narrated that *N. sativa* seed stimulates body's energy and helps recovery from fatigue and dispiritedness [9].

*N. sativa* seed and its oil are known to contain many active components to include: thymoquinone, thymohydroquinone, dithymoquinone, thymol, carvacrol, nigellimine-N-oxide, nigellicine, nigellidine and alpha-hederin. Moreover, *N. sativa* is reported to possess numerous pharmacological properties, like immune stimulation, anti-inflammatory, hypoglycemic, antihypertensive, antiasthmatic, antimicrobial, antiparasitic, antioxidant and anticancer, which have been reviewed by Randhawa and Alghamdi, Ali and Blunden, Salem, Padhye et al. and Ahmed et al. [10-14). In acute and chronic toxicity studies conducted on the laboratory animals, *N. sativa* seed, its oil and thymoquinone, its major active component, were found to be quite safe, particularly when given orally [15-17]. In the review articles mentioned above more stress is laid upon the antiiflammatory, anticancer, antioxidant and cytoprotective properties of the *N. sativa* and its active components. The pharmacological actions and the therapeutic potential pertaining to the central nervous system, particularly effects on psychiatric and neurological dysfunctions, are not adequately described. Besides, a lot more studies have been reported since then regarding neuropsychiatric potential of *N. sativa*.

Therefore, the present manuscript is intended to review and update the scientific knowledge about this precious natural herbal remedy relevant to the neurological and psychiatric illnesses. It is hoped that the present work would be of particular interest to the neurologists and psychiatrists and also benefit general physicians, medical students and the community.

## Methods

An online search was conducted for the published articles related to studies on the effects of *N. sativa* seed, its oil and active components on various clinical conditions concerning the central nervous system and abstracts and full articles in English were included for the preparation of this review. An effort was made to include all available information in the literature pertaining to neurological and psychiatric effects of *N. sativa*. However, it is not possible to cover everything in this short manuscript, therefore, authors apologize for any shortcomings. For the convenience of readers, various effects have been categorized as follows: Analgesic and antipyretic, anti-Parkinsonism, anticonvulsant, antidepressant, antianxiety and neuroprotective effects, as well as effects on tolerance and dependence, learning and memory and encephalitis.

### Analgesic and antipyretic effects

Pain is an important symptom that draws the attention of a patient to get treatment. The sensation of pain has both peripheral and central mechanisms. The peripheral component involves the synthesis of chemical mediators like bradykinin, prostaglandins, thromboxanes and leukotrienes, etc., via activation of cyclooxygenase and lipooxygenase enzymes by the noxious stimuli. These chemical mediators then stimulate the pain receptors in the periphery. The central mechanisms involve the pain transmission via sensory neurons and then its perception in the sensory cortex. Some of the analgesic drugs, like non-steroidal anti-inflammatory drugs (e.g. aspirin), operate through decrease in the synthesis of chemical mediators in the periphery by the inhibition of the enzymes involved in their synthesis. Whereas, others like opioid analgesics (e.g. morphine), operate through the activation of pain modulation pathways, which are closely associated with the pain transmission pathways in the central nervous system. These analgesics act like natural opiopeptins on the spinal and supraspinal κ-, μ- and δ-opioid receptors, present at the level of sensory relay centers, thalamus and sensory cortex in the pain modulation system; thus decrease the pain transmission and perception by the sensory neurons [18,19].

In Saudi Arabia and neighboring countries *N. sativa* oil is used as a topical treatment for pain and stiffness in joints. Fixed oil of *N. sativa* and thymoquinone were demonstrated to block cycloxygenase and 5-lipooxygenase pathways of arachidonate metabolism in the rat peritoneal leukocytes via dose-dependent inhibition of the formation of thromboxane B2 and leukotriene B4, synthesized by the activation of these enzymes, thus confirming its traditional use in arthritic conditions [20]. Later, volatile oil of *N. sativa* and the aqueous suspension of its crushed seeds were shown to inhibit carrageenan induced pain and edema in the hind paw of rats and the analgesic and anti-inflammatory effects were comparable to those of indomethacin and aspirin [21,22]. The results of these studies indicate the participation of the peripheral mechanisms in the control of pain by the *N. sativa*.

Besides the involvement of peripheral mechanisms in the control of pain, some investigators have also reported the possible involvement of the central mechanisms for the antinociceptive effects of *N. sativa*. The oral administration of *N. sativa* oil (50-400 mg/kg) dose-dependently suppressed the nociceptive response in the hot-plate test, tail-pinch test, acetic acid-induced writhing test and in the early phase of the formalin test. The systemic administration (2.5-10 mg/kg oral and 1-6 mg/kg intraperitoneal) and the intracavernous injection (1-4 μg/mouse) of thymoquinone attenuated the nociceptive response in not only the early phase but also the late phase of the formalin test. Naloxone (μ, κ and δ receptor antagonist) injected subcutaneously (1 mg/kg) significantly blocked *N. sativa* oil- and thymoquinone-induced antinociception in the early phase of the formalin test. Moreover, the intracavernous injection of naloxone (10 μg/mouse), the μ1-opioid receptor antagonist, naloxonazine (1-5 μg/mouse), or the κ-opioid receptor antagonist, nor-binaltorphimine (1-5 μg/mouse), significantly reversed thymoquinone-induced antinociception in the early phase of the formalin test, whereas the δ-opioid receptor antagonist, naltrindole (1-5 ng/mouse, intracavernous), had no effect on either phase. The antinociceptive effect of morphine was significantly reduced in thymoquinone and *N. sativa* oil tolerant mice These experiments suggest that the black seed oil and its active component, thymoquinone, produced antinociceptive effects through the central pain modulation pathways (via activation of the supraspinal μ- and κ-opioid receptor subtypes), besides peripheral analgesic and anti-inflammatory effects [23].

Another study also demonstrated potent central nervous system and analgesic activities of the aqueous and methanolic extracts of *N. sativa* seed. The analgesic activity was tested using two different assay procedures, hot-plate test and pressure test. Both extracts induced significant effects on reaction time in the hot-plate and pressure tests. The methanolic extract showed an increase in analgesic activity with respect to time, reaching a maximum effect at 180 min after the intraperitoneal administration. The aqueous extract recorded its maximum effect at 60 min from the time of administration. The same trend was observed with the pressure test. Moreover, the aqueous and methanolic extracts caused a significant decrease of normal body temperature after 30 min ($-3.15 \pm 0.35$ and $-2.18 \pm 0.41$, respectively) [24].

However, in some studies investigators could not demonstrate the involvement of opioid receptors. For example in one study black seed essential oil was found to produce a significant analgesic effect in acetic acid-induced writhing, formalin and light tail flick tests, but the opioid antagonist, naloxone, could not reverse the analgesic effect observed in the formalin test. In the same study oral administration of essential oil at doses of 100, 200 and 400 μL/kg did not exert a significant anti-inflammatory effect in the carrageenan test, however, intraperitoneal injection at the same doses significantly ($p<0.001$) inhibited carrageenan-induced paw edema. The essential oil at doses of 10 and 20 μL/ear also reduced croton oil-induced edema. The authors concluded that mechanism(s) other than opioid receptors are involved in the analgesic effect of essential oil since naloxone could not reverse this effect [25].

Similarly, in another study, oral and intraperitoneal administration of *N. sativa* polyphenols (NSP) significantly suppressed, in a dose-dependent manner, the nociceptive response in the early and late phases of the formalin test, and the effect on the late phase was more pronounced. Pretreatment with naloxone failed to reverse the analgesic activity of NSP in this test. In the acetic acid-induced writhing test, oral administration of NSP decreased the number of abdominal constrictions. NSP did not produce a significant analgesia in the light tail flick test in mice. Oral administration of NSP did not produce a significant reduction in carrageenan-induced paw edema, however, when injected intraperitoneally, NSP inhibited paw edema in a dose dependent manner. The authors concluded that NSP had analgesic and anti-inflammatory effects and the lack of analgesic effect of NSP in the light tail flick test and also the failure of naloxone to reverse the analgesia in the formalin test indicated that mechanisms other than stimulation of opioid receptors are involved [26].

The controversial results of the above mentioned studies, regarding the involvement of peripheral or central mechanisms for anti-nociceptive effects of *N. sativa*, are perhaps due to different types of extracts, chemical constituents, routes of administration and, particularly, doses used in these studies. Further investigations are required with more specific substances from the *N. sativa* seed and proper study designs to resolve these differences.

## Anticonvulsant effects

Epilepsy is known from ancient times and since then *N. sativa* seed and its oil have been used for its treatment. As mentioned above in the introduction also, the selection of black seed amongst the burial goods in the tomb of Tutinkhamun is perhaps related to epilepsy and cerebral malaria as the possible causes of his death at a relatively younger age [3-5]. The black seed was perhaps prescribed for the treatment in his life time and was included in the burial goods to continue its use in the life hereafter (as it was believed). Many studies, mentioned below, have confirmed the use of black seed for the treatment of epilepsy in the folk medicine.

Thymoquinone, the major constituent of *N. sativa* seed, was investigated for the anticonvulsant effects using pentylenetetrazole (PTZ) - and maximal electroshock (MES) - induced seizure models. In PTZ-induced seizures, thymoquinone given intraperitoneally (40 and 80 mg/kg), prolonged the onset and reduced the duration of myoclonic seizures. The protective effect of thymoquinone against mortality was 71.4% and 100% in these doses, respectively. In MES model, thymoquinone failed to reduce the duration of seizure, whereas exhibited a complete protection against mortality [27].

Similarly, pretreatment with *N. sativa* oil was tested for its ability to suppress the convulsive and lethal effects of PTZ in kindled mice (anti-epileptogenic effect) and to attenuate the PTZ-induced oxidative injury in the brain tissue (antioxidant effect). Valproate, a major antiepileptic drug, was also tested for comparison. Both substances significantly decreased oxidative injury in the mouse brain tissue, however, *N. sativa* oil was found to be more effective than valproate in preventing PTZ-induced seizures [28]. Likewise, aqueous extract of *N. sativa* seeds suppressed penicillin- induced epileptic activity in rats, which was possibly due to selectively altering the monoamine level in different regions of brain [7].

Despite the availability and use of numerous antiepileptic drugs, nearly 15% of childhood epilepsy cases are reported to be resistant to treatment. Knowing that the *N. sativa* ameliorated fits in the experimental models of epilepsy, a double-blind crossover placebo controlled clinical trial was conducted in children (13 months to 13 years) with refractory epilepsy. The aqueous extract of black seed (40 mg/kg/8 h), or placebo were administered as an adjunct therapy for four weeks. The frequency of seizures significantly decreased in the children receiving *N. sativa* extract compared to placebo ($p<0.05$). The authors concluded that the water extract of *N. sativa* had antiepileptic effects in children with refractory seizures [29].

Later, in another study, aqueous extract, fixed oil and volatile oil of black seed and its major active constituents (thymoquinone, α-pinene and p-cymene) were investigated against PTZ and maximal electroshock (MES)-induced convulsions. The potential of these constituents to induce minimal neurological deficit (MND) was also evaluated by using chimney test. All of the black seed constituents protected mice effectively against PTZ-induced convulsions except fixed oil. Volatile oil and its component p-cymene effectively suppressed convulsions induced by MES. All of the *N. sativa* seed constituents induced varying degrees of MND in the chimney test. In the same study, exploration on the role of receptors suggested that picrotoxin and bicuculline-sensitive GABA receptors, most probably GABA-A receptors, mediated an increase in GABA-ergic response. Moreover, thymoquinone potentiated the effect of valproate in both PTZ and MES models [30].

Recently, antioxidant and antiepileptic effects of curcumin, *N. sativa* oil and valproate in the pilocarpine-induced animal model of chronic epilepsy were also studied. The animals were treated with curcumin, *N. sativa* oil or valproate for 21 days and there was reversal of the levels of malondialdehyde, nitric oxide and reduced glutathione and restoration of the activities of CAT, Na+, K+-ATPase and acetylcholinesterase in the hippocampus, as well as the reduction of seizures [31].

## Antipakinsonism effects

Parkinson's disease is a slowly progressive neurodegenerative disorder caused by the damage to a small group of brain cells in the basal ganglia that control body movements. The available drug treatments for Parkinson's disease effectively control the symptoms but have many adverse effects. Natural herbal products could be better and safer substitutes for the management of Parkinsonism. Recently, some studies were carried out to evaluate the anti Parkinsonian activity of *N. sativa*. For example, the ethanolic extract of *N. sativa* seed (200 and 400 mg/kg orally) was investigated in chlorpromazine induced experimental animal model of catalepsy, besides the assessment of its effects on chemical parameters (TBARS, GSH, Nitrite and Total Protein). The cataleptic score was significantly reduced ($P<0.001$) with *N. sativa*. *N. sativa* also improved the depleted levels of reduced glutathione (GSH) ($P<0.001$) and total protein ($P<0.001$) and decreased the elevated levels of TBARS ($P<0.001$) and Nitrite ($P<0.001$) [32].

It is known that α-synuclein (αSN) induces synaptic toxicity and was reported to decrease the level of synaptophysin, a protein used as an indicator of synaptic density, in cultured hippocampal and hiPSC-derived neurons. Simultaneous treatment with αSN and thymoquinone protected neurons against αSN-induced synapstic damage, as revealed by immunostaining. Moreover, administration of thymoquinone efficiently induced protection in these cells against αSN-induced inhibition of synaptic vesicle recycling in hippocampal and hiPSC-derived neurons as well as against mutated P123H β-synuclein (βSN) neurons, as revealed by experiments using the fluorescent dye FM1-43. It was further demonstrated that thymoquinone reversed aSN-induced reduction in spontaneous firing activity. These results suggested that thymoquinone protected cultured rat primary hippocampal and hiPSC-derived neurons against αSN-induced synaptic toxicity and could be a promising therapeutic agent for patients with Parkinson's disease and dementia with Lewy bodies [33].

Thymoquinone was also shown to improve behavioral and cellular abnormalities and markers of oxidative stress in an experimental model of early Parkinson's disease in rats. In this study unilateral intrastriatal 6-hydroxydopamine (6-OHDA)-lesioned rats were pretreated with oral thymoquinone at doses of 5 and/or 10 mg/Kg three times daily for one week. Thymoquinone pretreatment significantly improved turning behavior, prevented loss of neurons in substantia nigra and lowered level of MDA. These results suggested that TQ could afford neuroprotection in neuro-degenerative disorders including Parkinson's disease [34].

## Neuroprotective effects

Besides the protection of neurons related to Parkinsonism, mentioned above, *N. sativa* extracts and its active components were also shown to prevent damage to spinal cord and other brain cells from trauma and various nerve toxins.

Possible beneficial effects of *N. sativa* in comparison to methylprednisolone were investigated on experimental spinal cord injury (SCI) in rats. SCI was performed by placing an aneurysm clip extradurally at the level of T11-12. SCI significantly increased the spinal cord tissue malondialdehyde (MDA) and protein carbonyl (PC) levels, however, SCI decreased superoxide dismutase (SOD), glutathione peroxidase (GSH-Px), and catalase (CAT) enzyme activities compared to the control. Methylprednisolone and *N. sativa* treatment decreased tissue MDA and PC levels and prevented inhibition of SOD, GSH-Px and CAT enzymes in the tissues [35].

Toluene is a common industrial solvent and long term exposure can cause damage to brain cells. The neuroprotective effect of *N. sativa* and thymoquinone were investigated in hippocampus after chronic toluene exposure in rats. The rats were randomly allotted into one of four experimental groups: Control, toluene treated, toluene with *N. sativa* extract and toluene with thymoquinone. Chronic toluene exposure caused severe degenerative changes, shrunken cytoplasm, slightly dilated cisternae of endoplasmic reticulum, markedly swollen mitochondria with degenerated cristae and nuclear membrane breakdown with chromatin disorganization in neurons of the hippocampus. The distorted nerve cells were mainly absent in thymoquinone and *N. sativa* extract treated rats [36].

Propoxur is a broad spectrum carbamate, widely used as a household insecticide and can cause neurotoxicity. The black seed oil significantly reversed the abnormalities induced by propoxur in the lipid peroxidation, protein carbonyl content, acetylcholine esterase activity and demonstrated antioxidant activities in different parts of rat brain [37].

Cerebral ischemia or stroke is a common cause of mortality and requires development of new drugs for its prevention and treatment. Recently, aqueous, hydroalcoholic, chloroform and petroleum ether extracts of *N. sativa* seeds (400 mg/kg, orally for 7 days) were evaluated for their neuroprotective role in cerebral ischemia induced by middle cerebral artery (MCA) occlusion in rats. Pretreatment with various extracts of *N. sativa* improved locomotor activity and grip strength of animals as compared to controls. Changes in the level of thiobarbituric acid reactive substance (TBARS), glutathione (GSH), superoxide dismutase (SOD) and catalase levels produced by MCA occlusion were also reversed. Authors concluded that the neuroprotective effects of *N. sativa* were due to its antioxidant, free radical scavenging and anti-inflammatory properties [38, 39].

Moreover, metformin and thymoquinone were reported to have strong protective effect against ethanol-induced neuronal apoptosis in primary rat cortical neurons, as they inhibited the apoptotic cascade by increasing Bcl-2 expression, repressed the activation of caspase-9 and caspase-3, reduced the cleavage of PARP-1 and prevented morphological changes [40].

## Antidepressant effects

In the folk medicine *N. sativa* seeds are reported to be used for the feeling of wellbeing, stimulate energy and recovery from fatigue and dispiritedness [9]. Recently, hydro-alcoholic extract of *N. sativa* and thymoquinone were investigated for their effect on lipopolysaccharide-induced depression like behavior in rats using forced swimming test and open field test. Forced swimming test was performed 3 times, on alternate days, for all groups: Passive controls (only saline), active controls (lipopolysaccharide 100 μg/kg, intraperitoneally 2 hours before test) and treated groups (receiving different doses of *N. sativa* extract or thymoquinone before lipopolysaccharide), and the immobility time was recorded each time. The immobility time in the active control (lipopolysaccharide group) was higher than that of control group (saline alone) in all 3 times, whereas, the groups pretreated with *N. sativa* extract or thymoquinone lowered immobility times as compared to active controls. In the open- field test, the peripheral crossing number was higher in active controls than passive controls; while in the animals pretreated with *N. sativa* extract or thymoquinone it was lower than active controls. Furthermore, the central crossing number was lower in the lipopolysaccharide group than that of saline controls, whereas, in animals pretreated with *N. sativa* extract or thymoquinone, the central crossing number was higher than that of active controls. The results indicated that hydro-alcoholic extract of *N. sativa* and its active principle, thymoquinone, could prevent lipopolysaccharide-induced depression like behavior in rats [41].

Considering the beneficial effects of *N. sativa* in the prevention of depression and relief of anxiety in animal studies a placebo controlled randomized clinical trial was carried out at a boarding school on young healthy adolescent human volunteers to investigate the effect of *N. sativa* seed on mood and anxiety. The assessment of mood was done with Bond-Lader scale and anxiety with State-Trait Anxiety Inventory, at the beginning and after four weeks of ingestion of 500mg once daily of either placebo (Group A) or *N. sativa* seed (Group B). Although the results for the evaluation of mood and anxiety were statistically not significantly different between group A and B, but there was statistically significant variation within group B and no variation within group A in both parameters. The authors suggested that the use of *N. sativa* seed as a nutritional supplement had positive effect on mood and anxiety [42].

## Antianxiety effects

Hole-Board test is frequently used for the validation of the anxiety in small animals. The number of holes explored in a specified time is counted after the administration of the test drug. The increased exploration capacity is considered to be an index of anxiety, but it is difficult to separate it from motor activity. A significant decrease in exploratory conduct in the mice was produced by the aqueous and methanolic extracts of *N. sativa*, using hole-board test. The effect of these extracts on spontaneous motor activity and motor coordination was also observed. The spontaneous motility was recorded in a photoactometer, whereas the motor coordination was examined by

Rota-Rod test. Both of these extracts caused a significant decrease in the spontaneous motility as well as motor coordination [24].

Benzodiazepines are commonly used for the management of anxiety and they also produce muscle relaxation and motor incoordination in higher doses [43]. If proper dose-response curves are constructed for the antianxiety effect and for the motor in coordination with the *N. sativa* extract, perhaps, we can differentiate between the therapeutic doses relieving anxiety and the toxic doses causing motor incoordination.

In another study, antianxiety effect of *N. sativa* oil was studied in rats, using open field and elevated plus maze models. After the oral administration of *N. sativa* oil for 4 weeks, the rats exhibited an increase in open field activity. The oil also produced anti-anxiety effect in rats when tested in elevated plus maze. There was an increase in the brain levels of 5-HT (5-hydroxy-trytamine, or Serotonin), but the levels of brain 5-HIAA (hydroxyindole acetic acid), a metabolite of 5-HT, decreased significantly. Brain and plasma levels of tryptophan also increased significantly. Therefore, it was suggested that *N. sativa* oil is a useful choice for the treatment of anxiety [44]. Although by different mechanism, perhaps by decreasing the metabolism of 5-HT, these changes in 5-HT levels produced by *N. sativa* oil are similar to changes produced by Serotonin Specific Reuptake Inhibitors (SSRIs), used in the treatment of anxiety and depression.

Moreover, the toxicity of methanolic extract of *N. sativa* on cultured rat cortical neurons and its influence on the release of excitatory (glutamate and aspartate) and inhibitory (gamma-aminobutyric acid and glycine) neurotransmitters in these neurons was also investigated. The cultured neurons were exposed to different times and concentrations of dried methanolic extract and cell viability was then determined by a quantitative colorimetric method. The extract did not induce any toxic effects on these neurons. However, the extract modulated amino acid release in the cultured neurons: GABA was significantly increased whereas secretion of glutamate, aspartate, and glycine were decreased. These findings suggest that the sedative and antianxiety effects of methanolic extract of *N. sativa* are related to changes in the inhibitory and excitatory amino acids levels [45].

Furthermore, the antianxiety effect of thymoquinone and its effect on the modulation of GABA and NO levels in brain were investigated in both the unstressed and stressed mice (mice subjected to 6 h immobilization). Thymoquinone (10 and 20 mg/kg), methylene blue (1 mg/kg) and diazepam (2 mg/kg) were administered intraperitoneally, followed by behavioral testing using an elevated plus maze, the light/dark test and the social interaction test in both unstressed and stressed mice. The effects of the above-mentioned drugs on plasma nitrite, a stable metabolite of nitric oxide and brain GABA content were also studied. Thymoquinone (10 and 20 mg/kg) produced significant antianxiety effects in unstressed mice without altering nitrite levels, but only the higher dose (20 mg/kg) of thymoquinone increased the GABA content in unstressed mice. In stressed mice, TQ (20 mg/kg) showed anxiolytic effects, with a significant decrease in plasma nitrite and reversal of the decreased brain GABA content. Pre-treatment with methylene blue enhanced the antianxiety effect of thymoquinone in both unstressed and stressed mice. It was concluded that NO-cGMP and GABA-ergic pathways are involved in the anxiolytic-like activity of thymoquinone [46]. Benzodiazepines are well known to relieve anxiety by GABA-mimetic effects [43].

## Effects on learning and memory

A long term administration of *N. sativa* increased 5-HT levels in brain and improved learning memory in rats [47]. Considering the experimental evidences for the beneficial effects of *N. sativa* seed on improvement of memory and learning, a randomized placebo controlled study was designed to investigate the effects of *N. sativa* seed on memory, attention and cognition in healthy elderly volunteers. The study group A received 500 mg *N. sativa* seed capsule twice daily for nine weeks and group B received placebo in the similar manner. There was significant difference ($p<0.05$) in the score of logical memory test-I and II, total score of digit span, 30 min delayed-recall, percent score in Rey-Osterrieth complex figure test, time taken to complete letter cancellation test, time taken in trail making test-A and test-B, score in part C of stroop test between two groups. The biochemical markers of cardiac, liver and kidney functions remained normal in both groups throughout the study period. It was concluded that *N. sativa* enhances memory, attention and cognition and thus could be considered as potential food supplement for the prevention of Alzheimer disease in elderly. However, for the treatment of Alzheimer disease and cognitive disorders further long term studies are recommended [48].

In another study, the effect of *N. sativa* on cognition in adolescent human males was examined at a boarding school in Bangladesh, besides the effect on mood and anxiety mentioned above. Two groups of recruited volunteers, A and B, received capsule of 500 mg placebo and 500 mg *N. sativa* seed, respectively, once daily for four weeks. All the volunteers were assessed for cognition with modified California verbal learning test-II (CVLT-II) at the beginning and after four weeks of either *N. sativa* or placebo ingestion. In the beginning of the study all parameters showed statistically similar results between group A and B. After 4 weeks of treatment CVLT II revealed that there was significant variation within group B in immediate short-term recall at trial 4 and 5 whereas this difference was found only in case of trial 5 between group A and B. However, long-term free recall and long-term cued recall had statistical differences between group A and B. The results indicated positive effect on the mood and anxiety [49].

Recently, a study was conducted to evaluate the effect of hydro-alcoholic extract of *N. sativa* on memory performance and its possible mechanisms in scopolamine-induced spatial memory impairment model using Morris water maze test. The time latency and path length in the Scopolamine treated group were significantly higher than in the passive controls receiving saline ($P<0.01$), while the *N. sativa* treated group showed a significantly shorter travel path and time latency compared to the active control receiving Scopolamine ($P<0.01$). Acetycholinestrase activity in the cortical tissues of the Scopolamine group was significantly higher than the passive control group ($P<0.01$), while Acetycholinestrase activity in the *N. sativa* treated groups was lower than the Scopolamine group ($P<0.01$). Moreover, pretreatment of the animals with *N. sativa* decreased the malondialdehyde concentration in hippocampal tissues and increased the thiol content compared to control group ($p<0.001$). The results revealed that the hydro-alcoholic extract of *N. sativa* prevented scopolamine-induced spatial memory deficits and decreased the Acetycholinestrase activity and oxidative stress induced by scopolamine in rats [50]. A similar study also demonstrated positive effects on learning and memory of rats after feeding of hydro-alcoholic extract of *N. sativa* during neonatal and juvenile growth [51].

## Effects on tolerance and dependence

Drug dependence is one of the major social and psychiatric problems of society. The drug abusers usually report to seek the treatment of withdrawal effects of drugs of dependence. The withdrawal effects are mostly controlled with the replacement therapy of a similar drug, which is usually longer acting. For example, withdrawal effects due to opioid drugs (Morphine and heroin) are controlled with a longer acting opioid, methadone.

In a clinical study *N. sativa* was shown to control the withdrawal effects of opioid dependence and its long term use prevented its abuse as well. No changes were observed in the physiological parameters (Blood pressure, pulse rate and respiration, etc.). The appetite increased but there was no significant weight gain. Besides the control of opioid dependence, *N. sativa* also treated the infections and weakness, from which the majority of addicts suffered [52].

An animal study was conducted to elucidate the possible mechanism of action of protective effect of *N. sativa* oil against tramadol-induced tolerance and dependence in mice by the hot plate test. Naloxone, a potent opioid antagonist (5 mg/kg, intraperitoneally), was shown to precipitate the withdrawal manifestations. Black seed oil also inhibited nitric oxide overproduction and increase in brain malondialdehyde level induced by repeated administration of tramadol to mice or by administration of naloxone to tramadol-dependent mice. The inhibitory effect of *N. sativa* oil on tramadol-induced tolerance and dependence was enhanced by concurrent intraperitonial administration of the NMDA receptor antagonist, dizocilpine (0.25mg/kg). Also, the inhibitory effect of the oil on naloxone-induced biochemical alterations in tramadol-dependent mice was enhanced by concurrent administration of dizocilpine. Similarly, concurrent administration of the NO synthase inhibitor, L-N (G)-nitroarginine methyl ester (10mg/kg) or the antioxidant, N-acetylcysteine (50mg/kg) enhanced these inhibitory effects of *N. sativa* oil. On the other hand, these effects were antagonized by concurrent administration of NO precursor, L-arginine (300 mg/kg). These results provide evidence that *N. sativa* oil appears to have a therapeutic potential in tramadol tolerance and dependence through blockade of NO overproduction and oxidative stress induced by the drug [53].

## Effect on encephalitis

**Toxoplasmosis:** *Toxoplasma gondii* is an intracellular protozoan parasite, with a worldwide distribution and causes opportunistic infection in humans and animals. Toxoplasmosis is a risk for newborns and for immunocompromized individuals, such as HIV carriers and patients receiving anticancer or immunesuppressant drugs. Infection of an immunocompetent human host leaves the subject with a life-long latent infection in the form of quiescent tissue cysts present mainly in the brain and muscles [54]. Combination of pyrimethamine and sulphadiazine is commonly used for treatment and prophylaxis of most clinical presentations of toxoplasmosis. However, this combination is not always suitable for prolonged treatment because of the appearance of adverse side effects.

Black seed oil (BSO) has been reported to show promising prophylactic and therapeutic effects against *T. gondii* in a murine model of infection. The mice were orally inoculated with *T. gondii* (Me49 strain) to cause brain cysts and divided into 3 groups: prophylactic group (given BSO for two weeks before *T. gondii* infection), treated group (given BSO on day 4 post infection) and control group (infected untreated). The effect of BSO was evaluated by the assessment of survival rate and brain cyst burden, brain histopathological lesions and immunohistochemical expression of inducible nitric oxide synthase (iNOS). In prophylactic or therapeutic groups BSO significantly enhanced protection of infected mice against death ($P=0.01$) and reduced brain cyst burdens at 5, 7 and 12 weeks post infection ($P<0.05$) compared to the infected untreated control. The brains of BSO prophylactic or therapeutic groups showed milder meningitis, encephalitis and perivascular cuffing compared to the infected untreated control ($P<0.05$). Moreover, expression of iNOS was significantly enhanced in both BSO prophylactic and therapeutic groups compared to the untreated infected control [55].

**Malaria:** Malaria is a significant public health problem in many countries of the world and causes substantial morbidity and mortality. *Plasmodium falciparum* is notorious to cause organ damage including brain and causes cerebral symptoms. The oxidative stress is an important factor in the pathophysiology of malaria, is mainly due to the generation of oxygen-nitrogen reactive species and causes further damage. The use of antioxidant supplements of synthetic or natural origin would constitute an effective adjuvant antimalarial therapy to prevent damage to the host and control cerebral symptoms [56]. *N. sativa* has been demonstrated to possess both the antimalarial and antioxidant properties and is a suitable potential remedy for cerebral malaria. *N. sativa* seeds extract when examined *in vitro* for antimalarial activity against schizonts maturation of *Plasmodium falciparum*, showed 100% inhibition of the parasite growth at a concentration of 50 mug/ml [57]. Methanolic extract of *N. sativa* seed was reported to possess both antimalarial and antioxidant activities against *Plasmodium yoelli nigeriensis* (*P. yoelli*) infection in mice. The extract, at a dose of 1.25 g/kg body weight not only suppressed *P. yoelli* infection in the mice, but also reversed the increase in levels of red cell and hepatic malondialdehyde (MDA) and the decrease in activities of superoxide dismutase, catalase, glutathione-S-transferase and the level of reduced glutathione in tissues of the mice [58]. In another study also the water extract of *N. sativa* seed was shown to have both anti-malarial and antioxidant effects and significantly reduced parasitaemia count and level of nitric oxide and increased survival rates of *Plasmodium berghei* NK65 infected mice [59]. Earlier, ethanol, chloroform and aqueous seed extracts of *N. sativa* were also demonstrated to possess anti-malarial properties against *Plasmodium berghei* in mice [6]. In a recent study, *N. sativa* seed or oil in feed in combination with chloroquine was shown to produce complete parasitaemia clearance and 100% survival rate in mice infected with chloroquine sensitive *Plasmodium berghei*, NK65 strain. Parasitaemia clearance and survival rate produced by these combinations were greater than *N. sativa* seed in feed or *N. sativa* oil extract in feed or chloroquine alone [60].

## Conclusions

*N. sativa* is known to possess a wide variety of medicinal properties and has been used as a natural remedy for many diseases since ancient times. In the present article neuropsychiatric effects are reviewed separately for the first time. In many animal experiments and few clinical trials it was found to be effective in the control of pain, fever, epilepsy, Parkinsonism, anxiety, depression, toxoplasmosis, malaria and to improve memory, mood and feeling of good health. Further basic and clinical investigations are needed to confirm these observations. Isolation of the active principles and preparation of more remedies from their derivatives are, perhaps, the future targets for the development of new drugs for neurological and psychiatric diseases.

## References


1. https://en.wikipedia.org/wiki/Nigella Sativa.
2. Zohary D, Hopf M (2000). Domestication of plants in the Old World (3rd edn).Oxford University Press. p. 206.
3. Roberts, M (16 February 2010).'Malaria' killed King Tutankhamun', BBC News. Retrieved 12 March 2010.
4. Hawass Z, Gad YZ, Ismail S, Khairat R, Fathalla D, et al. (2010) Ancestry and pathology in King Tutankhamun's family. JAMA 303: 638-647.
5. Rosenbaum, M (14 September 2012). "Mystery of King Tut's death solved?". ABC News. Retrieved 21 October 2013.
6. Abdulelah H, Zainal-Abidin B (2007) In vivo anti-malarial tests of Nigella Sativa (Black seed) different extracts. Am J Pharmacol Toxicol 2: 46-50.
7. Guha D, Biswas D, Purkayastha S (2005) Suppression of penicillin-induced epileptiform activity by Nigella Sativa: possible mediation by neurotransmitters. Biogenic Amines 19: 309-321.
8. El-Kadi A, Kandil O (1986) Effect of Nigella Sativa (the black seed) on immunity. Proceedings of the Fourth International Conference on Islamic Medicine, Kuwait.
9. Al-Jishi SAA (2000) Study of Nigella Sativa on blood hemostatic functions. MSc Thesis, King Faisal University, Dammam, Saudi Arabia.
10. Randhawa MA and Alghamdi MS (2002) A review of the pharmaco-therapeutic effects of Nigella Sativa. Pak J Med Res 41: 77-83.
11. Ali BH, Blunden G (2003) Pharmacological and toxicological properties of Nigella sativa. Phytother Res 17: 299-305.
12. Salem ML (2005) Immunomodulatory and therapeutic properties of the Nigella sativa L. seed. Int Immunopharmacol 5: 1749-1770.
13. Padhye S, Banerjee S, Ahmad A, Mohammad R, Sarkar FH (2008) From here to eternity - the secret of Pharaohs: Therapeutic potential of black cumin seeds and beyond. Cancer Ther 6: 495-510.
14. Ahmad A, Husain A, Mujeeb M, Khan SA, Najmi AK, et al. (2013) A review on therapeutic potential of Nigella sativa: A miracle herb. Asian Pac J Trop Biomed 3: 337-352.
15. Badary OA, Al-Shabana OA, Nagi MN, Al-Bekairi AM, Elmazar MMA (1998) Acute and subchronic toxicity of thymoquinone in mice. Drug Develop Res 44: 56-61.
16. Mansour MA, Ginwai OT, El-Hadiya T, ElKhatib AS, Al-Shabanah OA, et al. (2001) Effects of volatile oil constituents of Nigella Sativa on carbon tetrachloride-hepatotoxicity in mice: evidence for antioxidant effects of thymoquinone. Res Commun Mol Pathol Pharmacol 110: 239-251.
17. Al-Ali A, Alkhawajah AA, Randhawa MA, Shaikh NA (2008) Oral and intraperitoneal LD50 of thymoquinone, an active principle of Nigella sativa, in mice and rats. J Ayub Med Coll Abbottabad 20: 25-27.
18. Katzung BG, Masters SB, Trevor AJ (2009) Chapter 36, NSAIDs. Basic and Clinical Pharmacology (11thedn) Mc Graw Hill, LANGE Medical Books, New York, p622-623.
19. Katzung BG, Masters SB, Trevor AJ (2009) Chapter 31, Opioid Analgesics. Basic and Clinical Pharmacology (11thedn) Mc Graw Hill, LANGE Medical Books, New York, p534-537.
20. Houghton PJ, Zarka R, de lasHeras B, Hoult JR (1995) Fixed oil of Nigella Sativa and derived thymoquinone inhibit eicosanoid generation in leukocytes and membrane lipid peroxidation. Planta Med. 61: 33-36.
21. Mutabagani A, El-Mahdy SAM (1997) A study of the anti-inflammatory activity of Nigella Sativa L and thymoquinone in rats. Saudi Pharm J 5 : 110-113.
22. Al-Ghamdi MS (2001) The anti-inflammatory, analgesic and antipyretic activity of Nigella sativa. J Ethnopharmacol 76: 45-48.
23. Abdel-Fattah AM, Matsumoto K, Watanabe H (2000) Antinociceptive effects of Nigella sativa oil and its major component, thymoquinone, in mice. in Eur J Pharmacol 400: 89-97.
24. Al-Naggar TB, Gómez-Serranillos MP, Carretero ME, Villar AM (2003) Neuropharmacological activity of Nigella sativa L. extracts. in J Ethnopharmacol 88: 63-68.
25. Hajhashemi V, Ghannadi A, Jafarabadi H (2004) Black cumin seed essential oil, as a potent analgesic and antiinflammatory drug. Phytother Res 18: 195-199.
26. Ghannadi A, Hajhashemi V, Jafarabadi H (2005) An investigation of the analgesic and anti-inflammatory effects of Nigella sativa seed polyphenols. J Med Food 8: 488-493.
27. Hosseinzadeh H, Parvardeh S (2004) Anticonvulsant effects of thymoquinone, the major constituent of Nigella sativa seeds, in mice. Phytomedicine 11: 56-64.
28. Ilhan A, Gurel A, Armutcu F, Kamisli S, Iraz M (2005) Antiepileptogenic and antioxidant effects of Nigella sativa oil against pentylenetetrazol-induced kindling in mice. Neuropharmacology 49: 456-464.
29. Akhondian J, Parsa A, Rakhshande H (2007) The effect of Nigella sativa L. (black cumin seed) on intractable pediatric seizures. Med Sci Monit 13: CR555-559.
30. Raza M, Alghasham AA, Alorainy MS, El-Hadiyah TM (2008) Potentiation of Valproate-induced Anticonvulsant Response by Nigella sativa Seed Constituents: The Role of GABA Receptors. Int J Health Sci (Qassim) 2: 15-25.
31. Ezz HS, Khadrawy YA, Noor NA (2011) The neuroprotective effect of curcumin and Nigella sativa oil against oxidative stress in the pilocarpine model of epilepsy: a comparison with valproate. Neurochem Res 36: 2195-2204.
32. Sandhu K, Rana A (2013) Evaluation of antiparkinson's activity of Nigela sativa (Kalonji) seeds in chlorpromazine induced experimental animal model. Int J Pharm Pharm Sci 5: 884-888.
33. Alhebshi AH, Odawara A, Gotoh M, Suzuki I (2013) Thymoquinone protects cultured hippocampal and human induced pluripotent stem cells-derived neurons against a-synuclein-induced synapse damage. NeurosciLett.
34. Sedaghat R, Roghani M, Khalili M (2014) Neuroprotective effect of thymoquinone, the nigella sativa bioactive compound, in 6-hydroxydopamine-induced hemi-parkinsonian rat model. Iran J Pharm Res 13: 227-234.
35. Kanter M, Coskun O, Kalayci M, Buyukbas S, Cagavi F (2006) Neuroprotective effects of Nigella sativa on experimental spinal cord injury in rats. Hum Exp Toxicol 25: 127-133.
36. Kanter M (2008) Nigella Sativa and derived thymoquinone prevents hippocampal neurodegeneration after chronic toluene exposure in rats. Neurochem. Res 33: 579-588.
37. Mohamadin AM, Sheikh B, Abdel-Aal AA, Elberry AA, Al-Abbasie FA (2010) Protective effects of Nigella Sativa oil on propoxur-induced toxicityand oxidative stress in rat brain regions. Pesticide Biochemistry and Physiology 98: 128-134.
38. Akhtar M, Maikiyo AM, Khanam R, Mujeeb M, Aqil M, et al. (2012) Ameliorating effects of two extracts of Nigella sativa in middle cerebral artery occluded rat. J Pharm Bioallied Sci. 4: 70–75.
39. Akhtar M, Maikiyo AM, Najmi AK, Khanam R, Mujeeb M, et al. (2013) Neuroprotective effects of chloroform and petroleum ether extracts of Nigella sativa seeds in stroke model of rat. J Pharm Bioallied Sci 5: 119–125.
40. Ikram-Ullah, Najeeb-Ullah, Naseer MI, Le HY, Myeong OK (2012) Neuroprotection with metformin and thymoquinone against ethanol-induced apoptotic neurodegeneration in prenatal rat cortical neurons. BMC Neuroscience 13:11.
41. Hosseini M, Zakeri S, Khoshdast S, Yousefian FT, Rastegar M, et al. (2012) The effects of Nigella sativa hydro-alcoholic extract and thymoquinone on lipopolysaccharide - induced depression like behavior in rats. J Pharm Bioallied Sci 4: 219-225.
42. Bin Sayeed MS, Shams T, Fahim Hossain S, Rahman MR, Mostofa A, et al. (2014) Nigella sativa L. seeds modulate mood, anxiety and cognition in healthy adolescent males. J Ethnopharmacol 152: 156-162.
43. Katzung BG, Masters SB, Trevor AJ (2009) Chapter 22, Sedatives and antianxiety drugs. Basic and Clinical Pharmacology (11thedn) Mc Graw Hill, LANGE Medical Books, New York, 359-360.

44. Perveen T, Haider S, Kanwal S, Haleem DJ (2009) Repeated administration of Nigella sativa decreases 5-HT turnover and produces anxiolytic effects in rats. Pak J Pharm Sci 22: 139-144.
45. El-Naggar T, Gómez-Serranillos MP, Palomino OM, Arce C, Carretero ME (2010) Nigella sativa L. seed extract modulates the neurotransmitter amino acids release in cultured neurons in vitro. J Biomed Biotechnol 2010: 398312.
46. Gilhotra N, Dhingra D (2011) Thymoquinone produced antianxiety-like effects in mice through modulation of GABA and NO levels. Pharmacol Rep 63: 660-669.
47. Perveen T, Abdullah A, Haider S, Sonia B, Munawar AS, et al. (2008) Long-term administration of Nigella Sativa effects nociceotion and improves learning and memory in rats. Pak J Biochem Mol Biol 41: 141-143.
48. Bin Sayeed MS, Asaduzzaman M, Morshed H, Hossain MM, Kadir MF, et al. (2013) The effect of Nigella sativa Linn. seed on memory, attention and cognition in healthy human volunteers. J Ethnopharmacol 148: 780-786.
49. Bin Sayeed MS, Shams T, Fahim Hossain S, Rahman MR, Mostofa A, et al. (2014) Nigella sativa L. seeds modulate mood, anxiety and cognition in healthy adolescent males. J Ethnopharmacol 152: 156-162.
50. Hosseini M, Mohammadpour T, Karami R, Rajaei Z, Sadeghnia HR, et al. (2015) Effects of the hydro-alcoholic extract of Nigella Sativa on scopolamine-induced spatial memory impairment in rats and its possible mechanism. Chinese Journal of Integrative Medicine 21: 438-444.
51. Beheshti F, Hosseini M , Vafaee F, Shafei MN, Soukhtanloo M. (2015) Feeding of Nigella Sativa during neonatal and juvenile growth improves learning and memory of rats. Journal of Traditional and Complementary Medicine.
52. Sangi S, Ahmed SP, Channa MA, Ashfaq M, Mastoi SM (2008) A new and novel treatment of opioid dependence: Nigella sativa 500 mg. J Ayub Med Coll Abbottabad 20: 118-124.
53. Abdel-Zaher AO, Abdel-Rahman MS, Elwasei FM (2011) Protective effect of Nigella Sativa oil against tramadol-induced tolerance and dependence in mice: role of nitric oxide and oxidative stress. Neurotoxicology 32: 725-733.
54. da Silva RC, Langoni H (2009) Toxoplasma gondii: host-parasite interaction and behavior manipulation. Parasitol Res 105: 893-898.
55. Rayan HZ, Heba M, Wagih HM, Atwa MM (2011) Efficacy of Black Seed Oil from Nigella Sativa against Murine Infection with Cysts of Me49 Strain of Toxoplasma gondii. PUJ 4: 165-176.
56. Percário S, Moreira DR, Gomes BA, Ferreira ME, Gonçalves AC, et al. (2012) Oxidative stress in malaria. Int J Mol Sci 13: 16346-16372.
57. Ahmed el-HM, Nour BY, Mohammed YG, Khalid HS (2010) Antiplasmodial Activity of Some Medicinal Plants Used in Sudanese Folk-medicine. Environ Health Insights 4: 1-6
58. Okeola VO, Adaramoye OA, Nneji CM, Falade CO, Farombi EO, et al. (2011) Antimalarial and antioxidant activities of methanolic extract of Nigella Sativa seeds (black cumin) in mice infected with Plasmodium yoelli nigeriensis. Parasitology Research 108: 1507-1512.
59. Sosiawan TI, Linda W, Etty W (2012) Anti-Malaria Study of Nigella Sativa L. Seed Water Extract in Mus musculus Mice Balb C Strain In Vivo. Makara Journal of Science 16: 192-196.
60. Emeka PM, Badger-Emeka LI, Eneh CM, Khan TM (2014) Dietary supplementation of chloroquine with nigella sativa seed and oil extracts in the treatment of malaria induced in mice with plasmodium berghei.Pharmacogn Mag 10: S357-362.

# 14

# Ethnomedicinal Studies of Lalmohan Thana in Bhola District, Bangladesh

**Sohel MDD[1,2*], Kawsar MDH[2], Sumon MDHU[3] and Sultana T[1,2]**

[1]*Department of Pharmacy, State University of Bangladesh, Dhanmondi, Dhaka-1205, Bangladesh*

[2]*Incepta Pharmaceuticals Ltd, Dewan Idris Road, Zirabo, Savar, Dhaka, Bangladesh*

[3]*Department of Pharmacy, University of Asia Pacific, Dhanmondi, Dhaka-1209, Bangladesh*

[*]**Corresponding author:** Sohel MDD, Department of Pharmacy, State University of Bangladesh, Dhanmondi, Dhaka-1205, Bangladesh, E-mail: sohelphr15@gmail.com

**Abstract**

The purpose of the present study was to document the medicinal plants of a Unani folk medicinal practitioner in Lalmohan Thana that located in Bhola district in Bangladesh. There is very narrow information about plants used by traditional healers and general people in Bhola District in Bangladesh, for treating general ailments. An ethnomedicinal survey conducted among folk medicinal herbalists of one village in Bhola district resulted in the finding of 146 plants distributed into 64 families used by the herbalists. The various plants were used for treatment of ailments like Urinary Disorders, Contraceptive, Diuretics, Fever, Constipation, Menoxenia, Jaundice, Respiratory Disorders (Coughs, Mucus), Leprosy, Tuberculosis, Sexual disorders, Gastrointestinal Disorders (Dysentery, Diarrhea, Indigestion, Constipation), Vomiting, Helminthiasis, Jaundice, Infections, Heart Disorders, Skin Disorders, Gonorrhea, Urinary Problems, Edema, Typhoid, Liver Disorders, Blood Poisoning, Eye Disorders, Memory Loss, Ovarian Problems, Vaginitis, and Hypertension.

This study could play an important role for future phytochemical and pharmacological investigation.

**Keywords:** Ethno medicinal; Lalmohan Thana; Bhola district; Folk medicine; Bangladesh

## Introduction

In Greece the Unani system of medicine originated. Hippocrates is the father of this system of medicine. Disease is a usually caused by imbalance of the humors. Pharmacotherapy is resorted the balance of the humors. At present, Unani medicine is practiced in the Indian sub-continent countries of India, Bangladesh and Pakistan, the practitioners being known as Hakims. Traditional medicine in Bangladesh is a unique blend of different ethnomedicinal combination [1]. Folk medicinal practitioners (Kavirajes) form the primary health-care providers to a significant section of the rural and urban population of Bangladesh. They exploit a variety of medicinal plants for treatment of different ailments. Folk medicine possibly is the most common form of these traditional medicinal practices, and folk medicinal practitioners (FMPs) can be found in every village, towns and cities within the country. From ancient time, the tradition of ethno-medicine practice has been established in Bangladesh and such medicine practitioners are known as Kavirajes. According to the WHO, about 80% of the world's population relies on traditional medicine for their primary health care [2,3]. About 80% of more than 4,000 million inhabitants of the world rely chiefly on traditional medicines for their primary health care needs [4]. Lalmohan is located in Bhola District. Bhola district is an administrative district in southwestern part of Bangladesh, which includes Bhola Island. Bhola Island is the largest island of Bangladesh. The objective of the present study was to document the medicinal plants used by FMPs in one villages of Lalmohan Thana in Bhola district, Bangladesh [5]. Rural people are heavily depend on natural resources due to lack of modern medical knowledge [6]. Thus, over time, a practitioner can build up quite extensive knowledge on the medicinal properties of any given plant species [7]. The development of western medicine is believed to have been influenced by the writing of Greek philosophers, in particular, Hippocrates (460-377 BC) and Aristotle (384-322 BC) [8]. The folk medicinal practitioners do not have their own medicinal books or follow any standardized custom [9]. Medicinal plants play a significant role in the primary healthcare systems for the majority of the rural population. The ethomedicinal knowledge about the use of medicinal plants can be a resource for the scientist to identify potential drugs, thus, proper documentation of this knowledge overtime is very essential to protect them from extinction [10]. It has been estimated that about 64% of the total global population still remains dependent on traditional medicines for healthcare needs [11].

## Materials and Methods

The survey was carried out in the villages of Purbophara 3No. Ward, Lalmohan Thana, which is located in Bhola district in Bangladesh. It is a part of Lalmohan Thana. The villages had one medicinal practitioner, who practiced folk medicine. However, his name is Hakeem Md. Jamal Uddin (M. M, D.U.M.S) the Hakeem title suggesting that his selection of medicinal plants was influenced by the ancient Unani system of medicine. Actual interviews were conducted with the help of a semi-structured questionnaire and the guided field-walk method of Martin and Maundu. Briefly, in this method, the practitioners took the interviewers on guided field-walks through areas from where they collected medicinal plants, pointed out the plants, and as interviewers belonged to the mainstream Bengali-speaking population [12,13]. The interviews were conducted among the locals of different age groups, mostly between 25 to 65 years, including herbal practitioners (Kabiraj).

The interviews focused on basic questions concerning the informant's knowledge of the uses of local plants and there different characteristics. A typical question would be: which local plants do you know and/or use? How many people in your area use the plant as medicine? [14]. In this method, the Hakim took the interviewers on guided field-walks through areas from where he collected his medicinal plants, pointed out the plants, and described their uses [15] (Table 1).

| Botanical Name | Local Name | Family | Plant parts used | Uses |
|---|---|---|---|---|
| *Abelmoschus esculentus* | Bhindi | Malvaceae | Seed | Gastric Disorders |
| *Abelmoschus moschatus* | Muskdana | Malvaceae | Seed | Tonics, Urinary Discharge |
| *Abroma augusta L.* | Ulatkambal | Sterculiaceae | Leaf, Root | Amenorrhoea and Dysmenorrhoea, Regulates Irregular Menses Pain and Gonorrhea |
| *Abrus precatorius L.* | Kunch | Leguminosae | Seed, Leaf, Root | Contraceptive, Aphrodisiac |
| *Acacia farnesiana (L.) Willd* | Belatibabul | Fabaceae | Leaf, Bark | Diuretic, Treat Antiulcer, Anti-Pyritic |
| *Acacia nilotica (Linn.)* | Babul | Leguminosae | Leaf, Gum | Diarrhea, Fever |
| *Acalypha indica L.* | Muktajhuri, Biralhatchi | Euphorbiaceae | Leaf | Rheumatism, Constipation, Kill Worms In Sores |
| *Acanthus illicifolis L.* | Harkuch Kanta | Acanthaceae | Root, Plant | Diuretics |
| *Achyranthes Aspera L.* | Apang | Amaranthaceae | Whole Plant | Prolonged Menstrual Flow, Menoxenia (Abnormal Menses), Habitual Abortion, Jaundice |
| *Adhatoda vasica Nees* | Basak. | Acanthaceae | Root, Bark and Leaves | Cough, Asthma |
| *Adina cordifolia Benth & Hook* | Kelikadam | Malvaceae | Seed | Kill Worms In Sores |
| *Aegle marmelos L.* | Bael | Rutacae | Fruit, Leaves | Constipation, Cough |
| *Albizia lebbeck (L.) Benth.* | Sirish | Leguminosae | Leaf | Leprosy, Diarrhoea |
| *Albizia procera (Roxb.) Benth.* | Koroi | Leguminosae | Leaf | The leaves are insecticidal; made into poultice they are applied to ulcer. |
| *Allium cepa Linn.* | Pyaj | Liliaceae | Bulb | Aphrodisiac, Rheumatism |
| *Alocasia Indica (Roxb.) Schott.* | Mankachu | Araceae | Roots | Rheumatism, leprosy |
| *Aloe Indica Wild.* | Ghritakumari | Liliaceae | Skin of Fruit, Leaf | Digestive problems such as constipation, colitis and irritable bowel syndrome Kidney stones, Menstrual discomfort |
| *Alstonia scholaris (L.) R. Br.* | Chattim | Apocynaceae | Bark | Anthelmintic, Antipyretic, Antimalarial |
| *Amaranthus spinosus Linn.* | Kantanotya | Amaranthaceae | Leaf, Root | Diuretic, Gonorrhoea |
| *Amaranthus tricolor L.* | Lalshak. | Amaranthaceae | Leaves | Diuretics |
| *Amomum aromaticum Roxb.* | Morang elachi | Zingiberaceae | Fruit | Appetizer |
| *Amorphophallus campanulatus (Roxb.) Bl. Ex. Decne.* | Olkachu | Araceae | Tuber | Rheumatism, Abdominal Pain, Elephantiasis |
| *Anacardium occidentale L.* | Cashew Nut | Anacardiaceae | Fruit | Anti-diabetic, anti-bacterial |
| *Ananas Sativus schult. F.* | Anaras | Bromeliaceae | Leaf, fruit | Anthelmintic, diuretic, abortifacient |

| | | | | |
|---|---|---|---|---|
| *Annona reticulata L.* | Nona Ata | Annonaceae | Leaves and seeds | Anthelmintic, Insecticidal |
| *Anthocephalus indicus* | Kadam | Rubiaceae | Leaf | Anthelmintic |
| *Aphanamixis polystachya (Wall.) R.N. Parker.* | Royena | Meliaceae | Bark, Seed Oil | Spleen and Liver Diseases, Edema, Stimulating Liniment In Rheumatism |
| *Arachis hypogaea L.* | Mata kalai | Leguminosae | Fruit | Gonorrhea, Nutritious |
| *Areca catechth L,* | Supari | Palmae | Fruit | Anthelmintic, Rheumatism, Aphrodisiac |
| *Argyreia nervosa* | Bijarka | Convolvulaceae | Leaf, Fruit | Rheumatism, Diuretics |
| *Aristolochia indica L.* | Iswarmul. | Aristolochiaceae | Root, Leaf | Fever, Stimulant |
| *Artocarpus heterophyllus Lamk.* | Kathal | Moraceae | Fruit | Skin diseases, Nutritious |
| *Asparagus racemosus L* | Shatamull | Liliaceae | Root | Diuretic, Aphrodisiac, Antidiarrhoeaic |
| *Averrhoa carrambola Linn* | Kamranga | Oxalidaceae | Fruit | Antipyretic and anthelmintic, Antioxidant |
| *Azadirachta indica A. Juss.* | Neem | Meliaceae | Leaf, Bark, Seed Oil | Bacterial, Fungal, Antipyretic and Antimalarial |
| *Bacopa moniera L.* | Brahmi | Serophulariaceae | Whole Plant | Reducing anxiety, Improving memory formation |
| *Barringtonia acutangula (L.) Gaertn.* | Hijal | Lacythidaceae | Seed, Bark, Leaf, Root | Diuretics, Fever, Headache |
| *Basella alba Linn.* | Puishak | Basellaceae | Leaf | Skin diseases, Sexual weakness, Ulcers and laxative |
| *Benincasa hispida (Thunb.) Cogn.* | Chalkumra | Cucurbitaceae | Seed, Fruit | Epilepsy and Nervous Diseases |
| *Blumea lacera (Burm.f.) DC.* | Kukurshinga | Asteraceae | Whole plant | Antiviral, Antipyretic |
| *Boerhaavia diffusa L.* | Punarnava | Nyctaginaceae | Whole plant | Diuretic, Edema |
| *Brassica campestris L.* | Sarisa shak | Cruciferae | Seed | Cough, Leprosy |
| *Bombax ceiba L.* | Shimul-Tula | Bombacaceae | Root | Increase Sex In Male, Gynecological And Urinogenitial Disorders |
| *Buettneria pilosa Roxb.* | Harjora | Sterculiaceae | stem with leaves | treatment of fractured bones |
| *Butea monosperma Roxb.* | Palas | Leguminosae | Seed, Gum | Astringent, anthelmintic |
| *Caesalpinia bonduc (L.) Roxb.* | Nata | Fabaceae | Fruit, Root, Bark, Leaves | Antipyretic, Antispasmodic, Anthelmintic, Kidney Troubles, Asthma |
| *Cajanus cajan (L.) Huth.* | Arhar | Fabaceae | Leaves | Jaundice and Pneumonia |
| *Calotropis Gigantea (L.) R. Br.* | Akanda | Asclepiadaceae | Root, Leaf, Bark | Asthma, Emetic, Leprosy, Rheumatism |
| *Capsicum annuum L* | Jhal marich | Solanaceae | Fruit | Carminative, Stimulant, Sores, Tonic |
| *Cerica papaya Linn* | Papay | Caricaceae | Fruit | Carminative, Eczema, Warts, Anthelmintic, Digestion problems |
| *Carum roxbunghianum Benth.* | Radhuni | Apiaceae | Seed | abdominal spasm (colic) |
| *Cassia alata (L.) Gaertn.* | Daud pata | Leguminosae | Leaf | Skin diseases, Microbial infections. |

| | | | | |
|---|---|---|---|---|
| *Cassia fistula L.* | Sonalu | Leguminosae | Leaf, Bark, Root, Fruit | Helminthiasis, Constipation, Rheumatism |
| *Cassia occidentalis Linn.* | Kasondi | Caesalpiniaceae | Leaf, Seed | Hepatotoxicity |
| *Cassia tora Linn.* | Chakunda | Caesalpiniaceae | Seed, Fruit | Skin diseases like ringworm and itching, Anthelmintic |
| *Catharanthus roseus L.* | Nyantara | Apocynaceae | Root, Leaf | Diabetes mellitus, Hypotensive |
| *Cayratia pedata (Lam.) Juss. Ex Gagnep.* | Goalilata | Vitaceae | Leaf | Astringent |
| *Centella asiatica L.* | Thankuni | Umbellifera e | Whole Plant, leaf | Dysentery, Stomach pain, Memory tonic, Diuretic |
| *Chenopodium album L.* | Bathu sag | Chenopodiaceae) | Seed, plant | Improves the appetite, Abdominal pain |
| *Chrysopogon aciculatus (Retz.) Trin* | Premkata | Poaceae | Root, Seed | Anthelmintic |
| *Cinnamomum tamals Nees* | Tejpata | Lauraceae | Leaf | Heart disease, Gastrointestinal disorders, Diarrhea |
| *Citrullus lanatus (Thunb.) Mats.* | Tarmuj | Cucurbitaceae | Seed, Rife fruit | Cooling, Refreshing and stomachic, Laxative, Diuretic, Tonic |
| *Citrus aurantifolia (Christm.) Swingle* | Lebu, Kaghzilebu | Rutaceae | Fruit, Leaves | Appetizer, Eczema |
| *Cleome viscosa L.* | Hurhuria | Capparidaceae | Seed | Stomachic, laxative, Diuretic |
| *Clerodendrum indicum L.* | Bamanhati, Banchat, | Verbenacea e | Root, Leaf, | Respiratory problems, Cough, Irregular menstruation, Irregular blood pressure |
| *Clerodendrum viscosum Vent.* | Vant, Ghetu | Verbenacea e | Leaf, Root, Fruit | Scabies, Fever, Anthelmintic, |
| *Coccinia grandis (L.) Voigt* | Telakucha | Cucurbitaceae | Leaf | Hypertension, Diabetes, Jaundice |
| *Cocos nucifera L.* | Narikel | Arecaceae | Leaf, Fruit | Diuretics, Keep head cool, diabetes. |
| *Corchorus capsularis L.* | Pat shakh | Tiliaceae | Leaf, Seed | Dysentry |
| *Coriandrum Sativum Linn.* | Dhonia | Apiaceae | Seed | Loss of appetite |
| *Crataeva nurvala Buch-Ham* | Barun | Capparidaceae | Leaf, Root, Bark | To promote appetite and decrease secretion of bile |
| *Cucumis sativus L.* | Khira | Cucurbitaceae | Fruit, Seed | Reduce cholesterol, Diuretics |
| *Cucurbita maxima Duch.* | Calakumro | Cucurbitaceae | Seed | Diuretics, Anthelmintic |
| *Cuminum cyminum Linn* | Jeera | Umbellifera e | Fruit | Astringent, Carminative |
| *Cucuma longa L.* | Kacha Holud | Zingiberaceae | Rhizomes | Allergy, Inflammation, Skin disease, Anthelmintic |
| *Cuscuta reflexa Roxb.* | Swarnalata | Cuscutacea e | Seed, Stem | Flatulence, stomach pain, constipation |
| *Cymbopogon citratus (Dc.) Stapf.* | Lebugandhi Ghas. | Graminae | leaves | Fever, Rheumatism, appetizer and Anthelmintic |
| *Cyperus rotundus Linn.* | Mutha Ghas | Cyperacea e | Rhizomes | Stimulant, Stomachic aromatic |

| | | | | |
|---|---|---|---|---|
| *Dalbergia bissoo Roxb.* | Shishu | Leguminosae | Leaf, bark, seed | Leprosy, scabies, Astringent |
| *Datura meta Linn.* | Dhutura | Solanaceae | Leaf, Root, Seed | Asthma, Rheumatism, Fever, pain |
| *Derris trifoliata Lour.* | Panlata | Fabaceae | Bark, Stem | Stimulant, Insecticides, Rheumatism |
| *Dillenia indica Linn* | Chalta | Dilleniaceae | Fruit, Leaves | tonic and laxative; used in diarrhoea |
| *Diospyros peregrine Gurke* | Desi gabh | Ebenaceae | Fruit | Dysentery and diarrhea, Diuretics |
| *Dioscorea bulbifera L.* | Pagla Alu | Dioscoreaceae | tubers | dysentery, diarrhea, stomachic |
| *Dolichos lablab linn.* | Shim | Leguminosae | Seed, Leaf | Astringent, Nausea, vomiting and abdominal pains |
| *Eclipta alba Hassk* | Kesuriya | Asteraceae | Whole Plant | Protect the liver, tonic, deobstruent in hepatic and splenic enlargements, jaundice |
| *Elaeocarpus robustus linn.* | Jalpai, Jalphui. | Elaeocarpaceae | Fruit, Leaf | Splenic enlargements, Lethargy to food |
| *Elettaria cardamomum (L.) Maton* | Elas | Zingiberaceae | Fruit | Remedy for impotence and low sexual response. abdominal pains, Appetizer |
| *Embelia ribes Burm F* | Biranga | Myrsinaceae | Seed | Anthelmintic |
| *Eryngium foetidum L.* | Bon dhonia | Apiaceae | Root, Leaf | Diuretics, colds, coughs, hypertension, Arithitis |
| *Erythrina variegate L* | Madar | Fabaceae | Leaf, Bark, Root | Fever, Anthelmintic, |
| *Eucalyptus citriodora Hook.* | Eucalyptus | Myrtaceae | Juice of leaves | anti-inflammatory and analgesic qualities and can be applied to wounds to help prevent infection |
| *Eugenia jambolana (Lam)* | Jum | Myrtaceae | Juice of young leaves | Dysentery and diarrhoea. |
| *Eupatorium odoratum Linn* | Japanilata | Compositae | Leaf | The juice of the leaf is applied on wounds to cheek Bleeding. |
| *Ficus benghalensis L.* | Bot | Moraceae | Bark, Gum, leaf, fruit, root | Gonorrhea, Venereal diseases, Abscess, astringent, aphrodisiac |
| *Ficus glomerata Roxb.* | Jagadumur | Moraceae | Fruit, Bark | Leucorrhoea, biliousness, burning sensation, fatigue, Diabetes, Dysentry, nose bleeding |
| *Ficus hispida Linn.* | Kakdumul | Moraceae | Bark, fruit, leaf, root | Galactagogue, emetic, anaemia, haemorrhoids |
| *Glinus oppositifolius L.* | Gima shak | Molluginaceae | Whole plant | Abdominal pain and jaundice, loss of appetite, indigestion |
| *Glycosmis pentaphylla (Retz.) A. Dc.* | Ashshaora, Datmajan, | Rufaceae | Root, Leaf, Stem, Fruit, Whole Plant, | Cough, Rheumatism, Anaemia And Jaundice, Eczema, Pimple, Rheumatism, Dysentery, Dental Caries |
| *Gmelina arborea L.* | Gamar | Verbenaceae | Bark, Root | Astringent, Tonic |
| *Hedyotis corymbosa (L.) Link.* | Khetpapra | Rubiaceae | Whole Plant | Jaundice, Liver Disease, Fever, Heat Eruption, |
| *Hygrophila auriculata (Schum.) Heyne.* | Kulekhara, Talmakhna. | Acanthaceae | Whole Plant | Diuretics, Jaundice, Gonorrhea, Urinary Discharges, Inflammations |
| *Imperata cylindrica Rausch.* | Ulu | Poaceae | Roots | Fever |
| *Ipomea aquatica Forsk.* | Kalmi, Kalmi Shak. | Convolvulaceae | Root, leaves | Plants are used in leucoderma, biliousness, carminative |
| *Ipomoea batatus (L.) Lamk.* | Misti Alu | Convolvulaceae | Tubers, Root | Nutritional Source, Diarrhoea |
| *Ipomoea mauritiana Jacq.* | Bhuikumra | Convolvulaceae | Root, Tubers | Sexual Disabilities, Galactagogue |

| | | | | |
|---|---|---|---|---|
| *Jatropha curcus Linn.* | Bagh Verenda, Ban Verenda | Euphorbiaceae | Seed, Leaf | Purgative |
| *Kalanchoe pinnata (Lam.)Pers.* | Patharkuchi; | Crassulaceae | Leaves | Diuretic |
| *Lagenaria siceraria (Mol.) Stan.* | Lau, Kadu | Cucurbitaceae | Fruit and seed | Diuretic, headache |
| *Lannea Coromandelica (Houtt.) Merr.* | Kamila | Anacardiaceae | Bark | Astringent, Jaundice |
| *Lawsonia inermis Linn.* | Mehedi, Mendi, | Lythraceae | Leaf, Bark | Arthritis, Skin disease, |
| *LENS culinaris Medik.* | Musuri | Fabaceae | Seeds | Constipation |
| *Lippia nodiflora (L.) Rich.* | Bhui Okar | Verbenaceae | Leaf, Plant | diuretic, stomachic, good for ulcers, wounds, asthma, bronchitis, diarrhoea |
| *Ludwigia Adscendens (L.) Hara.* | Kesardam | Onagraceae | leaf | Dysentery |
| *Lycopersicon lycopersicum (L.)* | Tomato, bilati beguna | Solanaceae | Fruit | Antioxidant |
| *Mangifera indica L.* | Aam | Anacardiaceae | Leaf, Fruit, Seed, | Toothache, Astringent, Diuretics |
| *Manilkara achras (Mill.) Fosberg* | Sofeda | Sapotaceae | Seed | Fever, tonic, diuretica |
| *Marsilea quadrifolia Linn.* | Sushni saag | Marseliaceae | Leaf | Hypnotic |
| *Melia sempervirens L.* | Ghoranim | Meliaceae | Bark | Diuretics, leprosy, Anthelmintic |
| *Mentha spicata Linn.* | Pudina | Labiatae | Whole plant | Abdomina; pain, Constipation |
| *Mimosa pudica Linn.* | 'Lojjaboti | Fabaceae | Whole plant | Diuretics, uterine complaints, inflammation, fatigue |
| *Momordica charantia Linn.* | Korolla | Cucurbitaceae | leaf | Diabetes, helminthiasis, Ulcer |
| *Momordica cochinchinensis (Lour) Spreng.* | Kakroal | Cucurbitaceae | Fruit | Diabetes, Abdominal pain, Stimulent |
| *Musa paradisiacal L.* | Kala | Musaceae | Root, tubers, Fruit | Dysentery, Astringent, BP |
| *Nerium indicum Mill.* | Korobi | Apocynaceae | Root, leaves | Skin disease, Leprosy |
| *Nigella sativa Linn.* | Kalojira, Kalijira | Ranunculaceae | Seed | Stimulant and diuretic. |
| *Nymphaea nouchali Burm.f* | Sapla | Nymphaeaceae | Flower | Dysentery, Diarrhea, Heart disease, |
| *Ocimum basilicum Linn.* | Babui Tulshi | Lamiaceae | Whole plant | Fever, carminative, |
| *Ocimum sanctum Linn.* | Tulshi | Lamiaceae | Leaf | Fever, cough |
| *Phoenix Sylvestris (L.)* | Khejur | Arecaceae | Fruit, Root | Toothache, Nutritious |
| *Phyllanthus emblica L.* | Amloki | Euphorbiaceae | Fruit | Vomiting, cough, indigestion, jaundice, Skin disease |
| *Piper nigrum L.* | Gol morich | piperaceae | Seed, Fruit | Chest and joint pain, hair loss, diuretics |
| *Piper betle L.* | Paan pata | piperaceae | leaf | Brest and prostate cancer, stomach disorder |
| *Psidium guajava Linn,* | Piyara | Myrtaceae | leaves | Scarby, menstrual problem, diarrhea |
| *Punica granatum L.* | Dalim | Punicaceae | Bark | Anaemia, anthelmintics |

| | | | | |
|---|---|---|---|---|
| *Raphanus Sativus Linn* | Mula | Cruciferae | Leaf, Seed, Root | Carminative, stimulant, increase digestion |
| *Rauwolfia serpentina (L.) Benth. ex Kurz* | Sarpogondha | Apocynaceae | Root | Root extract is directly feed to neutralize the snake venom |
| *Rosa damascena mill L* | Golap | Rosaceae | Flower | Carminative, Astringent, Tonic, Vaginal disease |
| *Rumex Maritimus L* | Ban Palang | Polygonaceae | Plant | Refrigerant |
| *Rumex vesicarius Linn.* | Chuka Sak | Polygonaceae | Leaf | Refrigerent, diuretics, Appetizer |
| *Sesanum indicum L.* | Til | Pedaliaceae | Leaf, Seed, oil | Dysentery |
| *Solanum melongena L.* | Begun | Solanaceae | Leaf, Seed, Fruit | Laxative, Cough |
| *Tamarindus indica Linn* | Tentul | Leguminosae | Seed | Constipation |
| *Terminalia arjuna* | Arjun | Combretaceae | Bark | Heart disease |
| *Zingiber officinale Rose.* | Ada | Zingiberaceae | Rhizomes | stomachic, appetiser, expectorant |
| *Zizyphus mauritiana Lamk.* | Boroi | Rhamnaceae | Fruit, Root | astringent, laxative, stomachic |

**Table 1:** Ethnomedicinal usesof medicinal plants in Lalmohan Thana, Bhola district.

## Results and Discussion

In our study, we found large number participants who are female. According to Ikhtiar Alam SM, in Developing countries, society is, in general, male dominated in terms of participation in household decision making [16]. In Bangladesh, the male villagers are more knowledgeable than female in term of medicinal knowledge. Again, aged person are more knowledgeable than younger one.

According to Dr. Abdul Ghani almost 455 medicinal plants name so far been enlisted as growing or available in Bangladesh [17] (Figure 1).

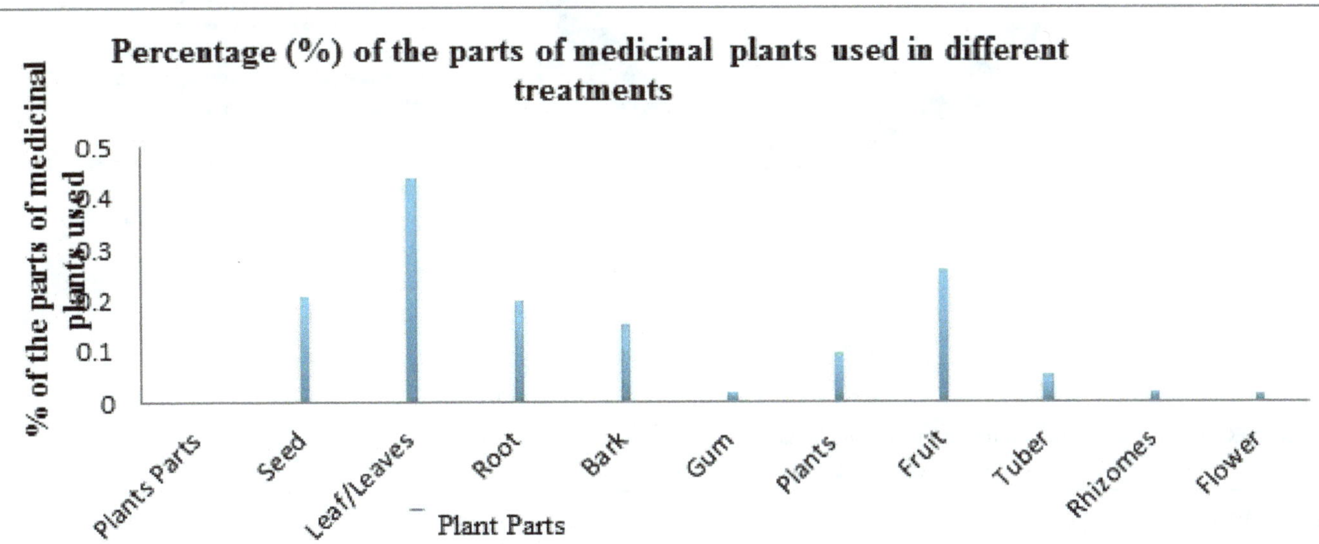


**Figure 1:** Parts of medicinal plants used in different preparations in the study area.

The Hakim was observed to use a total of almost 146 plants distributed into 64 families for different ailments. The percentage of medicinal plants parts Leaves (43.83%), Seed (20.55%), Root (19.86%), Bark (15.07%), Gum (2.05%), Plants (9.59%), Fruit (26.03%), Tuber

(5.48%), Rhizomes (2.05%), Flower (1.37%) are used for treatment of different ailments. The various plants were used for treatment of ailments like Urinary Disorders, Contraceptive, Diuretics, Fever, Constipation, Menoxenia, Jaundice, Respiratory Disorders (Coughs, Mucus), Leprosy, Tuberculosis, Sexual disorders, Gastrointestinal Disorders (Dysentery, Diarrhea, Indigestion, Constipation), Vomiting, Helminthiasis, Jaundice, Infections, Heart Disorders, Skin Disorders, Gonorrhea, Urinary Problems, Edema, Typhoid, Liver Disorders, Blood Poisoning, Eye Disorders, Memory Loss, Ovarian Problems, Vaginitis, and Hypertension (Figure 1).

Percentages were calculated as the ratio between the number of plants in which a certain part is used and the total number of plants.

**Data analysis**

The FC of the species of plants being utilized was evaluated using the formula: FC= (Number of times a particular species was mentioned/Total number of times that all species were mentioned) x 100 [18] (Figure 2).

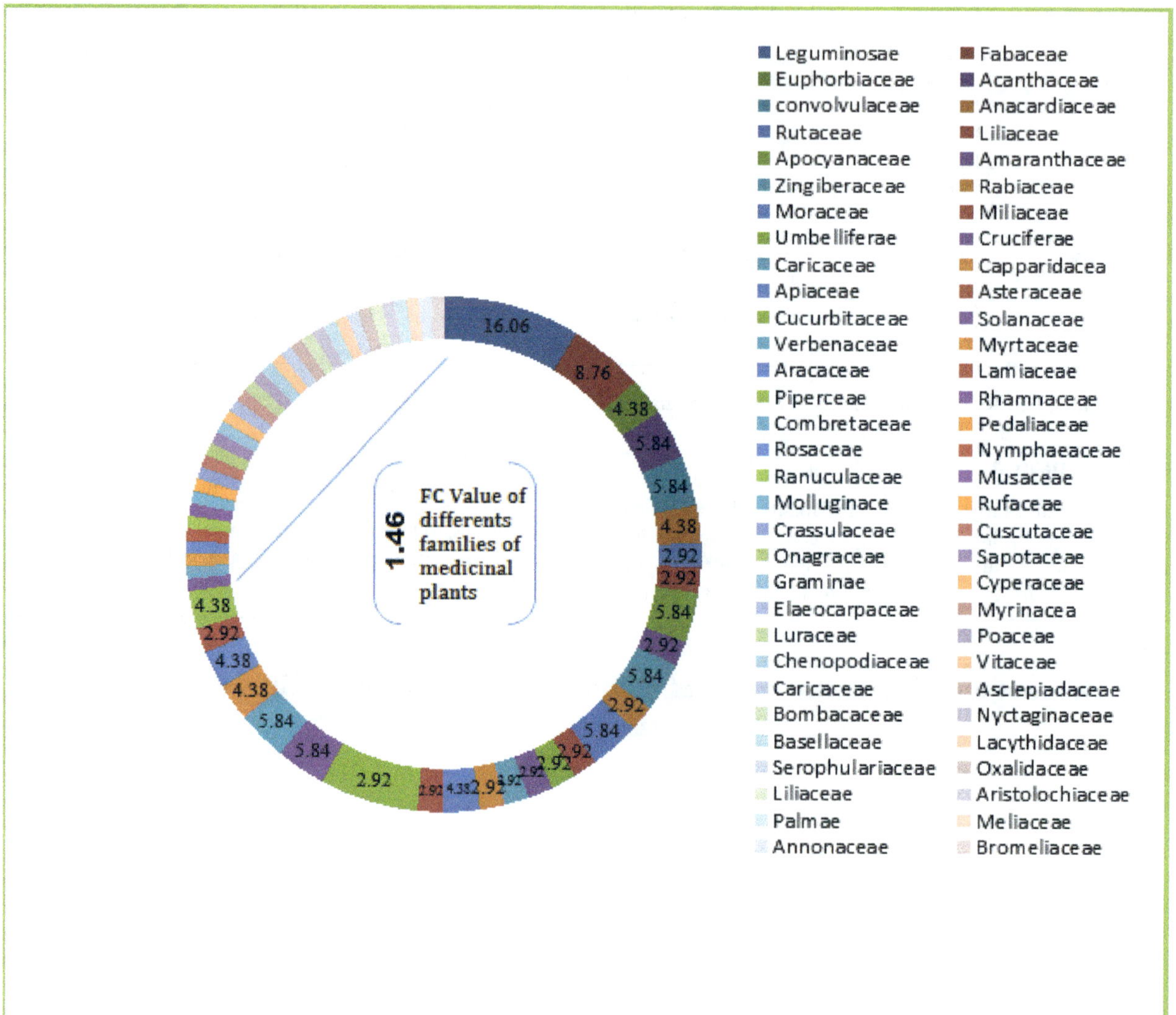


**Figure 2:** FC Value of different families of medicinal plants.

## Conclusion

Our study reveals that plants are still a major source of medicine for the local communities of most of the portions of our surveyed area, as modern health care facilities are still not sufficient. This report may represents a useful and long-lasting document, which can contribute to preserve knowledge on the use of medicinal plants in this region and also stimulate the interest of future generations on traditional healing practices. The information provided in the paper is limited and there is a scope to initiate further ethno botanical study among the communities to gather information as far as possible. The medicated claims incorporated in the study need to be evaluated through phytochemical and pharmacological investigations to discover their potentiality as drugs. It is urgent need for documenting these before such valuable knowledge becomes inaccessible and extinct.

## Acknowledgments

Authors would like to express gratitude and thanks to Traditional Health Practitioners and people involved in the interviews for providing information about the medicinal applications of the plants. The authors are also grateful to the Department of Pharmacy, State University of Bangladersh, for their suggestion and information during this research.

## References

1. Ocvirk S, Kistler M, Khan S, Talukder SH, Hauner H, et al. (2013) Traditional Medicinal Plants Used For The Treatment of Diabetes in Rural and Urban Areas of Dhaka, Bangladesh, An Ethnobotanical Survey. Journal of Ethnobiology and Ethnomedicine 9: 1-8.
2. Behera KK (2006) Ethnomedicinal plants used by the tribals of Similipal Bioreserve Orissa, India: a pilot studies. Ethnobotanical Leaflets 10:149-173.
3. Khisha T, Karim R, Chowdhury SR, Banoo R (2012) Ethnomedical Studies of Chakma Communities of Chittagong Hill Tracts, Bangladesh. Bangladesh Pharmaceutical Journal 15: 59-67.
4. Tumpa SI, Hossain Md. I, Ishika T (2014) Ethnomedicinal use of herbs by indigenous medicine practitioners of Jhenaidah district, Bangladesh. Journal of Pharmacognosy and Phytochemistry 3:23-33.
5. Afrin M, Rukaiya U, Sharmin S, Jannat K, Akter M, et al. (2015) Ethnomedicinal plants of three folk medicinal practitioners in two villages of Khulna district, Bangladesh. Journal of Chemical and Pharmaceutical Research 7:220-225.
6. Tariq A, Mussarat S, Adnan M, Abd_Allah EF, Hashem A, et al. (2015) Ethnomedicinal Evaluation of Medicinal Plants Used against Gastrointestinal Complaints. BioMed Research International Article ID 892947, 14.
7. Tuhin Md. IH, Asaduzzaman Md., Islam E, Khatun Z, Rahmatullah M (2013) Medicinal plants used by folk medicinal herbalists in seven villages of Bhola district, Bangladesh. American-Eurasian Journal of Sustainable Agriculture 7: 210-218.
8. Chikezie PC, Ojiako OA (2015) Herbal Medicine: Yesterday, Today and Tomorrow Altern Integr Med 4:1-5.
9. Rahmatullah M, Mollik Md. AH, Paul AK, Jahan R, Khatun Mst. A, et al. (2010)A Comparative Analysis of Medicinal Plants used to treat Gastrointestinal Disorders in two sub-districts of Great Khulna Division, Bangladesh. Advances in Natural and Applied Sciences 4: 22-28.
10. Bhowmik R, Saha MR, Rahman Md. A, Islam Md. Anwar Ul (2014) Ethnomedicinal Survey of Plants in the Southern District Noakhali, Bangladesh. Bangldesh Pharmaceutical Journal 17: 205-214.
11. Rahmatullah M, Mollik AH, Ali M, Abbas FB, Jahan R, et al. (2011) An Ethnomedicinal Survey of Vitbilia Village in Sujanagar Sub-District of Pabna District, Bangladesh. American-Eurasian J. Agric & Environ Sci 10: 106-111.
12. Martin GJ (1995) Ethnobotany: A 'People and Plants' Conservation Manual, Chapman and Hall, London; page 268.
13. Maundu P (1995).Methodology for collecting and sharing indigenous knowledge: a case study. Indigenous Knowledge and Development Monitor 3: 3-5.
14. Sajib NH, Uddin, SB (2015) Ethnomedicinal Study of Plants in Hathazari, Chittagong, Bangladesh. Pertanika J Trop Agric Sci 38: 197-210.
15. Muttaki AA, Ahmed Z, Islam Md. S, Opu SA, Sonda MK, et al. (2014) Medicinal plants and formulations of a Unani folk medicinal practitioner of Bhola district, Bangladesh. Journal of Chemical and Pharmaceutical Research 6:231-238.
16. Alam SMI (1998) Role of Women in Decision Making and Economic Contribution at Household Level. Journal of International Affairs 4: 13-15.
17. Ghani A (1998) Medicinal Plants: Chemical Constituents and Uses of the Medicinal Plants of Bangladesh.
18. Dey AK, Mamun OR, Rashid M, Millat MS, Rashid MM (2014) Ethnobotanical survey of medicinal plants used by traditional health practitioners and indigenous people in different districts of Chittagong division, Bangladesh. International Journal of Pharmaceutical Science 3: 01-07.

# 15

# Help-seeking Behavior among Adults in Riyadh, Saudi Arabia

**Sulaiman Abdullah Al Shammari[1*], Saleh Abdullah Alhaidar[2], Mazen Ayidh Alotaibi[2], Abdullah Alrayed Alanazi[2], Waleed Khalid Al Shammari[2], Abdulaziz Mashuj Alanazi[2], Hossam Khalid Alsahabi[2], Abdulmajeed Fahad Altammami[2] and Talal Mohammed Thaher[3]**

[1]*Department of Family and Community Medicine, Chair of Health Education and Health Promotion, King Saud University, Saudi Arabia*

[2]*College of Medicine, King Saud University, Saudi Arabia*

[3]*King Khalid General Hospital, Al Majmaah, Saudi Arabia*

[*]**Corresponding author:** Sulaiman Abdullah Al Shammari, Professor, Consultant Family Physician, Chairman of Health Education Center and Supervisor of Research Chair on Health Education and Health Promotion, Department of Family and Community Medicine, College of Medicine, King Saud University, P.O.Box 2925, Riyadh 11461, Saudi Arabia, E-mail: sulaiman@ksu.edu.sa

**Abstract**

**Background:** Management of people's health problems should be performed by qualified health professionals. However, an increasing number of individuals claim the ability to manage diseases despite not having received medical training. This study sought to identify the sociodemographic and socioeconomic characteristics of people seeking health-related assistance from nonprofessionals, their reasons for seeking help and sources of health information available to the public.

**Methods:** A cross-sectional descriptive study was conducted in Riyadh, Saudi Arabia, from September 2014 to March 2015. The sample size was 195 Saudi adults. An online survey consisting of a well-structured questionnaire was created using Google forms and distributed via a link to a website.

**Result:** A total of 269 participants met our criteria and completed the questionnaire. One hundred ninety-one participants (71%) were female and 152 (56.5%) were 30 years old or younger. The majority were unmarried 164 (61%) and 191 (71%) had a university education or higher. More than half of the participants (143; 53%) consulted a medical doctor (MD) and 100 (37%) relied on self-help or consulted relatives. The older the patient, the more likely he or she was to consult a physician rather than depend on self-help or advice from relatives. The majority of married participants consulted a physician (69; 65.7%); many of the unmarried participants (72; 43.9%) preferred self-help and consultation with relatives. Approximately half of the participants who preferred self-help and relatives' advice perceived a benefit; the other half did not notice a difference.

**Conclusion:** Our findings indicate that help-seeking behavior in the Saudi community requires improvement. Approximately half of the participants sought non-medical help. We hope this study will motivate investigators to research variety of help-seeking behaviors and their effects, such as the influence of the Internet on self-care.

**Keywords:** Help-seeking behavior; Riyadh; Traditional healer; Pharmacists; Self-help; Doctors

## List of Abbreviations:

ENT: Ear, Nose and Throat; GI: Gastrointestinal; HSB: Help-Seeking Behavior; KSA: Kingdom of Saudi Arabia; MD: Medical Doctor; MOH: Ministry of Health; PHC: Primary Health Care; SPSS: Statistical Package for the Social Sciences; TH: Traditional Healer; WHO: World Health Organization

## Introduction

Help-seeking behavior (HSB) is an appropriate way to seek a solution for a health problem and requires suitable interaction with a medically trained professional [1]. HSB has three main components: a health issue (physical or psychological), a person who needs help to address the health issue, and a source of help. For the purpose of the present study, we classified the source of help as a physician, pharmacist, or traditional healer (TH) or self-treatment. We defined a medical doctor (MD) as a person lawfully trained to practice medicine [2]. For "pharmacist" we used the World Health Organization (WHO) definition: professionals who "store, preserve, compound, and dispense medicinal products." Furthermore, they counsel patients on the proper use and adverse effects of drugs and medicines prescribed by MDs and other health professionals. Additionally, they contribute to researching, testing, preparing, prescribing, and monitoring medicinal therapies to optimize human health. Types of pharmacists include hospital, industrial, retail, and dispensing pharmacists [3]. Finally, self-treatment is an attempt to relieve one's own health problems using a treatment without professional supervision [4].

Traditional medicine professionals implement knowledge, skill, and practice gained through cultural experience. They typically examine patients and treat health problems (physical and psychological) and "research, develop and implement treatment plans using applications such as acupuncture, Ayurvedic, homeopathic and herbal" [3]. In the Saudi community, the THs are nonprofessionals as they do not have any certification and who base their therapies on traditional beliefs [5].

Finally, there are faith healers, who apply the traditions of the prophet Mohammad by reading the Holy Quran to alleviate illness [6].

The current study demonstrates the importance of HSB in the community. Cost and prevalence of diseases are reduced by treating the initial disease rather than correcting problems resulting from irresponsible interventions and poor practices of pharmacists and THs. In the Saudi community, misconceptions exist regarding pharmacists and THs. Furthermore, the availability of health centers is limited in some areas, which increases the likelihood that individuals will seek help from nonprofessionals or treat themselves.

The majority of people in Riyadh (79%) said they treated themselves; fewer individuals (21.4%) had received a specialist consultation, and 77.3% sought medically trained practitioners (3.8% pharmacists, 16.7% THs, and 2.2% self-treatment) [7]. Another study showed that 90.5% of mothers consulted physicians when their children less than two years of age were ill [8]. Furthermore, in Riyadh, most people who visited a TH were elderly (+60 years old), female, married or divorced, and illiterate. Common medical problems for which people sought help from a TH were abdominal pain, flatulence, low back pain, depression, and headache.

The most common reasons for visiting a TH were a belief in the success of alternative medicine and a preference for natural remedies [5]. More females (82%) than males (73%) sought help from medically trained practitioners. Five percent of males sought help from a pharmacist, compared with 2.2% of females. Twenty-one percent of males and 10% of females sought help from a TH [7]. Additionally, Chinese-American males were more likely than females to seek help from physicians but were less likely to seek help from friends [9].

Young men were less likely than women to suggest visiting a doctor for mental problems. In fact, only 16.4% of males thought that a severely depressed person should visit a doctor [10]. Another study showed that of women younger than 45 years, 76% sought help from a medically trained practitioner, 4.5% sought help from pharmacies, 17.3% sought help from a TH, and 2.2% used self-treatment. Moreover, for women older than 45 years, 89.5% sought help from a medically trained practitioner, 9.1% sought help from a TH, and 1.5% used self-treatment.

The same study found that for Saudis with a low education level, 85.7% sought help from a medically trained practitioner, 6.7% sought help from a TH and 6.7% practiced self-treatment. For Saudis with a higher education level, 77.3% sought help from a medically trained professional, 4.2% sought help from a pharmacist, 12.6% sought help from a TH, and 6.5% practiced self-treatment [7].

A Chinese-American study showed that negative life events and emotional distress reduced HSB, but it was higher in individuals with insurance coverage. Unemployed people were more likely to seek help from physicians [9]. Studies have shown that the most common reasons people cite for not seeking help for fecal incontinence are that they do not know how to ask for help and they feel embarrassment or shame. In addition, they said they thought that the situation was not serious or they lacked knowledge of treatment options [11].

Few Saudi studies of HSBs have been reported in the literature. The objectives of the current study were as follows: (1) to identify the sociodemographic and socioeconomic characteristics of people seeking the help of a nonprofessional, (2) to determine why patients seek help from non-professionals and (3) to identify sources of health information available to the public.

## Methods

A cross-sectional descriptive study was conducted in Riyadh, Saudi Arabia, from September 2014 to March 2015. The target population was Saudi adults with health problems in the eight weeks preceding the study who lived in Riyadh and used Internet services. We approached participants via Twitter, Facebook, Google Plus, and email. The inclusion criteria were being Saudi, Arabic-speaking, and over 18 years of age with access to a computer and Internet services and at least one account of the following type: Twitter, Facebook, Google Plus, or email. Both men and women were eligible. The exclusion criterion was chronic health problems for more than eight weeks (to avoid recall bias).

The estimated Saudi population over 18 years of age in Riyadh as of 2015 was 1,637,200 [12,13]. According to the Communication and Information Technology Commission, 97% of the population aged 12 years old and above in Riyadh use Internet services [14]. For the purpose of the present study, we conservatively estimated that 85% of people over 18 years old in Riyadh use Internet services. At a 95% confidence level, the estimation accuracy was 5%, and the estimated proportion was 85%. The target sample size was at least 195 Saudi adults.

Non-probability convenience sampling was used. Participants responded to our online survey, which consisted of a questionnaire randomly distributed via a link on Twitter, Facebook, or Google Plus or in email. Data were collected with an online questionnaire using Google Forms, which was partially taken from the published research of Al Shammari [7]. The questionnaire was in Arabic, which facilitated administration and completion by the general public. It included sociodemographic data such as age, gender, level of education, occupation, income, marital status, and source of medical knowledge. It also inquired about health problems in the preceding eight weeks, what type of practitioner was consulted, and the result of the consultation. Additionally, we asked why people sought help from a nonprofessional. We tested the questionnaire in a pilot study prior to the main study.

A total of 269 participants completed the questionnaires. We do not know the time taken by each participant to fill out the questionnaire. But, based on the pilot study, the time was less than 5 minutes. Statistical analyses were performed using the Statistical Package for the Social Sciences (SPSS), version 19 (SPSS Inc., Chicago, IL, USA). A chi square test or Fisher's exact test was used to compare the demographic characteristics with all the nominal variables. Statistically significant differences were assumed when the P value was less than 0.05.

The participants were asked to consent to the study after a clear explanation of the objectives and content of the questionnaire. The questionnaire stated that participation was voluntary and data would be used for research purposes. For confidentiality purposes, the questionnaire did not request the name of the respondent. Identifying information for Twitter, Facebook, Google Plus or email accounts was not recorded. The ethics review committee of the College of Medicine, King Saud University, Riyadh, approved this study.

## Results

The estimated sample size was 195 participants, but a total of 381 participants responded to the questionnaire. Only 269 people met the criteria and completed the study questionnaires. Therefore, a total of 269 complaints by the participants were analyzed in detail.

| Characteristics | N | MD | P | T | S | (P value) |
|---|---|---|---|---|---|---|
| **Gender** | | | | | | |
| Male | 78 (29%) | 40 (51.3% ) | 6 (7.7%) | 3 (3.8%) | 29 (37.2%) | 0.135 |
| female | 191 (71%) | 103 (53.9%) | 4 (2.1%) | 13 (6.8%) | 71 (37.2%) | |
| **Age** | | | | | | |
| 18-29 | 152 (56.5%) | 68 (44.7%) | 6 (4%) | 13 (8.5% ) | 65 (42.8% ) | 0.032 |
| 30-44 | 90 (33.5%) | 57 (63.3%) | 2 (2.2% ) | 2 (2.2%) | 29 (32.2% ) | |
| ≥45 | 27 (10%) | 18 (66.7% ) | 2 (7.4% ) | 1 (3.7%) | 6 (22.2% ) | |
| **Marital Status** | | | | | | |
| Un Married | 164 (61%) | 74 (45.1%) | 5 (3%) | 13 (7.9%) | 72 (44%) | 0.004 |
| Married | 105 (39%) | 69 (65.7%) | 5 (4.7%) | 3 (2.9%) | 28 (26.7%) | |
| **Level of Education** | | | | | | |
| Below Secondary school | 11 (4.1%) | 6 (54.5%) | 0 (0%) | 1 (9.1%) | 4 (36.4%) | 0.809 |
| Secondary school | 67 (24.9%) | 31 (46.2%) | 4 (6%) | 4 (6%) | 28 (41.8%) | |
| University | 191 (71%) | 106 (55.5%) | 6 (3.1%) | 11 (5.8%) | 68 (35.6%) | |
| **Occupation** | | | | | | |
| Do not work | 17 (6.3%) | 5 (29.4%) | 1 (5.9%) | 1 (5.9%) | 10 (58.8%) | NA |
| Housewives | 34 (12.6%) | 24 (70.5%) | 1 (3%) | 1 (3%) | 8 (23.5%) | |
| Students | 118 (43.9%) | 56 (47.4%) | 4 (3.4%) | 10 (8.5%) | 48 (40.7%) | |
| Teachers | 20 (7.4%) | 10 (50%) | 1 (5%) | 1 (5%) | 8 (40%) | |
| Administrative | 36 (13.4%) | 22 (61.1%) | 1 (2.8%) | 1 (2.8%) | 12 (33.3%) | |
| Military | 13 (4.8%) | 8 (61.5%) | 0 (0%) | 1 (7.7%) | 4 (30.8%) | |
| Health workers | 10 (3.7%) | 5 (50%) | 0 (0%) | 0 (0%) | 5 (50%) | |
| Others | 21 (7.8%) | 13 (61.9%) | 2 (9.5%) | 1 (4.8%) | 5 (23.8%) | |
| **Income** | | | | | | |
| <3.000 SR | 90 (33.5%) | 43 (47.8%) | 2 (2.2%) | 9 (10%) | 36 (40%) | NA |
| 3.000-6.999 SR | 26 (9.7%) | 18 (69.2%) | 0 (0%) | 2 (7.7%) | 6 (23.1%) | |
| 7.000-13.999 SR | 56 (20.8%) | 31 (55.3%) | 2 (3.6%) | 1 (1.8%) | 22 (39.3%) | |
| 14.000 SR ≤ | 23 (8.5%) | 13 (56.5%) | 2 (8.7%) | 0 (0%) | 8 (34.8%) | |
| Other | 74 (27.5%) | 38 (51.3%) | 4 (5.4%) | 4 (5.4%) | 28 (37.8%) | |
| N: Number of Participants; MD: Medical Doctor; P: Pharmacist; T: Traditional Healers; S: Self-help + Relative, etc.; NA: Not Applicable | | | | | | |

**Table 1:** Sociodemographic characteristics of 269 participants, with respect to different consultations.

Table 1 shows the sociodemographic characteristics of the participants; 191 (71%) were female, and 152 (56.5%) were 30 years old or younger. The majority were unmarried 164 (61%), and approximately 191 (71%) had a university education or higher. Approximately 118 (43.9%) were students, 36 (13.4%) were administrative workers, and 34 (12.6%) were housewives. Approximately 116 (43.1%) of the participants had a monthly income below 7.000 SR; 74 (27.5%) did not specify their income or had no income. Six males (7.7%) consulted pharmacists, compared with 4 females (2.1%). By contrast, 13 (6.8%) females but only 3 (3.8%) males consulted a TH. Moreover, as the participant age increased, consultations of MDs became more frequent, while dependence on self-help and relative consultations decreased. The majority (69; 65.7%) of the married participants consulted an MD, whereas most (72; 72%)

of the unmarried participants preferred self-help and relative consultations ($p<0.05$).

A high percentage of participants without a university education preferred self-help (32; 41%), whereas the majority of individuals with a university education or higher (106; 55.5%) consulted an MD. Ten of the unemployed participants (58.8%) and 48 (40.7%) of the students depended on self-help. However, the majority of the housewives (24; 70.5%), administrative workers (22; 61.1%) and military personnel (8; 61.5%) consulted an MD. In the group with an income lower than 3,000 SR, 36 (40%) depended on self-help compared with 43 (47.8%) who consulted an MD.

| Diseases | N | Medically Trained Practitioner | Benefit | Non Medically Trained Practitioner | Benefit |
|---|---|---|---|---|---|
| Respiratory Tract Disorders | 36 (13.4%) | 25 (69.4%) | 11 (44%) | 11 (30.6%) | 7 (63.6%) |
| Gastrointestinal Tract Disorders | 21 (7.8%) | 18 (85.7%) | 10 (55.6%) | 3 (14.3%) | 1 (33.3%) |
| Musculo skeletal Disorders | 10 (3.7%) | 9 (90%) | 3 (33.3%) | 1 (10%) | - |
| Psychological Disorders | 65 (24.1%) | 14 (21.5%) | 5 (35.7%) | 51 (78.5%) | 23 (45.1%) |
| Neurological Disorders | 11 (4.1%) | 6 (54.5%) | 1 (16.7%) | 5 (45.5%) | 2 (40%) |
| Cardiovascular Disorders | 13 (4.8%) | 8 (61.5%) | 4 (50%) | 5 (38.5%) | 1 (20%) |
| Endocrine Disorders | 14 (5.2%) | 12 (85.7%) | 8 (66.7%) | 2 (14.3%) | 1 (50%) |
| Dermatological Disorders | 8 (3%) | 8 (100%) | 6 (75%) | - | - |
| Urogenital Disorders | 7 (2.6%) | 6 (85.7%) | 6 (100%) | 1 (14.3%) | - |
| Orthopedic Disorders | 5 (1.9%) | 5 (100%) | 3 (60%) | - | - |
| Obstetric and Gynecological Disorders | 3 (1.1%) | - | - | 3 (100%) | 1 (33.3%) |
| Ophthalmology Disorders | 1 (0.4%) | - | - | 1(100%) | - |
| Ear, Nose and Throat Disorders | 37 (13.8%) | 19 (51.4%) | 17 (89.5%) | 18 (48.6%) | 13 (72.2%) |
| Dental Disorders | 3 (1.1%) | 2 (66.7%) | 1 (50%) | 1(33.3%) | 1 (100%) |
| Oncology Disorders | 4 (1.5%) | 4 (100%) | 2 (50%) | - | - |
| Hematology Disorders | 6 (2.2%) | 4 (66.7%) | 1 (25%) | 2 (33.3%) | 1 (50%) |
| Not specific disease | 25 (9.3%) | 13 (52%) | 11 (84.6%) | 12 (48%) | 4 (33.3%) |
| Total | 269 | 153 | 89 | 116 | 55 |
| | 100% | 56.90% | 58.20% | 43.10% | 47.40% |

Medically Trained Practitioner: Medical Doctor and Pharmacist; Non Medically Trained Practitioner: Traditional Healers and Self-help + Relative; N: Number of Participants

**Table 2:** The health problem versus the types of health seeking services and it benefit.

Table 2 shows the diseases that participants reported and the distribution of consultations of medically and non-medically trained practitioners. Psychological disorders were reported most often (65 people; 24.1%).

The second and third most common problems reported were ear, nose and throat (ENT) and respiratory disorders, by 37 (13.8%) and 36 respondents (13.4%), respectively.

The lowest percentage was found for ophthalmology disorders, with 1 person (0.4%). Dental and oncology disorders were reported by 3 (1.1%) and 4 (1.5%) people, respectively.

Regarding the types of health-seeking services, the majority of the participants who reported gastrointestinal (GI) disorders (18; 85.7%) and 25 (69.4%) with respiratory tract disorders consulted a medically trained practitioner (pharmacist or MD).

However, the majority of the participants with psychological disorders (51; 78.5%) sought help from a non-medically trained practitioner.

Twenty-five participants (9.3%) had nonspecific disorders, of whom 13 (52%) consulted a medically trained practitioner. A high proportion of these participants (11; 84.6%) claimed to receive a benefit. However, only 4 (33.3%) of 12 (48%) participants who consulted a non-medically qualified practitioner noted any benefit.

Figure 1 shows the sources of HSB. Physicians were consulted most often (143; 53%) followed by self-help and relatives (100; 37%). Pharmacist and THs were consulted by only 26 (10%) participants.

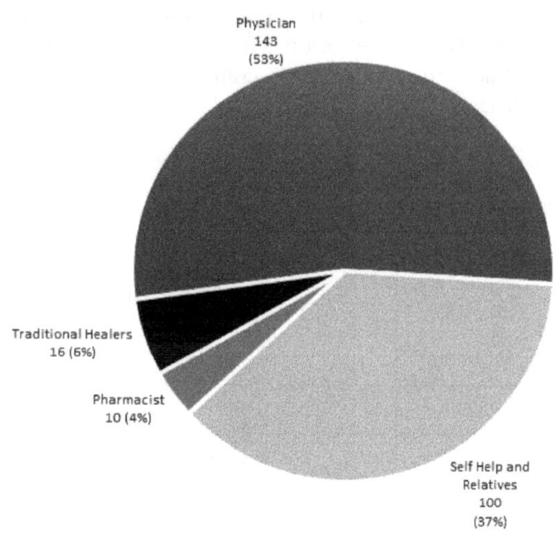


**Figure 1:** Source of help seeking behavior.

The 83 (58%) participants who consulted an MD reported a perceived benefit, but 58 (40.6%) did not notice a difference. Two (1.4%) participants felt they were harmed. However, approximately half of participants who preferred self-help and relative consultations reported a benefit; the other half noted no difference. Moreover, only 26 participants consulted a TH or pharmacist. Fourteen (53.8%) participants reported no difference, and 12 (46.2%) perceived a benefit (Figure 2).

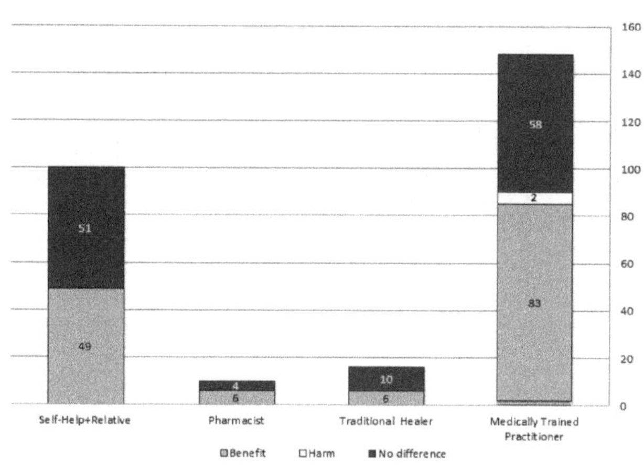


**Figure 2:** Source of help seeking behavior versus outcome perception.

The majority of the participants (55.6%) said they obtain health information from social media (WhatsApp, Twitter, and Facebook), followed by hospitals and health centers (54.7%). Websites and Web forums, TV and radio, and relatives and friends had similar rates of use, with 36%, 35.6% and 32.4%, respectively. Only 19.6% of participants received information via online newspapers, and 20.9% reported exposure to awareness campaigns and brochures.

The participants attributed their decision to seek help from nonprofessionals to the long delays for obtaining appointments at Ministry of Health hospital (MOH) (42.7%); the second most common reason given was difficulty accessing specialized health centers and long waiting times for medical consultations (40%). High health insurance costs also discouraged individuals from seeking advice from trained professionals (19.6%). Poorly equipped neighborhood health care centers led 17.3% of the participants to consult non-health professionals. However, easy access to pharmacists and THs were cited by 12.4% of the participants. Only 9.8% of the participants gave other reasons for seeking help from non-health professionals.

## Discussion

The most common disorders that caused participants to seek help from the various types of healthcare providers were psychiatric, ENT and respiratory disorders. Consistent with the WHO estimation that 25% of the world population suffers from mental illness, both in the developed and developing world's [15,16], approximately 24% of our participants complained of psychiatric disorders. Moreover, in Saudi Arabia, there are only 0.3 psychiatrists for every 10,000 individuals [17]. Thus, adequate professional health care is not readily available, which might contribute to the increased incidence or worsening of psychiatric disorders. ENT disorders comprised 13.8% of all complaints, which was associated with the season in which the study was conducted (winter). Furthermore, influenza-like illness epidemics occur with seasonal characteristics and marked winter peaks in most countries and regions [18]. Additionally, 13.4% of the complaints were respiratory disorders. An earlier study in Saudi Arabia showed that 18% of the subjects sought help for respiratory problems [7], which might be correlated with the dusty environment and smoking habits of the population [17]. A study in China showed that the degree of air pollution was closely associated with the number of patients with respiratory diseases [19].

Fifty-three percent of the subjects consulted an MD compared with 77% in a previous 1992 study [7]. Furthermore, it was surprising to find that the number of participants who reported self-treatment increased markedly, the previous rate was only 2%; it is now 37% [7]. The increase in self-treatment and decrease in MD consultations may be due to the increasing availability of medications without a prescription. It may reflect an increased access to knowledge through social media and the Internet. A recent report showed that the prevalence of using the Internet in Saudi Arabia rose from 5% in 2001 to approximately 55% of the population at the end of 2013 [20]. Additionally, the number of shops selling traditional therapy items has increased over the past three decades. The present study had some limitations, including that the majority of our study population was highly educated; 71% of the participants had a university education or higher. Thus, these individuals might be able to spend more on health care.

Age, marital status, play a significant role in HSB. In the present study, older participants consulted an MD more often than the younger participants. Additionally, married subjects more often consulted an MD (65.7%). As a previous study in Riyadh City showed, the majority of individuals over 45 years old consulted a medically trained practitioner (89.5%) and most of the married participants consulted a medically qualified practitioner (79.3%) [7]. However, it is common for an elderly patient to have multiple pathologies. The experience of older individuals has led them to recognize that their problems can only be solved by experts (i.e., MDs). Furthermore, family experiences led to increased consultations of medically qualified practitioners in antenatal and pediatric clinics by wives and children.

The primary source of health information for the participants was social media (55.6%). Earlier studies have shown that social media has a significant effect on promoting patient knowledge. Furthermore, obtaining health information helps patients overcome multiple barriers [21-23]. This platform opens an avenue for health decision makers to promote health.

The majority of the subjects reported benefits from seeking help from an MD. Moreover, 25 participants had vague symptoms, and they benefited from consulting medically (84.6%) and non-medically trained practitioners (33.3%). Medically trained practitioners are respected health care professionals who have at least six years of training. Therefore, they are trusted by the public, unlike nonprofessionals.

The reasons that people visited non-medically trained practitioners instead of MDs included lack of time and difficulty accessing specialized healthcare centers. Our results showed that health coverage by clinical services and the number of hospital beds was inadequate, which is recognized by the decision makers in the Kingdom of Saudi Arabia (KSA). WHO reports have cited 21 beds locally and 27 beds globally per 10,000 individuals, which illustrates the need for more hospitals and primary health care (PHC) centers [17]. Thus, the MOH plans to build vast medical complexes throughout the Kingdom to increase coverage. Furthermore, the MOH has adopted a new method to manage cases (i.e., one-day surgery), which has increased the bed turnover rate to approximately 4 per month [24]. In 2013, Riyadh City had 482 hospitals and PHC centers, an increase of 16.8% since 2006 [25].

## Conclusion/Recommendations

Based on the present study, approximately half of individuals seek non-medical help despite having a condition that requires medical help. Therefore, the HSB in the Saudi community is still in need of improvement. Because the use of the Internet has become common among the public, dependence on self-help treatment has increased. We hope this study will motivate researchers to examine different HSBs and their effects, such as the influence of the Internet on self-care. Furthermore, studies are needed to investigate participant claims of difficulty in accessing health care centers and coverage, the safety of THs, and the use of social media for rationalizing HSB.

## Acknowledgments

We thank all the participants. This study was supported by the College of Medicine Research Center and the Chair of Health Education and Health Promotion, the Deanship of Scientific Research, King Saud University, Riyadh, Saudi Arabia.

## References

1. Cornally N, McCarthy G (2011) Help-seeking behaviour: a concept analysis. Int J Nurs Pract 17: 280-288.
2. (2014) Dictionary.com
3. WHO (2010) Classifying health workers.
4. American Heritage® Dictionary of the English Language (2014) (5th edn.).
5. Al-Rowais N, Al-Faris E, Mohammad AG, Al-Rukban M, Abdulghani HM (2010) Traditional healers in Riyadh region: reasons and health problems for seeking their advice. A household survey. J Altern Complement Med 16: 199-204.
6. Alosaimi FD, Alshehri Y, Alfraih I, Alghamdi A, Aldahash S, et al. (2015) Psychosocial correlates of using faith healing services in Riyadh, Saudi Arabia: a comparative cross-sectional study. Int J Ment Health Syst 9: 8.
7. al-Shammari SA (1992) Help-seeking behavior of adults with health problems in Saudi Arabia. Fam Pract Res J 12: 75-82.
8. Al-Nahedh N (2004) Sociodemographic variables affecting the health seeking behaviour of mothers in a saudi community. J Family Community Med 11: 3-9.
9. Leung P, Cheung M, Tsui V (2012) Help-seeking behaviors among Chinese Americans with depressive symptoms. Soc Work 57: 61-71.
10. Klineberg E, Biddle L, Donovan J, Gunnell D (2011) Symptom recognition and help seeking for depression in young adults: a vignette study. Soc Psychiatry Psychiatr Epidemiol 46: 495-505.
11. Norton C, Dibley L (2013) Help-seeking for fecal incontinence in people with inflammatory bowel disease. J Wound Ostomy Continence Nurs 40: 631-638.
12. Ministry of economy and planning SA. Demographic Research (2007). In: CaIT (ed.) Commission.
13. Ministry of economy and planning SA. Population Estimates (2010). In: CDoSa (ed.) Information.
14. Communication and Information Technology Commission SA in cooperation with King Fahd University of petroleum and minerals. Individual reports, ICT Survey results in Saudi Arabia 2014.
15. WHO (2001) Mental disorders affect one in four people. Geneva.
16. Almutairi AF (2015) Mental illness in Saudi Arabia: an overview. Psychol Res Behav Manag 8: 47-49.
17. WHO (2015) World health statistics.
18. News. Sit (2014) The Reason for the Season: why flu strikes in winter.
19. Ping J (2015) Influence of hazy weather on patient presentation with respiratory diseases in Beijing, China. Asian Pac J Cancer Prev: APJCP 16: 607-611.
20. Communications and Information Technology Commission SA (2013). Annual report.
21. Mattingly TJ (2015) Innovative patient care practices using social media. J Am Pharm Assoc (2003) 55: 288-293.
22. Kofinas J, Varley A, Sapra K, Kanj RV, Chervenak FA, et al. (2014) Randomized controlled trial of adjunctive social media for more effective contraceptive counseling. Obstet Gynecol. 123: 107.
23. Greene JA, Choudhry NK, Kilabuk E, Shrank WH (2011) Online social networking by patients with diabetes: a qualitative evaluation of communication with Facebook. J Gen Intern Med 26: 287-292.
24. Ministry of Health KoSA (2012). MOH Sets Bed Occupancy Rate Plan for Hospitals.
25. Ministry of Health KoSA (2013). Health Statistical Annual book.

16

# Effect of Unani Formulation in Cervicitis (*Warme-unqur-rahm*)

**Shabnam Zahid**[1*], **Hina Rehman**[2], **Aysha Raza**[1], **Fahmida Kousar**[1]

*1Department of Ilmul Qabalat wa Niswan wa Atfal, Ayurvedic & Unani Tibbia College, Karol Bagh, New Delhi.*

*2 Research officer, Central research institute of Unani Medicine, Hyderabad, Telangana.*

***Corresponding author:** Shabnam Zahid, Research Scholar, Department of IlmulQabalatwaAmrazeNiswan (OBG), Ayurvedic and Unani Tibbia College, Karol Bagh, New Delhi, India, E-mail: shabnamparveen9@gmail.com

**Abstract**

**Objective:** To evaluate the efficacy and safety of Polyherbal Unani formulations (PHUFs) with placebo in *Warme-unqur-rahm* (Cervicitis).

**Methods:** A Randomized single-blind placebo controlled trial was designed to compare the efficacy of Unani formulations against placebo in diagnosed cases of cervicitis in the Department of Gynaecology of Ayurvedic & Unani Tibbia College, Delhi. Sixty married female participants with age group of 18-40 years having symptoms of cervicitis with no systemic illness and sexually transmitted diseases and not using oral or intrauterine contraceptives were randomly allocated to receive either test drug (n = 30) or placebo (n = 30) for three months.

In the test group, sufoofe sailan (PHUF) 5 gm orally was given twice daily and intravaginally humul (pessary) of isapghol (Isapgol: *Plantago ovata Forsk*) and alsi (Linseed: *Linum usitatissimum L.*) soaked in arqe gulab (rose water) was kept at mid-cycle for 10 days for three consecutive cycles and the placebo was given for same protocol. On the basis of improvement in subjective and objective parameters the response of treatment was graded as cured, improved and not cured. Results were analyzed by Chi-square/Fisher Exact test and Student t test.

**Results:** There was a significant improvement in the subjective and objective parameters in test group after treatment with $P < 0.001$. Cervical discharge, cervical erythema and cervical oedema were significantly reduced ($P < 0.001$) after three months of treatment. Interpretation and conclusion: Study revealed that test drug formulations were effective and safe in the management of cervicitis. Besides, the trial should be conducted on large sample size for effectiveness of drug.

**Keywords:** *Warme-unqur-rahm*; STDs; Cervicitis; Sufoofe sailan; Polyherbal Unani formulation

## Introduction

Gynaecological infections are common worldwide. Diseases of the cervix are common in almost all sexually active women as cervix is the most common site of genital infection [1]. The incidence of cervicitis is high about 30–45% in some STI clinic populations and sexually transmissible pathogens are present in most of the cases [2-3]. Cervicitis (*Warme-unqur-rahm*) is a clinical syndrome characterised with mucupurulent cervical discharge and signs of inflammation of cervix such as oedema and easily induced cervical bleeding (friability) [3,4].

Other subtle signs includes cervical ectopy with identification of ≥10 PMNLs per high power field in gram stained smear of cervical secretions [5,6]. The presence of above finding suggest either *Neisseria gonorrhoea* or Chalamydial infection but studies revealed that above organism are identified in only half or less than half of cases of cervicitis and causes of rest cases remain unknown [7,8].

*Mycoplasma genitalium, Mycoplasma hominis, Ureaplasma urealyticum, Bacterial vaginosis, Herpes simplex virus* (HSV), *Trichomonas vaginalis* etc. are organisms variably present in rest of cases and often called nonspecific cervicitis (NSC) [2,4,9].

Chronic cervicitis is more common, seen in about 35-85% of women with higher prevalent among parous [10,11]. Sacral backache, lower abdominal pain and dyspareunia are other symptoms of cervicitis. Unfortunately, infection of the cervix is often asymptomatic and represents a reservoir for sexual and perinatal transmission of pathogenic micro-organisms.

Hence, timely and correct diagnosis is essential as improper diagnosis and incorrect management can lead to serious consequences like PID, cervical neoplasias, infertility and adverse outcomes of pregnancy and new born [2,5]. It is also associated with increased shedding of HIV-1 from the cervix in the absence of chlamydial and gonococcal infection [12].

Centers for Disease Control and Prevention (CDC) recommends Chlamydia Trachomatis screening at least annually for all women aged 25 years of age and younger, because the majorities of infections in women are asymptomatic and do not usually cause visible signs of cervicitis [13].

Cervicitis affects many aspects of quality of life including reproductive ability and sexual functioning. Mental health and the ability to work and perform routine physical activities are also affected.

The initial therapy for cervicitis in conventional system is the use of antibiotics and antifungal drugs both orally and locally. Increase use of broad-spectrum antibiotic results in antibiotic resistance. Failure of medical treatment (after two or three attempts) further needs surgical interventions by diathermy, cauterization, cryotherapy, laser ablation, and others which cause further complications.

None of these treatments provides the definite efficacy in spite of high cost and side effects. Hence, there is a need for alternate therapy which is safe, effective, easily available and free from side effects.

Presently Complementary therapies are more accepted due to invidious effect of contemporary therapy. Research shows that almost half (49%) of women of reproductive age reported to use Complementary therapies [14]. One of complementary medicine is Unani system of medicine or Greco-Arab medicine, which was originated by Hippocrates (460-377 BC) and flourished by Arabs (9-13 AD) and Mughal physicians. Unani System of Medicine is bestowed with a number of single herb or formulations that have been in used for cervicitis since antiquity. Each and every part of the herbs are being used for a number of pharmacological actions and a range of herbal preparations are made by these including sufoof (powders), joshanda (decoction), arq (extract) and many more.

For present study Polyherbal formulation (PHF), "Sufoof" was selected as PHF have synergistic, agonistic and antagonistic actions that work to produce a wide range of therapeutic activity with fewer side effects. Intravaginally humul of Isapgol and Linseed for *warme-unqur-rahm* has been documented by eminent Unani scholars.

*Sufoofe sailan* has been mentioned to treat leucorrhoea in various classical texts but it has been clearly mentioned that the most common cause of leucorrhoea is *warme-unqu-rahm* [15-17]. Various ingredients of above formulation shown to have antimicrobial, [18-21] anti-inflammatory, [22-24] antioxidant, [25-26] analgesic, [22,24,26] immunomodulator [27] and wound healing properties [28]. Considering the aforementioned fact, the present study was carried out to evaluate the efficacy PHUFs in the management of cervicitis.

## Material and Methods

This was a single-centre, single-blind, placebo controlled and parallel group study with equal randomization (1:1). The study was conducted at Delhi, India.

### Participants

Sixty married participants between ages of 18–40 years having vaginal discharge, low backache, lower abdominal pain, dysuria, foul smell, pruritus vulvae, dyspareunia and post coital bleeding attending Obstetrics and Gynaecology OPD of Ayurvedic and Unani Tibbia College Hospital, Delhi during March 2013 to February 2014 were included in the study. Approval of study was taken from the Departmental Review Board. The subjects were randomly assigned in the test group (n = 30) and the control group (n = 30) using a computer generated randomization table.

Duly signed informed consents were obtained from all the patients prior to the initiation of the study. Patients with pelvic pathology, systemic illness, unmarried and pregnant women were excluded. Women using contraceptive measures (IUCD, OCPs) and having history of conisation, cryotherapy and cauterization were also excluded. All participants were thoroughly evaluated prior to study. Subjects having symptoms of cervicitis were underwent pelvic examination (in dorsal position). First vulva and perineum were examined for any discharge, erythema, excoriation, and any other skin changes. Speculum examination was done to note the condition of vagina and cervix (Edema, erythema, congestion, discharge, erosion) and bimanual examination was done to note the cervical texture, external os, hypertrophy, motion tenderness and uterine position (AV/RV). Simultaneously, Endocervical swab culture, Gram staining of endocervical secretion's smear and Pap smear were taken.

After a clinical diagnosis of cervicitis, all patients underwent certain investigations, including complete blood picture, erythrocyte sedimentation rates, random blood sugar, and complete urine analysis to exclude systemic illnesses. VDRL & HIV I & II to exclude STDs, pelvic ultrasound were done to exclude pelvic pathology and Pap smear to exclude malignancy.

### Intervention

Ingredients of *Sufoofe sailan* include; *Gul-e-Dhawa* (*Woodfordia fructicosa Kurz.*), *Gul-e-fufal* (*Areca catechu L.*), *Mochras (Salamalia malabarica Scholts & Endl.) and Gond-e-molasri (Mimusops elangi L.)*. Locally humul (pessary) of Isapgol (*Plantago ovata Forsk.*) and Alsi *(Linum usitatissimum L.)* were used. All the drugs were purchased from drug retailer of Delhi and were identified by taxonomist working in CSIR-NISCAIR (National Institute of Science Communication and Information Research), Dr. K.S. Krishnan Marg, New Delhi 11012.

The ingredients of *Sufoofe sailan* were finely powdered and filled in dry plastic packets and stored at cool and dry place while for placebo group capsules of wheat flour were made and filled in similar packets. For humul preparation, both Isapgol and Linseed were finely powdered and soaked in arq-e-gulab and this preparation was evenly applied on the humul and kept intravaginally at night in the mid-cycle under aseptic precautions.

In test group 5 gm of *sufoofe sailan* twice daily was given orally for 3 months and intravginally humool of Isapgol and Linseed was kept for 10 days after menses for three consecutive cycles. In placebo group 2 capsules of roasted flour twice daily were given orally, while intravaginally only humul of arq-e-gulab was given for the same protocol. The study duration was divided into 3 visits of follow-up of one month each at mid cycles (after menses) during treatment.

At each follow up patients were enquired about the signs and symptoms of cervicitis particularly about vaginal discharge, low backache, lower abdominal pain, dysuria, foul smell, pruritus vulvae, dyspareunia and post coital bleeding.

Pelvic examination was done at baseline, every month (mid cycles) and after three months of treatment to note the changes of cervix. Progression and regression of symptoms were recorded in case record form. Endocervical swab culture and Gram staining of endocervical secretion's smear were taken before and after treatment. Compliance to therapy was assessed at every follow-up by examining the packets in which medication was dispensed at previous visit. Participants were informed not to take any other concomitant treatment during study.

### Outcomes measures

Effectiveness of trial drugs were assessed by reduction in subjective and objectives parameters. Subjective parameter comprises symptoms of cervicitis (lowbackache, lower abdominal pain, discharge per vagina, dysuria, dyspareunia, post coital bleeding). Intensity of low backache and lower abdominal pain was assessed by Visual Analogue

Scale (VAS). VAS is commonly used validated scale due to its simplicity and reliability, containing a 10 cm line (0–10 defined as no pain to worst pain) [29].

Discharge per vaginum was graded from 0 to 4 grade: Score: 1-No discharge; 2-Mild (streak/spotting on undergarments); 3-Moderate (stain on undergarments); Score: 4-Severe (using pads) [12]. The other subjective parameters like dysuria, dyspareunia, and post coital bleeding were based on the arbitrary four point scale (0 = None, 1 = Mild, 2 = Moderate, 3 = Severe) and foul smell and pruritus vulvae were assessed by the presence (score 1) and absence (score 0). Objective Parameters was assessed by female genital infection grading system given by DAIDS as an addendum in 2009 [30].

It includes cervical discharge, cervical erythema, cervical oedema and friability and cervical motion tenderness. On the basis of improvement in subjective and objective parameters before, during and after the treatment, the response was graded as follows: Cured; Complete resolution of signs and symptoms with <10 WBCs per high power field and absence of bacteria on cervical gram stain and culture report should be negative.

Improved; Incomplete resolution of signs and symptoms with <10 WBCs per high power field and absence of bacteria on cervical gram stain and negative culture report. Or Complete resolution of signs and symptoms with = 10 WBCs per high power field with absence or presence of bacteria on cervical gram stain and negative culture report. Not cured; no apparent response or worsening of signs and symptoms and >10 WBCs per high power field and presence of bacteria on cervical gram stain and positive culture report.

## Adverse reactions or events

The safety of the drug was assessed by Serum Glutamic Oxaloacetic Transaminase (SGOT), Serum Glutamic Pyruvic Transaminase (SGPT), alkaline phosphatase, blood urea, serum creatinine and haemoglobin & ESR at baseline and after three months of treatment. All the participants were requested to report any adverse event during the trial.

## Statistical analysis

The Statistical software namely SAS 9.2, SPSS 15.0, Stata 10.1, MedCalc 9.0.1, Systat 12.0 and R environment ver.2.11.1 were used for the analysis of the data. Student t test (two tailed, independent) has been used to find the significance of study parameters on continuous scale between two groups (Inter group analysis) on metric parameters.

Mann Whitney U test has been used to find the significance between two groups for parameters on non-interval scale and Student t test (two tailed, dependent) has been used to find the significance of study parameters on continuous scale within each group. Chi-square/ Fisher Exact test has been used to find the significance of study parameters on categorical scale between two or more groups.

# Result

## Participants flow

A total of 131 participants of cervicitis were screened during the study period. Out of which 46 participants refused to participate; 25 were excluded and the rest of them (60) were randomized into experimental and placebo groups.

Two patients in the placebo group were drop out due to no improvement in symptoms of cervivcitis. The final analysis was conducted on 58 patients (Figure 1).

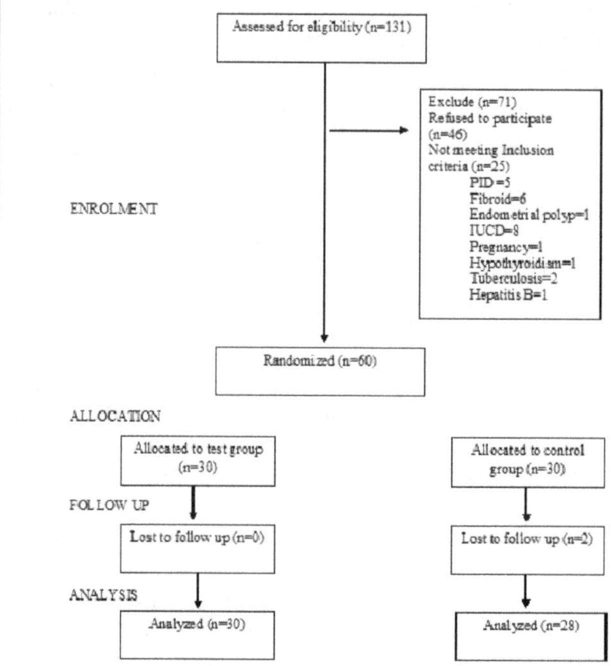


**Figure 1:** Flow diagram of participants.

## Baseline data

No significant difference was identified between the test and placebo groups with regard to basic demographic data (including age, education, socioeconomic status, menstrual and obstetric history and contraceptive measures) with P > 0.05 (Table 1). Thus the participants were homogenous before intervention.

The present study conducted on 60 patients of cervicitis aged between 18-40 years showed the highest incidence (53.3%) of cervicitis in the age group of 20-30 years. All patients have inflammatory changes in the Pap smear (18-mild, 38-moderate, 4-severe smear).

| Characteristic variables | Test group (n = 30) | Control group (n = 30) |
|---|---|---|
| Age in years | | |
| 20-30 | 16(53.3%) | 19(63.3%) |
| 31-40 | 14(46.7%) | 11(36.7%) |
| Mean ± SD | 31.27 ± 5.06 | 29.97 ± 5.48 |
| Socio economic status | | |
| Upper lower | 13(43.3%) | 14(46.7%) |
| Lowe middle | 12(40%) | 8(26.7%) |
| Upper middle | 5(16.7%) | 8(26.7%) |
| Education | | |

| Illiterate | 15(50%) | 14(46.7%) |
|---|---|---|
| Primary | 4(13.3%) | 0(0%) |
| Secondary | 3(10.0%) | 7(23.3%) |
| High school | 6(20%) | 6(20%) |
| Graduate or above | 0(0%) | 3(10.0%) |
| Occupation | | |
| Employee | 2(6.7%) | 4(13.3%) |
| Housewife | 28(93.3%) | 26(86.7%) |
| Obstetric History | | |
| Parity | | |
| 0 | 3(10%) | 1(3.3%) |
| 42401 | 10(33.3%) | 14(46.7%) |
| 42493 | 17(56.7%) | 14(46.7%) |
| >5 | 0(0%) | 1(3.3%) |
| Abortion | | |
| 0 | 22(73.3%) | 22(73.3%) |
| 42401 | 8(26.7%) | 8(26.7%) |
| Menstrual History | | |
| Age at menarche(yrs) | 12.83 ± 1.23 | 12.82 ± 1.11 |
| Duration of cycle (in days) | 27.83 ± 2.39 | 28.23 ± 2.3 |
| Duration of flow (in days) | 4.23 ± 1.57 | 4.23 ± 2.03 |
| Contraception | | |
| Nil | 10(33.3%) | 12(40%) |
| Condom | 16(53.3%) | 14(46.7%) |
| Tubectomy | 4(13.3%) | 4(13.3%) |
| Cytological pattern | | |
| Mild | 9(30%) | 9(30%) |
| Moderate | 19(63.3%) | 19(63.3%) |
| Severe | 2(6.7%) | 2(6.7%) |
| Data are presented as Mean ± SD and percentage. Analysis was done by Student t test (two tailed, independent) and Mann Whitney U test. P > 0.05; non-significant. | | |

**Table 1:** Comparison of basic variables of patients in test group and control group.

## Subjective parameters

The mean ± SD scores of both groups are shown in Table 2. In the test group, a significant difference was observed regarding the alleviation of vaginal discharge (P < 0.001), low backache (P < 0.001), lower abdominal pain (P < 0.001), dyspareunia (P < 0.001) after 3 months of intervention (Table 2).

| **Parameters** | **Test group (n = 30)** | | **P value** | **Control group (n = 30)** | | **P value** |
|---|---|---|---|---|---|---|
| | **Baseline** | **3 months** | | **Baseline** | **3 months** | |
| Vaginal discharge | 1.73 ± 0.45 | 0.30 ± 0.47 | <0.001** | 1.73 ± 0.44 | 1.71 ± 0.46 | 0.328 |
| Low backache | 5.03 ± 1.29 | 1.03 ± 1.06 | <0.001** | 5.07 ± 1.28 | 4.89 ± 1.29 | 0.050* |
| Lower Abdominal pain | 3.36 ± 0.67 | 0.03 ± 0.18 | <0.001** | 3.20 ± 0.41 | 3.14 ± 0.59 | 0.326 |
| Dysurea | 0.17 ± 0.38 | 0.00 ± 0.00 | 0.025* | 0.10 ± 0.31 | 0.11 ± 0.31 | 1.000 |
| Dyspareunia | 0.43 ± 0.50 | 0.00 ± 0.00 | <0.001** | 0.37 ± 0.49 | 0.39 ± 0.49 | 0.317 |
| Post coital bleeding | 0.13 ± 0.35 | 0.00 ± 0.00 | 0.046* | 0.00 ± 0.00 | 0.00 ± 0.00 | 1.000 |
| Nil | 26(86.7%) | 30(100%) | | 30(100%) | 30(100.0%) | |
| Yes | 4(13.3%) | 0(0%) | | 0(0%) | 0(0%) | |
| Foul smell | | | | | | |
| No | 5(16.7%) | 30(100%) | | 10(33.3%) | 12(40%) | |
| Yes | 25(83.3%) | 0(0%) | | 20(66.7%) | 16(53.3%) | |
| Pruritus vulvae | | | | | | |
| No | 18(60%) | 30(100%) | | 22(73.3%) | 24(80.0%) | |
| Yes | 12(40%) | 0(0%) | | 8(26.7%) | 6(20%) | |

Data are presented as Mean ± SD and percentage. Analysis was done by Student t test (two tailed, dependent). *Moderately significant (P value: 0.01 < P ≤ 0.05); **Strongly significant (P value: P ≤ 0.01).

**Table 2:** Effect of test drug and placebo on subjective parameters.

## Objective parameters

The Objective parameters (cervical discharge, cervical erythema, cervical oedema and friability and cervical motion tenderness) of the test group improved significantly after three months of treatment (P < 0.001). While non-significant difference was seen in placebo group. Gram negative bacteria were seen in smear of 24(80%) and 25(83.3%) patients in test group and control group respectively. 22 patients were improved and showed no bacteria in smear after treatment in test group. 7 patients in test and 5 in control group showed positive culture report. No causative pathogen was found in 23(76.7%) and 25(83.3%) in test and control group respectively (Table 3).

| Parameters | Test group (n = 30) | | P value | Control group (n = 30) | | P value |
|---|---|---|---|---|---|---|
| | Baseline | 3 months | | Baseline | 3 months | |
| Endocervical discharge | 1.70 ± 0.47 | 0.37 ± 0.49 | <0.001** | 1.67 ± 0.48 | 1.68 ± 0.48 | 1.000 |
| Cervical erythema | 1.27 ± 0.45 | 0.17 ± 0.38 | <0.001** | 1.07 ± 0.25 | 1.07 ± 0.26 | 1.000 |
| Cervical edema & friability | 1.07 ± 0.25 | 0.07 ± 0.25 | <0.001** | 1.17 ± 0.38 | 1.04 ± 0.19 | 0.043* |
| Cervical motion tenderness | 1.00 ± 0.45 | 0.03 ± 0.18 | <0.001** | 1.03 ± 0.18 | 1.00 ± 0.00 | 0.326 |
| WBCs | 26.07 ± 9.35 | 4.57 ± 4.79 | <0.001** | 25.77 ± 8.29 | 28.39 ± 10.18 | 0.056+ |
| Bacteria | | | | | | |
| Yes | 24(80%) | 2(6.7%) | | 25(83.3%) | 26(86.7%) | |
| No | 6(20%) | 28(93.3%) | | 5(16.7%) | 4(13.3%) | |
| Cervical swab (C&S) | | | | | | |
| Escherichia coli | 3(10%) | 1(3.3%) | | 1(3.3%) | 1(3.3%) | |
| Klebseilla | 1(3.3%) | 0(0%) | | 1(3.3%) | 0(0%) | |
| Stapylococcus | 3(10%) | 1(3.3%) | | 3(10%) | 3(10%) | |
| Sterile | 23 (76.67%) | - | | 25 (83.4%) | - | |

Data are presented as Mean ± SD and percentage. Analysis was done by Student 't' and test (two tailed, dependent). **Strongly significant (P value: P ≤ 0.01).

**Table 3:** Effect of test drug and placebo on objective parameters.

## Harms

All investigations were within normal range in test group after three months of intervention and no obnoxious effect were observed.

## Outcome

In the test group, out of 30 patients of cervicitis, 12(40%) were cured completely and 18(60%) were improved; while in control group no patients were cured completely but 4(13.3%) were improved. Comparison was done and it revealed that difference in cured and improved was strongly significant (P < 0.001) (Table 4).

| | Cured | Improved | Not cured |
|---|---|---|---|
| Test group (n = 30) | 12(40%) | 18(60%) | Nil (0%) |
| Control group (n = 30) | Nil (0%) | 4(13.3%) | 24(80%) |

Data presented as percentage; test used Chi square Fisher exact; P < 0.001 considered strongly significant.

**Table 4:** Therapeutic response of test formulations and placebo on cervicitis.

## Discussion

Cervicitis is probably the most frequent problem faced by gynaecologist, which is more complex because the inflammatory reaction in the cervix accompanies lesions of the corpus or the vagina. Cervicitis is commonly caused by STDs. It is a frequently asymptomatic inflammatory condition of the cervix [11,31-33]. Infective causes of acute and chronic cervicitis are more common than non-infective causes and include a wide spectrum ranging from bacterial, viral, protozoan and fungi micro-organisms commonly encountered in STIs [34].

According to Unani concept, there is defence power in the body known as *tabi'at-e-mudabbir-e-badan* which keeps body immune from certain microbial diseases. It guides the body to produces certain specific substances which constitute humors and thus maintain normal temperament of humors (blood, phlegm, bile and black bile). Any derangement in these humours either qualitatively or quantitatively leads to disease [35]. As Unani Scholars claimed that warme unqur rahm is caused by Ufunat and dominance of Khilt dam or Safra (blood or bile humour) [36-37] which belongs to *Warme har* disease. Hence, it should be treated with barid (cold) wa yabis (dry) drugs and requires the drug having dafe ta'fun (antimicrobial) and mohallil (resolvant) properties to relieve infections and associated symptoms of cervicitis [17]. The temperament of Gule dhawa, Supari, Mochras and Molsari is barid wa yabis (which are the ingredients of safofe sailan) and assumed that these drugs reduce the inflammation or dominance of khilt. Furthermore; improvement may also be due to various activities of the ingredients of PHUF. These herbs possess mohallil-e-warm (anti-inflammatory), dafe ta'fun (antimicrobial), mulattif (demulcent), mujaffif (desicant), munzij (concoctive) and qabiz (astringent) properties [38]. These herbs might have inhibited the proliferation and growth of microorganism and resolved the inflammatory process that led to the overall improvement in cervicitis. Recent studies also confirmed that these herbs possess antimicrobial, [18-21] anti-inflammatory, [22-24] antioxidant, [25-26] analgesic, [22,24,26] immunomodulator [27] and wound healing properties [28]. Study reveals Isapgol to have antimicrobial activity against *Staphylococcus aureus* [20] and *Escherichia coli* [39] while Linseeds have wide range of activity against *Staphylococcus aureus, Bacillus cereus, Klebsiella pneumonia* [21]. Tabasum et al. have conducted clinical trial on *Marham dakhlion* in chronic cervicitis and cervical erosion and the study revealed significant results in relieving the symptoms. Marham dakhlion is an ointment and Plantago ovate and *Linum usitatissimum* are one of the constituents of the formulation [40]. Similar results of these herbs were seen in our study.

This study demonstrates that the Unani formulations were effective in the improving symptoms of cervicitis. Sufoofe sailan, orally and intravaginally humool of Isapgol and Linseed was found to be beneficial in reducing the signs and symptoms of cervicitis. No obnoxious adverse effects were observed and the formulation was found safe and well accepted by the subjects. It can be concluded that Unani formulations were found to be effective and can serves an alternative therapy in cervicitis. Although the study showed remarkable response, its limitations include small population and lack of long term follow up. Therefore, studies with large sample size with long follow-up period need to be carried out for further exploration of efficacy and safety of Unani formulation.

## Acknowledgements

The authors are grateful to the head of institute Dr. K. K. Sijoria, for providing the facilities to carry out research. The authors are also grateful to Dr. K. P. Suresh, Scientist (Biostatistics), National Institute of Animal Nutrition and Physiology, Bangalore, for performing the statistical analysis.

## References

1. Durr-e-Nayab (2005) Reproductive tract infection among women in Pakistan. Pakistan Development Review 44: 2131-158.
2. Lusk MJ, Konecny P (2008) Cervicitis: a review. Current Opinion in Infectious Diseases 21: 49-55.
3. Marazo JM, Martin DH (2007) Management of Women with Cervicitis. Clinical Infectious Diseases 44: S102-S110.
4. Schwebke JR, Weiss HL (2002) Interrelationships of Bacterial Vaginosis and Cervical Inflammation. Sexually transmitted disease pp: 59-64.
5. Sweet RL (1998) The Enigmatic cervix. Dermatol Clin. 16: 739-745.
6. Myziuk L, Romanowski B, Brown M (2001) Endocervical gram stains smears & their usefulness in the diagnosis of chlamydia trachomatis. Sex Transm Infect 77: 103-106.
7. Paavonen J, Critchlow CW, De Reven I (1986) Etiology of cervical inflammation. American Journal of Obstetrics & Gynecology 154: 556-564.
8. Taylor SN, Lensing S, Schwebke J, Lillis R, Mena LA, et al (2013) Prevalence and Treatment Outcome of Cervicitis of Unknown Etiology. Sex Transm Dis 40: 379-385.
9. Gaydos C, Maldies NE, Hardick A, Hardick J, Quinn TC (2009) Mcycoplasma genitalium as a contributor to the multiple etiologies of cervicitis in women attending sexually transmitted diseases Clinics. Sex Transm Dis 36: 598-606.
10. Kumar P, Malhotra N (2008) Jeffcoate's Principles of Gynaecology (7th edn.). New Delhi, Jaypee Brother Medical Publishers (P) Ltd pp: 30-34, 54-55, 347-349.
11. Padubidri VG, Daftary SN (2011) Shaw's Textbook of Gynaecology (15th edn.). Reed Elsevier India (P) Ltd pp: 6-9, 128, 324.
12. Workowsi KA, Berman S (2010) Sexually Transmitted Diseases Treatment Guidelines. MMWR; 59(RR-12) pp: 1-110.
13. CDC (2012) Update to CDC's sexually transmitted diseases treatment guidelines, 2010: oral cephalosporins no longer recommended treatment for gonococcal infections. MMWR 61: 590-594.
14. Eisenberg DA, Davis RB, Ettner SL, Appel S, Wilky S, et al. (1998) Trends in alternative medicine use in the United States, 1990-1997: results of a follow up national survey. JAMA 280: 1569–1575.
15. Kabeeruddin M (YNM) Bayaz-e-Kabeer. Vol. II. Hikmat Book Dipo, Hyderabad Dakkin p: 72.
16. Anonymous (2006) National Formulary of Unani Medicine. Part I. New Delhi, Central Council of Research in Unani Medicine p: 242.
17. Kabeeruddin M (2003) Al-Akseer. Aejaz Publishing House, New Delhi pp: 1327-1332.
18. Parekh J, Chanda S (2007) In vitro antibacterial activity of the crude methanol extract of woodfordia fruticosa Kurz. Flower (Lythracea). Braz J Microbiol 38: 204-207.
19. Hada LS, Kakiuchi M, Hattori M, Namba T (1989) Identification of antibacterial principles against streptococcus mutans & inhibitory principles against glucosyltransferase from the seed of areca catechu L. Phytotherapy Research 3: 140-144.
20. Motamedi H, Darabpour E, Gholipour M, Seyyed Nejad SM (2010) Antibacterial effect of ethanolic & methanolic extracts of plantago ovate & oliveria decumbens Endemic in Iran against some pathogenic bacteria. International Journal of Pharmacology 6: 117-122.
21. Firas A, Al-Bayati (2007) Antibacterial activity of Linum Usitatissiumum L. seeds & active compound detection. Raj Journal Sci 18: 27-36.
22. Baravalia S, Vaghasiya YK, Chanda S (2012) Brine Shrimp Cytotoxicity, Antiinflammatory & Analgesic properties of woodfordia fruticosa Kurz flowers. Iran J Pharm Res 11: 851-861.
23. Fernandez-Banares F, Hinojosa J, Sanchez-Lombrana JL, Navarro E, Martínez-Salmerón JF, et al. (1999) Randomized clinical trial of plantago ovata seeds (dietary fiber) as compared with mesalamine in maintaining remission in ulcerative colitis. Am J Gastroenterol 94: 427-433.
24. Kaithwas G, Mukherjee A, Chaurasia AK, Majumdar DK (2011) Antiinflammatory analgesic & antipyretic activities of linum

usitatissimum L. (flaxseed/ linseed) fixed oil. Indian Journal of Experimental Biology 49: 932-938.

25. Lin ES, Li CC (2010) Evaluation of superoxide radical scavenging capacity & reducing power of areca flower extracts. Journal of Medicinal Plants Research 4: 975-981.
26. Dar A, Faizi S, Naqvi S, Roome T, Zikr-ur-Rehman S, et al. (2005) Analgesic & antioxidant activity of Mangiferin & its derivatives: the structure activity relationship. Biol Pharm Bull 28: 596-600.
27. Shah AS, Juvekar AR (2010) In vitro & in vivo immuno stimulatory activity of woodfordia fruticosa flowers on non specfic immunity. Pharma Biol 48: 1053-1058.
28. Gupta N, Jain VK (2011) Investigation of wound healing activity of methanolic extract of stem bark of mimusups elengi Linn. Afr J Tradit Complement Altern Med 8: 98-103.
29. Bijur PE, Silver W, Gallagher EJ (2001) Reliability of the Visual Analog Scale for Measurement of Acute Pain. Acad Emerg Med. 8: 1153-1157.
30. Anonymous (2004) Female Genital Grading Table for Use in Microbicide Studies. Addendum 1. Division of Aids Table For Grading The Severity of Adult And Pediatric Adverse Events. Version 1.0. November 2007 pp: 1-15.
31. Holmes KK, Stamm WE (1999) Lower genital tract infections in women. Sexually Transmitted Diseases (3rd edn.). New York, MC Graw-Hill pp: 761-781.
32. Falk L, Fredlend H, Jensen JS (2005) Signs & symptoms of urethritis & cervicitis among women with or without mycoplasma genitalium or chamydia tranchomatis infection. Sex Transm Infect 81: 73-78.
33. Donovan B (2004) Sexually transmissible infections other than HIV. Lancet 363: 545-556.
34. Nwachokor FN, Forae GD (2013) Morphological spectrum of non-neoplastic lesions of the uterine cervix in Warri, South-South, Nigeria. Nigerian Journal of Clinical Practice 16: 429-432.
35. Ahmed SI (1980) Introduction to Al-Umur Al-Tabi'yah. Saini Printers, Delhi pp: 15, 16, 40-42, 50-51, 76, 77.
36. Baghdadi IH (2007) Kitab Al-Makhtarat Fit-Tibb. (Urdu Translation). Vol. IV. New Delhi, CCRUM pp: 42-44.
37. Ibn Sina (2007) Al Qanoon. Vol. II Translated by Ghulam Husnain Kantoori. Delhi, Idara Kitabul Shifa p: 336, 337, 359.
38. Ghani N (YNM) Khazainul Advia. Part I-VI. Idara Kitab-us-Shifa pp: 229-230, 258-260, 700-701, 785-787, 1268, 1273-1274.
39. Ahmad N, Amir MK, Ayaz S, Ahmad S, Jan A, et al. (2012) Antimicrobial profile of the selected medicinal plants. International Journal of Chemical & Life Sciences 1: 1039-1041.
40. Latafat T, Siddiqui MMH, Jafri SAH (1992) A clinical study of Marham Dakhlion on Chronic cervictis and cervical erosion. Anc Sci Life 11: 158-162.

# 17

# Impact of a Novel Plant-based Treatment Option in Improving Pulmonary Function Markers in Patients with Chronic Obstructive Pulmonary Disease and Asthma

**Sachin A Shah**[1], **Ji Hyun Jamie Lee**[1], **Frank Son**[1], **Gloria St John**[1,2] **and Narinder Singh Parhar**[2*]

[1]*Thomas J Long School of Pharmacy and Health Sciences, University of the Pacific, Stockton, CA, USA*

[2]*Parhar Health Systems, Roseville, CA, USA*

[*]**Corresponding author:** Narinder Singh Parhar, MD, Sutter Independent Physician, Parhar Health Systems, 584 N. Sunrise Avenue, #100, Roseville, California 95661, Brazil, E-mail: Parharmd@gmail.com

**Abstract**

**Introduction:** COPD and asthma contribute to high morbidity and mortality along with a significant social and economic burden. Patients often turn to Nutraceuticals as adjunct therapy for disease management. Jeeva® is a novel plant based therapeutic option that integrates several nutraceuticals known to have immune-modulatory, anti-inflammatory and antioxidant properties. We sought to determine the magnitude of benefits of this novel integrative approach in patients having COPD ± asthma.

**Methods:** A retrospective evaluation of patient records was performed for all COPD and/or asthma patients who had consented to initiate Jeeva®. Demographic data, past medical history, and spirometry data (FEV1, FVC, FEV1/FVC, FEV1% predicted, FVC% predicted, FEV1/FVC% predicted) were collected. The primary endpoint was the maximum change in FEV1 and FVC pre-bronchodilator from baseline. A paired students' t-test was utilized to compare the maximum change post- Jeeva® from baseline. Intent-to-treat (ITT) analysis was performed using the last-observation carried forward methodology.

**Results:** A total of 24 patients were included for analyses. The average duration of Jeeva® consumption was 10.4 ± 5.5 months. There was a statistically significant change in FEV1 and FVC from baseline [1.72 ± 0.56 L to 1.98 ± 0.71 L; ($p < 0.001$) and 1.88 ± 0.72 L to 2.03 ± 0.70 L ($p = 0.004$) respectively]. All other endpoints also improved significantly from baseline.

**Conclusion:** Jeeva® improved pre-bronchodilator FEV1 and FVC by 264 mL and 314 ml from baseline. This is the first study suggesting significant improvements in objectively measured PFT markers after consumption of the plant-based nutraceutical Jeeva®. Further studies looking at Jeeva® in prospective, controlled settings are warranted.

**Keywords:** COPD; Asthma; Nutraceuticals

## Introduction

Chronic Obstructive Pulmonary Disease (COPD) and asthma are major causes of morbidity and mortality globally with COPD being the third leading cause of death [1]. COPD usually leads to persistent and progressive airflow limitations with enhanced chronic inflammatory responses and fibrosis in the airways that impacts activities of daily living and quality of life. According to the CDC, asthma accounts for one-quarter of all emergency room visits in the U.S. each year and over 3,000 deaths each year [2]. Although preventable to a certain degree and definitely manageable, COPD and asthma result in a significant social and economic burden [3].

The estimated total cost for the two conditions was approximately $68 billion in 2008 [4]. Starting in 2015, the Centers for Medicare and Medicaid Services (CMS) plans to expand its Hospital Readmission Reduction Program (HRRP) to include COPD. This is driven by the fact that 23% of COPD hospitalizations are subsequently readmitted within 30 days post discharge [5].

Current pharmacologic options for the management of COPD and asthma typically include short acting and long acting beta2-agonists, anticholinergics, and inhaled glucocorticoids. However, none of the existing medications or regimens have been conclusively shown to modify the long-term decline in lung function [6].

Nutraceuticals often provide an alternative or are complementary for the disease management for several disease states such as diabetes (Cinnamon, Aloe vera), dyslipidemia (Red yeast rice), the common cold (Echinacea), depression (St. John's Wort) [7-11].

Several plant based therapeutic options such as ginseng extract, yiqibushenhuoxue decoction, Bufei granules, and Weijing decoction have been purported to have pulmonary function improving properties [12-15]. Jeeva® is a novel plant based therapeutic option that integrates several nutraceuticals known to have immune-modulatory, anti-inflammatory and antioxidant properties (Table 1) [16-32].

It integrates Arabinogalactan, Acai berry, concentrated Aloe polysaccharides, Bilberry, Gum Acacia, Star Anise, and Turmeric Root in varying doses and is available in a capsule form [16].

Many patients claim to have improved disease related quality of life, but no systematic evaluation has been performed with Jeeva®. We completed the first retrospective assessment of patients having COPD and asthma treated with Jeeva® at a private physician's office.

| Ingredients | Antioxidant | Anti-inflammatory | Anti-microbial |
|---|---|---|---|
| Arabinogalactan [17,18]<br>*Larix decidua* | ✓ | | ✓ |
| Acai berry [19,20]<br>*Euterpe oleracea* | ✓ | ✓ | ✓ |
| Aloe Vera [21-23]<br>*Aloe barbadensis* | ✓ | ✓ | ✓ |
| Bilberry<br>*Vaccinium mytillus* | ✓ | ✓ | ✓ |
| Gum Acacia [27]<br>*Acacia senegal* | | ✓ | |
| Star Anise [28-30]<br>*Illicium verum* | ✓ | ✓ | ✓ |
| Turmeric Root [31,32]<br>*Curcuma longa* | ✓ | ✓ | |

**Table 1:** Biological activity of ingredients in Jeeva®.

## Methods

We performed a retrospective evaluation of patient records from 2012 to 2014 at a private physician's office in Roseville, California. The primary practitioner specializes in internal medicine and holds board certification in the practice of alternative medicine. All patients voluntarily signed an informed consent document before initiation of Jeeva®.

Patients were selected for analysis if having a diagnosis of COPD and/or asthma, and consumed Jeeva® (1-3 capsules daily based on clinical judgement) for at least 90 days in addition to standard of care.

Patients were only included if having baseline and at least 1 follow up visit with spirometry data (FEV1 and FVC measurements).

Forced expiratory volume in 1 second (FEV1), defines the volume of air that can be forced out in one second after taking a deep breath and forced vital capacity (FVC) measures the volume of air forcibly exhaled from the point of maximal inspiration both of which are accepted objective markers of pulmonary function. Those under 18 years of age were excluded. Patients were not excluded based on any co-morbidity.

A comprehensive chart review was conducted to collect demographic data, past medical history, and spirometry data. Medication history was collected but not tracked serially due to the limited availability of data.

Pulmonary function test parameters (FEV1, FVC, FEV1/FVC, FEV1% predicted, FVC% predicted, FEV1/FVC% predicted) were extracted at baseline and for each subsequent visit with available spirometry data.

The primary endpoint was the maximum change in FEV1 and FVC pre-bronchodilator from baseline. Secondary endpoints included the maximum change from baseline in FEV1 post-bronchodilator, FEV1% predicted pre-bronchodilator, FEV1% predicted post-bronchodilator, FVC post-bronchodilator, FVC% predicted pre-bronchodilator, FVC% predicted post-bronchodilator, FEV1/FVC pre-bronchodilator, FEV1/FVC post-bronchodilator, FEV1/FVC% predicted pre-bronchodilator, and FEV1/FVC% predicted post-bronchodilator.

A paired students' t-test was utilized to compare the baseline to the max change post- Jeeva® for all endpoints with a $p < 0.05$ considered significant. For patients with missing data, an intent-to-treat (ITT) analysis was performed using the last-observation carried forward methodology.

Since some patients had exaggerated effects, changes in FEV1 and FVC > 1L from baseline and >0.20 with FEV1/FVC from baseline were considered as outliers and excluded.

## Results

A total of 24 patients were included for analyses. Sixteen patients were male (66%) with eight (33%) were Female. The average age and weight were 72 ± 12 years and 84 ± 15 kg respectively. All had COPD with 13 (54%) having concomitant asthma. Seventeen (71%) were former smokers and one (4%) was a current smoker.

Fourteen patients (58%) had hypertension, six (25%) had diabetes and six (25%) had coronary artery disease. Relevant comorbid past medical history included allergic rhinitis (63%), anxiety (29%), and chronic sinusitis (13%). Twelve patients were on short acting beta-2 agonists (50%), eleven on a long acting beta-2 agonist and corticosteroid combination (46%), six on anticholinergics (25%), two on inhaled corticosteroids (8%), and one on a leukotriene modifier (4%). Average duration of Jeeva® consumption was 10.4 ± 5.5 months.

FEV1 pre-bronchodilator improved significantly from baseline (1.72 ± 0.56 L to 1.98 ± 0.71 L; $p < 0.001$) (Figure 1a). FEV1 post-bronchodilator improved significantly from 1.88 ± 0.72 L to 2.03 ± 0.70

L ($p = 0.004$). FEV1 % predicted pre- and post-bronchodilator also improved significantly (Table 1).

FVC pre-bronchodilator improved significantly from baseline (2.49 ± 0.66 L to 2.81 ± 0.73 L; $p < 0.001$) (Figure 1b). FVC post-bronchodilator improved significantly from 2.73 ± 0.82 L to 2.83 ± 0.81 L ($p = 0.006$). FVC% predicted pre and post-bronchodilator also improved significantly (Table 1).

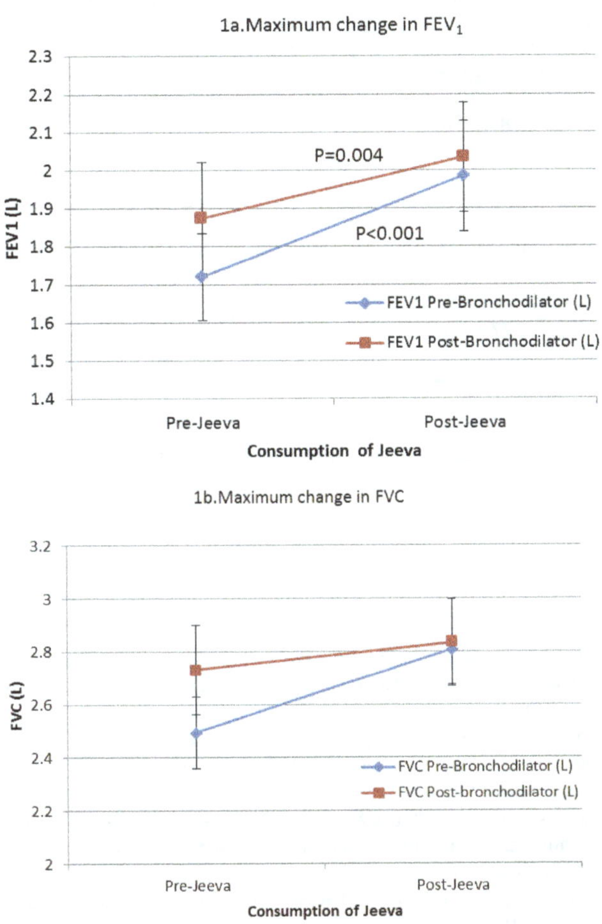


**Figure 1:** Maximum change in FEV1 and FVC.

FEV1/FVC pre-bronchodilator improved significantly from baseline (0.69 ± 0.16 to 0.77 ± 0.14; $p < 0.001$). FEV1/FVC post-bronchodilator improved significantly from 0.68 ± 0.14 to 0.74 ± 0.12 ($p < 0.001$). FEV1/FVC% predicted pre-bronchodilator improved significantly from baseline (94.3 ± 21.5 to 103.4 ± 20.9; $p < 0.001$). FEV1/FVC% predicted post-bronchodilator improved significantly from 93.2 ± 19.4 to 100.8 ± 16.1 ($p = 0.001$).

## Discussion

In our assessment of patients consuming Jeeva® for over 10 months, FEV1 and FVC pre-bronchodilator increased by 264 mL and 314 ml from baseline respectively. In a randomized, double-blind study by Murali et al., a proprietary product DCBT1234-Lung KR was compared to a salbutamol/theophylline/bromhexine combination and a lactose placebo [33]. After 6 months (n = 39) FEV1 changed significantly from 1.32 ± 0.61 L to 1.50 ± 0.72 L post DCBT1234-Lung KR. The comparator arms showed non-significant changes. In another study ginseng extract significantly increased FEV1 and FVC by 27% and 32.5% from baseline [12]. The impact of salmeterol, fluticasone, and salmeterol/fluticasone combination on pulmonary function parameters was compared in a randomized controlled trial [34]. After 12 months of treatment, the changes in FEV1 pre-bronchodilator from baseline were 78 ml, 41 ml, and 88 ml in the three groups respectively. Similarly, the mean improvements in FVC were 139 mL, 57 mL, and 57 mL after salmeterol, fluticasone, and salmeterol/fluticasone combination, respectively [34].

The respiratory system undergoes various physiological, immunological, and anatomical changes with age [35]. The estimated rate of decline in FEV1 is 25-30 mL/yr starting at age of 35-40 years and can double to 60 mL/yr after the age of 70 years [35]. FVC generally declines at approximately 22 mL/yr in healthy subjects (20 to 60 years) [36].

Chronic inflammation in the lungs can lead to narrowing of airways, destruction of parenchymal tissues, and other structural damages leading to a further decline in pulmonary function [36]. Jeeva® contains ingredients with anti-inflammatory, antioxidant, and immunomodulatory properties (Table 1) potentially explaining the mechanism behind the benefits seen in PFT markers. Based on some of the known literature on the ingredients, Jeeva® may be beneficial in long-term disease prognosis and reversibility of COPD.

There is a direct relationship between the severity of COPD and the cost of care justifying an accurate cost-benefit analysis of the available therapeutic options [37]. It is believed that the cost of estimated medical expenditure for COPD ($2507/year per patient) often under-represent the true costs [38]. Factoring in sociodemographic characteristics (age, race, education level, etc.) and indirect costs (care provided by family member), the true adjusted cost of COPD is anticipated to be much higher at $4932/year per patient [38].

In our analyses, Jeeva® posed benefits of similar magnitude (P FT parameters) and of clinical importance warranting further investigations. Whether Jeeva® used as monotherapy, or complementary to the current pharmacotherapeutic standard-of-care for COPD/asthma needs future evaluation.

Our analysis has several limitations worth noting. We could not evaluate changes in medications due to limited data. It is possible that the large magnitude of benefit seen in our results is compounded by concurrent changes in medications. A systematic assessment of patient symptoms and adverse effects was not extracted. Further, disease related hospital admissions were not assessed. Future studies should assess hospital readmission along with a standardized assessment of quality of life.

A lack of a control arm and a small sample size pose inherent limitations in data extrapolation and wide applicability. While Jeeva® is manufactured by an FDA approved manufacturer, the potency of herbal raw ingredients can vary based on the location and season of the harvest making it difficult to ascertain standardization in Jeeva® capsules [39]. Since the active moieties of the different herbal ingredients in Jeeva® need further discovery, an understanding of the pharmacokinetic profile remains unknown (Table 2).

| PFT parameters | Baseline | Max change | p-value |
|---|---|---|---|
| FEV1 (Liters) | 1.72 ± 0.56 | 1.98 ± 0.71 | $p < 0.001$ |
| FEV1 (Liters) [post-bronchodilator] | 1.88 ± 0.72 | 2.03 ± 0.70 | $p = 0.004$ |
| FEV1% predicted | 60.1 ± 14.0 | 68.1 ± 20.3 | $p = 0.002$ |
| FEV1% predicted [post-bronchodilator] | 66.67 ± 27.7 | 72.1 ± 26.1 | $p = 0.004$ |
| FVC (Liters) | 2.49 ± 0.66 | 2.81 ± 0.73 | $p < 0.001$ |
| FVC (Liters) [post-bronchodilator] | 2.73 ± 0.82 | 2.83 ± 0.81 | $p = 0.006$ |
| FVC% predicted | 65.1 ± 14.1 | 72.2 ± 13.9 | $p = 0.004$ |
| FVC% predicted [post-bronchodilator] | 65.1 ± 19.1 | 69.6 ± 19.2 | $p = 0.003$ |
| FEV1/FVC | 0.69 ± 0.16 | 0.77 ± 0.14 | $P < 0.001$ |
| FEV1/FVC [post-bronchodilator] | 0.68 ± 0.14 | 0.74 ± 0.12 | $P < 0.001$ |
| FEV1/FVC% predicted | 94.3 ± 21.5 | 103.4 ± 20.9 | $p < 0.001$ |
| FEV1/FVC% predicted [post-bronchodilator] | 93.2 ± 19.4 | 100.8 ± 16.1 | $p = 0.001$ |

**Table 2:** Impact of Jeeva® on PFT parameters.

## Conclusion

Jeeva® improved pre-bronchodilator FEV1 and FVC by 264 mL and 314 ml from baseline. This is the first study suggesting significant improvements in objectively measured PFT markers after consumption of the plant-based nutraceutical Jeeva®. Further studies looking at Jeeva® in prospective, controlled settings are warranted.

## References


1. World Health Report (2012) Geneva: World Health Organization.
2. Bousquet J, Bousquet PJ, Godard P, Daures JP (2005) The public health implications of asthma. Bull World Health Organ 83: 548-554.
3. The Global Burden of Disease (2004) World Health Organization.
4. National Heart, Lung, and Blood Institute (2010) Morbidity and mortality chartbook on cardiovascular, lung and blood disease. Bethesda, Maryland: US Department of Health and Human Services, Public Health Service, National Institutes of Health.
5. Jencks SF, Williams MV, Coleman EA (2009) Rehospitalizations among patients in the Medicare fee-for-service program. N Engl J Med 360: 1418-1428.
6. Anthonisen NR, Connett JE, Kiley JP, Altose MD, Bailey WC, et al. (1994) Effects of smoking intervention and the use of an inhaled anticholinergic bronchodilator on the rate of decline of FEV1. The Lung Health Study. JAMA 272: 1497-505.
7. Allen RW, Schwartzman E, Baker WL, Coleman CI, Phung OJ (2013) Cinnamon use in type 2 diabetes: an updated systematic review and meta-analysis. Ann Fam Med 11: 452-459.
8. Ngo MQ, Nguyen NN, Shah SA (2010) Oral aloe vera for treatment of diabetes mellitus and dyslipidemia. Am J Health Syst Pharm 67: 1804, 1806, 1808.
9. Li Y, Jiang L, Jia Z, Xin W, Yang S, et al. (2014) A meta-analysis of red yeast rice: an effective and relatively safe alternative approach for dyslipidemia. PLoS One 9: e98611.
10. Shah SA, Sander S, White CM, Rinaldi M, Coleman CI (2007) Evaluation of echinacea for the prevention and treatment of the common cold: a meta-analysis. Lancet Infect Dis 7: 473-480.
11. Bukhari IA, Dar A (2013) Behavioral profile of Hypericum perforatum (St. John's Wort) extract. A comparison with standard antidepressants in animal models of depression. Eur Rev Med Pharmacol Sci 17: 1082-1089.
12. Gross D, Shenkman Z, Bleiberg B, Dayan M, Gittelson M, et al. (2002) Ginseng improves pulmonary functions and exercise capacity in patients with COPD. Monaldi Arch Chest Dis 57: 242-246.
13. Liu J, Gao F, Li Z (2014) Effect of yiqibushenhuoxue decoction on chronic obstructive pulmonary disease measured by St. George's respiratory disease questionnaire scores and forced expiratory volume. J Tradit Chin Med 34: 445-449.
14. Guo S, Sun Z, Liu E, Feng J, Fu M, et al. (2014) Effect of bufei granule on stable chronic obstructive pulmonary disease: a randomized, double blinded, placebo-controlled, and multicenter clinical study. J Tradit Chin Med 34: 437-444.
15. Liu S, Shergis J, Chen X, Yu X, Guo X, et al. (2014) Chinese herbal medicine (weijing decoction) combined with pharmacotherapy for the treatment of acute exacerbations of chronic obstructive pulmonary disease. Evid Based Complement Alternat Med Epub 257012.
16. http://integrativepulmonarycarecenter.com/
17. Kelly GS (1999) Larch arabinogalactan: clinical relevance of a novel immune-enhancing polysaccharide. Altern Med Rev 4: 96-103.

18. Chatterjee UR, Ray S, Micard V, Ghosh D, Ghosh K, et al. (2014) Interaction with bovine serum albumin of an anti-oxidative pectic arabinogalactan from Andrographis paniculata. Carbohydr Polym 101: 342-348.
19. Domej W, Oettl K, Renner W (2014) Oxidative stress and free radicals in COPD--implications and relevance for treatment. Int J Chron Obstruct Pulmon Dis 9: 1207-1224.
20. Skyberg JA, Rollins MF, Holderness JS, Marlenee NL, Schepetkin AI, et al. (2012) Nasal Acai Polysaccharides Potentiate Innate Immunity to Protect against Pulmonary Francisella tularensis and Burkholderia pseudomallei Infections. PLoS Pathogens 8: e1002587.
21. Manvitha K, Bidya B (2014) Aloe vera: a wonder plant its history, cultivation and medicinal uses. J Pharmacognosy and Phytochemistry 2: 85-88
22. Zhong JS, Huang YY, Zhang TH, Liu YP, Ding WJ, et al. (2015) Natural phosphodiesterase-4 inhibitors from the leaf skin of Aloe barbadensis Miller. Fitoterapia 100: 68-74.
23. Habeeb F, Shakir E, Bradbury F, Cameron P, Taravati MR, et al. (2007) Screening methods used to determine the anti-microbial properties of Aloe vera inner gel. Methods 42: 315-320.
24. Hohtola A (2010) Bioactive compounds from northern plants. Adv Exp Med Biol 698: 99-109.
25. Burdulis D, Sarkinas A, Jasutiene I (2009) Comparative study of anthocyanin composition, antimicrobial and antioxidant activity in bilberry (Vaccinium myrtillus L.) and blueberry (Vaccinium corymbosum L.) fruits. Acta Poloniae Pharmaceutica 66: 399-408.
26. Braga PC, Antonacci R, Wang YY, Lattuada N, Sasso DM, et al. (2013) Comparative antioxidant activity of cultivated and wild Vaccinium species investigated by EPR, human neutrophil burst and COMET assay. European Review of Medical and Pharmacological Sciences 17: 1987-1999.
27. Ali BH, Ziada A, Blunden G (2009) Biological effects of gum arabic: a review of some recent research. Food Chem Toxicol 47: 1-8.
28. Benmalek Y, Yahia OA, Belkebir A, Fardeau ML (2013) Anti-microbial and anti-oxidant activities of Illicium verum, Crataegus oxyacantha ssp monogyna and Allium cepa red and white varieties. Bioengineered 4: 244-248.
29. De M, De AK, Sen P, Banerjee AB (2002) Antimicrobial properties of star anise (Illicium verum Hook f). Phytother Res 16: 94-95.
30. Kang P, Kim KY, Lee HS, Min SS, Seol GH, et al. (2013) Anti-inflammatory effects of anethole in lipopolysaccharide-induced acute lung injury in mice. Life Sci 93: 955-961.
31. Shishodia S, Sethi G, Aggarwal BB (2005) Curcumin: getting back to the roots. Ann N Y Acad Sci 1056: 206-217.
32. Bengmark S, Mesa MD, Gil A (2009) Plant-derived health: the effects of turmeric and curcuminoids. Nutr Hosp 24: 273-281.
33. Murali PM, Rajasekaran S, Paramesh P, Krishnarahashekar OR, Vasudevan S, et al. (2006) Plant based formulation in the management of chronic obstructive pulmonary disease: A randomized double-blind study. Respiratory Med 100: 39-45.
34. Calverley P, Pauwels R, Vestbo J, Jones P, Pride N, et al. (2003) Combined salmeterol and fluticasone in the treatment of chronic obstructive pulmonary disease: a randomised controlled trial. Lancet 361: 449-456.
35. Sharma G, Goodwin J (2006) Effect of aging on respiratory system physiology and immunology. Clin Interv Aging 1: 253-260.
36. Swanney MP, Stanton JD, O'Reilly-Nugent A (2014) Natural decline in FEV1 and FVC: Self versus reference equations. ERJ 42: 1787.
37. Jansson SA, Andersson F, Borg S, Ericsson A, Jönsson E, et al. (2002) Costs of COPD in Sweden according to disease severity. Chest 122: 1994-2002.
38. Miller JD, Foster T, Boulanger L, Chace M, Russell MW, et al. (2005) Direct costs of COPD in the U.S.: an analysis of Medical Expenditure Panel Survey (MEPS) data. COPD 2: 311-318.
39. Fong HH (2002) Integration of herbal medicine into modern medical practices: issues and prospects. Integr Cancer Ther 1: 287-293.

18

# One- And Two-year Outcomes of Treating Preschool Children with Autism with a Qigong Massage Protocol

**Louisa MT Silva*, Mark Schalock, Kristen R Gabrielsen and Gretchen HD**

[1]Teaching Research Institute, Western Oregon University, USA
[2]Associate Research Professor, Teaching Research Institute, Western Oregon University, USA
[3]MPH, Project Director, Consultant for Teaching Research Institute, Western Oregon University, USA
[4]Consultant/Project Manager, Teaching Research Institute, Western Oregon University, USA

**Abstract**

**Background:** Randomized controlled trials have repeatedly demonstrated that treatment with a five-month qigong massage protocol significantly reduces the severity of autism. The treatment protocol is known as Qigong Sensory Training (QST) autism massage and is given daily by parents and weekly by therapists for five months. Treatment reduces the tactile abnormalities that are universal in young children with autism and results in improved social skills, language and behavior. At five months, tactile abnormalities are reduced by 1/2, autistic behavior is reduced by 1/3, autism severity is reduced by 16%, and 6% of children have moved off the spectrum. What has not yet been done is to measure outcomes with longer-term treatment. This observational study investigates outcomes with up to 24 months of treatment.

**Methods:** 75 children entered this observational study upon completion of five months of treatment with the QST protocol. They received daily parent treatment and monthly therapist treatment for the balance of the first year, and daily parent treatment without therapist support for the second year. Sequential evaluations were conducted at baseline (n=75), five months (n=75), 12 months (n=67) and 24 months (n=31).

**Results:** Continued treatment resulted in continued improvement. At 12 and 24 months, mean tactile responses normalized by 57% and 72%, with 24% and 32% falling into the normal range; mean autism severity decreased by 27% and 44%, with 12% and 26% of children moving out of autistic range.

**Conclusions:** Results demonstrated that longer-term treatment resulted in resolution of tactile impairment and continued improvement of social skills, language and behavior. The rate of coming off the spectrum (1 in 4 children by year-2) was far higher than the natural history of ASD would predict. Results support earlier recommendations to treat tactile abnormalities at the time of autism diagnosis in order to improve autism outcomes.

**Keywords:** Autism treatment; Tactile anormalities; Qigong; QST massage

**Abbreviations:** ASD: Autism Spectrum Disorder; CARS: Childhood Autism Rating Scale; ABC: Autism Behavior Checklist; SSC: Sense and Self-Regulation Checklist; PLS: Preschool Language Scale; QST: Qigong Sensory Treatment; EIBI: Early Intensive Behavioral Intervention; ABA: Applied Behavioral Analysis

## Introduction

Autism is the most common developmental disability in the United States and is currently estimated to affect 1 in 45 children [1]. Its cause remains unknown. Clinically, it is defined by the appearance of social/language delay, unusual and repetitive behavior, and abnormal sensory responses by the age of three [2]. Autism occurs on a spectrum of severity in the lack of social/communication skills, behavioral flexibility, and cognitive ability. As of yet there is no clear explanation for why autism occurs on a spectrum of severity, and no research-based treatment that reliably improves all symptoms of autism across the spectrum [3].

A new direction for autism research and treatment was opened in 2013 when abnormal sensory responses were reclassified from co-morbid symptoms to core diagnostic autism symptoms [2]. At that point, it was recognized that abnormal responses to touch are among the earliest and most prevalent of sensory symptoms [4,5], that severity of tactile abnormalities is related to severity of autism [6], and that the sense of touch had not been proven to be intact in autism. Research as to the specific nature of tactile abnormalities in autism is ongoing. Children with autism were first described by Kanner to lack interest in affective/affiliative touch [7]. Since then, qualitative research has shown that children with autism are distinguished by a pattern of abnormal responses to light touch and pain [8]. New research from mammalian studies indicates that affectionate/affiliative touch is mediated by small unmyelinated tactile fibers (known as C-tactile fibers), and that loss of fibers presents as discomfort with light touch and decreased pain responsivity [9,10]. Diagnosis of small fiber tactile loss is by skin biopsy and specialized staining [11]. This year, the first four biopsies reported in children with autism demonstrated 50% loss of small fibers [12]. This was the first study to report skin biopsy results in children with autism and much work remains to be done to definitively diagnose the cause of tactile abnormalities in autism.

In tandem with research investigating the nature of tactile abnormalities in autism, randomized control studies investigating the effect of qigong massage treatment on severity of tactile abnormalities and severity of autism were conducted [13-15]. The protocol known as Qigong Sensory

***Corresponding author:** Louisa MT Silva, Visiting Professor ,Teaching Research Institute, Western Oregon University, Post Office Box 92, McMinnville, OR 97128, USA, E-mail: lmtsilva@qsti.org

Treatment (QST) massage for autism, is based on Chinese medicine. Treatment is delivered daily by parents and weekly by trained therapists.

The QST intervention has a defined theory and methods described in a manual. Autism is theorized to be due, at least in part, to early partial loss of the sense of touch. Loss of the affective/affiliative component of touch in the early developmental period is theorized to explain the specific social/communication delay and abnormal behaviors characteristic of autism. Treatment uses a massage protocol to stimulate recovery and growth of tactile fibers by increasing circulation to the skin. The effectiveness of Chinese medical approaches to increasing skin circulation has been previously documented [16,17].

This is the second arm of a three-year study that replicated and extended earlier studies investigating the effect of qigong massage on children with autism. The first arm replicated results reported by earlier RCTs in 103 preschool children with autism: at five months, tactile responses had normalized by 49% (based on the Sense and Self-regulation Checklist [18], autistic behavior was reduced by 32% (based on the Autism Behavior Checklist [19], and severity of autism, as measured by a stable measure of autism (based on the Childhood Autism Rating Scale [20] was reduced by 12% [21]. Improvements occurred across the spectrum of autism severity.

With confirmation that five months of the qigong massage intervention is powerfully effective on measures of autism, we wished to determine the effect of longer-term treatment. The literature assessing the natural history of autism indicates that the severity of core autism features can be expected to remain stable in childhood with only a small percentage of children improving slightly and a similar small percentage of children worsening slightly over 8-12 years [22-24]. This second study arm was an observational follow-along study investigating the effect of one and two years of treatment on tactile abnormalities and severity of autism in children who participated in the first study arm. In addition, we investigated factors influencing parent fidelity with daily treatment, and whether longer-term outcomes were influenced by initial severity of tactile abnormalities. The main research questions included:

1. How do tactile abnormalities and severity of autism change over time in response to QST massage treatment?

2. How does behavior and general development change over time in response to QST massage treatment?

3. How does intensity of the parent support program influence parent fidelity (adherence to the massage protocol)? What reasons do parents give for missing treatment?

4. How does parent fidelity with ongoing treatment influence outcomes over time?

5. Does pre-treatment severity of tactile impairment influence treatment outcomes over time?

Additional research questions include:

6. Do parents perceive a change in their children's affective and affiliative responses to touch?

7. How do cost and efficacy of this intervention compare with more widely known early intervention for autism?

## Materials and Methods

### Study design

This study was the second arm of a two-part study. The first arm was a five-month replication study that evaluated efficacy of the QST massage protocol [21]. This second study arm was a 19-month observational follow-along study of children who participated in the first study and completed the five-month treatment protocol. There was no control group for the second study arm.

Standardized assessments of autism, language, and development were carried out pre-treatment and at five, 12 and 24 months post onset of treatment by three qualified professionals Additional evaluations were conducted with validated parent/caregiver questionnaires.

### Participants and recruitment

Inclusion/exclusion criteria for entry into the study included age of 2-5 years; formal diagnosis of autism; no additional chronic disability; no psychoactive medication or pharmaceutical chelation therapy; and not receiving intensive Applied Behavioral Analysis (ABA) treatment for autism. Two study participants were identified as receiving non-intensive ABA treatment at 8 and 10 hours/week, respectively. Parents agreed to give their children the daily massage treatment for the duration of the study and to follow through with training and support visits. Parents were asked about additional interventions for autism at the one-year and two-year assessments.

### Verifying and confirming the diagnosis of autism

Children were required to have a diagnosis of autism by formal autism evaluation as a condition of entry into the study. Records were reviewed and diagnoses confirmed by neurodevelopmental pediatricians using DSM-IV criteria.

### Demographic information

At post-treatment the average age of participants was 57.7 months. At 12 months the average age was 64.1 months and at 24 months the average age was 78 months. Boys made up 90% of the sample at 12 months and 87% of the sample at 24 months. Overall prevalence of autism in boys is 4.5 times that of girls [25]. Lower income families were 33% of the participants at 12 months and 36% at 24 months. Families of cultural minorities were 28% of the participants at 12 months and 39% at 24 months. Eighty percent of parents involved had no previous experience with massage or Chinese medicine. Families who withdrew from the study did not have different demographics.

### Study completion

A total of 75 children entered this follow-along study. Of these 75 children, 67 participated in the year 1 post-testing, and 31 completed the year 2 post-testing.

### The tactile stimulation protocol

The QST massage protocol is a whole body protocol that takes about 15 minutes and is usually done at bedtime. It is formalized in a parent training manual and DVD with flexible constraints [26]. The parent is taught not to avoid areas that are uncomfortable but instead to adjust the techniques to the child's responses within the comfort zone of the child. Over the course of treatment, tactile responses undergo predictable changes from hyposensitive to hypersensitive to normosensitive. The protocol requires adjustment of manual technique with each transition.

The protocol has 12 parts that follow the acupuncture channels down the front and back of the body. Massage is carried out towards the hands and feet in the direction of capillary blood flow. Both patting and pressure are used according to the child's response. Generally, a quicker, lighter, patting technique is used to begin with, especially in areas of numbness. In areas where the child withdraws from touch or is ticklish, slower pressing techniques are used. Additional options are available when neither patting nor pressure resolves the difficulty. For a summary of the massage movements, go to http://qsti.org/wp-content/uploads/2014/06/12MovementsAutism.pdf.

Therapists providing the parent training and support program graduated from a 60-hour training and supervision [27,28]. At support visits, therapists provided treatment, coached parents in the massage and evaluated parent fidelity with massage implementation. During the first five months, weekly therapist visits were provided. For the balance of the first year monthly visits were provided. No therapist visits were provided in the second year.

### Measures

The following measures were used to evaluate baseline, five-month, 12 months, and 24 months outcomes.

**Childhood Autism Rating Scale, 2nd edition, standard version (CARS):** The CARS is a reliable and widely used rating scale for the diagnosis of autism. CARS scores do not vary significantly by age between toddler and preschool-aged children indicating that it is a stable, repeated-outcomes measure in that age range [20,24]. The CARS rates children on 15 core components of autism, and yields a composite score ranging from non-autistic to mildly, moderately, or severely autistic. Studies indicate that the CARS demonstrates high concordance with clinical diagnosis by DSM-IV criteria [29]. Independent psychometric support for the CARS reports high criterion-related validity, interrater and test-retest reliability, and internal consistency. A score of 25.5 serves as the cutoff for a diagnosis of autism on the mild end of the autism spectrum; 30 to 36 is scored as moderate; 36 and higher is scored as severe [30]. A decrease in score represents a decrease in severity of autism. The pre-treatment median score of 39 was used as the criteria in the analyses to determine effects on language development by level of severity. The CARS was administered by blinded professional examiners.

**Preschool Language Scale, 5th edition (PLS):** The PLS is a measure of global language skills and standardized subscales evaluating relative ability in receptive and expressive language in children under seven years old. Internal consistency (split-half reliability) ranges from 0.91 to 0.93 for the subscale scores and 0.95 for the total score. Independent psychometric support for the PLS indicates high criterion-related validity, interrater and test–retest reliability, and that it is a valid measure of language in children with ASD [31,32]. An increase in score represents improved language skills. The PLS was administered by blinded professional examiners.

**Vineland adaptive behavior scales, 2nd edition (Vineland-II):** The Vineland is a validated parent interview that assesses socialization, communication, motor skills, and daily living skills. Cronbach's alpha is 0.97 for the composite scale and ranges from 0.83 to 0.95 for the domains. An increase in score represents an increase in developmental skills and abilities. The Vineland parent interview was conducted by blinded professional examiners [33].

**Autism Behavior Checklist (ABC):** The ABC is a validated measure of autism and a component of the Autism Screening Instrument for Educational Planning. The ABC is a sensitive measure of change in response to classroom interventions [19]. It measures behaviors typical of autism in multiple domains: sensory, relating, body and object use, language, social and self-help. Crohbach's alpha is 0.89. The mean value for typically developing children is reported at 17.81 [34]. A decrease in scores represents a reduction in autistic behavior. The Autism Behavior Checklist was completed by parents.

**Sense and Self-regulation Checklist (SSC):** The SSC is a validated parent/caregiver measure of sensory and self-regulatory difficulties and delays in children with autism [18]. It evaluates signs of peripheral impairment of touch (pain and numbness) by location and severity, and confirms severity of tactile impairment by evaluating touch-dependent self-regulatory delay. Cronbach's alpha is 0.83. SSC scores differentiate between children with ASD and typical development; mean scores are 39.6 (SD 10.6) and 18.4 (SD 9.5), respectively. Mean oral/tactile scores for ASD and typical children are 29.2 (SD 7.9) and 14.5 (SD 7.2). Mean "Other Sensory" scores for ASD and typical children are 17.5 (SD 6.1) and 6.9 (SD 5.0). Mean self-regulatory difficulty scores for ASD and typical children are 56.8 (SD 14.1) and 25.8 (SD 11.3). The overall SSC mean scores for ASD and typical children are 89.5 (SD 21.4) and 38.4 (SD 18.0). A decrease in scores represents a decrease in sensory abnormalities and self-regulatory difficulties.

**Fidelity and social validation testing** : Therapists monitored parent fidelity with massage procedures. For the first year of treatment, parents completed a daily log recording fidelity with daily massage, reasons for missing the massage, and problems or concerns. In addition, parents completed surveys at 12 months and 24 months with open-ended questions related to implementation of the treatment and observed changes in their child.

### Data collection

Pre- and post-intervention data collection was conducted within a one-month window both prior to beginning of treatment and after the 5 month protocol was completed. Twelve months and 24 months data collection also was conducted within a one-month window. Trained professionals administered the Vineland, CARS and PLS in the home.

Parents completed an online set of surveys and background questionnaires that included the Sense and Self-Regulation Checklist and the Autism Behavior Checklist. Parents offer the singular advantage of providing information about specific types of behaviors, in a variety of settings and over a much longer time than is available to the examiner during the typical evaluation [35]. Parent reports on specific behavioral and developmental responses have been found to be valid and reliable when compared with professional evaluations [36,37].

### Data analysis

Initial analyses were conducted to detect any potential attrition bias at 12 months and 24 months testing using 2-way ANOVA and MANOVA on outcome measures. To test whether the treatment effects maintain, intensify or recede over time when parents continue to provide treatment, within group one-way repeated measures ANOVAs were conducted on dependent measures at pre-treatment, post-treatment, one-year follow-up and two-year follow-up. Post-hoc pairwise Bonferroni-corrected comparisons were conducted to further test the nature of effects over time on each outcome measure. Separate unbalanced two-way repeated measure ANOVAs were conducted on pre-post follow-up scores to determine whether important differences in longitudinal effects by level of continued treatment fidelity or initial tactile abnormalities occur. Separate repeated measure ANOVA analyses were conducted and reported on the two intact cohorts of pre-post-12 months assessments (n=67) and the pre-post-12 months-24 months assessments (n=31).

## Results

### Sample size adequacy and power analysis

Power analyses to determine adequacy of sample size for this study were conducted using pre- to post-treatment published outcomes. Using the least significant treatment effects as a conservative effect size, power was estimated for both within-group repeated measures ANOVA and within-between group repeated measure ANOVA analyses. Allowing for attrition, a final n of 24 and a $p<0.05$, a power analysis yielded a power of 0.96 on both within and within-between interaction repeated measure ANOVAs. The cohort sizes of 67 and 31 provide adequate power.

### Attrition bias

Based on two-way ANOVA and MANOVA no differences were found between completers and non-completers at post-treatment or at 12 months. F values ranged from 0.018 to 3.57 at post and 0.002 and 1.47 at 12 months, with associated p. values ranging from 0.979 to 0.057. At 24 months, completers had higher levels of abnormal sensory response at baseline than did those who did not complete two-year testing.

### Longitudinal effects of intervention

**Tactile abnormalities and severity of autism:** Results from the repeated measures ANOVA for pre-post and one-year assessments are shown in Table 1. Overall there were significant reductions in tactile abnormalities and severity of autism from the pre-treatment to one-year assessments. In both cases, there was a significant change from pre- to post-treatment. Significant changes from post to one-year testing were also seen in severity of autism as measured by the CARS.

From pre-treatment to 12 months, the decrease in tactile abnormalities from 28.5 to 20.5 represented a mean normalization of 56.9%; that is, the decrease from 28.5 to 20.5 represents 56.9% of the improvement toward the score of 14.49 of typically developing children. Almost one quarter of the children (23.9%) obtained a score of 14 or lower on tactile abnormalities by the end of 12 months. The decrease in autism severity as measured by the CARS scores represented a mean normalization of 26.8% toward the score of 25.5. Overall, 12.3% of children reached the score of 25.5 which represents the threshold for autism on the CARS by the end of 12 months.

**Behavior and general development:** Overall significant positive differences were found for all outcomes except Other Sensory responses. Significant changes from post to one-year testing were seen on measures of self-regulation, language development, social development and in daily living skills. As can be seen in Table 1, the decrease on the ABC from 77.9 to 57.1 represented a 34.7% mean normalization toward the score of 17.81 for typically developing children. By the end of year one, more than one in eight (13.4%) of the children reached the typical score of 17.81. The decrease in self-regulation scores also represented a 36.9% mean normalization toward the score of 25.8. Six percent of children reached this score by the end of 12 months.

Results from the repeated measures ANOVA from pre-treatment to 24 months are shown in Table 2. Looking across two years, stronger trends emerge, with continued significant improvements on all outcomes. Scores improve significantly from pre- to post-treatment, from post to 12 months and then from 12 months to 24 months.

From pre-treatment to 24 months, the decrease in tactile abnormalities from 29.8 to 18.7 represented a mean normalization of 72.3%. Almost one third of the children (32.3%) obtained a score of 14 or lower on tactile abnormalities response by the end of two years. The decrease in autism severity as measured by the CARS scores represented a mean normalization of 43.8% toward the score of 25.5, which represents the threshold for autism on the CARS. Overall, 25.8% of children reached the score of 25.5 by two years. The decrease on the ABC represented a 48.5% mean normalization toward the score of 17.81 for typically developing children. Overall 12.9% of the children reached the typical score of 17.81 by two years. The decrease in self-regulation scores also represented a 49.1% mean normalization toward the score of 25.8. Nearly one in ten (9.7%) of children reached this score by the end of two years (Figure 1).

**Fidelity:** Fidelity data for the first five months is reported in a previous article [21]. Twelve months after the parents were trained to give their children the massage, therapists once again tested parents on the 12 massage movements using a checklist. Sixty-one percent of parents demonstrated full fidelity with massage procedures. Twenty percent needed correction on one or two of the 12 parts of the massage. Eighteen percent of parents needed correction on three or more of the movements.

**Influence of intensity of the parent support program on parent fidelity:** Idelity was strongly related to the frequency of the therapist home visits F (2,29)=41.1, $p<0.000$. High or full fidelity was defined as receiving the massage 6-7 times a week. Fidelity remained high during the first five-months due to the weekly therapist home visits: 80% of children received the treatment 6-7 times a week and the remainder received the massage 4-5 times a week. When therapist home visits decreased to once a month during the remainder of the first year, overall fidelity dropped: 34% children received the treatment 6-7 times per week and the remainder received the massage 5 or less times a week. When therapist home visits were discontinued in the second year, fidelity dropped again: 33% received the treatment 4 or more times a week and the remainder received the treatment 3 or fewer times a week.

**Effects of treatment fidelity on treatment outcomes:** Fidelity effects were evaluated by defining full versus less than full fidelity at 5, 12 months and 24 months. At 12 months, children who experienced full fidelity (n=22) saw improved outcomes over children experiencing less than full fidelity (n=45). The most apparent effects were observed in addressing abnormal tactile response. As can be seen in Figure 2, abnormal tactile response decreased from 29.5 to 17.5 with full fidelity and from 30.1 to 23.9 with less than full fidelity. Full fidelity represented an 80.2% change toward normalization of touch while less than full implementation represented a 39.3% change toward normalization of touch. Severity of autism declined from 37.5 to 33.5 (33.3% normalization) with full fidelity and from 39.2 to 35.3 (28.4% normalization) with less than full fidelity.

At 24 months the differences were more pronounced for touch and severity of autism. Children who experienced full fidelity (n=10) saw improved outcomes over children experiencing less than full fidelity (n=21). Abnormal tactile response decreased from 29.5 to 16.3 with full fidelity and from 30.1 to 20.5 with less than full fidelity. Full fidelity represented an 87.8% change toward normalization of touch while less than full implementation represented a 61.4% change toward normalization of touch. Severity of autism declined from 37.5 to 30.9 (54.8% normalization) with full fidelity and from 39.2 to 34.2 (36.8% normalization) with less than full fidelity. These results are shown in Figure 2.

At the end of two years, 60% of children with full fidelity achieved normal touch compared to 23.8% of children with less than full fidelity. Thirty percent of participants with full fidelity achieved scores on the CARS consistent with neurotypical development compared to 23.8% of

| Pre-post-12 month Outcomes (N = 67) | Pre-treatment Mean (SD) | Post-treatment Mean (SD) | 12 months Mean (SD) | F (2,65) | p | Partial $\eta^2$ | Tukey's HSD |
|---|---|---|---|---|---|---|---|
| Abnormal Oral-Tactile Response | 28.5 (8.1) | 22.1 (8.2) | 20.5 (9.5) | 41.2 | <0.000 | 0.559 | 1>2,3 |
| Other Sensory | 10.3 4.3 | 11.0 5.6 | 12.3 6.2 | 4.9 | 0.010 | 0.132 | 1<3 |
| Childhood Autism Rating Scale | 38.5 (7.2) | 36.9 (7.2) | 35.0 (7.9) | 17.7 | <0.000 | 0.360 | 1>2,3<br>2>3 |
| Autism Behavior Checklist | 77.9 (26.8) | 60.0 (29.6) | 57.1 (29.2) | 30.5 | <0.000 | 0.484 | 1>2,3 |
| Self-Regulation | 55.8 (13.9) | 44.8 (13.0) | 41.6 (14.5) | 46.8 | <0.000 | 0.590 | 1>2,3<br>2>3 |
| PLS-Receptive Communication | 29.0 14.3 | 33.1 14.5 | 35.7 16.5 | 37.2 | <0.000 | 0.541 | 1<2,3<br>2<3 |
| PLS-Expressive Communication | 29.3 13.3 | 32.7 13.3 | 35.9 15.5 | 48.8 | <0.000 | 0.608 | 1<2,3<br>2<3 |
| Vineland Socialization | 42.0 19.8 | 51.5 22.0 | 60.4 27.6 | 55.6 | <0.000 | 0.638 | 1<2,3<br>2<3 |
| Vineland Daily Living Skills | 39.8 23.0 | 48.2 24.7 | 58.3 31.5 | 60.4 | <0.000 | 0.657 | 1<2,3<br>2<3 |

**Table 1:** Repeated measures ANOVA results for pre-post treatment and 12 month follow-up.

| Pre-Post-12 month-24 month Outcomes | Pre Mean (SD) | 6 months Mean (SD) | 12 month Mean (SD) | 24 month Mean (SD) | F (3,28) | p | $\eta^2$ | Tukey's HSD |
|---|---|---|---|---|---|---|---|---|
| Abnormal Oral-Tactile Response | 29.8 (7.9) | 22.9 (9.2) | 21.2 (10.5) | 18.7 (8.8) | 16.16 | <0.000 | 0.634 | 1>2,3,4<br>2>4<br>3>4 |
| Other Sensory | 11.2 4.9 | 11.4 5.0 | 13.6 6.1 | 11.5 5.8 | 3.6 | 0.027 | 0.277 | NA |
| Childhood Autism Rating Scale | 38.5 (8.1) | 37.1 (8.0) | 34.6 (8.7) | 32.8 (9.1) | 11.79 | <0.000 | 0.558 | 1>2,3,4<br>2>3,4<br>3>4 |
| Autism Behavior Checklist | 81.1 (28.3) | 60.3 (31.4) | 59.6 (31.8) | 50.4 (29.2) | 10.42 | <0.000 | 0.528 | 1>2,3,4<br>2>4<br>3>4 |
| Self-Regulation | 58.2 14.9 | 46.1 14.9 | 42.0 17.7 | 38.1 16.3 | 18.1 | <0.000 | 0.660 | 1>2,3,4<br>2>4 |
| PLS-Receptive Communication | 29.0 15.6 | 32.9 15.8 | 35.4 17.4 | 41.3 17.6 | 23.1 | <0.000 | 0.712 | 1<2,3,4<br>2<4<br>3<4 |
| PLS-Expressive Communication | 30.1 13.5 | 32.9 13.3 | 35.4 15.8 | 40.8 17.4 | 25.5 | <0.000 | 0.732 | 1<2,3,4<br>2<3,4<br>3<4 |
| Vineland Socialization | 42.6 21.2 | 51.3 22.9 | 58.1 28.0 | 75.5 31.1 | 27.3 | <0.000 | 0.745 | 1<2,3,4<br>2<3,4<br>3<4 |
| Vineland Daily Living Skills | 39.9 23.5 | 47.4 24.9 | 58.8 33.9 | 76.4 40.2 | 23.6 | <0.000 | 0.716 | 1<2,3,4<br>2<3,4<br>3<4 |

**Table 2:** Repeated measures ANOVA results for pre-/post-treatment (6-months), 12 month and 24 month follow-up.

participants with less than full fidelity. Level of fidelity was seen to have the most direct and significant effect on improving abnormal touch.

### Effects of pre-treatment severity of tactile impairment on outcomes

Children with varying levels of tactile abnormality at pre-treatment made significant improvements in touch, severity of autism, as well as autistic behaviors, as seen in Table 3. Pre-treatment groups based on severity of abnormal tactile response were created by simply splitting the sample in half based on tactile abnormality score. The

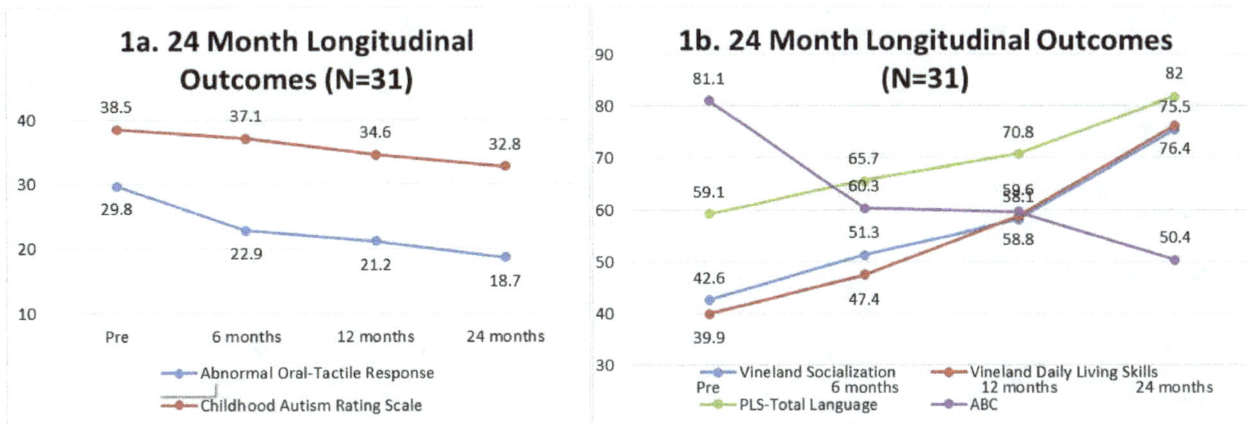


**Figure 1:** Overall changes in treatment outcomes for 24 month cohort.

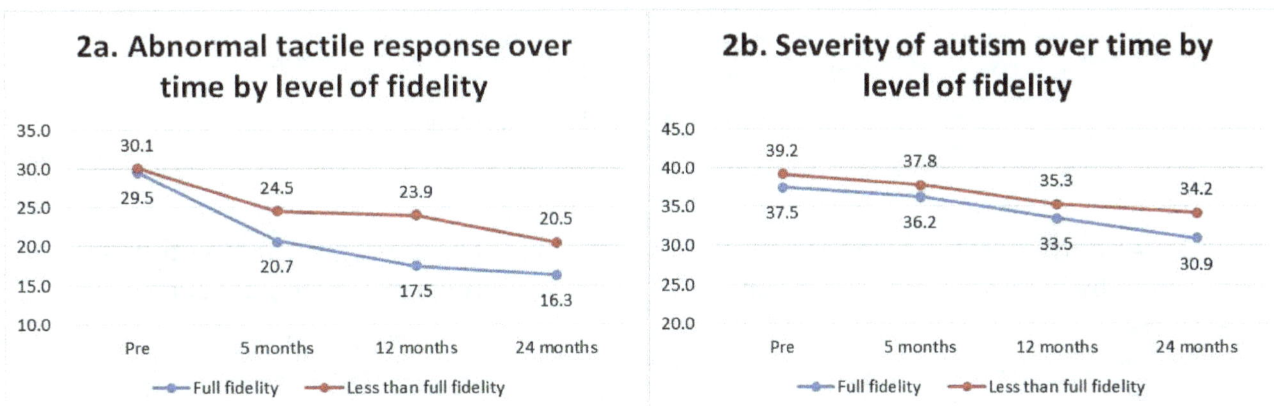


**Figure 2:** Changes in treatment outcomes for 24 month cohort by level of treatment fidelity.

absolute magnitude of improvement in touch was larger in the more severe group while children with less severe touch experienced larger decreases in severity of autism and autistic behaviors. Severity of tactile abnormalities differentiated severity of autism and autistic behaviors prior to treatment. These differences were maintained over time.

As can be seen in Figure 3, the observed differences in scores were significant at each assessment period for abnormal tactile response, autistic behavior and language development on independent samples t-tests. Scores for severity of autism differed significantly post treatment and at 24 months using the same tests.

At 24 months the differences are pronounced between children with severe tactile abnormalities prior to treatment and those with milder tactile abnormalities. Mean abnormal tactile response decreased from 23.5 to 14.4 with milder tactile abnormalities and from 35.1 to 22.3 with more severe tactile abnormalities. On average this represents a 100% change to normalization with half the children reaching normalized touch for those starting with milder tactile issues and a 62% normalization and 17.6% of the children reaching normalized touch for those with more severe tactile issues.

Severity of autism scores for children with milder tactile issues normalized by 72.8%, with 42.9% of children reaching neurotypical development. Scores for children with more severe tactile issues normalized by 27% with 17.6% of children reaching neurotypical development. Changes in autistic behavior scores followed a similar pattern. Scores for children with milder tactile issues normalized by 64.5%, with 21.4% of children reaching normalized behavior. Scores for children with more severe tactile issues normalized by 39.7% with 5.9% of children reaching normalized behavior.

Changes in overall language development also followed this pattern. Scores for children with milder tactile issues normalized by 54.8%, with 50.0% of children reaching normalized language. Scores for children with more severe tactile issues normalized by 23.6% with 5.9% of children reaching normalized language.

### Parents' perception of a change in children's affective and affiliative responses to touch

Parents' narrative responses to the following questions were analyzed:

1) Do you see any differences in your relationship with your child, compared to a year ago? and,

2) What differences, if any, did you notice about your child's development during the last year? Parents reported an increase in child-initiated touch and bonding more frequently than any other

| Pre-post-12 month-24 month Outcomes | Pre Mean (SD) | Post Mean (SD) | 12 months Mean (SD) | 24 months Mean (SD) | F (3,14) F (3,11) | p | $\eta^2$ | Tukey's HSD |
|---|---|---|---|---|---|---|---|---|
| Abnormal Oral-Tactile Response: More severe | 35.1 (4.1) | 27.7 (7.9) | 26.2 (9.0) | 22.3 (7.7) | 15.0 | <0.000 | 0.762 | 1>2,3,4 2>4 |
| Abnormal Oral-Tactile Response : Less Severe | 23.5 (6.7) | 17.1 (7.1) | 15.2 (9.1) | 14.4 (8.4) | 4.3 | 0.031 | 0.540 | 1>2,3,4 |
| Behavior: More severe | 92.4 (23.5) | 77.0 (28.1) | 74.0 (28.1) | 62.8 (29.1) | 4.1 | 0.027 | 0.470 | 1>4 |
| Behavior: Less Severe | 67.3 (28.3) | 40.0 (22.2) | 42.0 (27.6) | 35.4 (22.0) | 9.3 | 0.002 | 0.717 | 1>2,3,4 |
| Severity of Autism: More Severe | 40.7 (9.1) | 39.2 (8.7) | 37.7 (9.4) | 36.6 (9.3) | 3.5 | 0.044 | 0.429 | 1>4 |
| Severity of Autism: Less Severe | 35.8 (6.0) | 34.5 (6.0) | 30.8 (6.4) | 28.3 (6.7) | 10.1 | 0.002 | 0.734 | 1>3,4 2>4 3>4 |
| Language (PLS): More Severe | 47.9 (22.4) | 53.7 (23.6) | 56.2 (28.8) | 66.1 (29.2) | 11.5 | <0.000 | 0.711 | 1<2,3,4 2<4 3<4 |
| Language (PLS): Less Severe | 72.8 (30.6) | 80.4 (28.5) | 88.5 (29.4) | 101.4 (31.4) | 24.8 | <0.000 | 0.871 | 1<2,3,4 2<3,4 3<4 |

**Table 3:** Longitudinal outcomes by severity of touch.

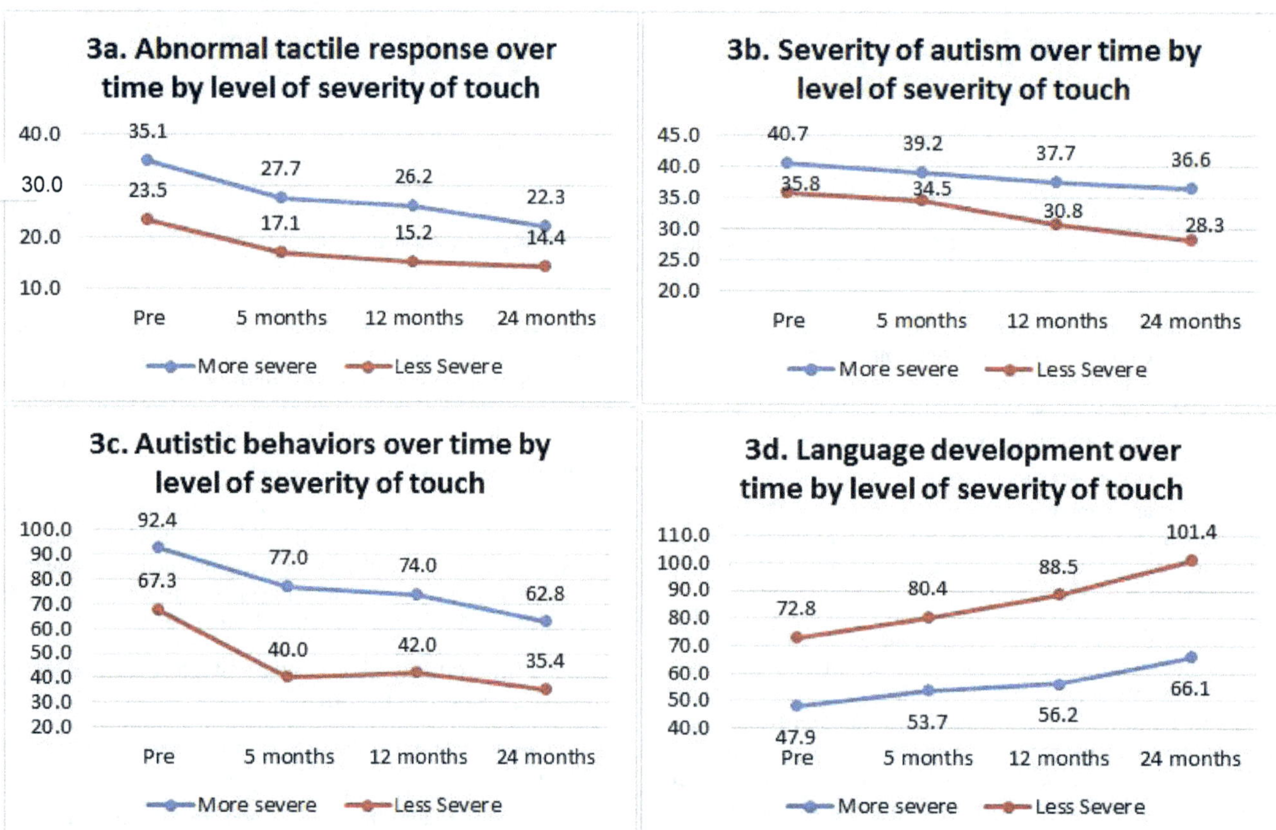


**Figure 3:** Effects of severity of tactile abnormalities over time.

developmental change. One hundred percent of parents reported an increase in bonding with their children at the end of year one. As such, this was by far the most consistent finding in the 1-year parent outcomes data. During year one and year two, nearly three-fourths of parents reported that the child-to-parent bond continued to increase. See Table 4 for examples of parent comments.

## Comparison of cost and efficacy of QST massage

In Table 5 we compare QST Massage and a widely known intervention for autism, early intensive behavioral intervention (EIBI) [38]. For this comparison, we use hours per week required for implementation as our measure of cost in order to avoid confusion with regional variations in cost. Professional and parent hours per week for implementation, efficacy on core autism symptoms, and areas where efficacy is limited are also compared.

## Adverse effects

There were no adverse effects reported in children.

# Discussion

The intention of this follow-along study was to observe the effects of 12 months and 24 months of treatment with QST massage on tactile abnormalities and measures of autism. With regards to tactile abnormalities, results indicate that longer-term treatment resulted in further improvement of tactile responses up to the point of full normalization in a number of children. Improvement was progressive and encompassed not only decreased pain and numbness, but also increased affectionate/affiliative touch. By 12 months, mean tactile responses had normalized by over one-half, and about one-quarter of children had scores within the normal range. At 24 months, mean tactile responses had normalized by about three-fourths; one-third of children scored in the normal range. This is the first report that full normalization of tactile abnormalities is possible with QST massage treatment. Severity of initial tactile abnormalities did not appear to pose a barrier to recovery, and although milder children recovered faster, a number of more severe children also had normalization of scores.

| Comments from Parents |
|---|
| We are closer. |
| We are much closer now as father and son. |
| She is a lot more cuddly. |
| He is more cuddly and affectionate. |
| He often asks for massage. |
| He wants us to touch him more. |
| He hugs me if he thinks that I am sad. |
| He hugs his sister. |
| He will climb up on my lap and give hugs and kisses. |
| He seeks us for comfort. |
| He has more empathy. He displays spontaneous affection. |

**Table 4:** Changes in affective and affiliative touch.

| | Early Intensive Behavioral Intervention | QST Massage for Autism |
|---|---|---|
| Total # professional hrs/ week | 20-40 hrs/week | 1.5 hrs/week |
| Total # parent hrs/week | Optional | 1.75 hrs/week |
| Expected duration of intervention | 2 years | 1-4 years |
| Efficacy on core autism symptoms | Language delay | Language delay<br>Social delay<br>Sensory abnormalities |
| Limited efficacy in some sub-groups of children | Limited efficacy in 50% of children; efficacy tends to be better in higher-functioning children [34] | Efficacy with both higher and lower-functioning groups |

**Table 5:** Cost-efficacy comparison.

Touch is the most important sense informing early childhood development [39]. Parent/caregiver touch stimulates orientation to face and facilitates learning the nonverbal communication skills upon which verbal communication rests [40]. The rewarding and bonding properties of touch provide the primary positive reinforcement for social engagement [41]. And the engaging and soothing properties of touch are necessary for the development of early self-regulation skills relative to attention and self-soothing [42]. Thus it was not surprising that progressive normalization of tactile responses was associated with progressive improvement of language, social skills, and behavioral self-regulation.

As might be expected, normalization of the individual components of autism was associated with a significant decrease in autism severity overall, as measured by the CARS. By 12 months, the mean severity of autism had decreased by 25% and 12% of children scored within the neurotypical range. By 24 months, the mean severity of autism had decreased by 44% and 25% of children scored within the neurotypical range. Children with less severe autism based on the CARS (a score of under 37) were the first to drop into the normal range for CARS scores with 22.6% of children achieving normalization at the end of 12 months, and 57.1% of children at the end of two years. Initial severity of autism (a score of 37 or greater) was not a complete barrier to more severe children reaching the neurotypical range; 2.9% achieved normalization by 12 months, and 5.6% of children by 24 months. This is the first time that full normalization of CARS scores has been reported in response to treatment with QST massage for autism.

The analysis of treatment outcomes by severity of tactile abnormalities indicates that initial severity of tactile abnormalities was a good predictor of whether children reached the normal range for language skills. At 24 months, 50% of less severe children scored in the neurotypical range for language in contrast with 6% for the group with more severe tactile abnormalities. The finding can be explained on the basis of the importance of touch to the development of nonverbal communication skills, and the impact of a barrier to touch on development of these skills. It is noteworthy that to date there has been no consistently accurate early predictor of which children will eventually acquire language [43,44]. Initial severity of tactile abnormalities also predicted comparable differences in outcome on severity of autism as measured by the CARS and the ABC. Thus, if we define higher functioning autism as relatively more language, less autistic behavior, and less severity on CARS scores, then initial severity of tactile impairment would appear to have predicted the emergence of higher versus lower functioning groups in this study. During this follow-along study, fidelity was influenced by frequency of therapist visits. As therapist support visits decreased from weekly, to monthly, to none at all, fidelity also fell. And when fidelity diminished, treatment effects did also. Interestingly, Figure 2 illuminate what is essentially a dose-response curve in treatment outcomes with the lesser dose of treatment resulting in a lesser treatment effect on touch and severity of autism. Treatment outcomes were considerably better in children who received full fidelity, the full "dose" of treatment. Practically speaking, the ongoing therapist visit was a gentle reminder to parents to keep the home program going, although not all parents required ongoing therapist visits for full fidelity.

How then to take the results of this follow-along study into consideration and design a parent support program to optimize outcomes? The results indicate that the goal of treatment can be established as full normalization of tactile responses. Fidelity with treatment can be monitored with a daily parent log. Response to treatment can be monitored with biannual testing of tactile responses with the SSC. Regular therapist visits are recommended until treatment goals are met, with flexibility to increase frequency of visits if fidelity falls. In more severe children, we estimate therapist visits once or twice a month for the remainder of the first year will protect fidelity. In less severe children, we estimate monthly visits will be sufficient. In the second year, we suggest monthly therapist visits for both groups.

## Limitations of the Study

The main limitation of this study is that it was an observational study rather than an experimental study. A true control group would have provided experimental evidence that longer-term treatment resulted in additional improvement. However, a true control group would have required that treatment be deferred for two years. This was ethically problematic because it is best practice in pediatrics to treat sensory loss as early as possible in order to protect developmental outcomes, and there is now strong experimental evidence that QST massage effectively treats tactile abnormalities and substantially improves developmental outcomes. Two factors strengthened the validity of the observational evidence in this study:

1) The magnitude and direction of results across the multiple measures were consistent with results reported in the experimental studies; and

2) The dose-response relationship in the fidelity data argued against confounding variables. As noted earlier, the natural history of autism in childhood is one of stability of autism severity, and does not account for a 44% decrease in severity of autism, or 1 in four children coming off the spectrum after two years.

## Conclusions

These longer-term observational results lend support to the recommendations made in the preceding randomized controlled trial: that QST massage is an effective treatment for tactile abnormalities in children with autism; that treatment results in decreased severity of behavioral, social, and language components of autism as well as a autism severity overall; and that treatment of tactile abnormalities should be recommended at the time of autism diagnosis in order to enhance developmental outcomes [21]. Longer-term treatment resulted in continued improvement up to the point of full normalization of tactile and CARS scores in some children. Initial severity of tactile impairment was a good predictor of which children ended in the higher and lower functioning groups. Finally, this study provided useful information for structuring the parent support program to optimize treatment outcomes.

## Directions for Future Research

A five-year study to identify the point of maximum benefit from the intervention is planned in preschool children under conditions optimizing parent fidelity with daily treatment. Measures of autism as well as measures of classroom success will be evaluated. Further exploration of the nature of tactile abnormalities in autism is underway, and biopsies for a case-control comparing C-tactile fiber counts in autistic and neurotypical children have been taken. A clinical study evaluating skin biopsies before and after treatment is also planned.

## Acknowledgements

This study was supported by Grant R40 MC 24945 from the Maternal and Child Health Research Program, Maternal and Child Health Bureau, Health Resources and Services Administration, and Department of Health and Human Services. We wish to thank the project's QST therapists and blind-to-group assessors for the time and effort they put into this study.

## References

1. Zablotsky B, Black L, Maenner M, Shieve L, Blumberg S (2015) Estimated prevalence of autism and other developmental disabilities following questionnaire changes in the 2014 National Health Interview Survey. National Health Statistics.
2. American Psychiatric Association (2013) Diagnostic and Statistical Manual of Mental Disorders (5th edn.) Author, Washington DC.
3. Camarata S (2014) Early identification and early intervention in autism spectrum disorders: Accurate and effective? International Journal of Speech-Language Pathology 16: 1-10.
4. Baranek GT (1999) Autism during infancy: a retrospective video analysis of sensory-motor and social behaviors at 9-12 months of age. J Autism Dev Disord 29: 213-224.
5. Tomchek SD, Dunn W (2007) Sensory processing in children with and without autism: a comparative study using the short sensory profile. Am J Occup Ther 61: 190-200.
6. Foss-Feig JH, Heacock JL, Cascio CJ (2012) Tactile responsiveness patterns and their association with core features in autism spectrum disorders. Res Autism Spectr Disord 6: 337-344.
7. Kanner L (1943) Autistic disturbances of affective contact. Nervous Child 2: 217-250.
8. Silva LM, Schalock M, Gabrielsen KR (2015) About Face: Evaluating and Managing Tactile Impairment at the Time of Autism Diagnosis. Autism Res Treat 2015: 612507.
9. McGlone F, Wessberg J, Olausson H (2014) Discriminative and affective touch: sensing and feeling. Neuron 82: 737-755.
10. Liljencrantz J, Björnsdotter M, Morrison I, Bergstrand S, Ceko M, et al. (2013) Altered C-tactile processing in human dynamic tactile allodynia. Pain 154: 227-234.
11. Lauria G, Hsieh S, Johansson O (2010) European Federation of Neurological Societies/Peripheral Nerve Society Guideline on the use of skin biopsy in the diagnosis of small fiber neuropathy: Report of a joint task force of the European Federation of Neurological Societies and the Peripheral Nerve Society. European Journal of Neurology 17: 903-991, e44-e49.
12. Silva LMT, Schalock M (in press) First skin biopsy reports in children with autism show loss of C-tactile fiber. Journal of Neurological Disorders.
13. Silva LMT, Cignolini A, Warren R, Skowron-Gooch A, Budden S (2007) Improvement in sensory impairment and social interaction in young children with autism following treatment with an original Qigong massage methodology. The American Journal of Chinese Medicine 35: 393-406.
14. Silva LMT, Schalock M, Ayres R, Bunse C, Budden S (2009) Qigong massage treatment for sensory and self-regulation problems in young children with autism: A randomized controlled trial. American Journal of Occupational Therapy 63: 423-432
15. Silva LMT, Schalock M, Gabrielsen K (2011) Early intervention for autism with a parent-delivered qigong massage program: A randomized controlled trial. American Journal of Occupational Therapy 65: 550-559.
16. Tian Y, Wang G, Huang T, Jia S, Zhang Y, et al. (2013) Impacts on skin blood flow under moving cupping along meridians in different directions [article in Chinese]. Zhongguo Zhen Jiu [Chinese Acupuncture and Moxibustion] 33: 247-251.

17. Zhang W, Wang L, Huang T, Tian Y, Xu Y, et al. (2008) Laser Doppler perfusion imaging for assessment of skin blood perfusion after acupuncture. Medical Acupuncture 20: 109-118.

18. Silva LMT, Schalock M (2012) Sense and self-regulation checklist, a measure of comorbid autism symptoms: Initial psychometric evidence. American Journal of Occupational Therapy 66: 177-186.

19. Krug D, Arick J, Almond P (2008) Autism screening instrument for educational planning (3rd edn.) Pro-Ed, Austin, Texas.

20. Schopler E, Reichler R, Renner B (2013) Childhood Autism Rating Scale (2nd edn.) Western Psychological Services, Los Angeles, CA.

21. Silva LMT, Schalock M, Gabrielsen K, Budden S, Buenrostro M, et al. (2015) Early intervention with a parent-delivered massage protocol directed at tactile abnormalities decreases severity of autism and improves child-to-parent interactions: A replication study. Autism Research and Treatment.

22. Gotham K, Pickles A, Lord C (2012) Trajectories of autism severity in children using standardized ADOS scores. Pediatrics 130: e1278-e1284.

23. Rutter M, Couteur AL, Lord C (2003) Autism Diagnostic Interview-Revised. Torrance, CA: Western Psychological Services.

24. Chlebowski C, Green JA, Barton ML, Fein D (2010) Using the childhood autism rating scale to diagnose autism spectrum disorders. J Autism Dev Disord 40: 787-799.

25. Christensen D (2016). Prevalence and characteristics of autism spectrum disorder among children aged 8 years—Autism and developmental disabilities monitoring network, 11 sites, United States, 2012. MMWR. Surveillance Summaries 65.

26. Silva LMT (2011) Qigong massage for your child with autism: A home program from Chinese medicine. Singing Dragon, London; Philadelphia.

27. Silva LM, Ayres R, Schalock M (2008) Outcomes of a pilot training program in a qigong massage intervention for young children with autism. Am J Occup Ther 62: 538-546.

28. Touch-based Treatment for Autism with Qigong Massage: Training for Parents and Professionals.

29. Rellini E, Tortolani D, Trillo S, Carbone S, Montecchi F (2004) Childhood Autism Rating Scale (CARS) and Autism Behavior Checklist (ABC) correspondence and conflicts with DSM-IV criteria in diagnosis of autism. Journal of Autism and Developmental Disorders 34: 703-708.

30. Perry A, Condillac RA, Freeman NL, Dunn-Geier J, Belair J (2005) Multi-site study of the Childhood Autism Rating Scale (CARS) in five clinical groups of young children. J Autism Dev Disord 35: 625-634.

31. Zimmerman I, Steiner V, Pond R (2011) Preschool Language Scale (5th edn.) Pearson, San Antonio, Texas.

32. Friberg J (2010) Considerations for test selection: How do validity and reliability impact diagnostic decisions? Child Language Teaching and Therapy 26: 77-92.

33. Parrow S, Cicchetti D, Balla D (2005) Vineland Adaptive Behavior Scales (2nd edn.) Pearson, San Antonio, Texas.

34. Marteleto MR, Pedromônico MR (2005) Validity of Autism Behavior Checklist (ABC): preliminary study. Rev Bras Psiquiatr 27: 295-301.

35. Bagnato S, Munson S, Neisworth J (1989) Linking developmental assessment and early intervention: Curriculum-based prescriptions. Aspen Publishers.

36. Squires J, Nickel R, Bricker D (1990) Use of parent-completed developmental questionnaires for child-find and screening. Infants and Young Children 3: 46-57.

37. Limbos MM, Joyce DP (2011) Comparison of the ASQ and PEDS in screening for developmental delay in children presenting for primary care. J Dev Behav Pediatr 32: 499-511.

38. Reichow B (2012) Overview of meta-analyses on early intensive behavioral intervention for young children with autism spectrum disorders. J Autism Dev Disord 42: 512-520.

39. Ardiel EL, Rankin CH (2010) The importance of touch in development. Paediatr Child Health 15: 153-156.

40. Dawson G, Meltzoff AN, Osterling J, Rinaldi J, Brown E (1998) Children with autism fail to orient to naturally occurring social stimuli. J Autism Dev Disord 28: 479-485.

41. Dunbar RI (2010) The social role of touch in humans and primates: behavioural function and neurobiological mechanisms. Neurosci Biobehav Rev 34: 260-268.

42. Kopp C (1982) Antecedents of self-regulation: A developmental perspective. Developmental Psychology 18: 199.

43. Vivanti G, Prior M, Williams K, Dissanayake C (2014) Predictors of outcomes in autism early intervention: why don't we know more? Front Pediatr 2: 58.

44. Thurm A, Lord C, Lee LC, Newschaffer C (2007) Predictors of language acquisition in preschool children with autism spectrum disorders. J Autism Dev Disord 37: 1721-1734.

# 19

# The Effect of Wet Cupping on Blood Haemoglobin Level

**Samiha A. Mourad**[1*] **and Soad K. Al-Jaouni**[2]

[1]*Prophetic Medicine Research Clinic, King Abdulaziz University, Jeddah, Saudi Arabia*

[2]*Department of Hematology, Faculty of Medicine, King Abdulaziz University, Jeddah, Saudi Arabia*

[*]**Corresponding author:** Samiha A. Mourad, Prophetic Medicine Research Clinic, King Abdulaziz University, Jeddah, Saudi Arabia, E-mail: dr.samiha-mourad@hotmail.com

**Abstract**

Although wet cupping is quite a popular procedure that is practised worldwide, there is not enough evidence that it may cause anaemia as a side effect. In this observational retrospective pre–post study, we looked through the previously recorded data of patients who received wet cupping at King Abdulaziz University Hospital. We included in the study all those who had their complete blood count done before and immediately after the procedure (n=364). Then, we recorded their blood haemoglobin, red blood cell count, mean corpuscular volume, mean corpuscular haemoglobin and haematocrit before wet cupping, immediately after it, within 3 months after it, then, finally, from 3 months to 6 months after it. Three comparisons took place for each blood test by comparing the pre-reading with each one of the three post-readings. There was no statistically significant difference in any of the pre–post comparisons of those blood tests. However, after excluding those who were not anaemic and keeping only the anaemic patients, the comparison showed statistically significant improvement, but not clinically significant, when comparing the red blood cell count and the haematocrit before and immediately after wet cupping — p value was 0.000 for both. The mean difference for red blood cell count was –0.80 million cells/μL (–0.12 to –0.39) while the haematocrit mean difference was –0.64% (–0.96 to –0.33). In conclusion, anaemia was not found as a side effect of wet cupping.

**Keywords:** Wet cupping, Safety, Haemoglobin, Anemia, Prophetic medicine, Saudi Arabia

## Introduction

Cupping is a well-known traditional healing remedy in many parts of the world. Wet cupping is defined as "the process of using a vacuum at different points on the body but with incisions in order to remove 'harmful' blood which lies just beneath the surface of the skin" [1]. It is known in Arabic language as hijama. For Muslims, it has special importance because it was recommended by the Prophet Mohammed (peace be upon him) on many occasions. For example, he said, "Indeed the best of remedies you have is hijama (cupping)" [1].

Although wet cupping has been a well-known treatment procedure for many years, there is no clear evidence regarding its safety on patients' haemoglobin levels. This study should help to build a solid, safe base for future wet-cupping studies and clinical practice on anaemic patients. The objectives of this study are to determine the effect of wet cupping on blood haemoglobin level, and measure the risk of anaemia caused by this procedure. Furthermore, the study will assess the effect of wet cupping on haemoglobin level within the subgroup of anaemic patients by comparing it before and after the procedure.

## Literature Review

Few studies have investigated the effect of wet cupping on blood haemoglobin level. The most relevant one is a study conducted in Iran in 2009 by Mahdavi et al. [1], who performed wet cupping on 56 healthy men between 20 and 40 years old, on one point between the two scapulae on the back, opposite T2-T5. They did many blood tests before the procedure and 2 weeks after it, including complete blood count. The mean haemoglobin level before wet cupping was 15.67 ± 1.2, and after cupping it was 15.12 ± 1.25. The p value was 0.045, which was a statistically significant difference, but, apparently, a clinically nonsignificant difference. But we cannot generalise those results because it was a small sample size and they included only healthy, young men.

A number of case reports testify that patients performed excessive wet cupping for a long period and then developed anaemia. We have found six such case reports in the literature with similar stories of a patient who developed anaemia and even some had anaemia with complications following an excessive course of wet cupping—and, in one case, dry cupping. Five of those case reports or case series were for Korean patients [2-5] and one was from Turkey [6]. All those cases had a common history of performing what was described as repeated, excessive, or long-duration cupping. The sessions were performed very frequently; for example, two to three times per week as described in one study [3]. The duration of treatment was long in all of those studies ranging from 2 months [2] to more than 10 years [4]. Logically, the very frequent cupping and the long duration might have caused the severe anaemia in those cases, but this cannot be conclusively determined by only those case reports. On the other hand, this still cannot answer the question if the performance of less frequent wet-cupping sessions for a shorter duration can have the same effect on haemoglobin or not.

## Methods

The design of this study is an observational retrospective pre–post study to investigate the effect of wet cupping on different blood parameters and answer the question if wet cupping or hijama causes anaemia. The study was performed at King Abdulaziz University Hospital in Jeddah in the Prophetic Medicine Clinic, which is funded and supervised by the Y.A. Jameel, Scientific Chair of Prophetic Medical Applications. This clinic mainly provides wet-cupping therapy for patients referred from other clinics in the hospital who ask for hijama for different reasons. The data were taken from the records of the patients who attended that clinic during January 2013 to December 2013. We included all the patients who attended the clinic during that period and excluded those who did not have a complete blood count (CBC) before receiving hijama. We also excluded those who had no CBC done immediately after hijama. After excluding those patients, the sample size was 364 participants.

All participants who received wet cupping at the Prophetic Medicine Clinic signed a consent form indicating that their data would be used in multiple studies funded by the scientific chair. Confidentiality of data was ensured throughout the study.

The usual hijama procedure in the Prophetic Medicine Clinic involves cleaning the target area with an alcohol swab, placing the cup over the area and starting suction. The cup is then gently removed and five very superficial incisions, about 0.3 cm to 0.7 cm in length and 0.2 mm in depth, are made parallel to each other. After creating the incisions, the cup is placed over the same area and the suctioning is repeated. This procedure is performed on all or most target hijama sites at the same time. The amount of blood extracted per session is about 50 mL to 100 mL from all sites in the body. After that, the areas are cleaned and dressed. Usually, there is at least a month gap before the next hijama session at the clinic.

The investigations used for comparison are haemoglobin (HB), haematocrit (HCT), red blood cell (RBC) count, mean corpuscular volume (MCV) and mean corpuscular haemoglobin (MCH). Those investigations' readings were taken at different time points: before hijama, immediately after hijama, within 3 months after hijama and between 3 months and 6 months after hijama. Some patients had no measurements taken within 6 months, other than that done immediately after hijama, so those were included only in the first comparison and excluded from the following ones.

Statistical analysis was done using SPSS program version 16.0. Baseline categorical variables are presented in frequencies and ratios, while baseline continuous variables are presented in means and standard deviations. Student's t-test analyses will be used to compare mean HB, HCT, RBC count, MCV and MCH before wet cupping and immediately after it, before wet cupping and within 3 months after it, and before wet cupping and from 3 months to 6 months after it. The diversity of the patients included in the study is the reason for not using ANCOVA (discussed in the "Results" section). Moreover, we repeated the same set of comparisons within the subgroup of anaemic patients to assess if hijama is safe to be performed among them.

## Results

The patients who were chosen for this study had a wide age range, from 14 to 86 years, but most of them were within the adults' range of 18 and 65 years old. Most of the participants were female, with a ratio of about 1 male to 3 females. The mean values of the participants' HB, RBC, MCV, MCH and HCT were all within the normal ranges. The majority of the participants had more than one hijama session on different days, and the average number of hijama sites in each session was about nine sites of wet cupping. Unfortunately, there were no data available for the average amount of blood extracted from the patients in each hijama session. Table 1 shows more details about the baseline characteristics of the participants.

| Baseline characteristic | n | Result | Range (if applicable) |
|---|---|---|---|
| Mean age, years (± SD) | 363 | 44.4 (± 13.9) | 14 to 86 years |
| Male: female ratio | 364 | 92:272 | – |
| Smoker: non-smoker ratio | 364 | 38:320 | – |
| Mean HB level (± SD) | 364 | 12.9(± 1.8) | 4.5 to 17.9 |
| Mean RBC (± SD) | 364 | 4.7 (± 0.6) | 3.0 to 6.7 |
| Mean MCV (± SD) | 322 | 82.2 (± 6.8) | 55.9 to 113.5 |
| Mean MCH (± SD) | 322 | 27.8 (± 5.0) | 15.2 to 86.8 |
| Mean HCT (± SD) | 364 | 50.3 (± 203.6) | 16.9 to 3907.0 |
| Mean number of hijama sessions | 328 | 2.8 (± 1.7) | 1 to 14 |
| Mean number of hijama sites per session | 323 | 9.3 (± 4.3) | 2 to 37 |

**Table 1:** Baseline characteristics of participants before hijama.

The majority of the patients who were referred to the Prophetic Medicine Clinic had pain as their main complaint. Nevertheless, many of them reported to the clinic with more than one complaint; 120 of the 364 included in the study had multiple complaints. Table 2 gives the full description of all the complaints that the patients had, with the frequency of each complaint.

| The complaint of the participant | The frequency of the complaint* |
|---|---|
| Back pain | 136 |
| Shoulder pain | 48 |
| Knee pain | 40 |
| Other pain | 87 |
| Headache and migraine | 66 |
| Hypertension | 28 |
| Infertility | 25 |

| | |
|---|---|
| Diabetes Mellitus | 10 |
| Hormonal disturbance | 8 |
| Allergy | 8 |
| Chronic fatigue | 8 |
| Rheumatoid arthritis | 7 |
| Psychological problem | 5 |
| Other complaints | 37 |
| No complaint** | 81 |
| * Note that many participants had more than one complaint.<br>** Some people receive hijama for general well-being, without having a specific complaint or disease. | |

**Table 2:** Participant complaints.

Many comparisons were drawn from the participants' results to show the difference between their blood results before and immediately after hijama, then before and within 3 months after hijama and finally before and from 3 to 6 months after hijama. The after-hijama readings were taken after the final hijama session, because most of the participants had more than one hijama session. Each comparison was displayed in mean difference with p values and confidence intervals. In general, there were no statistical differences between any of the readings before and after hijama. Table 3 shows those comparisons in depth.

| Comparison | Comparison between baseline and results immediately after hijama | Comparison between baseline and results within 3 months after hijama | Comparison between baseline and results within 6 months after hijama |
|---|---|---|---|
| Haemoglobin (HB) | | | |
| Number of cases | 364 | 193 | 78 |
| Mean HB before hijama (± SD) | 12.9 (± 1.8) | 12.6 (± 1.8) | 12.3 (± 1.8) |
| Mean HB after hijama (± SD) | 12.9 (± 1.8) | 12.5 (± 1.8) | 12.2 (± 1.8) |
| Mean difference (95% CI) | 0.02 (–0.06 to 0.08) | 0.10 (0 to 0.19) | 0.03 (–0.18 to 0.24) |
| p value | 0.689 | 0.055 | 0.764 |
| Red blood cell (RBC) count | | | |
| Number of cases | 364 | 194 | 78 |
| Mean RBC before hijama (± SD) | 4.7 (± 0.6) | 4.7 (± 0.5) | 4.6 (± 0.6) |
| Mean RBC after hijama (± SD) | 4.7 (± 0.5) | 4.6 (± 0.6) | 4.6 (± 0.6) |
| Mean difference (95% CI) | –0.01 (–0.03 to 0.02) | 0.02 (–0.01 to 0.05) | –0.01 (–0.07 to 0.05) |
| p value | 0.639 | 0.152 | 0.79 |
| Haematocrit (HCT) | | | |
| Number of cases | 364 | 193 | 78 |
| Mean HCT before hijama (± SD) | 50.3 (± 203.6) | 12.6 (± 25.8) | 37.8 (± 7.1) |
| Mean HCT after hijama (± SD) | 38.8 (± 4.4) | 12.5 (± 4.8) | 36.8 (± 5.2) |
| Mean difference (95% CI) | 11.54 (–9.43 to 32.50) | 0.10 (0.00 to 0.19) | 0.98 (–0.47 to 2.42) |

| p value | 0.28 | 0.196 | 0.183 |
|---|---|---|---|
| Mean corpuscular volume (MCV) | | | |
| Number of cases | 321 | 190 | 78 |
| Mean MCV before hijama (± SD) | 82.2 (± 6.8) | 81.7 (± 7.0) | 80.5 (± 7.3) |
| Mean MCV after hijama (± SD) | 82.2 (± 7.3) | 81.7 (± 7.2) | 79.8 (± 1.0) |
| Mean difference (95% CI) | 0.02 (–0.28 to 0.33) | –0.02 (–0.26 to 0.22) | 0.69 (–0.47 to 1.84) |
| p value | 0.884 | 0.872 | 0.241 |
| Mean corpuscular haemoglobin (MCH) | | | |
| Number of cases | 321 | 190 | 78 |
| Mean MCH before hijama (± SD) | 27.8 (± 5.0) | 27.7 (± 6.1) | 27.1 (± 0.7) |
| Mean MCH after hijama (± SD) | 27.9 (± 5.8) | 27.7 (± 6.6) | 27.1 (± 6.8) |
| Mean difference (95% CI) | –0.15 (–0.49 to 0.18) | 0.04 (–0.72 to 0.80) | 0.04 (–1.85 to 1.94) |
| p value | 0.361 | 0.923 | 0.966 |

**Table 3:** Comparison between the HB, RBC, HCT, MCV and MCH levels before and within 3 and 6 months after hijama.

The same method of comparison was repeated for only the participants who initially had anaemia before the first session of hijama. The definition of anaemia by the World Health Organization is less than 13 g/dL for males and less than 12 g/dL for females [7]. This definition was followed in the selection of the anaemic patients. Although the results showed a statistically significant increase in the RBC and HCT when comparing their mean values before and immediately after hijama, it was not a clinically significant difference. For the RBC, the mean value before hijama was 4.4 million cells/μL (± 0.5) and after hijama was 4.5 million cells/μL (± 0.6). For the HCT, the mean value before hijama was 33.6% (± 3.2) and after hijama was 34.3% (± 3.8). In the following comparisons, this difference disappeared during the 3-month and the 6-month follow-up investigations. However, we need to point out here that there were fewer participants this subgroup than the total number of participants that we started with, which decreases the power of the results. In Table 4, more details are shown regarding this subgroup.

| **Comparison** | **Comparison between baseline and results immediately after hijama** | **Comparison between baseline and results within 3 months after hijama** | **Comparison between baseline and results within 6 months after hijama** |
|---|---|---|---|
| Haemoglobin (HB) | | | |
| Number of cases | 99 | 58 | 31 |
| Mean HB before hijama (± SD) | 10.8 (± 1.3) | 10.7 (± 1.4) | 10.6 (± 1.6) |
| Mean HB after hijama (± SD) | 10.9 (± 1.5) | 10.7 (± 1.7) | 10.8 (± 1.5) |
| Mean difference (95% CI) | –0.12 (–0.33 to 0.07) | –0.06 (–0.25 to 0.13) | –0.17 (–0.55 to 0.20) |
| p value | 0.198 | 0.553 | 0.355 |
| Red blood cell (RBC) count | | | |
| Number of cases | 99 | 58 | 31 |
| Mean RBC before hijama (± SD) | 4.4 (± 0.5) | 4.4 (± 0.6) | 4.4 (± 0.6) |
| Mean RBC after hijama (± SD) | 4.5 (± 0.6) | 4.4 (± 0.6) | 4.5 (± 0.6) |
| Mean difference (95% CI) | –0.80 (–0.12 to –0.39) | –0.04 (–0.10 to 0.02) | –0.04 (–0.17 to 0.08) |
| p value | 0.000 | 0.214 | 0.495 |

| Haematocrit (HCT) | | | |
|---|---|---|---|
| Number of cases | 99 | 58 | 31 |
| Mean HCT before hijama (± SD) | 33.6 (± 3.2) | 33.4 (± 3.7) | 33.3 (± 4.1) |
| Mean HCT after hijama (± SD) | 34.3 (± 3.8) | 33.7 (± 4.4) | 33.7 (± 4.1) |
| Mean difference (95% CI) | −0.64 (−0.96 to −0.33) | −0.30 (−0.79 to 0.19) | −0.45 (−1.44 to 0.54) |
| p value | 0.000 | 0.226 | 0.359 |
| Mean corpuscular volume (MCV) | | | |
| Number of cases | 88 | 56 | 30 |
| Mean MCV before hijama (± SD) | 77.3 (± 7.5) | 76.6 (± 7.5) | 75.6 (± 7.4) |
| Mean MCV after hijama (± SD) | 77.5 (± 7.6) | 76.6 (± 7.8) | 75.9 (± 7.1) |
| Mean difference (95% CI) | −0.19 (−0.45 to 0.07) | −0.002 (−0.569 to 0.566) | −0.29 (−1.34 to −0.57) |
| p value | 0.148 | 0.995 | 0.570 |
| Mean corpuscular haemoglobin (MCH) | | | |
| Number of cases | 88 | 56 | 30 |
| Mean MCH before hijama (± SD) | 25.4 (± 5.8) | 25.3 (± 6.9) | 25.6 (± 9.1) |
| Mean MCH after hijama (± SD) | 25.5 (± 5.8) | 24.4 (± 3.4) | 24.2 (± 3.1) |
| Mean difference (95% CI) | −0.06 (−0.18 to 0.05) | 0.93 (−0.83 to 2.70) | 1.46 (−1.91 to 4.83) |
| p value | 0.287 | 0.294 | 0.384 |

**Table 4:** Comparison between the HB, RBC, HCT, MCV and MCH levels before and within 3 and 6 months after hijama, among anaemic participants only.

## Discussion

All the results prove that anaemia is not a side effect of wet cupping, or hijama. The diversity of the patients included in the study gives it more strength and easier generalisability, because it contains a wide spectrum of age and a wide variety of different complaints. On the other hand, it would be better if we had a consistent number of patients in all of the follow-up results comparisons to have similar powers in all of them, but that was not possible because of the fact that it was a retrospective observational study and we had no control or choice on the investigations done—a drawback of using a retrospective design. We recommend that future studies use a prospective design. It will also be beneficial to accurately measure the amount of blood extracted in each session, as this might affect the outcome.

If we compared the results of this study with the previously mentioned studies, we can say that the results are consistent with the study by Mahdavi et al. [1]. Clearly those results are different from the case reports that were listed previously. They all reported very frequent wet or dry cupping for a long duration followed by the patients suffering from anaemia [2-6]. Therefore, the anaemia might be due to the unusual excessive cupping sessions that were done in those reports. This is unlikely to happen with the usual wet-cupping procedure as we described here. Although some hijama practitioners claim that hijama might be a treatment for anaemia, it was clear in this study that such a treatment did not improve the HB levels in those who were anaemic at the beginning of the study.

## Conclusion

Wet cupping does not cause anaemia, and it is safe for anaemic patients; however, it is yet to be proven as a valid treatment for anaemia.

## Acknowledgements

This study was funded by Y.A. Jameel, Scientific Chair of Prophetic Medical Applications in King Abdulaziz University (Jeddah, Saudi Arabia). We acknowledge all the staff who work in the Prophetic Medicine Clinic in King Abdulaziz University Hospital, Dr. Anhar Gazaz, Dr. Manal Dahlawi, Mrs. Zakeia Abdulsattar, Mrs. Sabria Kholy, Mrs. Fatmah Ahmed, Dr. Iman Al-Feqy and Ms. Rasha Ramadan. Special thanks to Mrs. Khadija Lokman for the data entry and Dr. Nouran Aleyeidi for her help in the data analysis and research writing.

## References

1. Mahdavi MR, Ghazanfari T, Aghajani M, Danyali F, Naseri M (2011) Evaluation of the Effects of Traditional Cupping on the Biochemical, Hematological and Immunological Factors of Human Venous Blood. In: Bhattacharya A, editor. A Compendium of Essays on Alternative Therapy. Rijeka: InTech, Croatia, pp. 67–88.
2. Kim KH, Kim TH, Hwangbo M, Yang GY (2012) Anaemia and skin pigmentation after excessive cupping therapy by an unqualified therapist in Korea: a case report. Acupunct Med 30: 227-228.

3. Lee SJ, Suh YS, Lee YJ, Cho DG, Lee MJ, et al. (2011) Iron Deficiency Anemia due to Long-time Bloodletting Using Cupping. Korean J Fam Med 32: 56-59.
4. Sohn IS, Jin ES, Cho JM, Kim CJ, Bae JH, et al. (2008) Bloodletting-induced cardiomyopathy: reversible cardiac hypertrophy in severe chronic anaemia from long-term bloodletting with cupping. Eur J Echocardiogr 9: 585-586.
5. Lee HJ, Park NH, Yun HJ, Kim S, Jo DY (2008) Cupping Therapy-induced Iron Deficiency Anemia in a Healthy Man. Am J Med 121: e5-e6.
6. Akdogan RA, Akdogan E (2011) An unusual cause of iron deficiency anemia in a healthy man: Hijamah. Turk J Hematol 28: 254-256.
7. WHO (2011) Haemoglobin concentrations for the diagnosis of anaemia and assessment of severity. Vitamin and Mineral Nutrition Information System. WHO/NMH/NHD/MNM/11.1.

# 20

# Cost-Effectiveness Analysis of Complementary and Alternative Medicine in Treating Anxiety Disorders

**Matthew Kutch***

*Department of Economics, Ohio Northern University, USA*

***Corresponding author:** Matthew Kutch, Department of Economics, Ohio Northern University, USA, E-mail: m-kutch@onu.edu

**Abstract**

**Objectives:** Using survey data, this study produces estimates of the cost, effectiveness, and cost-effectiveness of complementary and alternative medicine combined with traditional therapies (pharmacotherapy and/or psychotherapy) in the treatment of anxiety disorders. Unlike past cost-effectiveness analyses that use a narrow definition or randomized controlled trials, this study uses a broad definition of complementary and alternative medicines and survey data to assess the cost-effectiveness.

**Study Desi and Outcome Measures:** This analysis uses the Medical Expenditure Panel Survey (MEPS), an overlapping panel survey of medical use, expenditure, and health status for the civilian non-institutionalized U.S. population to identity economic costs and effects for individuals with anxiety disorders. The primary measure of effect is based on self-perceived mental health status. Cost-effectiveness is determined by estimation of incremental net benefit method. Potential self-selection bias is investigated using observable characteristics and inverse propensity score weighting.

**Results:** Complementary and alternative medicine users with an anxiety disorder showed a statistically insignificant decrease in costs compared to nonusers (\$458.95 versus \$467.03; p-value 0.920). Complementary and alternative medicine expenditures were offset by a statistically significant decrease in office-based and pharmaceutical costs. Complementary and alternative medicine users showed an increase in the probability of steady or improved mental health compared to nonusers (0.7549 versus 0.6912; p-value 0.190) resulting in an incremental cost-effectiveness ratio of -\$12.70 per 10% increase in the probability of steady or increased mental health. The evidence suggests a high probability that complementary and alternative medicine is cost-effective for large values of effect for anxiety disorders (p-value 0.080 for WTP of \$5000).

**Conclusions:** This survey data indicates complementary and alternative medicine users with anxiety disorders had slightly lower costs and improved outcomes. Limitations are considered.

**Keywords:** Cost; Cost-effectiveness; Economic evaluation; Anxiety

## Abbreviations:

CAM: Complementary and Alternative Medicine; MEPS: Medical Expenditure Panel Survey; ICER: Incremental Cost-Effectiveness Ratio; INB: Incremental Net Benefit; WTP: Willingness-to-Pay

## Introduction

Anxiety and depression have a significant global prevalence (22.0%) and are associated with some of the most significant impacts on quality of life [1]. A large-scale nationally representative survey estimated 12-month prevalence for any mental health disorder at over 25% of the US adult population with anxiety disorders and mood disorders (depression disorder and bipolar disorder) with particularly high rates of prevalence (18.1% and 9.5% respectively) [2]. US Spending on mental health and substance abuse is projected to reach \$281 billion by 2020, representing 6.5% of all health spending [3].

Conventional treatments for anxiety disorders include medication or cognitive-behavioral therapy (CBT). Medications cannot cure anxiety disorders, but can keep them under control while receiving psychotherapy [4]. In CBT patients change their thinking patterns that support their fears and change the way they react to anxiety-provoking situations. Similar to many Complementary and alternative medicine (CAM) modalities, CBT may often incorporate deep-breathing exercises to relieve anxiety and encourage relaxation.

Complementary and alternative medicines (CAM) are forms of treatment that are used in addition to (complementary) or instead of (alternative) standard treatment and can include a wide array of treatments, from acupuncture and massage therapy to herbal remedies and hypnosis. Complementary and alternative medicine (CAM) covers a heterogeneous spectrum of ancient to new-age approaches that purport to prevent or treat disease [5]. Practices are considered unconventional when they are either not widely taught in medical schools or when they are not widely practiced in hospitals or outpatient facilities [6].

Many individuals use CAM to improve health and well-being, including the relief of symptoms associated with chronic illness or the side-effects to conventional treatment. A previous study used the 2007 National Health Interview Survey (NHIS) to describe patterns of CAM users' characteristics and use, finding 38% of adults had used complementary and alternative medicine in the previous 12 month, most commonly nonvitamin, nonmineral, natural products, deep breathing exercises, meditation, chiropractic or osteopathic manipulation, massage therapy, and yoga [5]. Common diseases and conditions for which people use CAM includes back, neck, or joint pain, arthritis, and mental health disorders (anxiety, depression, ADHA/ADD) [5].

Past studies demonstrate the increased use of CAM for individuals with mental health disorders. Kessler et al. [6] using a 1997-1998 nationally representative survey suggests that the majority of people in the United States with self-defined anxiety attacks or severe depression use some form of CAM as a component of treatment. This assumes a broadly drawn definition of CAM that includes prayer as spiritual healing, relaxation techniques, and imagery. The authors find no statistical difference in the observable characteristics of individuals with anxiety attacks or severe depression who use CAM and individuals without anxiety attacks or severe depression who use of CAM.

Unützer et al. [7] similarly found individuals who reported use of alternative medicine were more likely to meet diagnostic criteria for at least one of the mental disorders under consideration (depression, dysthymia, panic disorder, generalized anxiety disorder, bipolar disorder, or psychosis). In the 1997 update of their seminal nationally representative estimates of complementary and alternative care use, Eisenberg et al. [8] found that 40.9% of individuals reporting severe depression and 42.7% of individuals with anxiety attacks used alternative therapy in the previous year. They estimated total expenditure on CAM for 1997 at $21.2 billion, with estimated out-of-pocket expenditures totaling $9.1 billion [9].

Grzywacz et al. [9] found that while CAM use was higher for the elderly with anxiety disorders, a majority did not use CAM to treat anxiety disorders. Su and Li [10] found CAM use was more likely among racial and ethnic minorities and when conventional treatment is more difficult. A number of meta-analyses have considered specific modality of CAM evaluated in a RCT structure. Chiesa and Serretti [11] found mindfulness-based stress reduction reduced ruminative thinking and trait anxiety, as well as increase empathy and self-compassion. Manzoni et al. [12] found relaxation training showed a medium-large effect size in treatment in anxiety with higher efficacy for meditation and for longer treatments. Nestoriuc et al. [13] found biofeedback had significant effects in diminishing symptoms of anxiety and depression. Past cost-effectiveness analyses use randomized controlled trials or other quasi-experimental settings to examine the efficacy of specific complementary and alternative treatments or a narrow definition of CAM, finding generally favorable, but mixed results [14-16].

Bar-Sela et al. [17] use a pre-test and post-test design to assess the impact of CAM on a depression, anxiety, and fatigue in cancer patients undergoing oncology treatment, finding positive results on all dimensions. McPherson and McGraw [18] also used a pre-test and post-test design to assess the impact of CAM use on Generalized Anxiety Disorder for members of the military. Anxiety symptoms were improved for the study participants who completed the 6-week program.

## Objective

The objective of this study is to assess the cost-effectiveness of complementary and alternative medicine (broadly defined) as addition to traditional treatments (drug therapy and psychotherapy) for anxiety disorders as measured by self-reported mental health status. Past cost-effectiveness analyses have used randomized controlled trials (RCTs) to examine the efficacy of specific complementary and alternative treatments or a narrow definition of CAM.

This study uses the 1998 Medical Expenditure Panel Survey (MEPS), a panel survey of medical use, expenditure, and health status for the civilian non-institutionalized US population to investigate the outcomes for complementary and alternative medicine.

While past studies used this data to estimate use for different groups, none tried to estimate the cost-effectiveness. Davis and Darden examine the patterns of CAM use by children [19]. Ritchie et al. [20] examined the predictors of CAM use for a specific health concern. Neither of these studies documented differences in cost of effect of CAM use.

Unlike past studies of CAM that rely on an experimental (or quasi-experimental design), this study uses panel data combined with propensity score matching and inverse propensity score weighting in the incremental net benefit framework to estimate cost-effectiveness to uncover potential self-selection bias. The results demonstrate a minor impact on the cost-effectiveness estimates when adjusting for individual heterogeneity.

## Methods

### Study design

Data for the economic evaluation comes from the 1998 Medical Expenditure Panel Survey (MEPS), a nationally representative stratified random survey of the civilian noninstitutionalized population of the United States.

The MEPS is conducted by the Agency for Healthcare Research and Quality (AHRQ), part of the U.S. Department of Health and Human Services. The survey includes demographic characteristics, health conditions, health status, use of medical care services, charges and payments, access to care, satisfaction with care, health insurance coverage, income, and employment. Each household in a MEPS panel is interviewed for five rounds covering a two year period. Panel 2 covers calendar years 1997 and 1998 and panel 3 covers calendar years 1998 and 1999.

The Medical Expenditure Panel Survey (MEPS) uses a set of condition identifiers which aggregates clinically similar conditions by 5-digit DSM-IV TR Codes. The Anxiety Disorder condition identifier includes many different types of Anxiety Disorders. Perceived health status and perceived mental health status are both self-reported on a 5-point Likert scale (1-Excellent, 2-Very Good, 3-Good, 4-Fair, and 5-Poor). The MEPS also collects secondary, more specific measures of health status, including social limitations and cognitive limitations. This analysis considers an anxiety condition identifier based on clinically related DSM-IV-TR diagnosis of anxiety.

The 1998 MEPS includes a section of questions about complementary and alternative medicine (CAM). The MEPS definition of complementary and alternative medicine includes acupuncture, nutritional advice, massage therapy, herbal remedies, bio-feedback, imagery or relaxation techniques, homeopathic treatments, spiritual healing or prayer, hypnosis, or traditional medicine such as Chinese or American Indian medicine. Follow-up questions assess interaction with physician, use for specific problems, and spending and financing issues.

## Cost Measurement

The measure of cost for this analysis includes the direct total charges associated anxiety disorder. The four main sources of charges considered in this analysis are pharmacotherapy charges, office-based charges, outpatient-based charges, emergency room charges, and complementary and alternative medicine charges. Only the pharmacotherapy, office-based, emergency room-based, and outpatient-based charges linked to the specific anxiety condition identifier are considered under this analysis.

This analysis uses the measure of total charges in the Medical Expenditure Panel Survey (MEPS). As recommended, this is the broadest measure of cost, i.e., a societal measure of cost [21]. Direct costs are the primary measures of cost. Given limitations of the data available and evidence of similarities between CAM users and nonusers, the indirect costs associated with work incapacity were assumed negligible.

The MEPS identifies other sources of charges that are not considered as part of this analysis. The other sources of charges include home health-based charges, and dental visit-based charges, among others. Charges with mental health disorders from these sources would not represent typical treatment for the common mental health disorders under consideration, and thus, are excluded from this analysis.

## Outcome Measurement

The primary measure of effectiveness of mental health treatment for this analysis is a global measure of self-reported mental health status. This global mental health measure would include changes in both physical and emotional health from the mental health disorders. The self-reported measure of mental health on a 5-point Likert scale (1-Excellent, 2-Very Good, 3-Good, 4-Fair, and 5-Poor) considers any self-reported health status of "Good" or better as good mental health and "Fair" or "Poor" mental health are considered not good mental health. This dichotomous collapse of the 5-point self-reported mental health status is similar past research [22,23].

Secondary measures of mental health status for this analysis include self-reported limitations on instrumental activities of daily living, functional limitations, social limitations, and cognitive limitations. Limitations on the instrumental activities of daily living are measured by difficulty with using the telephone, paying bills, taking medication, preparing light meals, laundry, or shopping. Functional limitations are measured by difficulties walking, climbing stairs, grasping objects, reaching overhead, lifting, bending, stooping, or standing for long periods. Cogitative limitations are measured by confusion or memory loss, problems making decisions, to the point that it interferes with daily activities or requiring supervision for one's own safety. Social limitations are measured by limitations participating in social, recreational, or family activities.

There is a question of how meaningful self-reported global health measures are in terms of capturing clinically- or epidemiologically-meaningful aspects of health.

In a review of studies related to the validity of self-rating of health, 23 of 27 studies found self-rating of health reliably predicted survival in populations even while accounting for known health risk factors [24]. Idler et al. [25] subsequently found self-rated health also predicts mortality and functions limitations using NHANES data.

Ried et al. [26] found that self-reported health status was moderately correlated with subjective well-being =0.41, t=11.3, p<0.0001), but the two were different constructs. Collapsing both measures to dichotomous variables also showed a statistically significant correlation (0.63, p<0.0001), but a difference in construct.

Global health measures include the Short Form-36 (SF-36) and the abridged Short Form-12 (SF-12). The SF-36 and SF-12 were surveys designed to capture significant variation in health domains. The eight domains of health in the SF-36 and SF-12 Index scores include physical functioning, role limitations because of physical health problems, bodily pain, social functioning, general mental health (psychological distress and psychological well-being), role limitations (from emotional problems), vitality (energy/fatigue), and general health perceptions.

The mental health scales of the SF-36 and SF-12 Index scores are based on the five-item Mental Health Inventory (MHI) that best predict summary score for the 38-item MHI, covering four major mental health dimensions (anxiety, depression, loss of behavioral or emotional control, and psychological well-being) [27]. The MHI has been successfully evaluated in clinical trials comparing quality of life outcomes and compared favorably with emotional reactions score from the Nottingham Health Profile and the summary SIP Psychosocial scale. The MHI discriminates psychiatric patients from those with other medical conditions [27].

The validity of the SF-36 Index score was investigated early in its development [28]. The authors found a good basis for establishing guidelines for the interpretation of score differences for each scale as a measure of physical and/or mental health effects. When observed differences are found in the physical functioning and mental health scales are found, physical or mental causes can be attributed with a high degree of confidence [28].

McCollum et al. [29] linked the SF-12 Index score to the self-reported health status measure used in this research for patients with diabetes and minor depression. Using the 2001 MEPS, they found that diabetes patients with minor depression had a lower mental health summary score (from SF-12), greater cognitive limitation, and lower mental health status as measured by a 5-point Likert scale controlling for relevant demographics and underlying health.

## Cost-effectiveness Assessment

Cost-effectiveness analysis was calculated with the incremental cost-effectiveness ratio (ICER) where the difference in cost ($\mu_{\Delta C}$) between CAM users and CAM nonusers is normalized by the difference in effect between CAM users and CAM non users ($\mu_{\Delta E}$).

$$ICER = \frac{meancosts_{CAM} - meancosts_{NoCAM}}{meaneffect_{CAM} - meaneffect_{NoCAM}}$$

$$ICER = \frac{\mu_{\Delta C}}{\mu_{\Delta E}}$$

A useful reformulation of the problem defines the incremental net benefit as the monetized difference in effect less the difference in the cost where $\lambda$ is the value of a unit of effect (either gained or lost) [30].

$$INB(\lambda) = \lambda * \mu_{\Delta E} - \mu_{\Delta C}$$

A positive incremental net benefit is equivalent to a treatment being cost-effective and is evidence to support the adoption of the new treatment in place of the control. The Cost-Effectiveness Acceptability Curve (CEAC) is a one way to convey the uncertainty of the cost-effectiveness of treatment. Estimates of the CEAC can be obtained both through nonparametric bootstrapping repeated samples or using the p-values on the treatment coefficient from estimation of the incremental net benefit. The mirror image of the p-value (i.e., 1-(p-value)) of the hypothesis test on a positive coefficient on the treatment dummy yields an estimate of the cost-effectiveness-acceptability curves that is asymptotically equivalent to the nonparametric bootstrapping approach [31]. Formally, the CEAC is defined as:

$$CEAC(\lambda) = Prob(ICER \langle \lambda|\mu_{\Delta E} > 0) + Prob(ICER \langle \lambda|\mu_{\Delta E} < 0)$$

The cost-effectiveness acceptability curve is interpreted as conditional probability of cost-effective CAM for a given value of effect.

## Investigating Self-Selection Bias

Past cost-effectiveness analyses use randomized controlled trials to examine the efficacy of specific complementary and alternative treatments or a narrow definition of CAM. Unlike past cost-effectiveness analyses that use randomized control trials, this analysis uses observational data to estimate cost-effectiveness. Individuals are not randomly assigned to either the control or treatment group, rather, they self-select into either control or treatment group. If the unobserved heterogeneity of the individual is correlated with the decision to select into either treatment or control group, then the estimates of differences in costs and effects (and, thus, incremental cost-effectiveness ratios) will be biased.

This research investigates the potential self-selection bias in two ways: inclusion of observable characteristics and inverse propensity score weighting. All are incorporated into the incremental net benefit framework. A simple extension of the basic incremental net benefit method includes a vector of observable characteristics ($X_i$):

$$NB_i(\lambda) = \beta_0 + \beta_1 CAM_i + \Gamma X_i + \varepsilon_i$$

Statistical differences in observable characteristics may be related to the unobservable heterogeneity that influences selection into either treatment or control. Propensity score method is recognized as a semi-parametric approach to mitigate partially the effect of self-selection bias in non-experimental data [32]. All observations of CAM and CAM nonusers are used to estimate the predicted probability of treatment as a function of observable characteristics. The predicted probabilities of treatment for observations in the CAM group are matched to similar predicted probabilities of treatment for observation in the CAM nonuser group with a similar predicted probability using one-to-one nearest neighbor matching. Inverse propensity score weighting is similar to propensity score matching with the advantage that all observations of the sample are considered in the estimation of incremental net benefit. All observations in the CAM user and nonuser groups are used to estimate the predicted probability of treatment as a function of observable characteristics. The predicted probability of seeking treatment for an observation ($PS_i$) is used to construct the weight for that observation according to the following:

$$w_i = \frac{1}{PS_i}$$

For observation i in the CAM group

$$w_i = \frac{1}{1 - PS_i}$$ For observation i in the CAM nonuser group

Using inverse propensity score weighting in the estimation of incremental net benefit decreases the probability that CAM is cost-effective for higher values of a unit of effect, except for the psychotherapy use sample. For low values of a unit of effect, using inverse propensity score weighting increases the probability that CAM is cost-effective.

## Statistical Analysis

Baseline characteristics were analyzed using traditional Student t-tests for comparing differences in continuous variables and a chi-squared test for categorical variables. Incremental cost-effectiveness ratios and cost-effectiveness acceptability curves were estimated with multiple regressions including inverse propensity score weighting as described above. The significance level of 0.05 (two-sided) was used on baseline characteristics. SAS version 9.2 was used for estimation and bootstrapping cost-effectiveness analysis and the cost-effectiveness acceptability curves.

## Results

### Baseline characteristics

A total of 808 individuals with anxiety disorders were identified. Of those, 12.62% (102) were CAM users and 87.38% (706) were CAM nonusers.

As shown in Table 1, CAM users were more likely to be female and white, live in the west, be employed, and have at least some college.

Table 1 also presents the baseline characteristics of CAM users and nonusers. There are no statistically significant differences in baseline health characteristics between the two groups. CAM users are more likely to be female, white, live in the Northeast or West, and be employed. There were no statistically significant differences in income.

| | CAM users | (n=102) | CAM nonusers | (n=706) | |
|---|---|---|---|---|---|
| | MEAN | SD | MEAN | SD | p-Value |
| **Baseline Health Characteristics** | | | | | |
| Initial Overall Health (5pt Scale) | 2.70 | 1.21 | 2.87[b] | 1.19 | 0.184 |
| Initial Overall Mental Health (5pt Scale) | 2.64 | 1.12 | 2.66[b] | 1.14 | 0.823 |
| Initial IADL Limitations | 0.0693[a] | 0.2552 | 0.0939[c] | 0.2919 | 0.850 |

| | | | | | |
|---|---|---|---|---|---|
| Initial Functional Limitations | 0.2255 | 0.4200 | 0.2340[d] | 0.4236 | 0.422 |
| Initial Social Limitations | 0.1584[a] | 0.3670 | 0.1280[c] | 0.3344 | 0.399 |
| Initial Cognitive Limitations | 0.1275 | 0.3351 | 0.1264[e] | 0.3326 | 0.977 |
| **Demographic Characteristics** | | | | | |
| Age | 43.67 | 13.78 | 47.53 | 15.86 | 0.196 |
| Male | 0.1765 | 0.3831 | 0.3116 | 0.4635 | 0.005 |
| White (Not Hispanic) | 0.8039 | 0.3990 | 0.7068 | 0.4556 | 0.041 |
| Black (Not Hispanic) | 0.0588 | 0.2365 | 0.0949 | 0.2933 | 0.235 |
| Hispanic | 0.1176 | 0.3238 | 0.1799 | 0.3844 | 0.120 |
| Other Race (Not Hispanic) | 0.0196 | 0.1393 | 0.0184 | 0.1345 | 0.933 |
| Northeast | 0.0686 | 0.2541 | 0.1856 | 0.3890 | 0.003 |
| Midwest | 0.1765 | 0.3831 | 0.1926 | 0.3946 | 0.698 |
| South | 0.3137 | 0.4663 | 0.3399 | 0.4740 | 0.600 |
| West | 0.4412 | 0.4990 | 0.2819 | 0.4502 | 0.001 |
| **Socioeconomic Characteristics** | | | | | |
| Personal Income | 27776 | 26402 | 24269 | 25637 | 0.211 |
| Employed | 0.6961 | 0.4622 | 0.5793 | 0.4940 | 0.025 |
| College Graduate | 0.2353 | 0.4263 | 0.1856 | 0.3890 | 0.233 |
| Other Degree | 0.0980 | 0.2988 | 0.0793 | 0.2704 | 0.519 |
| Some College | 0.2157 | 0.4133 | 0.1827 | 0.3867 | 0.425 |
| HS or Less | 0.4412 | 0.4990 | 0.5496 | 0.4979 | 0.040 |
| [a]n=101; [b]n = 705; [c]n=703; [d]n=701; [e]n=704 | | | | | |

**Table 1:** Descriptive statistics for baseline characteristics.

## Cost Measurement

Table 2 presents measures of cost and effectiveness between CAM users and nonusers. Office-based charges represent the largest source of traditional cost for both CAM users and nonusers ($141.29 and $258.58, respectively), followed by pharmaceutical costs ($112.30 and $167.11, respectively). CAM users have statistically significant lower levels of both office-based costs (p-value 0.022) and pharmaceutical costs (p-value 0.048) than CAM nonusers. The overall anxiety-related costs are not statistically difference ($458.95 versus $467.03, p-value 0.920); this evidence implies that CAM users with anxiety disorders are substituting CAM treatment for both pharmacotherapy and psychotherapy treatment. (Table 3).

| | CAM users | (n=102) | CAM nonusers | (n=706) | |
|---|---|---|---|---|---|
| | **MEAN** | **SD** | **MEAN** | **SD** | **p-Value** |
| **Outcomes** | | | | | |
| Overall Mental Health Status (5pt Scale) | 2.58 | 1.1383 | 2.70 | 1.1406 | 0.324 |
| Probability [Good Mental Health] | 0.8039 | 0.3990 | 0.7720 | 0.4199 | 0.469 |
| Probability [Steady or Improved Mental Health] | 0.7549 | 0.4323 | 0.6912 | 0.4623 | 0.190 |
| **Overall Costs (in $US)** | | | | | |

| Office-Based Costs | 141.29 | 323.14 | 258.58 | 1059.51 | 0.022 |
|---|---|---|---|---|---|
| Outpatient-Based Costs | 0.64 | 6.44 | 21.18 | 320.31 | 0.089 |
| ER-Based Costs | 2.21 | 20.45 | 20.16 | 169.10 | 0.007 |
| Pharmaceutical Costs | 112.30 | 241.86 | 167.11 | 360.62 | 0.048 |
| CAM Costs | 202.70 | 461.33 | 0.00 | 0.00 | <0.001 |
| Total Costs | 458.95 | 657.56 | 467.03 | 1271.46 | 0.920 |

**Table 2:** Measures of effectiveness and costs.

| | CAM users | CAM nonusers | Group Differences | p-Value |
|---|---|---|---|---|
| Effect (in Pr[MH>=0]) | 0.7549 | 0.6912 | 0.0637 | 0.190 |
| Anxiety-Related Costs (mean) | 458.95 | 467.03 | -8.08 | 0.920 |
| **ICER** | | | | |
| Estimated ICER (mean) | -1.27 | | | |
| Quadrant | IV (ΔE>0, ΔC<0) | | | |
| Estimated ICER (median) | 24.06 | | | |
| Quadrant | I (ΔE>0, ΔC>0) | | | |
| WTP | Pr[CE\|WTP] | Pr[CE\|WTP,X] | Pr[CE] w/ IPW | |
| 0 | 0.548 | 0.433 | 0.706 | |
| 1000 | 0.786 | 0.706 | 0.885 | |
| 2000 | 0.878 | 0.822 | 0.922 | |
| 3000 | 0.909 | 0.862 | 0.930 | |
| 4000 | 0.917 | 0.879 | 0.930 | |
| 5000 | 0.920 | 0.887 | 0.931 | |

**Table 3:** Incremental cost-effectiveness results.

## Outcome Measurement

Three measures of effectiveness are considered. Average overall self-reported mental health on a 5-point Likert scale indicated CAM users ended with improved mental health (2.58 versus 2.70; p-value 0.324).

The probability of ending with good mental health over the study period was higher for CAM users than for CAM nonusers (0.8039 versus 0.7720; p-value 0.469).

The probability of steady or improved mental health over the study period was higher for CAM users than for CAM nonusers (0.7549 versus 0.6912; p-value 0.190). A more ideal measure of effectiveness, Quality Adjusted Life Years (QALYs) would be used; unfortunately, this is not possible given the limitations of the data.

## Cost-Effectiveness Assessment

This economic analysis shows that for those with anxiety, CAM users have slightly lower costs with higher effect than CAM nonusers, resulting in an ICER of -$1.27 per 1% increase in the probability of steady or improved mental health. The difference in cost between groups is small, and not statistically significant.

The average difference in cost and effect between CAM users and nonusers is located in the quadrant IV of the incremental cost-incremental effectiveness plane (Figure 1).

These averages represent an increase in effectiveness (0.0637; p-value 0.190) and a decrease in cost (-$8.08; p-value 0.920). Using median cost, the estimated ICER is $24.06 per 1% increase in the probability of steady or improved mental health.

This difference in median cost would be located in quadrant I of the incremental cost-incremental effectiveness plane, with an increased effectiveness but also an increased cost.

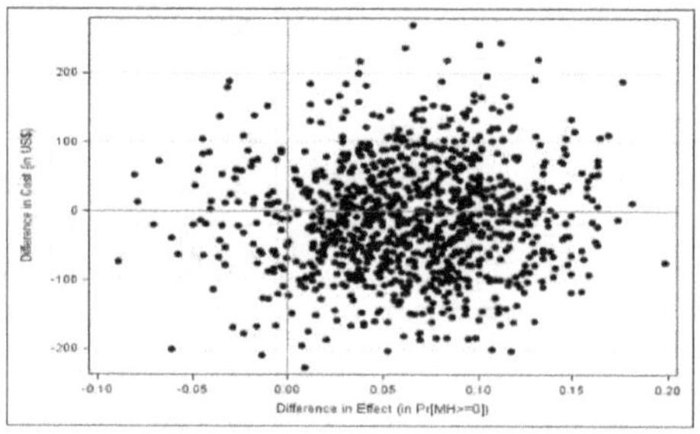

Figure 1: Bootstrap replicates of the difference in cost and effect in the incremental cost-incremental effectiveness space for CAM users versus nonusers. A significant portion are in quadrants I (ΔC>0, ΔE>0) and IV (ΔC<0, ΔE>0).

To assess the uncertainty of the incremental cost-effectiveness ratio, Figure 1 shows 1000 bootstrapped replicates of the cost and effectiveness data. While individually, neither cost nor effectiveness is statistically significant at traditional levels of significance, it is clear that a substantial number of the replicates represent cost-effectiveness for a wide range of values of willingness-to-pay (WTP) for the effect. The cost-effectiveness acceptability curves based on the bootstrap replicates are a method to quantify the uncertainty of the incremental cost-effectiveness ratios. Figure 2 shows the cost-effectiveness acceptability curve for a range of values. The probability of a treatment being cost-effective for a given value of a unit of effect is estimated as the proportion of the 1,000 bootstraps that are cost-effective (i.e., below the value of a unit of effect line in the incremental cost-incremental effectiveness space). Values of a unit of effect (either the willingness-to-pay for greater effect or willingness-to-accept a lower level of effect) are measured on the horizontal axis and the probability that treatment is cost-effective is measured on the vertical axis.

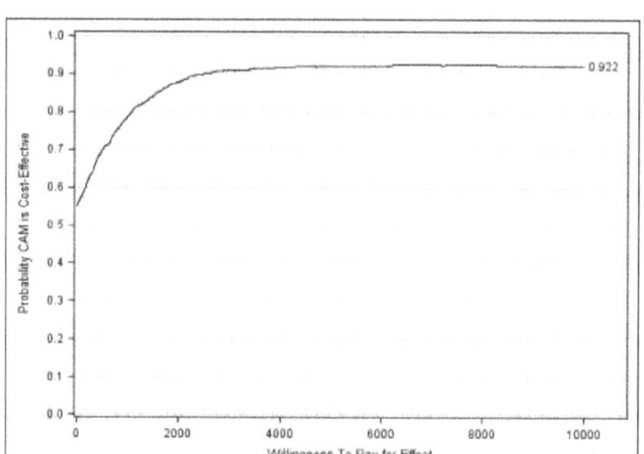


Figure 2: Cost-effectiveness acceptability curve showing probability CAM is cost-effective for a given willingness to pay for a unit of effect.

Including additional demographic controls into the estimation of incremental net benefit only slightly reduces the probability of cost-effectiveness (0.920 reduced to 0.887 for WTP=5000 for example). Additionally, using inverse propensity score weighting in the estimation of incremental net benefit slightly increases the probability that CAM is cost-effective for higher values of a unit of effect (0.931 versus 0.920 for WTP=5000 for example) (Figure 3).

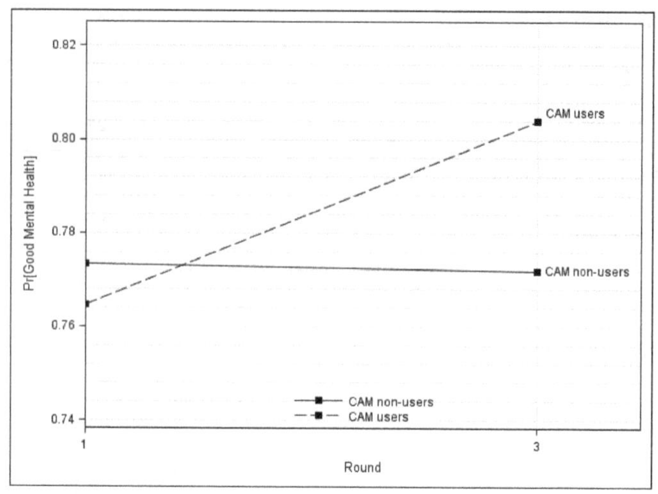


Figure 3: Probability of good mental health from initial measurement (0.7647 versus 0.7734; p-value 0.825) to final measurement (0.8039 versus 0.7720; p-value 0.469) for CAM users and nonusers.

## Discussion

This research provides information on a very specific research question: Is complementary and alternative medicine (broadly defined) a cost-effective addition to traditional treatment for anxiety disorders the measures of the probability of good self-reported mental health status using observational data on patient treatment and characteristics? This research investigates potential self-selection bias of observational data in the estimates of the net benefit.

The most significant limitation of this current study is the age of the data. The current study extends the use the 1998 MEPS using current methods of cost-effectiveness analysis. However, if patterns of CAM use, patterns of anxiety treatment, and associated costs change significantly, then the current study should be interpreted as historical economic analysis describing the state of complementary and alternative medicine around the turn of the century. Su and Li [10] found an increase in CAM use in more current NHIS data, especially for chiropractics, massage, and acupuncture. While the extent to which the results apply to current CAM practices may be limited, these results still provide insight into the baseline of an analysis of CAM practices. If CAM costs increase at a faster rate than other forms of traditional therapy, the current results could represent a lower bound on the cost-effectiveness of CAM.

A second limitation of the current data concerns the definition of modalities included. The 1998 MEPS did not include prayer, spiritual beliefs, vitamins or supplements in the CAM definition. This explains the very significant difference in CAM use in this data compared to previous national estimates [5-8].

Another potential limitation of the current study is the use of self-reported mental health as a measure of effectiveness. While it is questionable if self-reported mental health status is reliable enough in measuring clinically significant changes in patients with anxiety, the direction of these results were statistically related in other MEPS years to improvement in other outcomes measures, specifically the EQ-5D

Index Score, the SF-12 Index Score, the probability of long-term work missed, and number of days missed.

Overall, these results suggest only a slight upward bias in the initial unconditional estimates of incremental net benefit for anxiety disorders. A positive correlation between seeking CAM treatment and the individual heterogeneity would produce this upward bias. If an individual knows that CAM will work better for them, they would be more likely to seek CAM treatment. If that individual heterogeneity is related to the observable characteristics, then controlling for them in the estimation of incremental net benefit will reduce this self-selection bias. The estimation of incremental net benefit using propensity matching is nearly identical to the unconditional estimation of incremental net benefit. These results suggest a slight bias in the initial unconditional estimates of incremental net benefit for anxiety disorder.

For anxiety disorders, there is some evidence to suggest that CAM is cost-effective for large values of a unit of effect. It should be noted that the values of a WTP associated with statistical significant of cost-effectiveness may be too large, in practice, to justify; the opportunity cost of scarce healthcare dollars is not explicitly models and could, most likely, adversely impact the results. Efforts to investigate potential self-selection bias in the data show an upward bias in the initial, unconditional estimates of incremental net benefit.

This analysis also assumes that the use of charges instead of the cost of production does not bias the results in a systematic way. Implicitly, producer mark-up over the cost of production is assumed zero for both traditional and CAM treatment. Given the use of patent-protected pharmacotherapy treatments and the lack of perfectly competitive markets for each form of treatment, this assumption is questionable. However, it is not possible to assign an a priori expectation to this potential bias. Given the available data in the MEPS, there is not a feasible method for addressing this potential source of bias.

This analysis assumes that there is no difference in the level of direct nonmonetary resources and the indirect impact of treatment for CAM users and nonusers. The MEPS does include information regarding employment and compensation. If information on treatment acquisition time was available, it would be possible to construct a proxy for nonmonetary resource cost for this analysis. Most likely, acquisition time would vary by the of CAM treatment. Given the lack of detailed information on specific CAM treatment use, the lack of precise treatment acquisition time, and the limitations of employment compensation as a measure of time cost, this extension does not seem feasible for the current dataset.

Another possible route to investigate potential self-selection bias in observational data is with estimating net benefit with instrumental variables. This would require an instrument that is correlated with the decision to seek CAM treatment that is uncorrelated with the outcome of CAM treatment. State-level differences in reimbursement rates could serve as another potential instrument in future research. However, state identifiers are not available in the publically available MEPS used in this analysis.

## Conclusion

In conclusion, this observational study indicates for patients with anxiety disorders CAM users have improved outcomes and slightly lower costs with a high probability of cost-effectiveness. While these findings working with the best available tools in the 1998 MEPS are interesting, certainly additional research is warranted, especially given the data limitations and shortcomings. Future research would benefit from collecting cost information alongside RCTs of different CAM modalities with better established measurements of anxiety disorders.

## Acknowledgement

This work was begun as part of a dissertation requirement. The author thanks Alvin Headen, Stephen Margolis, Tamah Morant, and Melinda Morrill for helpful feedback throughout the stages of this project. All errors are the author's own. The author would also like to thank the anonymous reviewers for their helpful feedback.

## References

1. Grimaldi-Bensouda L, Begaud B, Lert F, Rouillon F, Massol J, et al. (2011) Benchmarking the burden of 100 diseases: results of a nationwide representative survey within general practices. BMJ Open 1: e000215.
2. Kessler RC, Chiu WT, Demler O, Merikangas KR, Walters EE (2005) Prevalence, severity, and comorbidity of 12-month DSM-IV disorders in the National Comorbidity Survey Replication. Arch Gen Psychiatry 62: 617-627.
3. Mark TL, Levit KR, Yee T, Chow CM (2014) Spending on mental and substance use disorders projected to grow more slowly than all health spending through 2020. Health Aff (Millwood) 33: 1407-1415.
4. National Institute of Mental Health (2016) Anxiety disorders.
5. Barnes PM, Bloom B, Nahin RL (2008) Complementary and alternative medicine use among adults and children: United States, 2007. Natl Health Stat Report 1-23.
6. Kessler RC, Soukup J, Davis RB, Foster DF, Wilkey SA, et al. (2001) The use of complementary and alternative therapies to treat anxiety and depression in the United States. Am J Psychiatry 158: 289-294.
7. Unützer J, Klap R, Sturm R, Young AS, Marmon T, et al. (2000) Mental disorders and the use of alternative medicine: results from a national survey. Am J Psychiatry 157: 1851-1857.
8. Eisenberg DM, Davis RB, Ettner SL, Appel S, Wilkey S, et al. (1998) Trends in alternative medicine use in the United States, 1990-1997: results of a follow-up national survey. JAMA 280: 1569-1575.
9. Grzywacz JG, Suerken CK, Quandt SA, Bell RA, Lang W, et al (2006) Older adults' use of complementary and alternative medicine for mental health: findings from the 2002 National Health Interview Survey. J Altern Complement Med 12: 467-473.
10. Su D, Li L (2011) Trends in the use of complementary and alternative medicine in the United States: 2002-2007. J Health Care Poor Underserved 22: 296-310.
11. Chiesa A, Serretti A (2009) Mindfulness-based stress reduction for stress management in healthy people: a review and meta-analysis. J Altern Complement Med 15: 593-600.
12. Manzoni GM, Pagnini F, Castelnuovo G, Molinari E (2008) Relaxation training for anxiety: a ten-years systematic review with meta-analysis. BMC Psychiatry 8: 41.
13. Nestoriuc Y, Martin A, Rief W, Andrasik F (2008) Biofeedback treatment for headache disorders: a comprehensive efficacy review. Appl Psychophysiol Biofeedback 33: 125-140.
14. Solomon D, Adams J, Graves N (2013) Economic evaluation of St. John's wort (Hypericum perforatum) for the treatment of mild to moderate depression. J Affect Disord 148: 228-234.
15. Canter PH, Coon JT, Ernst E (2005) Cost effectiveness of complementary treatments in the United Kingdom: systematic review. BMJ 331: 880-881.
16. Herman PM, Poindexter BL, Witt CM, Eisenberg DM (2012) Are complementary therapies and integrative care cost-effective? A systematic review of economic evaluations. BMJ Open 2: e001046.
17. Bar-Sela G, Danos S, Visel B, Mashiach T, Mitnik I (2015) The effect of complementary and alternative medicine on quality of life, depression,

anxiety, and fatigue levels among cancer patients during active oncology treatment: phase II study. Support Care Cancer 23: 1979-1985.

18. McPherson F, McGraw L (2013) Treating generalized anxiety disorder using complementary and alternative medicine. Altern Ther Health Med 19: 45-50.
19. Davis MP, Darden PM (2003) Use of complementary and alternative medicine by children in the United States. Arch Pediatr Adolesc Med 157: 393-396.
20. Ritchie CS, Gohmann SF, McKinney WP (2005) Does use of CAM for specific health problems increase with reduced access to care? J Med Syst 29: 143-153.
21. Gold M, Siegel J, Russell L, Weinstein M (1996) Cost-effectiveness in health and medicine. New York: Oxford University Press, USA.
22. Spinks J, Hollingsworth B (2012) Policy implications of complementary and alternative medicine use in Australia: data from the National Health Survey. J Altern Complement Med 18: 371-378.
23. Tait EM, Laditka JN, Laditka SB, Nies MA, Racine EF, et al (2013) Reasons why older americans use complementary and alternative medicine: Costly or ineffective conventional medicine and recommendations from health care providers, family, and friends. Educ Gerontol 39: 684-700.
24. Idler EL, Benyamini Y (1997) Self-rated health and mortality: a review of twenty-seven community studies. J Health Soc Behav 38: 21-37.
25. Idler EL, Russell LB, Davis D (2000) Survival, functional limitations, and self-rated health in the NHANES I Epidemiologic Follow-up Study, 1992. First National Health and Nutrition Examination Survey. Am J Epidemiol 152: 874-883.
26. Ried LD, Tueth MJ, Handberg E, Nyanteh H (2006) Validating a self-report measure of global subjective well-being to predict adverse clinical outcomes. Qual Life Res 15: 675-686.
27. Ware J, Sherbourne C (1992) The MOS 36-item short-form health survey (SF-36) I: Conceptual framework and item selection. Med Care 30: 473-483.
28. McHorney CA, Ware JE Jr, Raczek AE (1993) The MOS 36-Item Short-Form Health Survey (SF-36): II. Psychometric and clinical tests of validity in measuring physical and mental health constructs. Med Care 31: 247-263.
29. McCollum M, Hansen LB, Ghushchyan V, Sullivan PW (2007) Inconsistent health perceptions for US women and men with diabetes. J Womens Health (Larchmt) 16: 1421-1428.
30. Stinnett AA, Mullahy J (1998) Net health benefits: a new framework for the analysis of uncertainty in cost-effectiveness analysis. Med Decis Making 18: S68-S80.
31. Fenwick E, O'Brien B, Briggs A (2004) Cost-effectiveness acceptability curves - facts, fallacies, and frequently asked questions. Health Econ 13: 405-415.
32. Dehejia R, Wahba S (2002) Propensity score-matching methods for nonexperimental causal studies. Rev Econ Stat 84: 151-161.

# Anti-Haemorrhagic Activity of Polyherbal Formulation in Menorrhagia

**Danish Jahan[1*], Wajeeha Begum[2], Mariyam Roqaiya[2], Yousuf Khalil Hussaini[3]**

[1]*National Institute of Unani Medicine, Kottigepalya, Bengaluru, Karnataka, India*

[2]*Luqman Unani Medical College, Hospital & Research Centre, 12 Naubag, Bijapur, Karnataka, India*

[3]*Jamia Tibbiya Deoband, Uttar Pradesh, India.*

[*]**Correspondant author:** Danish Jahan, National Institute of Unani Medicine, Kottigepalya, Bengaluru, Karnataka, India, E-mail: dr.danishjahan@gmail.com

**Abstract**

**Background:** Menorrhagia i.e., excessive menstrual blood loss is a common problem that interferes with women's physical, emotional, social and material quality of life. Unani physicians have mentioned so many herbal formulations to treat menorrhagia. This study was aimed to compare the efficacy of polyherbal unani formulation and tranexamic acid on menorrhagia.

**Materials & Methods:** This prospective randomized single blind standard controlled trial was conducted in Department of Niswan wa Qabala, National Institute of Unani Medicine. 40 patients were assigned to test (20) and control (20) groups. Both the test as well as control was given orally for five days from first day of menstrual cycle for two consecutive cycles. Assessment of efficacy was based on pictorial blood loss assessment chart (PBAC) to assess the amount of blood loss. Hb% and quality of life were also assessed as secondary outcome. Chi-square/ Fisher Exact test has been used to find the significance of study parameters on categorical scale between groups.

**Results:** There was no significant difference found between the groups on all parameters assessed which shows that the test drug can be an alternative for tranexamic acid after clinical trial on large sample size and for longer duration.

**Conclusion:** Test drug has been found having equal effect with tranexamic acid. There is need for further study on large sample size.

**Keywords:** Menorrhagia; Polyherbal; Anti-haemorrhagic

## Introduction

Heavy flow during periods is called menorrhagia or kasrate tams and it is one of the most common reasons for women to be referred to gynecologists. It is the main presenting problem in at least half of those who undergo hysterectomies [1]. Prevalence of menorrhagia is approximately 10% to 15% in women of reproductive age [2]. It has two conditions, either flow increases in amount or duration [3,4].

Indeed, the associated discomfort, anxiety and impaired quality of life lead many women to surgical procedures, ranging from endometrial ablation to hysterectomy, often in the absence of any detectable pathology [5]. Several drug classes are recommended for the treatment of heavy menstrual bleeding (HMB); however, most of them are not accepted by patients because of either failure in controlling the bleeding or side-effects [6].

Unani physicians have stated that in kasrate tams excessive flow of blood is mainly due to two causes that is weakness in quwate masika (retentive power) or increase in quwate dafiya (excretory power) or both. Cause of weakness of quwate dafiya is any type of sue mizaj (abnormal temperament), mainly sue mizaj haar yabis (hot & dry), which causes weakness of uterus and its vessels and leads to opening of mouth of vessels and rupture of vessels.

Cause of excess functioning of quwate dafiya (excretory power) is due to khilt lazaa, hararat and hiddat (excess heat) of blood. This hiddat and lazaa again causes opening of mouth of blood vessels [7,8].

In unani literature numbers of drugs are available single as well as in compound form to treat haemorrhage. Almost same drugs have also been mentioned for menorrhagia. These drugs are effective to control bleeding by having its haemostatic and astringent property e.g., anjabar, geru, sange jarahat, dammul akhwain, etc. [9,10]. A polyherbal unani formulation sharbate anjbar is the most popular and most common composition to treat haemorrhage [11-13].

Sharbate anjbar is available with different formulations which are being used from many years for haemorrhage. So considering the above fact, the present study was carried out in Dept. of Ilmul Qabalat wa Amraze Niswan, NIUM Hospital, Bangalore, to scientifically evaluate the efficacy of sharbate anjbar in the management of menorrhagia.

Sharbate anjbar is having four drugs beekhe anjabr (*Polygonum bistorata*), aqaqia (*Acacia arabica*), sandal surkh, sandal sufaid (*Santalum album*) [12,13]. These drugs have habis (hemostatic) and qabiz (astringent) properties.

## Materials and Methods

A prospective single blind randomized standard controlled study was conducted in the Dept. of Ilmul Qabalat wa Amraze Niswan, NIUM Hospital, Bangaluru from November 2014 to March 2015 to compare the efficacy of polyherbal unani formulation and tranexamic acid on menorrhagia. The study protocol was approved by Institutional Ethical Committee, NIUM Bangalore.

Inclusion criteria were married as well as unmarried women of reproductive age group complaining of heavy menses with regular cycles. Patients with irregular and inter-menstrual bleeding, patient suffering from systemic illness, blood dyscrasias, malignancy and severe anaemia (Hb% less than 7.5 g), unwillingness or inability to comply the requirements of the protocol were excluded from the study.

In each patient, history was evaluated and a complete physical examination including breast and abdominal examination and per vaginal (in married patients) examination was performed. Personal details, history, clinical features and investigations were recorded in the case record form (CRF) structured for the study.

Following thorough evaluation of patient by history and clinical examination, patients were advised for necessary investigations. Complete blood picture with ESR, BT, CT, Platelet count, Random blood sugar, Complete urine examination, Blood urea, serum creatinine, SGOT, SGPT, alkaline phosphatise, Whole abdomen scan Thyroid profile, Pap smear (in married patients) were investigated.

After a control cycle, (Figure 1) total of 40 patients meeting the inclusion criteria were randomly assigned to test (20 patients) and control (20 patients) groups after explaining the study in detail and receiving the informed consent. Randomization was done by using computer generated random table.

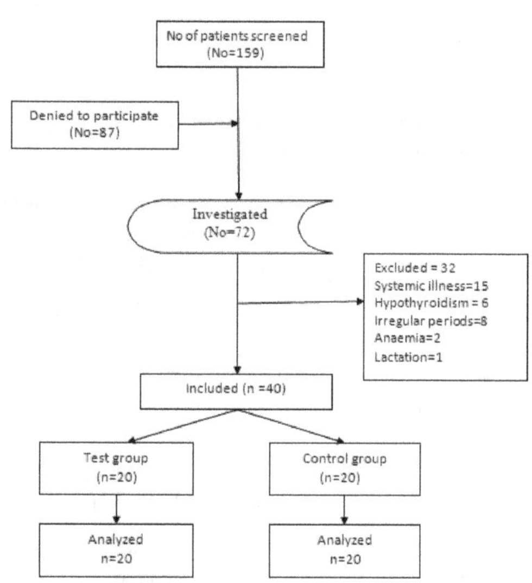


**Figure 1:** Flow diagram of the participants.

For the test group a polyherbal syrup formulation *sharbate anjbar* was selected which contains *beekhe anjbar, aqaqia,* sandal surkh, and sandal sufaid. These drugs were purchased from local drug retailer of Bangalore by purchase committee and were identified by Dept. of Pharmacology, NIUM.

Syrup was prepared in pharmacy of this institute according to the standard unani method of preparation and given in the dose of 25 ml BD for 5 days during menses from the first day of menstrual cycle for two consecutive cycles. In the control group standard drug tranexamic acid 500 mg BD was also given for 5 days from the first day of menstrual cycle for two cycles. Assessment of blood loss during periods was done by PBAC score and assessment in improvement of quality of life was done by SF-36 score.

Patients were assessed for two consecutive cycles during the treatment and one cycle after the treatment. During treatment amount of bleeding were assessed by asking duration of cycle, amount of flow which was assessed by calculating the total no. of pads used in one cycle and duration of flow from both the groups.

Apart from that improvement in quality of life was assessed by using SF-36 questionnaire before and after treatment. Effectiveness of trial drugs were assessed by Pictorial blood loss assessment chart (PBAC score) to assess the amount of blood loss, SF-36 score to asses quality of life and improvement in Hb%.

Chi-square/Fisher Exact test has been used to find the significance of study parameters on categorical scale between groups.

## Results and Discussion

Baseline demographic profile was same between the two groups with p value >0.05 (Table 1). As shown in Table 2, baseline PBAC score in test group was 496.55 ± 256.37 and in control score was 595.70 ± 379.76 which is not significant between the groups with p value of 0.339. During first treatment cycle score was calculated as 160.30 ± 54.20 in test group and 257.25 ± 257.77 in control group with p value of 0.108. During second cycle 124.65 ± 46.57 score was calculated in test group and 220.95 ± 246.06 in control group which is statistically significant between the groups with p value of 0.094. During after treatment follow up cycle the score was calculated as 109.50 ± 38.50 in test group and 291.85 ± 483.95 in control group which is not significant with p value 0.101. Mean difference in groups were found 387.05 in test group and 303.85 in control group.

| Characteristic | Test group | | Control group | | P value |
|---|---|---|---|---|---|
| | No | % | No | % | |
| **Age (years)** | | | | | |
| Nov-20 | 5 | 25 | 3 | 15 | |
| 21-30 | 9 | 45 | 8 | 40 | |
| 31-40 | 4 | 20 | 7 | 35 | P=0.787 |
| 41-50 | 2 | 10 | 2 | 10 | |
| Total | 20 | 100 | 20 | 100 | |
| **Marital status** | | | | | |
| Married | 11 | 55 | 14 | 70 | |
| Unmarried | 9 | 45 | 6 | 30 | P=0.327 |
| Total | 20 | 100 | 20 | 100 | |
| **Occupation** | | | | | |
| Employed | 1 | 5 | 1 | 5 | |

| House wife | 10 | 50 | 16 | 80 | |
|---|---|---|---|---|---|
| Student | 9 | 45 | 3 | 15 | P=0.100 |
| Total | 20 | 100 | 20 | 100 | |
| **SES** | | | | | |
| Lower | 0 | 0 | 1 | 5 | |
| Lower middle | 9 | 45 | 5 | 25 | |
| Upper lower | 5 | 25 | 8 | 40 | P=0.699 |
| Upper middle | 5 | 25 | 5 | 25 | |
| Upper | 1 | 5 | 1 | 5 | |
| Total | 20 | 100 | 20 | 100 | |
| **Habitat** | | | | | |
| Rural | 1 | 5 | 2 | 10 | |
| Urban | 19 | 95 | 18 | 90 | P=1.000 |
| Total | 20 | 100 | 20 | 100 | |
| **Diet** | | | | | |
| Mixed | 17 | 85 | 18 | 90 | |
| Veg. | 3 | 15 | 2 | 10 | P=0.633 |
| Total | 20 | 100 | 20 | 100 | |

**Table 1:** Baseline demographic of the patients with menorrhagia in test and control group.

| PBAC Score | Test group | Control group | P value |
|---|---|---|---|
| Baseline | 496.55 ± 256.37 | 595.70 ± 379.76 | 0.339 |
| First cycle | 160.30 ± 54.20 | 257.25 ± 257.77 | 0.108 |
| Second cycle | 124.65 ± 46.57 | 220.95 ± 246.06 | 0.094+ |
| After treatment follow up | 109.50 ± 38.50 | 291.85 ± 483.95 | 0.101 |
| Difference | 387.05 | 303.85 | - |
| P value (Before – After) | <0.001** | <0.001** | - |

**Table 2:** PBAC Score of patients studied.

In present study it is obvious that the test drug has almost equal effect with control drug in improvement of PBAC score. PBAC score to assess the menstrual blood loss has been used in various previous studies conducted. Jaisamrarn et al. [14] has showed a significant decrease in PBAC score from 350.5 to 178.6 with 49% decrease in mean menstrual blood flow after two cycles which was significant. One more study conducted by Lee et al. [15] showed significant reduction in PBAC score from 262.0 to 125.0 with 47.4% decrease in mean menstrual blood flow.

Significant improvement in PBAC score in test group is attributed due to haemostatic property of sharbate anjbar by which it reduces bleeding [11-13]. Ingredients of sharbate anjbar contains tannin, gallic acid, ellagic acid and flavonoids which are potential styptic and astringent there by reduces heavy menstrual blood loss [7,10,16-19]. *Acacia arbica* one of the ingredients has also been studied for its coagulation property in the mice [20]. Another study has shown that *Acacia arabica* along with *Moringa oleifera* are haemostatic and hasten blood coagulation [21].

| SF-36 Score | Test group | Control group | P value |
|---|---|---|---|
| Before treatment | 233.75 ± 90.42 | 185.55 ± 61.06 | 0.055+ |
| After treatment | 777.70 ± 35.65 | 697.15 ± 161.89 | 0.036* |
| Difference | 543.95 | 511.6 | - |
| P value (Before – After) | <0.001** | <0.001** | - |

**Table 3:** SF-36 Score of patients studied.

Table 3 shows mean SF-36 score. Before treatment it is 233.75 ± 90.42 in test group and 185.55 ± 61.06 in control group with a p value of 0.055 and after treatment it is calculated as 777.70 ± 35.65 in test group and 697.15 ± 161.89 in control group with p value of 0.036. Mean difference is 543.95 in test group and 511.60 in control group. On inter group comparison before treatment findings were suggestive significant (p value: $0.05<p<0.10$) in both the groups. After treatment findings were moderately significant with p value of (p value: $0.01<p \leq 0.05$). In test group drug was found more effective in improving quality of life than control group.

Menorrhagia is a common gynecological condition that has a significant impact on the wellbeing and quality of life of many women's. In present study SF-36 questionnaire was used to evaluate the impact of treatment on women's quality of life and it is obvious that test drug is significant in improving women's quality of life. These findings are similar with the studies conducted by Pattison et al. [22] and Marjoribanks et al. [23]. In these studies, significant improvement in quality of life was observed after treatment.

| SF-36 Score | Test group | Control group | P value |
|---|---|---|---|
| Before treatment | 233.75 ± 90.42 | 185.55 ± 61.06 | 0.055+ |
| After treatment | 777.70 ± 35.65 | 697.15 ± 161.89 | 0.036* |
| Difference | 543.95 | 511.60 | - |
| P value (Before –After) | <0.001** | <0.001** | - |

**Table 4:** Hemoglobin % of patients studied.

Table 4 is showing improvement in Hb% in mean ± SD. Baseline Hb % was found 11.71 ± 1.45 in test group and 11.66 ± 1.54 in control group with p value of 0.908 and after two treatment cycles it was found 11.96 ± 1.43 in test group and 11.56 ± 1.68 in control group with p value of 0.428. On intergroup comparison after treatment findings were not significant (p>0.05). On intra group comparison findings were also not significant (p>0.05) but in test group drug was found more effective in improving Hb% than control group. Besides these no adverse effect was found in both the groups.

## Limitation of the study

Small sample size.

## Conclusion

Present study shows that sharbate anjabar is found to have almost equal effect with tranexamic acid on all the parameters studied but sample size was small so study on large sample size is needed before keeping it as an alternative for menorrhagia.

## References


1. https://www.york.ac.uk/media/crd/ehc19.pdf
2. Asgari Z, Hoseinzadeh F, Hoseinzadeh A, Hafizi L (2014) Evaluation of the success rate of Endometrial Ablation by Cavaterm™ plus technique. J Minim Invasive Surg Sci. 3: e12431.
3. Jurjani I (1903) Tarjuma Zakheerae Khawarzum Shahi, Vol 6. Munshi Nawal Kishore, Lucknow, pp. 590-597.
4. Sina I (2007) Al-Qanoon Fit-Tib. Idarae Kitabus Shifa, New Dehli, pp. 1089-1091, 1065.
5. Borgatta L (2009) Heavy menstrual bleeding assessing impact, evaluating management options. Boston University.
6. Goshtasebi A, Mazari Z, Gandevani SB, Naseri M (2015) Anti-hemorrhagic activity of Punica granatum L. flower (Persian Golnar) against heavy menstrual bleeding of endometrial origin: a double-blind, randomized controlled trial. Med J Islam Repub Iran 29: 199.
7. Rushd I (1987) Kitabul Kulliyat. 2nd edn. CCRUM, New Delhi. pp. 114-117.
8. Majoosi ABA. Kamilus Sana. Idarae Kitab-us-Shifa, New Delhi, pp. 784,785.
9. Kabeeruddin M. Makhzanul Mufradat. Ejaz Publication House, New Delhi, pp. 82, 96, 396.
10. Hakeem MAH (2002) Bustanul Mufradat. Idarae Kitab-ul-Shifa, New Delhi, pp. 75, 82, 96, 396.
11. Said HM (1997) Hamdard pharmacopeia of eastern medicine. Sri Satya Guru Publications, New Delhi, pp. 173, 353.
12. Jilani G (1995) Mukhzinul murakkabat. Ejaz Publishing House, New Delhi, pp. 198.
13. Khan S (2006) Bayaze Khas al Maruful Ilaj. Ejaz Publishing House, New Delhi, pp. 269.
14. Jaisamrarn U, Srinil S (2005) Treatment of idiopathic menorrhagia with tranexamic acid. J Med Assoc Thai 88: 1-6.
15. Lee JY, Hahn PM, Van JP, Reid RL (2007) Treatment of menorrhagia with Tranaxaemic acid. J Obstet Gynaecol Can 22: 1-5.
16. Jeelani G (1996) Makhzanul Hikmat. Vol.II. Ejaz Publishing House, New Delhi, pp. 793-797.
17. Arzani A (1903) Tibbe Akbar. Faisal Publication, Deoband, pp. 594-597.
18. Dutta DC (2005) Textbook of gynecology. New Central Book Agency, Kolkata, pp.74, 175, 270, 355, 421, 431.
19. Arunkumara KKIU, Walpola BC, Subasingh S, Yoon MH (2011) Pterocarpus santalinus Linn. (Rath hadum) A review of its botany, uses, phytochemistry and pharmacology. JKSABC 54: 495-500.
20. Raaof AW, Al-Naqqash ZA, Jawad ALM, Muhsan SM (2013) Evaluation of the Activity of Crude Alkaloids Extracts of Zingiber officinale Roscoe., Thymus vulgaris L. and Acacia arabica L. as Coagulant Agent in Lab Mice. Biomed Biotechnol 1: 11-16.
21. Bhatnagar M, Parwani L, Sharma V, Ganguli J, Bhatnagar A (2013) Hemostatic, antibacterial biopolymers from Acacia arabica (Lam.) Willd. And Moringa oleifera (Lam.) as potential wound dressing materials. Indian J Exp Biol 51: 804-810.
22. Pattison H, Danniels J, Kai J, Gupta JK (2011) The measurement properties of the menorrhagia multi attribute quality of life scale: A pscycometric analysis. BJOG 1528-1531.
23. Marjoribanks J, Lethaby A, Farquhar C (2010) Surgery verses medical therapy for heavy menstrual bleeding, Newzealand. The Cochrane Collaboration, pp. 2-18.

# 22

# Assessment of Timing of First Antenatal Care Visit and Associated Factors Among Pregnant Women Attending Antenatal Care in Dilla Town Governmental Health Institutions, Southern Ethiopia

**Tadele Girum***

*Department of Public Health, Arba Minch College of Health Sciences, Arba Minch, Ethiopia*

***Corresponding author:** Girum T, Department of Public Health, Arba Minch College of Health Sciences, Arba Minch, Ethiopia. E-mail: girumtadele@yahoo.com

**Abstract**

**Introduction:** The new focused antenatal care model recognizes that every pregnant woman is at risk for complications and four antenatal care visits are recommended for most pregnant women; the first one being early in the first trimester. When pregnant women attend antenatal care late they miss the cares being provided in the first 16 weeks. Therefore it is important to assess timing of first antenatal care visit and identify associated factors for late coming for the sake of intervention.

**Methods:** Institutional based cross-sectional study was conducted among 362 randomly selected pregnant women from April to June 2014 in Dilla town, Southern Ethiopia. The data had been entered in to Epi Info version 7 and analyzed through SPSS version 20. Bivariate analysis was run to look for the association between dependent and explanatory variables; and using variables which have p-value ≤ 0.25 binary logistic regressions was fitted. Association presented in odds ratio with 95% confidence interval and significance determined at P-value less than 0.05.

**Results:** The mean time of first antenatal care visit was found to be 15.9 (SD 3.7) weeks and the proportion of women who visit their first antenatal care within the recommended time (before or at 16 weeks of gestation) was 49.7%; nearly equal to late presentation. Rural residence (AOR=3.6, 95% CI (1.72, 6.62)), low monthly income (AOR=3.20, 95% CI (1.5, 6.74)), illiteracy (AOR=1.48, 95% CI (1.12, 3.04)), not being advised on timing of visit (AOR=4.64, 95% CI (2.32, 8.17) and unplanned pregnancy (AOR=5.02, 95% CI (2.21, 8.95)) were independent predictors of late presentation for first antenatal care.

**Conclusion:** Even though, half of pregnant women started antenatal care attendance during the first trimester the finding was not satisfactory. Hence, further activities are needed through health education and promotion.

**Keywords:** Antenatal care; Timing; First antenatal care booking

## Introduction

Globally, more than half a million women are still dying annually as a result of complications of pregnancy and childbirth [1]. Ninety-nine percent of these occur in developing countries, of these deaths 50% occurred in Sub-Saharan Africa (SSA) [2]. Thus a woman in Africa may face a lifetime risk of death during pregnancy and childbirth as high as one in 26, compared with only one in 7300 in developed regions [3]. Ethiopia is one of the countries with the highest maternal mortality, with 420 mother's death per 100,000 live birth and much more morbidities were there [4]. With the appropriate care, maternal mortality is in fact a very rare event. The care provided at pregnancy, delivery and postpartum periods markedly reduce maternal mortality [1-3].

Pregnancy is a very important event from both social and medical points of view. Therefore, pregnant women should receive special care and attention from the family, community and from the health care system. The objective of antenatal care (ANC) is to assure that every pregnancy culminates in the delivery of a healthy baby without impairing the health of the mother [5] which includes prevention, identification and treatment of conditions as well as help a woman approach pregnancy and birth as a positive experiences through health promotion and disease prevention, early detection and treatment of complications and existing diseases, birth preparedness and complication readiness planning programs.

World health organization (WHO) recommends that, pregnant women should seek ANC within the first three months of pregnancy. Early antenatal care attendance during the first three months of gestation plays a major role in detecting and treating some complications of pregnancy and forms a good basis for appropriate management during delivery and after childbirth. Failure to attend antenatal care early results in the potential for complications during pregnancy, delivery and puerperium [6,7]. However, existing evidence from developing countries including Ethiopia indicates that few women seek antenatal care at early stage of their pregnancy [8,9].

Studies have identified several factors that influence the utilization of antenatal care in developing countries, although there are few studies regarding factors affecting the timing of first ANC attendance. These factors include, among others, maternal education, and husband's education, availability of health service, cost, household income, women's employment, media exposure, and having a history of obstetric complications [10-12].

Therefore, timely ANC is generally acknowledged to be an effective method of preventing adverse outcomes of pregnancy. Thus this study aimed to assess timing of first antenatal care visit and associated factors among pregnant women attending ANC clinics in Dilla town governmental health institutions, 2014.

## Materials and Methods

### Study design and settings

This cross-sectional study was conducted from April 01 to June 30, 2014 at public health facilities of Dilla town, Southern Ethiopia. The town has a total population of 96,920 of which 47,394 are males & the rest 49,526 are females organized in three sub cities. There are two public health centers and one referral hospital which offer ANC service and other maternal health packages.

### Study population and sampling technique

The study population was pregnant women who attended ANC service in Dilla town public health institutions. The sample size was calculated using single population proportion formula $n=(Z\ \alpha/2)^2\ P\ (1-P)/d^2$ based on the following assumptions: proportion of timely ANC visit is taken 31% from [8], significant level at $\alpha=0.05$, at 95% confidence interval, margin of error is 5% and 10% nonresponse rate, the minimum sample size became 362 pregnant women. The sample was allocated proportionally for the three health facilities and collected with a systematic random sampling technique. Annual performance report of the health institutions the year before the study period was taken as reference to estimate the client load in each health institution. Based on the information proportion to sample for each institution under the study was allocated. Therefore, 63% (228) of the sample size was allocated to hospital and the rest to health centers. Systematic random sampling technique was used and every second pregnant mother was selected for an exit interview. The first study subject was determined randomly.

All pregnant women who were attending antenatal care service in Dilla town that came to health institution during data collection period were eligible for the interview and pregnant women who were unable to hear and speak were excluded.

### Data collection procedure and data quality control

The data collection tool was first prepared in English after reviewing related literatures and then translated to Amharic language. Exit interview technique was used to collect data with structured and pretested questionnaire. Data were collected by four midwives after trained for a day and supervised by the principal investigator. The check list sought information on: socio-demographic characteristics, obstetric history, past experiences and physical findings. The data were collected by three nurses after getting training.

### Study variables and data analysis

The dependent variables is timing of first ANC which is dichotomized as late initiation (after 16 week of gestation) which is coded zero and other wise as early; and the independent variables were characteristics, obstetric history, past experiences and physical findings. After data collection, each questionnaire was checked for completeness and consistency. Data was cleaned, coded and entered into Epi-info version 7 and exported to SPSS version 20 for Windows, then exploratory data analysis carried out to check the levels of missing values, presence of influential outliers, independence of errors, multi-collinearity and normality.

Binary and multiple logistic regressions were run to assess the association of various factors with late presentation. Variables significant at $P<0.25$ level in the bivariate analysis were included in the final binary logistic regression analysis, to identify independent predictors. The forward stepwise regression method was applied to get a list of best predictors and any statistical test is considered significant at P level less than 0.05 in the final model. Covariates were checked for interaction effect. Finally the fitness of the model was checked by Hosmer and Lemeshow test. The results were presented in the form of tables, texts and figure. The strength of association of predictor variables were assessed using odds ratio and significance of variables were reported by using 95% confidence interval and p-values <0.05.

### Ethical statement

Ethical clearance was obtained from institutional review office of Arba Minch University. Permission to conduct the study also was obtained from town administration selected institutes. Informed consent was obtained from each study participants. Each respondents were informed about the purpose of the study and also that all data obtained from them were kept confidential by using codes instead of any personal identifiers.

## Result

### Socio-demographic characteristics of study participants

Over all 362 pregnant women who were attending antenatal care service at public health facilities were interviewed and none of them have refused to respond for the interview. The respondents' age ranged from 16 to 36 years with a mean age of 25.46 (SD 6 years). More than half of the respondents were in the age group 25-34 years and 170 (47%) were attended grade 12 and above in their educational level. The majority 158 (43.6%) of women were private workers and all were married (Table 1).

| **Characteristics** | **N (%)** |
|---|---|
| **Residence** | |
| Rural | 75 (20.7) |
| Urban | 287 (79.3) |
| **Age** | |
| 15-24 | 149 (41) |
| 25-34 | 170 (47) |
| 35 and above | 43 (12) |
| **Educational status** | |
| No formal school | 73 (20) |
| Primary | 107 (29.6) |
| Secondary | 103 (28.5) |

| Grade 12+ | 79 (21.9) |
|---|---|
| **Monthly income** | |
| < 1000 ETB | 175 (48.3) |
| ≥ 1000 ETB | 187 (51.7) |
| **Occupational status** | |
| Government employer | 108 (29.8) |
| Private/NGO | 158 (43.6) |
| No job | 88 (24.3) |
| Other | 8 (2.2) |

**Table1:** Socio demographic characteristics of the pregnant women in Dilla town public health facilities, South Ethiopia, 2014.

## Obstetric history and current pregnancy

Majority of the respondents (71.4%) were multiparas and among the pregnant women who ever gave birth, most of them (58.9%) have gave birth to one child. The mean gestational age of the pregnant women during the interview time was 15.9 (SD 3.7) weeks. Majorities (47%) had one and more ANC visits at the time of data collection. Among those respondents, having more than one pregnancy 80.3% had antenatal follow up in their previous pregnancies. Among those who are currently pregnant 74.86% was planned. Majority of them 63.8% knows their pregnancy after missing period while the rest by urine test. Of those who are currently pregnant 18% of them faced pregnancy associated complication (Table 2).

| Characteristics | | N (%) |
|---|---|---|
| History of still birth (321) | Yes | 8 (2.5) |
| History of abortion (321) | Yes | 65 (20.2) |
| Last pregnancy complication (321) | Yes | 208 (64.8) |
| ANC visit for last pregnancy (321) | Yes | 229 (71.3) |
| have advised on ANC (362) | Yes | 259 (71.55) |
| pregnancy planned (362) | Yes | 271 (74.9) |
| check for pregnancy (362) | Missed period | 231 (63.8) |
| pregnancy related medical complication | Yes | 65 (18) |

**Table 2:** Obstetrics and current pregnancy related response among pregnant women in Dilla town public health facilities, South Ethiopia, 2014.

## Timing of first ANC attendance

Based on mothers recall and record, review the proportion of mothers who made their first ANC visit later than the 16 week; beyond the recommended time were 182 (50.3%). Similarly equivalent proportion of mothers visited in the recommended time (within 16 weeks of gestation). Timing of first ANC attendance ranges from 4$^{th}$ week to 36$^{th}$ week during pregnancy; with mean gestational age of 15.9 (SD 3.7) weeks. Two hundred fifty nine (71.55) pregnant women were received advice about ANC use from any one before their first ANC visit, majorly from health extension workers and community voluntaries. In addition 83% of pregnant women were aware about danger signs during pregnancy; they mention one danger sign of pregnancy.

## Factors associated with late first antenatal care attendance

The effects of each independent variable on the late initiation of first ANC were tested using binary logistic regression analysis. Among the variables place of residence, educational status, monthly household income, still birth, gravidity, advice status and pregnancy plan status were associated in bivariate analysis but others failed to show significant association.

The final multivariable model was built by using variables having P-values less than 0.25 in bivariate analysis with forward step wise method. After controlling the effect of other variables in the final multivariate model rural residence, no formal education, lower household income, not being advised and unplanned pregnancy were significantly associated with the outcome variable; late ANC booking for first visit.

Pregnant women who are living in rural areas were around four times (AOR=3.6, 95% CI (1.72, 6.62)) more likely to be late for first ANC attendance as compared to women of urban dwellers. The odds of pregnant women with monthly income of <1000 ETB to delay ANC booking were three times (AOR=3.20, 95%CI (1.5, 6.74)) higher compared to high monthly income family. Similarly the odds of late registration is 1.48 (1.12, 3.04) times higher for illiterates than literate mothers.

Pregnant women who was not advised the recommended time were 4.64 (2.32, 8.17) more likely to book late for their first ANC as compared to their counterparts who received advice on recommended time.

Pregnant women with unplanned pregnancy were five times (AOR=5.02, 95%CI (2.21, 8.95)) more likely to book late for their first ANC as compared to their counterparts with planned pregnancy (Table 3).

| Variables (n=362) | First ANC attendance | | Crude OR (95% CI) | Adjusted OR (95% CI) |
|---|---|---|---|---|
| | Late | Early | | |
| **Place of Residence** | | | | |
| Rural | 60 | 15 | 5.4 (3.2, 7.5) | 3.6 (1.72, 6.62)* |
| Urban | 122 | 14 | 1 | 1 |

| Educational status | | | | |
|---|---|---|---|---|
| No formal educat. | 51 | 22 | 2.8 (1.33, 5.10) | 1.48 (1.12, 3.04)* |
| Formal education | 131 | 158 | 1 | 1 |
| **Occupational status** | | | | |
| No job | 45 | 42 | 1.19 (0.24-3.56)** | |
| Have job | 130 | 145 | 1 | |
| **Monthly income** | | | | |
| <100 ETB | 108 | 70 | 2.3 (1.22, 3.41) | 3.20 (1.5, 6.74)* |
| ≥ 1000 ETB | 74 | 110 | 1 | 1 |
| **Gravida** | | | | |
| One | 20 | 21 | 1.01 (0.12, 2.16)** | |
| Two & above | 156 | 165 | 1 | |
| **Advised** | | | | |
| No | 72 | 31 | 3.14 (1.93, 5.78) | 4.64 (2.32, 8.17)* |
| Yes | 110 | 149 | 1 | 1 |
| **Plan of pregnancy** | | | | |
| Un Planned | 64 | 27 | 3 (1.8, 4.32) | 5.02 (2.21, 8.95)* |
| Planned | 118 | 153 | 1 | 1 |
| **History of still birth** | | | | |
| No | 5 | 3 | 1.68 (1.05, 9.45)** | 1.1 (0.46, 5.32) |
| Yes | 176 | 178 | 1 | 1 |
| ** Not significant at p.value ≤ 0.25 in COR, * significant at p.value ≤ 0.05 in AOR | | | | |

**Table 3:** Factors associated with timing of first ANC attendance among pregnant women in Dilla town public health facilities, South Ethiopia, 2014.

## Discussion

This study assessed timing of first antenatal care visit and identified associated factors for late coming among pregnant women attending antenatal care in Dilla town public health institutions This study identified that the mean time to visit ANC for the first booking was 15.9 (SD 3.7) weeks and 50.3% of the pregnant women initiated antenatal care later than the recommended time (after 16 weeks). This finding is lower than studies conducted in Addis Ababa (Ethiopia), Western Kenya and South Western Nigeria in which the prevalence of late booking was 60%, 87% and 82.6% respectively [13-15]. This might be due to the time, socio-demographic, economic, and cultural differences as evidenced by our study was conducted after health promotion was advocated in the last two years and participants are mainly urban dwellers. However the prevalence of late booking is higher than a study conducted in Kassala (Eastern Sudan) and similar to a study conducted in Durban, South Africa [16,17].

After controlling the effect of other variables rural residence, no formal education, lower household income, not being advised and unplanned pregnancy were significantly associated with late presentation for first ANC visit. Rural women were 3.6 times more likely to be booked late for their first ANC visit than urban dweller women. This finding is supported by a study conducted in Hadiya, SNNP in which late ANC service utilization is two times higher in rural than urban residents [18]. This could be due to the fact that urban residents are nearer to health facilities, are educated and knowledgeable. Furthermore illiterate women were 1.48 more likely to be late for ANC visit than women who have formal education. It is also in line with other studies [16,18].

Similarly pregnant women who had low household monthly income were 3.2 times more likely to be booked late for their first ANC booking as compared to their counterparts with high monthly income. This finding is in line with a study conducted in Hadiya Zone (Ethiopia), Holeta town (Ethiopia), and Nigeria [12,15,18]. This could be because of the fact that those who have better income are more educated and income increase the ability to pay for health care services, transportation, and other indirect costs.

The other factor that significantly associated with late antenatal care entry in this study was not getting advice about timing of first ANC.

This study found that pregnant women who did not receive advice on recommended time were 4.64 times more likely to be registered late for their first ANC as compared mothers who ever received an advice. This was in line with studies conducted in Addis Ababa and Uganda, in which women were more likely to visit earlier when they were advised up on their pregnancies [13,19]. Accordingly having unplanned pregnancy was found to be a significantly associated with late booking of ANC. In this study it was found that women with unplanned pregnancy were 5 times more likely visit late for their first ANC as compared to their counterparts. This finding is in line with studies conducted in south west Nigeria and Kenya [14,15].

Even though this study has come up with important finding with respect to late registration for first ANC visit, there are certain limitations worth mentioning here. Due to cross- sectional nature of the study temporal relationship could not be ascertained. The other concern was pregnant women who attend antenatal care at private health facilities are not included in the study. Moreover, gestational age was determined based on women's reports of their last menstrual period (LMNP). However, it can be applicable to similar population.

## Conclusion and Recommendation

The study showed that nearly half of women initiated their first ANC booking later than the recommended time and the mean time for the record was 15.9 (SD 3.7) weeks. Being rural resident, having lower monthly income, not received advice on when to start antenatal care visits, No formal education and unplanned pregnancy were factors significantly associated with late first antenatal care booking. Therefore addressing rural women through health extension workers, giving an advice, improving economic capacity and avoiding unplanned pregnancy through family planning are important measures to overcome the problem.

## Acknowledgments

I would like to sincerely thank Head of the health institutions, data collectors and study participants.

## References

1. WHO (2014) Trends in Maternal mortality 1990–2013, Estimates by WHO, UNICEF, UNFPA, the World Bank, and the United Nations Population Division, World Health Organization, Geneva, Switzerland.
2. Hogan MC, Foreman KJ, Naghavi M (2010) Maternal mortality for 181 countries, 1980–2008: a systematic analysis of progress towards millennium development goal 5. The Lancet 375: 1609-1623.
3. Hill K, Thomas K, Zahr CA, Walker N, Say L, et al. (2007) Estimates of maternal mortality worldwide between 1990 and 2005. The Lancet 370: 1311-1319.
4. Central Statistical Agency (2014) Mini Ethiopia Demographic and Health Survey 2014, Central Statistical Agency, Addis Ababa, Ethiopia.
5. Villar J, Bergsj P (2002) Manual for the implementation of new model, WHO Antenatal Care Randomized Trial, World Health Organization. Geneva.
6. Carroli G, Rooney C, Villar J (2001) How effective is antenatal care in preventing maternal mortality and serious morbidity? An overview of the evidence. Paediatr Perinat Epidemiol 15: 1-42.
7. WHO (2005) The World Health Report 2005: Make Every Mother and Child Count, World Health Organization, Geneva, Switzerland.
8. Central Statistical Agency [Ethiopia] and ICF International (2012) Ethiopia Demographic and Health Survey 2011. Addis Ababa, Ethiopia and Calverton, Maryland, USA.
9. Wado YD, Afework MF, Hindin MJ (2013) Unintended pregnancies and the use of maternal health services in S.W. Ethiopia. BMC Int Health Hum Rights 13: 36.
10. Simkhada B, Teijlingen ER, Porter M, Simkhada P (2008) Factors affecting the utilization of antenatal care in developing countries: systematic review of the literature. J Adv Nurs 61: 2440-260.
11. Tsegay Y, Gebrehiwot T, Goicolea I, Edin K, Lemma H, et al. (2013) Determinants of antenatal and delivery care utilization in Tigray region, Ethiopia: a cross-sectional study. Int J Equity Health 12: 30.
12. Birmeta K, Dibaba Y, Woldeyohannes D (2013) Determinants of maternal health care utilization in Holeta town, central Ethiopia. BMC Health Services Research 13: 256.
13. Tariku A, Melkamu Y, Kebede Z (2010) Previous utilization of service does not improve timely booking in antenatal care: Cross sectional study on timing of antenatal care booking at public health facilities in Addis Ababa. Ethiop. J Health Dev 3: 226-33.
14. Anna E, Hanneke M, Frank O (2006) Use of antenatal services and delivery care among women in rural western Kenya: a community based survey. Reprod Health 3: 2.
15. Adekanle D, Isawumi A (2008) Late antenatal care booking and Its predictors among pregnant women In South Western Nigeria. Online J Health Allied Sci 7: 4.
16. Abdel AA, Mohammed O, Ameer A (2010) Use of antenatal care services in Kassala, eastern Sudan. BMC Pregnancy Childbirth 10: 3.
17. Sibeko S, MBCh B (2006) Healthcare attendance patterns by pregnant women in Durban, South Africa. SA Fam Pract 48: 17.
18. Zeine A, Mirkuzie W, Shimeles O (2010) Facors influencing antenatal care service utlization in Hadya zone Ethiopia. J Health Sci 20: 75-82.
19. Lynn A, Florence M, Nazarius M (2008) Adolescent and adult first time mothers' health seeking practices during pregnancy and early motherhood in Wakiso district, central Uganda. Reprod Health 5: 13.

# 23

# The Use of *Streptococcus salivarius* K12 in Attenuating PFAPA Syndrome

**Di Pierro Francesco[1*], Campana Andrea[2], Panatta Maria Laura[2], Antenucci Valeria[2] and De Vincentiis Giovanni[2]**

[1]*Velleja Research, Milan, Italy*

[2]*Ospedale Pediatrico Bambino Gesù, Rome, Italy*

[*]**Corresponding author:** Francesco Di Pierro, Velleja Research, Viale Lunigiana 23, 20125, Milano, Italy, E-mail: f.dipierro@vellejaresearch.com

**Abstract**

PFAPA (Periodic Fever with Aphthous stomatitis, Pharyngitis, and Adenitis) syndrome is a rare, poorly understood, clinical entity characterized by a sudden onset of fever, aphthous stomatitis, pharyngitis, and cervical adenitis. PFAPA affects mainly children and generally resolves before puberty with no subsequent consequences for the patient. Use of acetaminophen (APAP), anti-inflammatory drugs, corticosteroids and tonsillectomy are considered potential treatment options. *Streptococcus salivarius* K12 is a perfectly tolerated, oral-colonizing probiotic strain that releases two lantibiotics (salivaricins A2 and B) known to antagonize the *in vitro* and *in situ* growth of many oral pathogenic streptococci, as well as being endowed with anti-viral and anti-inflammatory capabilities. As demonstrated in our study the 90-day administration of strain K12 appears to have reduced specific signs of PFAPA, leading also to a reduction in drug use. Larger prospective and controlled studies are now indicated to more definitively establish the relevance of our assumption and the importance of these preliminary observations.

**Keywords:** PFAPA syndrome; *Streptococcus salivarius* K12; IL-8; Inflammatory cytokines; Children

## Introduction

Periodic fever with aphthous stomatitis, pharyngitis, and adenitis (PFAPA) represents the most common periodic fever syndrome of childhood. The etiology is poorly understood. No genetic defects have yet been identified and the incidence of the syndrome has not been accurately established [1]. The condition is characterized by a sudden onset of fever and can be accompanied by aphthous stomatitis, pharyngitis, and cervical adenitis with less common symptoms including headache, rash, and gastrointestinal disturbances. PFAPA episodes normally recur every 3 to 8 weeks and resolve within 6-7 days of onset [2]. Even if published supportive evidence is limited and its precise role has yet to be clarified, tonsillectomy appears to have been the most common option for management of PFAPA syndrome when symptoms markedly interfere with the child's quality of life and/or other strategies, such as treatment with acetaminophen and anti-inflammatory drugs, has failed [3]. Although the pathogenesis remains obscure, the disease displays characteristics of an inflammatory reaction. During PFAPA attacks, complement, IL-1-related and IFN-induced genes are significantly overexpressed. PFAPA flares are also accompanied by significantly increased serum levels of chemokines for activated T lymphocytes, GM-CSF, G-CSF, and pro-inflammatory cytokines such IL-1β, IL-6 and IL-8 [4,5]. The probiotic bacterium *Streptococcus salivarius* K12 produces the lantibiotic bacteriocins, named salivaricin A2 and salivaricin B [6]. These bacteriocins interfere with the growth of *Streptococcus pyogenes, Haemophilus influenza, Streptococcus pneumoniae* and *Moraxella catarrhalis,* bacteria commonly involved in the pathogenesis of bacterial pharyngo-tonsillitis and/or acute otitis media (AOM) [7]. Recent clinical trials, conducted in children have demonstrated that treatment with probiotic K12 reduces the occurrence of episodes of pharyngo-tonsillitis and AOM [8-10] without modifying the levels of either IL-1β or TNF-α, but with considerable reduction of IL-8 release [7]. We have therefore assumed that the strain K12, being endowed with anti-pharyngitis, anti-tonsillitis and anti-inflammatory properties, could counteracts PFAPA syndrome. Indeed, some anecdotal reports of parents of PFAPA-affected children that the characteristic symptoms of PFAPA appeared to have abated while their children were taking probiotic K12 has encouraged us to propose the hypothesis of a possible anti-PFAPA effect played by the strain K12.

## Methods

*Streptococcus salivarius* K12 (BLIS Technologies, Dunedin, New Zealand), was formulated as slowly-dissolving oral tablets by SIIT (Trezzano S/N, Milan, Italy) and notified as nutritional supplement to the Italian Ministry of Health as Bactoblis® by Omeopiacenza (Pontenure, Italy), according to the provisions of law 169 of 2004, on July 5, 2011 (notification number: 53435). The preparation of Bactoblis® used contained no less than 1 billion colony-forming units (CFU)/tablet of *Streptococcus salivarius* K12. Starting from T=0 to T=90, 1 tablet of Bactoblis® was administered to each subject every night, just before sleep. The tablet was allowed to slowly dissolve in the oral cavity, without biting or swallowing. Saliva production is typically reduced in the evening hours and this improves the effectiveness of oral colonization. Only for the very first treatment, the administration of the tablet was preceded, about 30 minutes before, by the use of a chlorhexidine-based (0.2%) mouthwash. This procedure improves the efficacy of oral colonization by creating bacteria-depleted niches in the oral tissues. In order to evaluate the level of subject adherence to the established protocol, the subjects were asked to return any unused product boxes and tablets. Acceptable adherence was considered to be the administration of not less than 95% of the allocated tablets. Our study concerning the PFAPA-affected children treated with the strain K12 has been performed with both ethical committee positive opinion and parental consent. Because of the small number of subjects tested, no statistical analysis has been performed.

## Results

The four children evaluated in our work and diagnosed with PFAFA syndrome were all outpatients of the Pediatric Department at Bambino Gesù Hospital (Rome, Italy).

As shown in Table 1 their principal PFAPA-relevant features were: 1) one fever episode, with temperature of about 39°C, per month; 2) one pharyngitis episode per month; 3) possible presence of aphthous stomatitis and/or cervical adenitis; 4) possible use of cortisone and/or ibuprofen and/or acetaminophen; 5) poor quality of life and sleep. As shown in Table 2, three subjects out of four had no episodes of fever, aphthous stomatitis, pharyngitis or lymphadenopathy during 90-days treatment with the strain K12. Consequently, no drugs were administered during this period. According to their parents, for these three subjects both quality of life and sleep also improved substantially. Just a bit different results were reported for a fourth subject (Table 3) with no signs consistent with those of PFAPA syndrome occurring during the second and the third month of treatment with strain K12. For this subject one day of fever occurred during the first month of treatment and one day of fever occurred during the following 30-day wash out period. Also for this fourth subject, both life and sleep quality were reported by the parents to be improved. This fourth case seems to be a very infrequent presentation of PFAPA syndrome and might be differently explained, especially as related to the impressive amount of medication (apparently ineffective) prescribed during the first month of observation.

| Subject; age (years) and sex | PFAPA diagnosis (month/year) | Fever episodes (per month); maximum temperature; duration of fever | Presence of apthous stomatitis | Pharyngitis episodes per month; duration of pharyngitis | Presence of cervical adenitis | Cortisone use | APAP use; times per day | Ibuprofen use; times per day | Quality of Life (1-10) | Quality of Sleep (1-10) |
|---|---|---|---|---|---|---|---|---|---|---|
| 1; 5; male°° | 01/2015 | 1.0; 39.5°C; 4 days | yes | 1.0; 3 days | no | no | yes; 4 | yes; 4 | 2 | 2 |
| 2; 10; male^ | 11/2013 | 1.5; 39.0°C; 4 days | no | 1.0; 1 day | yes | yes | yes; 4 | yes; 4 | 3 | 3 |
| 3; 6; male° | 09/2014 | 1.0; 39.0°C; 4 days | no | 1.0; 4 days | yes | no | yes; 4 | yes; 4 | 5 | 7 |
| 4; 7; male* | 01/2014 | 1.0; 39.5°C; 5 days | yes | 1.0; 4.5 days | yes | yes | yes; 3-4 | yes; 3-4 | 2 | 2 |

°° APAP: 250 mg/dose; Ibuprofen 150 mg/dose; ^Deflazacort 32 mg/dose/die; APAP 500 mg/dose; Ibuprofen 200 mg/dose; °APAP 250 mg/dose; Ibuprofen 150 mg/dose; *Deflazacort 30 mg/dose; APAP 500 mg/dose; Ibuprofen 200 mg/dose

**Table 1:** Clinical conditions and parameters of the four cases of PFAFA prior to their use of probiotic K12.

| Parameters | 1°month with K12 | 2° month with K12 | 3° month with K12 | 4° month (wash out) |
|---|---|---|---|---|
| Fever episodes; maximum temperature; duration of fever | No fever | No fever | No fever | No fever |
| Presence of apthous stomatitis | No lesions | No lesions | No lesions | No lesions |
| Pharyngitis episodes; duration of pharyngitis | No pharyngitis | No pharyngitis | No pharyngitis | No pharyngitis |
| Presence of cervical adenitis | No lymphadenopathy | No lymphadenopathy | No lymphadenopathy | No lymphadenopathy |
| Use of cortisone | No use | No use | No use | No use |
| Use of APAP | No use | No use | No use | No use |
| Use of Ibuprofen | No use | No use | No use | No use |
| Quality of Life (1-10)° | 7.0 ± 1.0 | 8.0 ± 1.5 | 10.0 ± 0.0 | 9.0 ± 0.5 |
| Quality of Sleep (1-10)° | 7.0 ± 1.0 | 7.0 ± 1.0 | 7.0 ± 1.0 | 7.0 ± 0.5 |

° average values ± standard deviation are given

**Table 2:** Signs and symptoms trends in subjects 1, 2 and 3 during the 90 days treatment with probiotic K12.

| Parameters | 1° month with K12 | 2° month with K12 | 3° month with K12 | 4° month wash out |
|---|---|---|---|---|
| Fever episodes; maximum temperature; duration of fever | 1; 40°C; 2 days | No fever | No fever | 1; 39°C; 1 day |
| Presence of apthous stomatitis | No lesions | No lesions | No lesions | No lesions |
| Pharyngitis episodes; duration of pharyngitis | 1; 4 days | No pharyngitis | No pharyngitis | 1; 1 day |
| Presence of cervical adenitis | No lymphadenopathy | No lymphadenopathy | No lymphadenopathy | No lymphadenopathy |
| Use of cortisone* | 1 day | No use | No use | 1 day |
| Use of APAP° | 2 days | No use | No use | No use |
| Use of Ibuprofen^ | 2 days | No use | No use | No use |
| Quality of Life (1-10) | 4 | 7 | 8 | 8 |
| Quality of Sleep (1-10) | 4 | 7 | 7 | 7 |
| *Deflazacort: 30 mg/dose/die; °APAP: 500 mg x 3-4 doses/die; ^Ibuprofen 200 mg x 3-4 doses/die | | | | |

**Table 3:** Signs and symptoms trends in subject 4 during the 90 days treatment with probiotic K12.

## Discussion

Although the pathogenesis of the PFAPA syndrome has not been clarified it appears to be associated with the onset of an inflammatory cytokine cascade. *Streptococcus salivarius* K12, also identified as ATCC BAA-1024, in addition to being effective in counteracting some of the bacteria and viruses implicated in pharyngo-tonsillitis and OMA, has also been shown to be effective in reducing the levels of some cytokines, such as IL-8, that are involved in the development of the inflammatory response and possibly in the pathogenesis of PFAPA. We have anecdotally observed that the use of the strain K12 seems to interfere with the development of signs and symptoms of PFAPA syndrome, thereby limiting the use of drugs and improving the quality of life and sleep of children having a diagnosis of PFAPA syndrome. Nevertheless PFAPA syndrome is not yet precisely defined but even presents aspects so polymorphic in their repetitiveness (duration of febrile episodes, age of onset, associated symptoms) to be easily confused with other conditions such as recurrent infections related to life in community, recurrent bacterial infections favored by recent viral infections, cyclic neutropenia or transient IgA deficiency. These results seem to confirm our hypothesis and suggest a possible option that can result in the reduction of the use of non-steroidal anti-inflammatory drugs, steroids and/or antibiotics, as well as possibly eliminate the use of tonsillectomy for a disease that beyond the discomfort for the patient and for the family is anyways absolutely benign. Since PFAPA syndrome is a disease with hyper-immune responses involving different tissues, the most probable starting point would be the involvement of tonsillar lymphoid tissue which is possibly stimulated by bacterial and viral infections. We predict that prolonged use of *Streptococcus salivarius* K12 would have a favorable effect. Our observations are very preliminary but provide encouragement for further investigation of the use of probiotic K12 for the control of this syndrome. Considering the absolute tolerability of the product, double-blind, randomized, prospective, placebo-controlled studies are now indicated to systematically evaluate the efficacy of probiotic K12 in the control of PFAPA syndrome.

## Conflict of interest

FDP, as Velleja Research Scientific & Research Director, is the formulator responsible of the finished product containing the strain K12. The other Authors report no conflict of interest.

## Acknowledgment

The Authors reports no sources of support.

## References

1. Esposito S, Bianchini S, Fattizzo M, Baggi E, Marchisio P, et al. (2014) The enigma of periodic fever, aphthous stomatitis, pharyngitis and adenitis syndrome. Pediatr Infect Dis J 33: 650-652.
2. Vigo G, Zulian F (2012) Periodic fevers with aphthous stomatitis, pharyngitis, and adenitis (PFAPA). Autoimmun Rev 12: 52-55.
3. Garavello W, Pignataro L, Gaini L, Torretta S, Somigliana E, et al. (2011) Tonsillectomy in children with periodic fever with aphthous stomatitis, pharyngitis and adenitis syndrome. J Pediatr 159: 138-142.
4. Stojanov S, Lapidus S, Chitkara P, Feder H, Salazar JC, et al. (2011) Periodic fever, aphthous stomatitis, pharyngitis, and adenitis (PFAPA) is a disorder of innate immunity and Th1 activation responsive to IL-1 blockade. Proc Natl Acad Sci U S A 108: 7148-7153.
5. Ling E, Israeli M, Klein T, Amir J, Harel L (2014) Periodic fever, aphthous stomatitis, pharyngitis and cervical adenopathy syndrome is associated with activation of GM-CSF and burst-like expression of IL-8 in peripheral blood. Mod Rheumatol 24: 997-1000.
6. Hyink O, Wescombe PA, Upton M, Ragland N, Burton JP, et al. (2007) Salivaricin A2 and the novel lantibiotic salivaricin B are encoded at adjacent loci on a 190-kilobase transmissible megaplasmid in the oral probiotic strain Streptococcus salivarius K12. Appl Environ Microbiol 73: 1107-1113.
7. Wescombe PA, Hale JD, Heng NC, Tagg JR (2012) Developing oral probiotics from Streptococcus salivarius. Future Microbiol 7: 1355-1371.
8. Di Pierro F, Donato G, Fomia F, Adami T, Careddu D, et al. (2012) Preliminary pediatric clinical evaluation of the oral probiotic Streptococcus salivarius K12 in preventing recurrent pharyngitis and/or

tonsillitis caused by Streptococcus pyogenes and recurrent acute otitis media. Int J Gen Med 5: 991-997.

9. Di Pierro F, Colombo M, Zanvit A, Risso P, Rottoli AS (2014) Use of Streptococcus salivarius K12 in the prevention of streptococcal and viral pharyngo-tonsillitis in children. Drug Healthc Patient Saf 6: 15-20.

10. Gregori G, Righi O, Risso P, Boiardi G, Demuru G, et al. (2016) Reduction of group A beta-hemolytic streptococcus pharyngo-tonsillar infections associated with use of the oral probiotic Streptococcus salivarius K12: a retrospective observational study. Ther Clin Risk Manag 12: 87-92.

# Efficacy of Oral Supplementation with Silymarin and S-Adenosyl-L-Methionine in Patients with Non Alcoholic Fatty Liver Disease

**Ilaria Giangrandi[1,2], Monica Dinu[1,2*], Giuditta Pagliai[1,2], Francesco Sofi[1,2,3] and Alessandro Casini[1,2]**

[1]*Department of Experimental and Clinical Medicine, University of Florence, Italy*

[2]*Unit of Clinical Nutrition, University Hospital of Careggi, Florence, Italy*

[3]*Don Carlo Gnocchi Foundation Italy, Onlus IRCCS, Florence, Italy*

[*]**Corresponding author:** Monica Dinu, Department of Experimental and Clinical Medicine, University of Florence, Largo Brambilla 3, Florence-50134, Italy, E-mail: mdinu@uni i.it

## Abstract

**Background and Aim:** Non-alcoholic fatty liver disease (NAFLD) is the most common liver disease worldwide, affecting up to one-third of the population in industrialized countries. Silymarin and S-Adenosyl-L-Methionine (SAMe) have therapeutic potential for treatment of liver disease. The aim of the present pilot study was to evaluate the possible effect of a supplementation with Silymarin and SAMe in NAFLD patients.

**Methods:** Fifteen NAFLD patients (mean age: 46.3 ± 15 years) confirmed by ultra-sonographic findings were subjected to a 12-month oral supplementation with Silymarin and SAMe. Anthropometric measurements, biochemical parameters, liver function and hepatic fat content were assessed at baseline, at 6 months and at the end of treatment.

**Results:** After a 12-months' oral supplementation a significant improvement ($p<0.05$) in several biochemical parameters such as total cholesterol (mean reduction: -8.67 mg/dL), insulin (-1.34 U/L) and HOMA-IR (-1.35) was observed. Similarly, serum levels of alanine aminotransferase (ALT) and alkaline phosphatase (ALP) significantly decreased by 13% (-3.87 U/L and -10.4 U/L respectively), with a small but significant amelioration in the risk profile. Finally, the ultrasonography examination revealed an improvement in liver echo-texture and a regression of the degree of hepatic steatosis, associated with a 22% increase of the Doppler Perfusion Index (DPI), which corresponds to better liver hemodynamic.

**Conclusion:** Our findings suggest that a prolonged Silymarin and SAMe supplementation could be used as an adjunctive therapy to improve metabolic risk profile and hepatic steatosis in patients with NAFLD. Further research is needed to confirm these preliminary results.

**Keywords:** Silymarin; S-adenosyl-L-methionine; NAFLD

## Introduction

Non-alcoholic fatty liver disease (NAFLD) is the most common liver disease in the industrialized countries [1]. Its prevalence increased from less than 10% in the 1980s, through 10% to 20% in the 1990s, to current rates of 15% to 30% or higher [1]. NAFLD represents the outcome of genetically-determined interactions between a changing environment and a susceptible host. The environmental factors include an excess of energy intake, particularly in the form of cheap, highly processed simple carbohydrates and saturated fats, and reduced levels of physical fitness resulting from a sedentary lifestyle [2]. NAFLD embraces a pathological spectrum of liver disease, from cases of steatosis with virtually no evidence of hepatocellular injury or liver inflammation, often referred to as simple steatosis through steatohepatitis (NASH), to cases with cirrhosis [3]. Individuals with only hepatic steatosis (simple steatosis) infrequently show signs of any histologic progression, and are not at significant long-term risk of liver-related death [4], but those with advanced hepatic fibrosis are likely to experience liver-related complications (ascites, variceal bleeding, and/or hepatocellular carcinoma) [5].

Furthermore, hepatic necroinflammatory activity in patients with NAFLD is able to increase the risk of future cardiovascular disease [6], and confers a higher risk of unfavorable liver-related outcomes by promoting development of hepatic fibrosis. The lipid molecules that accumulate, together with triglycerides, in some NAFLD livers can participate directly in pathogenesis of the necroinflammatory element of NASH [7]. From the scientific literature it is known that high intracellular levels of Silymarin and S-Adenosyl-L-Methionine (SAMe) act in: reducing the uptake of exogenous toxic substances, increasing membrane fluidity, detoxifying the hepatic cell, preventing the depletion of glutathione and thereby increasing its availability, having anti-inflammatory activity and in promoting the regeneration of liver cells [8,9]. The aim of the present intervention study was to evaluate the possible effect of an oral supplementation of Silymarin and SAMe in NAFLD patients.

## Material and Methods

### Study population

Fifteen patients with a diagnosis of NAFLD referred to the Unit of Clinical Nutrition of the University Hospital of Careggi, Florence, Italy, and characterized by ultrasonography features indicative of NAFLD were eligible for enrolment. Written informed consent was obtained from all patients. The study protocol followed the ethical guidelines of the Declaration of Helsinki and was approved by our departmental Ethics Committee.

The inclusion criteria were as follows: age >18 years, lack of excessive alcohol consumption (<20 g/d), ultrasound examination demonstrating fatty liver, negative diagnostic tests for viral hepatitis and absence of other causes of liver disease. Exclusion criteria included a history of alcohol intake >20 g/d, use of drugs known to be associated with liver steatosis, undernutrition, chronic viral hepatitis and chronic liver disease of other causes (autoimmune hepatitis, primary biliary cirrhosis, primary sclerosing cholangitis, hereditary haemochromatosis, Wilson's disease, a1-anti-trypsin deficiency, coeliac disease). Pregnant and breastfeeding women were also excluded.

## Study design

All patients were subjected to a 12-months' oral supplementation with 1 tablet per day of Duoliver (Biocure Srl, Milan), a food supplement containing Silymarin (140 mg) and SAMe (200 mg) without dietary guidelines or other lifestyle changes. The products were packed in labelled boxes. Compliance was verified by counting the empty boxes on return. A medical examination with measurement of body mass index (BMI), blood tests and liver ultrasonography was performed at baseline, at 6 months and at the end of the treatment. BMI was calculated as weight (kg)/height ($m^2$).

The laboratory evaluation included total cholesterol, LDL-cholesterol, HDL-cholesterol, triglycerides, fasting glucose blood levels, insulin blood levels, insulin resistance index (HOMA-IR), aspartate aminotransferase (AST), alanine aminotransferase (ALT), gamma glutamyl transferase (γ-GT), alkaline phosphatase (ALP), and total and fractionated bilirubin. All subjects were interviewed by means of an ad hoc questionnaire for the frequency and quantity of recreational activities performed during the preceding year. Hence, physical activity was graded into qualitative terms such as absent or light (i.e. inactive or either occasional walking or recreational activity only), moderate (i.e. frequent recreational activities, regular walking for 30 minutes three to five times per week or sporting exercise at least once a week) and intense (i.e. sporting activity at least twice a week, plus frequent recreational activities or walking, or frequent sporting activities only). The dietary profile of the study patients was evaluated by an experienced clinical dietician with the aid of software specific for the analysis of food habits and the estimation of nutrient and caloric intake.

## Fatty liver evaluation

B-mode ultrasound and duplex Doppler investigation were performed by the same expert operator using a high-quality ultrasound device equipped with a 5 MHz Convex array transducer (Voluson 530 DMT; Kretz Technik AG, Zipf, Austria). The patients fasted for at least 12 h and underwent scanning in a supine position; data were obtained during suspended inspiration. In a B-mode imaging evaluation, the liver echo-texture was scored on a four-grade scale, by comparing it with the right kidney cortical echogenicity: Grade 0, absent steatosis; Grade 1, mild steatosis (lightly and homogeneously increased liver echo-texture, with patent intrahepatic vascular pattern; absent posterior attenuation); Grade 2, moderate steatosis (moderate increase of liver echo-texture; partial dimming of the vessels; early posterior attenuation); and Grade 3, severe steatosis (diffuse increase of liver echogenicity, with no longer visible intrahepatic vessels; heavy posterior attenuation). Duplex Doppler ultrasound allowed a semi-quantitative measurement of fatty storage on the basis of the Doppler Perfusion Index (DPI) (i.e. the ratio between hepatic artery blood flow and total liver blood flow).

## Laboratory parameters

Venous blood samples anticoagulated with 0.129 M sodium citrate (ratio 9:1) were collected from the antecubital vein into evacuated plastic tubes (Vacutainer; BD, Milan, Italy), after overnight fasting. Whole venous blood was also collected in tubes without anticoagulant. Citrated and serum samples were centrifuged at 2,000× g for 10 min at 4°C, and supernatants were stored in aliquots at –80°C until assays. Lipid variables, blood glucose, insulin, and hepatic function tests were assessed by conventional methods, as well as the HOMA-IR.

## Statistical analysis

Statistical analysis was performed using the SPSS (Statistical Package for Social Sciences, Chicago, IL, USA) software for Macintosh (Version 20.0). Results were expressed as means ± standard deviation. The Chi-square test was used to identify statistically significant differences between categorical variables. The Wilcoxon test for related data was used to evaluate differences between two time-points. A general linear model for repeated measurements, with adjustments for age, sex and BMI change, was used to compare differences between baseline and the end of the intervention period. A P value ≤ 0.05 was considered significant for all the analyses.

# Results

Between January, 2015 and May, 2015 a total of 15 patients (11 females, 4 males; mean age: 46.3 ± 15 years) with NAFLD were included in the protocol. Participants received a Silymarin plus SAMe supplement for 12 months. None of them withdrew from the study during the research period and no adverse events were observed. At baseline, the average BMI was 30.9 ± 8.9 kg/$m^2$, with 7 (47%) patients categorized as obese or extremely obese and 4 (27%) patients classified as overweight. The assessment of liver steatosis showed a moderate/severe steatosis in 6 (40%) patients.

After 6 and 12 months of food supplementation with Silymarin and SAMe, BMI did not change significantly with respect to baseline (p=0.65). In order to analyse the changes in the biochemical variables after the intervention, a general linear model adjusted for age, sex and BMI change was performed. As reported in Table 1, supplementation was found to result in a significant reduction by 4% (mean reduction: -8.67 mg/dL; p=0.01) for total cholesterol levels with respect to baseline. Also insulin levels and HOMA-IR decreased significantly by 9% and 15%, respectively (-1.34 U/L; p<0.01 and -1.35; p=0.03) with an amelioration of the metabolic status of patients. Non-significant differences were observed for LDL-cholesterol, HDL-cholesterol and triglycerides.

With regard to the liver function tests, at the end of the study we observed a significant reduction by 13% in the levels of both ALT (-3.87 U/L; p=0.01) and ALP (-10.4 U/L; p=0.04), with non-significant changes in the other parameters (Table 2). The echo-Doppler examination revealed a 22% increase in the hepatic DPI, moving from a mean of 0.18 ± 0.07 at baseline to 0.22 ± 0.05 at the end of the treatment (normal value range: 0.20-0.30), although this was not significant (p=0.08). However, ultrasonography indicated a regression of steatosis in a consistent proportion of patients: after a 12-months' oral supplementation with Silymarin and SAMe, 5 patient out of 6 with moderate/severe steatosis regressed to mild steatosis (Figure 1).

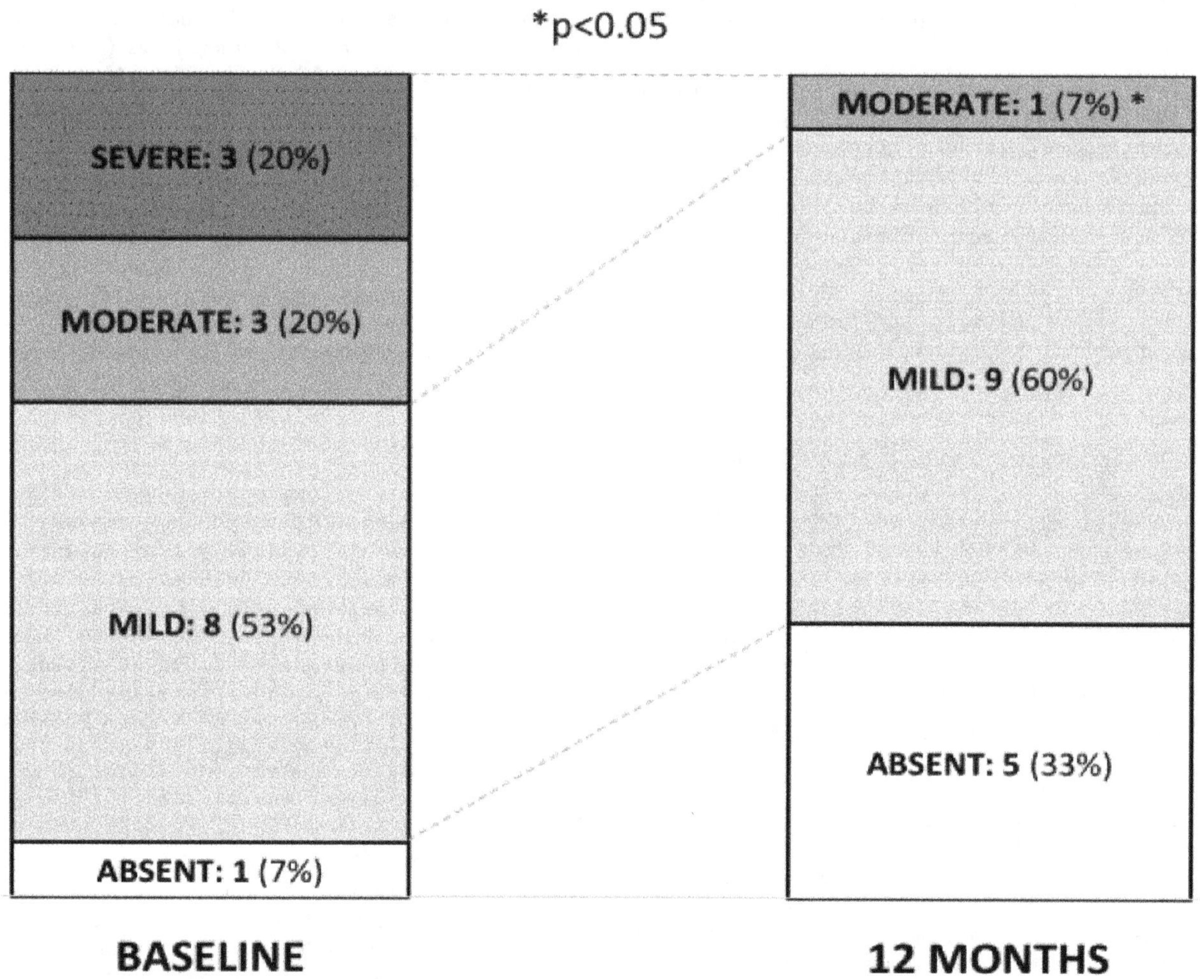


**Figure 1:** Modification of steatosis grade in enrolled subjects after a 12-months' oral supplementation with Silymarin plus SAMe.

| Variable | baseline (T0) | 6-months (T1) | 12-months (T2) | p value† |
|---|---|---|---|---|
| Cholesterol, mg/dL | 211.3 ± 31.5 | 204.0 ± 27.4 | 202.6 ± 30.6* | 0.014 |
| LDL-cholesterol, mg/dL | 143.9 ± 26.8 | 144.1 ± 24.1 | 140.7 ± 22.2 | 0.366 |
| HDL-cholesterol, mg/dL | 45.9 ± 9.51 | 47.0 ± 8.28 | 48.3 ± 8.84 | 0.246 |
| Triglycerides, mg/dL | 120.1 ± 53.6 | 116.3 ± 45.1 | 119.3 ± 44.5 | 0.93 |
| Glucose, mg/dL | 93.1 ± 10.9 | 90.8 ± 7.42 | 91.1 ± 6.80 | 0.352 |
| Insulin, mU/L | 16.1 ± 5.33 | 15.5 ± 4.9 | 14.7 ± 5.04* | 0.006 |
| HOMA-Index | 3.67 ± 1.75 | 3.39 ± 1.29 | 3.11 ± 1.15* | 0.025 |

Data are reported as mean and standard deviation,
HOMA=Homeostatic Model Assessment,
*p<0.05 for Wilcoxon signed-rank test (T0 *vs* T1 and T0 *vs* T2), †General linear model for repeated measurements adjusted for age, sex and BMI change.

**Table 1:** Modification of biochemical parameters in enrolled subjects after 6- and 12-months' oral supplementation with Silymarin plus SAMe.

| Variable | baseline (T0) | 6-months (T1) | 12-months (T2) | p value† |
|---|---|---|---|---|
| AST, U/L | 21.9 ± 7.30 | 21.3 ± 7.07 | 21.2 ± 6.71 | 0.443 |
| ALT, U/L | 30.0 ± 15.4 | 28.6 ± 13.3 | 26.1 ± 13.5* | 0.013 |
| γ-GT, U/L | 44.4 ± 39.9 | 45.7 ± 60.1 | 44.6 ± 59.1 | 0.974 |
| ALP, U/L | 80.7 ± 34.3 | 77.5 ± 31.6 | 70.3 ± 30.7* | 0.039 |
| Total bilirubin, mg/dL | 0.75 ± 0.23 | 0.70 ± 0.20 | 0.81 ± 0.16 | 0.235 |
| Direct bilirubin, mg/dL | 0.18 ± 0.08 | 0.21 ± 0.10 | 0.23 ± 0.09 | 0.097 |
| Indirect bilirubin, mg/dL | 0.57 ± 0.22 | 0.49 ± 0.22 | 0.57 ± 0.16 | 0.875 |

Data are reported as mean and standard deviation,
AST: Aspartate Aminotransferase; ALT: Alanine Aminotransferase; γ-GT: Gamma Glutamyl Transferase; ALP: Alkaline Phosphatase,
*$p<0.05$ for Wilcoxon signed-rank test (T0 *vs* T1 and T0 *vs* T2),
†General linear model for repeated measurements adjusted for age, sex and BMI change.

**Table 2:** Modification of hepatic function tests in enrolled subjects after 6- and 12-months' oral supplementation with Silymarin plus SAMe.

## Discussion

The current study reported a beneficial effect of an oral supplementation on the metabolic risk profile in patients with NAFLD. Indeed, after a 12-month oral supplementation, the ultrasonography examination revealed an improvement in liver echo-texture and a regression of the degree of hepatic steatosis, associated with a remarkable increase of DPI, which corresponds to better liver hemodynamic. Moreover, a significant improvement in several biochemical parameters such as total cholesterol, insulin, HOMA-IR, ALT and ALP was also observed after the intervention period.

To date, lifestyle modifications, healthy diet and physical activity are the most effective treatment for NAFLD, but for many people they are difficult to achieve and maintain [10]. Therefore, over the past years, several therapeutic proposals such as weight reducing, lipid-lowering, and insulin-sensitizing drugs have been proposed. These agents should act to reduce the link between adipose tissue and liver function by acting as anti-inflammatory and immunomodulatory agents. However, a validated and unique approach has not yet been obtained [10]. On the other hand, the use of complementary medicines, such as natural antioxidants, may have therapeutic potential. In fact, oxidative stress is thought to play a central role in the aetiology of NAFLD, as fatty acid oxidation produces reactive oxygen species, which cause direct cellular damage and activate pro-inflammatory cytokines. (1) Derived from the milk thistle plant (*Silybum marianum*), Silymarin is an example of a modern drug that arose from traditional medicine practices. The hepatic protection of this flavonoid complex has been attributed to its antioxidant, anti-inflammatory and antifibrotic properties [11].

This study is one of the few clinical trials that assessed the potential role of Silymarin and SAMe in the treatment of NAFLD. Supplementation with Silymarin alone has been investigated in two Iranian studies [12,13], exhibiting large effects on serum levels of ALT and AST. In parallel, an initial pilot study [14] and a subsequent large randomised placebo-control trial [15], conducted by Loguercio et al. [15], reported that a supplementation with Silybin (the major active constituent of Silymarin) combined with vitamin E and phosphatidylcholine improved insulin resistance and liver histology in patients with NAFLD. In a further clinical trial, food supplement containing vitamin E, L-glutathione, L-cysteine, L-methionine and *Silybum marianum*, given twice a day for 3 months in 72 subjects with NAFLD, reduced the biochemical, inflammatory and ultrasonic indices of hepatic steatosis [16]. Similar results were obtained in three studies [17-19] where the addition of Silymarin improved the efficacy of the lifestyle intervention. Conversely, Sorrentino et al. [20] reported a significant improvement of biometric parameters and liver steatosis, but not a reduction of liver function tests after supplementation with Silymarin. Finally, one study [21] comparing disposition of silymarin between NAFLD and Hepatitis C (HCV) patients has found that the effects of silymarin on liver disease progression was greater in NAFLD patients than in HCV patients.

While the positive effect of Silymarin on biochemical parameters and liver function has been tested in several clinical trials, there are no human studies that currently address the effect of SAMe in NAFLD patients. Indeed, the evidence of a role for SAMe in the pathogenesis of NAFLD has mainly been based on the study of animal models. Current knowledge suggests that altered hepatic SAMe level may lead to NAFLD development as SAMe is a methyl donor in the synthesis of phosphatidylcholine, which is required for VLDL assembly and hepatic triglyceride export [20]. In addition, reduced SAMe levels seem to sensitize the liver to lipopolysaccharide-induced injury and promotes expression and release of pro-inflammatory cytokines [22].

Although results are promising, the number of participants represents a limitation. Further and larger studies are needed before drawing any firm conclusions. In addition, up to now, there is no evidence on the ideal quantity and duration of supplementation with Silymarin plus SAMe for NAFLD. We cannot exclude that a higher dosage and/or a prolonged intake could reach even better outcomes. A current problem of clinical trials conducted on NAFLD patients is how to measure the outcome [23]. In particular, routine laboratory tests are helpful but not sufficient to assay the effectiveness of treatment, while needle liver biopsy, that provides the most conclusive evaluation both for diagnosis and follow-up, cannot be carried out in all patients because of invasiveness and possible complications. In the present study, in order to improve the accuracy of the evaluation, besides the liver function tests we performed ultrasonography to assess the hepatic fat content, and duplex doppler ultrasound, which provides a quantitative, non-invasive evaluation of NAFLD by measuring hepatic artery and portal vein blood flow.

In conclusion, our findings suggest that a prolonged Silymarin plus SAMe oral supplementation might have positive effects in patients with NAFLD, improving hepatic steatosis and insulin resistance, and reducing cholesterol and liver enzymes level. In patients who fail to change their lifestyle, Silymarin and SAMe could be a valid alternative therapeutic option, where appropriate as a complementary treatment associated with other therapeutic programs. Further research is needed to confirm these preliminary results.

## Acknowledgments

This work was supported in part by a grant from Biocure S.r.l., Milan, Italy.

## References

1. Rinella ME (2015) Nonalcoholic fatty liver disease: a systematic review. JAMA 313: 2263-2273.
2. Thoma C, Day CP, Trenell MI (2012) Lifestyle interventions for the treatment of non-alcoholic fatty liver disease in adults: a systematic review. J Hepatol 56: 255-266.
3. Kleiner DE, Makhlouf HR (2016) Histology of Nonalcoholic Fatty Liver Disease and Nonalcoholic Steatohepatitis in Adults and Children. Clin Liver Dis 20: 293-312.
4. Dam-Larsen S, Franzmann M, Andersen IB, Christoffersen P, Jensen LB, et al. (2004) Long term prognosis of fatty liver: risk of chronic liver disease and death. Gut 53: 750-755.
5. Bhala N, Angulo P, van der Poorten D, Lee E, Hui JM, et al. (2011) The natural history of nonalcoholic fatty liver disease with advanced fibrosis or cirrhosis: an international collaborative study. Hepatology 54: 1208-1216.
6. Motamed N, Rabiee B, Poustchi H, Dehestani B, Hemasi GR, et al. (2016) Non-alcoholic fatty liver disease (NAFLD) and 10-year risk of cardiovascular diseases. Clin Res Hepatol Gastroenterol.
7. Goh GB, McCullough AJ (2016) Natural History of Nonalcoholic Fatty Liver Disease. Dig Dis Sci 61: 1226-1233.
8. Abenavoli L, Aviello G, Capasso R, Milic N, Capasso F (2011) Milk thistle treatment of nonalcoholic fatty liver disease. Hepat Mon 11: 173-177.
9. Anstee QM, Day CP (2012) S-adenosylmethionine (SAMe) therapy in liver disease: a review of current evidence and clinical utility. J Hepatol 57: 1097-1109.
10. Scherer A, Dufour JF (2016) Treatment of Non-Alcoholic Fatty Liver Disease. Dig Dis 34: 27-31.
11. Parmar M, Gandhi T (2008) Hepatoprotective herbal drug, silymarin from experimental pharmacology to clinical medicine-A review. Pharmacogn Rev 2: 102.
12. Hajaghamohammadi AA, Ziaee A, Rafiei R (2008) The Efficacy of Silymarin in Decreasing Transaminase Activities in Non-Alcoholic Fatty Liver Disease: A Randomized Controlled Clinical Trial. Hepat Mon 8: 191-195.
13. Hajiaghamohammadi AA, Ziaee A, Oveisi S, Masroor H (2012) Effects of metformin, pioglitazone, and silymarin treatment on non-alcoholic Fatty liver disease: a randomized controlled pilot study. Hepat Mon 12: e6099.
14. Loguercio C, Federico A, Trappoliere M, Tuccillo C, de Sio I, et al. (2007) The effect of a silybin-vitamin e-phospholipid complex on nonalcoholic fatty liver disease: a pilot study. Dig Dis Sci 52: 2387-2395.
15. Loguercio C, Andreone P, Brisc C, Brisc MC, Bugianesi E, et al. (2012) Silybin combined with phosphatidylcholine and vitamin E in patients with nonalcoholic fatty liver disease: a randomized controlled trial. Free Radic Biol Med 52: 1658-1665.
16. Cacciapuoti F, Scognamiglio A, Palumbo R, Forte R, Cacciapuoti F (2013) Silymarin in non alcoholic fatty liver disease. World J Hepatol 5: 109-113.
17. Aller R, Izaola O, Gómez S, Tafur C, González G, et al. (2015) Effect of silymarin plus vitamin E in patients with non-alcoholic fatty liver disease. A randomized clinical pilot study. Eur Rev Med Pharmacol Sci 19: 3118-3124.
18. Hashemi SJ, Hajiani E, Sardabi EH (2009) A placebo-controlled trial of silymarin in patients with nonalcoholic fatty liver disease. Hepat Mon 9: 265-270.
19. Abenavoli L, Greco M, Nazionale I, Peta V, Milic N, et al. (2015) Effects of Mediterranean diet supplemented with silybin-vitamin E-phospholipid complex in overweight patients with non-alcoholic fatty liver disease. Expert Rev Gastroenterol Hepatol 9: 519–527.
20. Sorrentino G, Crispino P, Coppola D, De Stefano G (2015) Efficacy of lifestyle changes in subjects with non-alcoholic liver steatosis and metabolic syndrome may be improved with an antioxidant nutraceutical: a controlled clinical study. Drugs R D 15: 21-25.
21. Schrieber SJ, Hawke RL, Wen Z, Smith PC, Reddy KR, et al. (2011) Differences in the disposition of silymarin between patients with nonalcoholic fatty liver disease and chronic hepatitis C. Drug Metab Dispos 39: 2182-2190.
22. Chawla RK, Bonkovsky HL, Galambos JT (1990) Biochemistry and pharmacology of S-adenosyl-L-methionine and rationale for its use in liver disease. Drugs 40: 98-110.
23. Sumida Y, Nakajima A, Itoh Y (2014) Limitations of liver biopsy and non-invasive diagnostic tests for the diagnosis of non-alcoholic fatty liver disease/non-alcoholic steatohepatitis. World J Gastroenterol 20: 475-485.

# 25

# A Study on the Mechanisms of Action of Jumihaidokuto for Patients with Acne: The Relationship between the Antioxidative Effect of Jumihaidokuto and Acne Improvement

**Mayumi Nomoto**[1,2*]

[1]Nomoto Mayumi Skincare Clinic, 1-3-7 Bandai, Chuo-ku, Niigata-shi, Niigata-ken, Japan

[2]Department of Clinical Pharmacology, Faculty of Pharmaceutical Sciences, Niigata University of Pharmacy and Applied Life Sciences, 265-1 Higashijima, Akiha-ku, Niigata, Japan

## Abstract

**Background:** Drugs with various mechanisms of action such as antimicrobial agents, adapalene, and benzoyl peroxide are used to treat acne worldwide. In Japan, Kampo medicines have also traditionally been used for acne, including the medicine Jumihaidokuto (JHT). The mechanisms of action of Kampo medicines such as JHT have not been fully clarified, but it has been pointed out that oxidative stress is involved in the development of acne. Therefore, the author focused on the antioxidative effect of JHT and examined its relationship with acne improvement.

**Methods:** JHT (9 g/day) was administered for 3 weeks to 53 patients with acne, followed by measuring the diacron-reactive oxygen metabolites (d-ROMs) value as an indicator of oxidative stress, the biological antioxidant potential (BAP) value as an indicator of antioxidative potency, and the numbers of inflammatory and non-inflammatory skin rashes occurring before and after JHT administration. After the administration of JHT, the following results were observed.

**Results:** 1) The d-ROMs values of subjects who had a high baseline d-ROMs value were significantly reduced and the BAP values of those who had a low baseline BAP value were significantly increased; 2) there were significant reductions in the numbers of inflammatory and non-inflammatory skin rashes; 3) there was a significant correlation between the d-ROMs value and the number of non-inflammatory skin rashes; 4) the d-ROMs values of patients who rated their acne as "improved" by questionnaire were significantly reduced.

**Conclusion:** The above results suggest that an antioxidative effect is one of the mechanisms by which JHT contributes to acne improvement.

**Keywords:** Jumihaidokuto (Shi-Wei-Bai-Du-Tang); Kampo medicine; Acne vulgaris; d-ROMs; BAP; Oxidative stress

## Introduction

Kampo medicine is a traditional Japanese medicine made by combining several kinds of medicinal herbs. It has spread widely as a treatment used in modern medical care in Japan and there are many Kampo medicines that are used for treating acne. On the other hand, drugs with various mechanisms of action such as antimicrobial agents, adapalene, and benzoyl peroxide have been developed as modern acne treatments and are being used around the world. However, the authors have come across patients whose acne was not improved by administration of such drugs. In our hospital, good results have been obtained by the oral intake of Jumihaidokuto (JHT) Kampo medicine in such cases [1]. Topically applied drugs are used as the basic treatments for acne, but it is considered that the oral administration of JHT has a systemic acne-improving effect that differs from the localized effects of topically applied drugs.

JHT is composed of 10 kinds of herbal medicines and can be widely applied to skin diseases such as acne, urticaria, and atopic dermatitis for its anti-inflammatory, antibacterial, pus discharging, and antipruritic actions. Previous research found that cherry bark, one of the constituent herbal medicines of JHT, had an estrogen production inducing effect, and suggested that estrogen healed acne by antagonizing testosterone, which is an exacerbator of sebum secretion [2]. The author uses JHT mainly to female acne patients, so that estrogen receptor expresses higher in female, and JHT is said to improve acne in female more effectively [3]. However, JHT is considered to have other mechanisms of action in addition to its estrogen production inducing effect, since it was observed to be equally effective in women of different ages and in menstruating and non-menstruating women in a previous survey conducted by the author [1]. Among these potential mechanisms of action, the authors focused on the antioxidative effect reported for antibacterial drugs such as minocycline [3] that are also taken orally as medicines for acne.

The involvement of oxidative stress in the development of acne has been pointed out before. Some reports have shown that xanthine oxidase, which mediates the generation of reactive oxygen species, and malondialdehyde, a marker of lipid peroxidation, were present at higher concentrations in the blood circulation of acne patients compared with healthy individuals [4,5]. In addition, the abundance of superoxide dismutase, an endogenous-antioxidant enzyme, was found to vary depending on the severity of acne [6]. These reports suggested that oxidative stress is a causative factor in the development and/or exacerbation of acne.

***Corresponding author:** Mayumi Nomoto, Department of Dermatology, Nomoto Mayumi Skincare Clinic, 1-3-7 Bandai, Chuo-ku, Niigata-shi, Niigata-ken-950-0088, Japan, E-mail: n.nomoto@beautifulskin.jp

Therefore, the authors focused on the involvement of oxidative stress in acne to reveal a new mechanism of action for JHT as a treatment for acne and studied the relationship between acne improvement and the antioxidative effect of JHT [7].

## Methods

### Participants

Fifty-three adult females aged 20-47 years (mean age 33 ± 8 years) with a diagnosed of acne vulgaris, participated in this study. The study was set at Nomoto Mayumi Skincare Clinic (Niigata-ken, Japan) between January 2014 and January 2015. The severity grade of acne by counting the inflammatory rashes [8] before the study was as follows: mild, 45 patients; moderate, 8 patients. Although these patients had only few rashes, they had strong inflammation and tend to recur. So, they are considered as a recalcitrant acne vulgaris patients who did not improve by standard acne treatments in other hospitals before.

The study was approved by the Ethics Committee of the Niigata University of Pharmacy and Applied Life Sciences (reference: H25-008). Data were collected from patients whose written consent was obtained after a complete explanation of the study procedures was provided to them.

### Intervention

A fine granular JHT extract obtained from Kracie Pharmaceutical, Ltd. was used as the study drug. The dose of 9 g/day, which corresponds to 1.5 times the normal dose, was divided into 3 administrations per day and was orally administered before or between meals for 3 weeks. The use of drugs other than JHT was prohibited for patients during the study. The author set the dose and duration with reference to the report of Takemura [9] which found that the dose of 9 g/day produced an improvement in the acne of patients with recalcitrant acne vulgaris for which the normal dose of JHT (6 g/day) was not sufficiently effective. In addition, a previous report by Nomoto [1] showed that administering 1.5 times the normal dose of JHT for 3 weeks resulted in an improvement in the acne of 79.5% (97/122) of cases with recalcitrant acne vulgaris.

Six grams of fine granular JHT extract contains 3.9 g of powdered extract obtained by hot water extraction after mixing the following 10 types of herbal medicines together: *Bupleurum* root (2.5 g), *Platycodon* root (2.5 g), *Cnidium* rhizome (2.5 g), *Poria* sclerotium (2.5 g), *Saposhnikovia* root (2.5 g), *Glycyrrhiza* root (1.5 g), Ginger (1.0 g), *Schizonepeta* spike (1.5 g), *Aralia* rhizome (1.5 g), and Pruni cortex (cherry bark) (2.5 g). The three-dimensional (3D) high performance liquid chromatography (HPLC) analysis of JHT is shown in Figure 1.

### Outcomes measures

The primary outcome for this study was to evaluate the effect of JHT on oxidative stress and antioxidative potency in acne patients. For secondary outcome, improvements of inflammatory and non-inflammatory rashes were evaluated.

Blood was collected at the start and end of the study, and then the diacron-reactive oxygen metabolites (d-ROMs) value of each sample

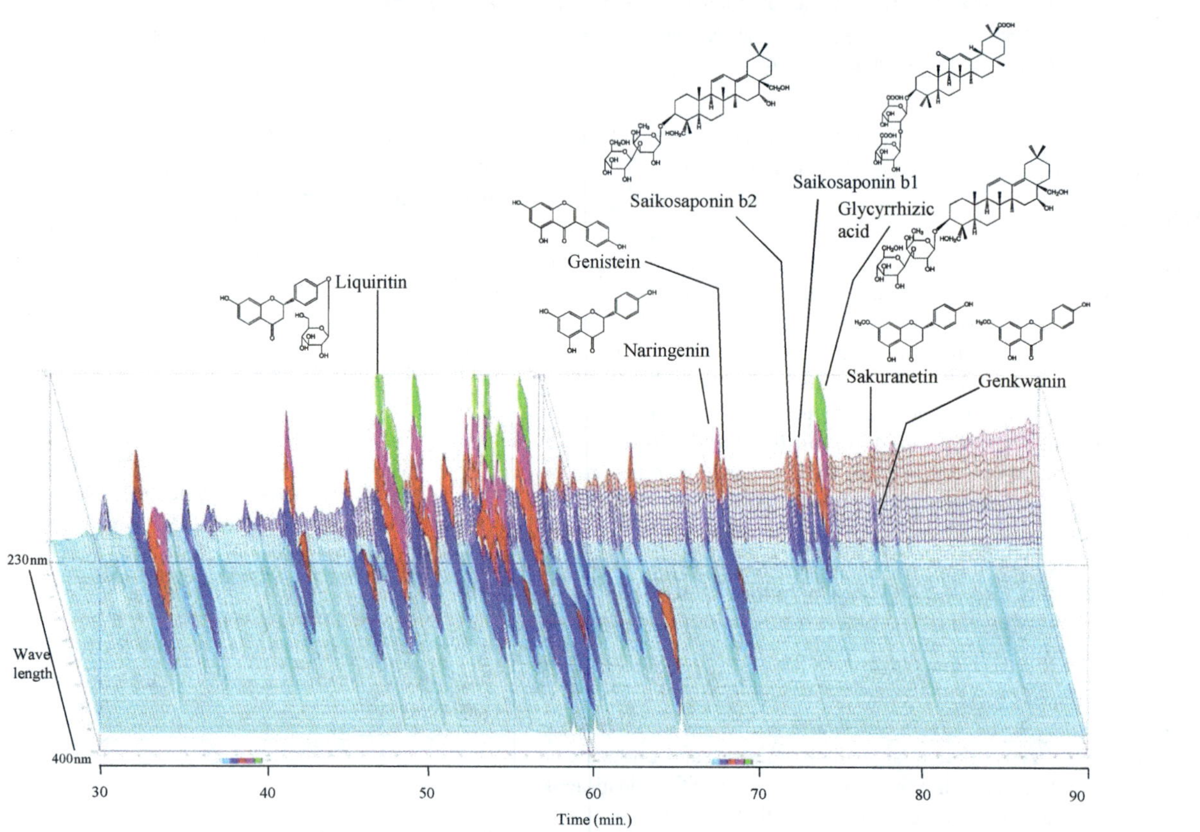


**Figure 1:** Typical 3D-HPLC chromatogram of JHT.

was measured as an indicator of oxidative stress and the biological antioxidant potential (BAP) value was measured as an indicator of antioxidative potency. The d-ROMs test measures the amount of hydroperoxide (R-OOH), which is a metabolite produced by active oxygen species and free radicals, in the sample via the colorimetric change of a chromogen. The d-ROMs value is represented by an arbitrary unit, U.CARR. The BAP test measures the ability of a sample to reduce trivalent iron ions ($Fe^{3+}$) to divalent iron ions ($Fe^{2+}$) and is represented by the unit μM. The degrees of oxidative stress corresponding to each range of d-ROMs values are as follows: normal, 200-300 U.CARR; borderline, 301-320 U.CARR; mild, 321-340 U.CARR; moderate, 341-400 U.CARR; high, 401-500 U.CARR; severe, ≥ 501 U.CARR [10]. The degrees of antioxidative potency corresponding to each range of BAP values are as follows: normal, ≥ 2200 μM; borderline, 2200 μM to 2000 μM; slightly low, 2000 μM to 1800 μM; low, 1800 μM to 1600 μM; very low, 1600 μM to 1400 μM; extremely low, ≤ 1400 μM [11]. Patients were classified into subgroups according to their d-ROMs and BAP values as follows. Based on their d-ROMs value at the start of the study, patients were divided into a d-ROMs normal group (≤ 320 U.CARR) and a d-ROMs high group (>320 U.CARR). Based on their BAP value at the start of the study, patients were also divided into a BAP normal group (>2000 μM) and a BAP low group (≤ 2000 μM).

Moreover, the numbers of inflammatory and non-inflammatory rashes at the start and end of the study were measured as an indicator of acne improvement. The changes in each measured value between the start and end of the study were indicated as "Δd-ROMs" for the change in d-ROMs value, "ΔBAP" for the change in BAP value, "Δnumber of inflammatory skin rashes" for the change in the number of inflammatory skin rashes, and "Δnumber of non-inflammatory skin rashes" for the change in the number of non-inflammatory skin rashes. Correlation analyses of Δd-ROMs and ΔBAP with Δnumber of inflammatory skin rashes and Δnumber of non-inflammatory skin rashes were performed to examine the relationships of the degree of oxidative stress and the degree of antioxidative potency with the improvement of acne rashes.

Furthermore, the patients were asked to grade their feelings about the changes in their acne symptoms by selecting from the choices of "improved", "no change", and "worsened" at the end of the study, compared with their feelings at the start of the study.

### Statistical analysis

Analysis was conducted based on non-parametric tests, since the data could not be confirmed to be normally distributed. All the results are represented by the median ± interquartile range. Utilizing Statcel 3 software (OMS Inc., Saitama, Japan) for statistical analysis, Wilcoxon's signed rank test was used for the evaluation of the d-ROMs values, BAP values, and the number of rashes before and after the administration of JHT, and Spearman's rank correlation test was used for correlation analyses. A probability value of less than 5% was considered significant.

## Results

### Patient characteristics

The patient characteristics are shown in Table 1.

### Effect of JHT administration on the d-ROMs and BAP values

**d-ROMs value:** In the analysis of all 53 cases, a significant reduction in the mean d-ROMs value was observed, with a change from 324 U.CARR at the start of the study to 313 U.CARR at the end of the study ($p<0.05$). The d-ROMs normal group showed no significant difference in the mean d-ROMs value between the start and end of the study, but the d-ROMs high group showed a significant reduction in the mean d-ROMs value at the end of the study compared with the value at the start of the study ($p<0.05$; Figure 2).

| Sex | No. of cases | % | Concomitant drugs | No. of cases | % |
|---|---|---|---|---|---|
| Male | 0 | 0 | Nil | 53 | 100 |
| Female | 53 | 100 | **Treatment history** | **No. of cases** | **%** |
| **Age** | **No. of cases** | **%** | Present | 11 | 20.8 |
| 20-29 | 24 | 45.3 | Nil | 42 | 79.2 |
| 30-39 | 14 | 26.4 | Tretinoin gel 0.05% | 3 | 5.7 |
| 40-49 | 15 | 28.3 | Adapalene gel 0.1% | 17 | 32.1 |
| **The main development site of acne** | **No. of cases** | **%** | Clindamycin phosphate lotion 1% | 12 | 22.6 |
| Entire face | 7 | 13.2 | Nadifloxacin cream 1% | 3 | 5.7 |
| Face line* | 27 | 50.9 | Clobetasone butyrate ointment 0.05% | 1 | 1.9 |
| Lower jaw | 16 | 30.2 | Sulfur and camphor lotion | 1 | 1.9 |
| Perioral | 7 | 13.2 | Minocycline | 25 | 47.2 |
| Buccal region | 9 | 17 | Clarithromycin | 4 | 7.5 |
| Forehead | 5 | 9.4 | Tosufloxacin | 2 | 3.8 |
| Nasal region | 2 | 3.8 | Doxycycline | 1 | 1.9 |
| Temple | 1 | 1.9 | Levofloxacin | 1 | 1.9 |
| Scalp | 1 | 1.9 | Roxithromycin | 1 | 1.9 |
| Chest | 2 | 3.8 | Vitamin C, calcium pantothenate formulation | 3 | 5.7 |
| Back | 4 | 7.5 | Tranexamic acid | 1 | 1.9 |
| *From the lower jaw to the neck | | | Low dose pill | 1 | 1.9 |
| | | | Tokishakuyakusan# | 2 | 3.8 |
| **The presence or absence of premenstrual worsening** | **No. of cases** | **%** | Keishibukuryogan# | 1 | 1.9 |
| Present | 26 | 49.1 | Keishibukuryogankayokuinin# | 1 | 1.9 |
| Nil | 12 | 22.6 | Jumihaidokuto# | 1 | 1.9 |
| Unknown | 15 | 28.3 | Seijobofuto# | 1 | 1.9 |
| | | | #These are Kampo medicines | | |

**Table 1:** Patient characteristics.

**BAP value:** In the analysis of all 53 cases, no significant difference in the mean BAP value was observed, with a change from 2117 μM at the start of the study to 2144 μM at the end of the study (p=0.6). The BAP normal group showed no significant difference in the mean BAP value between the start and end of the study, but the BAP low group showed a significant increase in the mean BAP value at the end of the study compared with that at the start of the study (p<0.05; Figure 3).

### Effect of JHT administration on the numbers of skin rashes

A significant decrease was observed in the numbers of inflammatory and non-inflammatory skin rashes at the end of the study, compared with the corresponding numbers at the start of the study (p<0.01 and p<0.05, respectively; Figure 4).

### Correlation analyses of the d-ROMs and BAP values with the numbers of skin rashes

A significant correlation was observed between Δd-ROMs and Δnumber of non-inflammatory skin rashes (rs=0.61, p<0.01; Table 2).

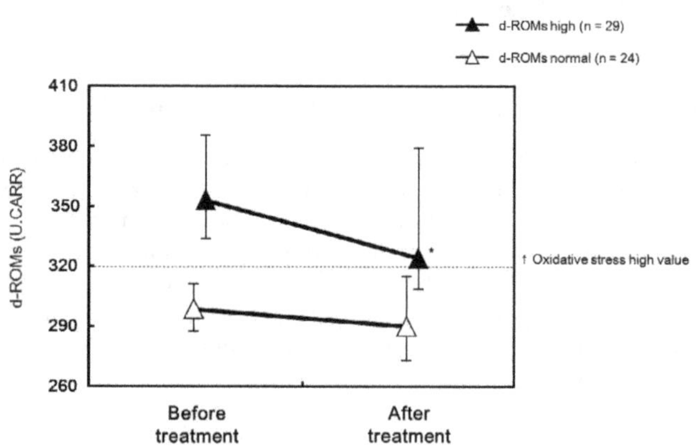


**Figure 2:** Effect of JHT administration on d-ROMs (oxidative stress). The cases were divided into 2 groups (d-ROMs high and d-ROMs normal) and were evaluated for change in the d-ROMs values before and after the administration of JHT. Results are presented as median ± interquartile range. Statistical analysis was performed using Wilcoxon's signed rank test (*p<0.05, *vs* before treatment).

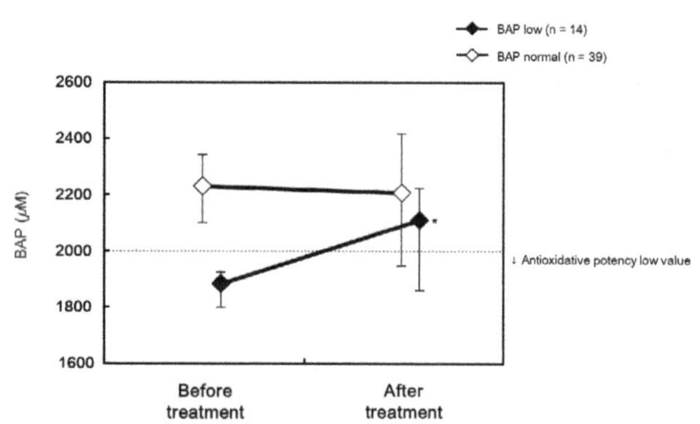


**Figure 3:** Effect of JHT administration on BAP (anti-oxidative potency). The cases were divided into 2 groups (BAP low and BAP normal) and were evaluated for change in the BAP values before and after the administration of JHT. Results are presented as median ± interquartile range. Statistical analysis was performed using Wilcoxon's signed rank test (*p<0.05, *vs* before treatment).

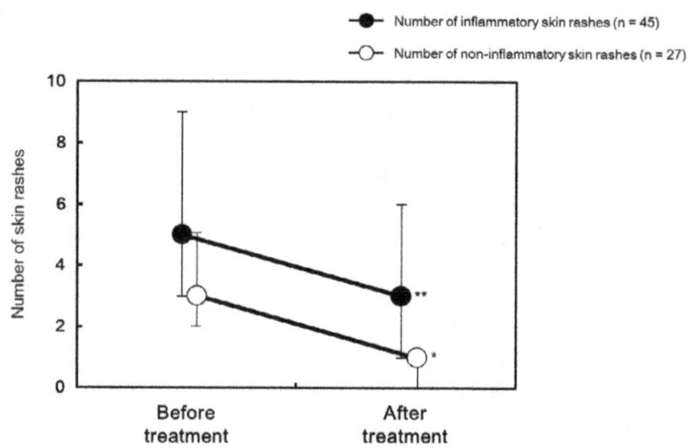


**Figure 4:** Effect of JHT administration on the numbers of skin rashes. The change of the number of inflammatory skin rashes and non-inflammatory rashes before and after the administration of JHT was evaluated. Results are presented as median ± interquartile range. Statistical analysis was performed using Wilcoxon's signed rank test (*p<0.05, **p<0.01, vs before treatment).

### Relationship between the subjective degree of improvement of acne and the d-ROMs value after the administration of JHT

Among all, 48 patients were able to evaluate their grade of feelings. The group of subjects who rated their acne as "improved" at the end of the study showed a significant decrease in the mean d-ROMs value at the end of the study, compared with that at the start of the study (p<0.01; Figure 5).

## Discussion

The antibacterial effect of JHT against *Propionibacterium acnes* (*P. acnes*) has been reported before [12], and it has been mainly used to treat acne due to its antibacterial property. Moreover, it has been reported that cherry bark, an herbal medicine that has recently begun to commonly be blended into JHT, has the ability to bind estrogen receptor β and can also enhance estradiol production by dermal fibroblasts [3,13]. That is, JHT blended with cherry bark locally enhances estrogen secretion in skin and acts antagonistically with respect to testosterone. There is a study that JHT and cherry bark suppressed the promotion of sebum secretion induced by testosterone *in vitro* [14]. Furthermore, clinical data was reported for 44 female patients with acne. In those cases, improvements in the symptoms of red papules, white papules, and pustules were observed after a 12-week combined treatment with JHT extract and a topical antimicrobial drug, resulting in a 77.3% cumulative improvement rate [3].

An effect that differs from those of the topical treatment drugs primarily used for acne treatment can be expected from JHT, since it is considered to be effective for acne due to its antibacterial effect and its systemic estrogen production inducing effect. One of the effects considered is a beneficial change in the constitution of subjects who are vulnerable to acne development [1]. The estrogen induction promoting effect of JHT might contribute to the inhibition of sebum secretion at the early stage of acne development, but JHT is considered to have other effects in addition to inducing estrogen production, since its effectiveness was observed regardless of the age and menstruation status of female subjects in a previous survey conducted by the authors [1].

Acne has a significant emotional impact in addition to its physical symptoms, since it tends to develop on the faces of the younger

| Spearman's rank correlation test | Δd-ROMs | ΔBAP |
|---|---|---|
| ΔNumber of inflammatory skin rashes | 0.07 | 0.04 |
| ΔNumber of non-inflammatory skin rashes | 0.61** | -0.24 |

**Table 2:** Correlation analyses of the d-ROMs and BAP values with the numbers of skin rashes. Correlation analyses of the changes in the d-ROMs and BAP values (Δd-ROMs and ΔBAP) and the changes in the numbers of inflammatory and non-inflammatory skin rashes (Δnumber of inflammatory skin rashes and Δnumber of non-inflammatory skin rashes) before and after administration of JHT. Statistical analysis was performed using Spearman's rank correlation test (**p<0.01, rs).

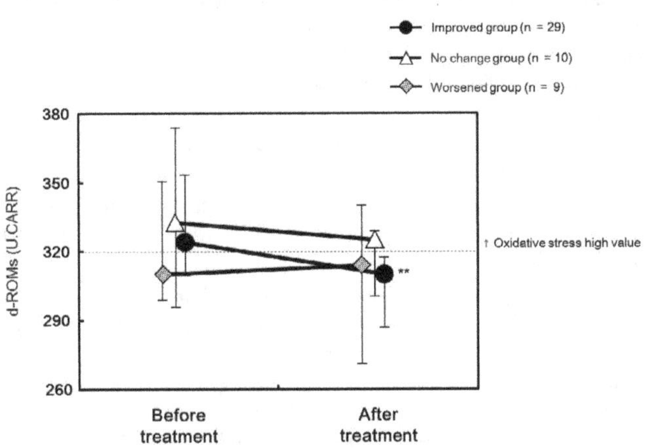


**Figure 5:** Relationship between the degree of subjective improvement of acne and the d-ROMs value after the administration of JHT. The patients were divided into 3 groups ("improved", "no change", and "worsened") based on their subjective ratings of the degree of improvement in their symptoms of acne, and the changes in their d-ROMs values before and after JHT administration were evaluated. Results are presented as median ± interquartile range. Statistical analysis was performed using Wilcoxon's signed rank test (**p<0.01, vs before treatment).

generation, who are concerned about their appearance [15]. It is considered that oxidative stress is closely related to acne since prolonged acne leads to psychological stress, which promotes the generation of active oxygen species [16] and reduces the activity of antioxidants [17].

The experience of the authors that JHT was effective for the treatment of acne in cases where the involvement of psychological stress was suggested indicates that JHT might correct the heightened oxidative stress typical of acne and contribute to acne improvement partly via a systemic antioxidative effect. Focusing on oxidative stress, this study produced the following results: the d-ROMs high group showed a significant reduction in the mean d-ROMs value after the administration of JHT, while the BAP low group showed a significant increase in the mean BAP value. Kampo medicines have traditionally been used to correct disturbances in immune function [18], the autonomic nervous system [19], and the endocrine balance of living organisms [20], and the present results suggest that JHT, via its antioxidative effect, can correct the heightened oxidative stress that typically occurs in patients with acne. JHT has previously been found to have an antioxidative effect by in vitro and in vivo studies [21,22]. According to the *in vivo* study, numerous polyphenols of JHT, such as genistein and liquiritigenin are prone to inhibit dermatitis via antioxidative effect [22]. However, the present study is the first to have revealed that JHT administration has an impact solely on patient groups in which abnormalities of oxidative stress level and antioxidative potency were observed in the blood circulation at baseline. On the other hand, no significant changes were observed in the d-ROMs normal and BAP normal groups between before and after JHT administration. However, acne vulgaris is a chronic inflammatory disease, and the degree of oxidative stress that people experience is expected to be constantly changing in modern society. Even if the degree of oxidative stress of a patient is normal when it is measured, continuous administration of JHT might help to control the fluctuations of oxidative stress that occur as a result of environmental stresses.

Another novel finding in this study was the observation of a significant correlation between the change in the d-ROMs value and the number of non-inflammatory skin rashes between before and after the administration of JHT. There have been some reports confirming a relationship between oxidative stress and inflammatory skin rashes [4,23], but the level of knowledge about the relationship between oxidative stress and non-inflammatory skin rashes is sparse. The accumulation of sebum in hair follicles that is observed with non-inflammatory skin rashes (pimples) involves several processes such as 1) enhancement of sebum secretion by testosterone, 2) reduction in the concentration of linolenic acid in sebum, 3) production of lipid peroxides by oxidation of sebum components such as squalene, 4) production of inflammatory cytokines such as interleukin (IL)-1α by lipid peroxides, and 5) dyskeratosis of the hair follicle funnel due to the effects of inflammatory cytokines [24,25]. In this series of processes, increased oxidative stress is suggested to be related to the oxidation of sebum components. For example, a previous report stated that squalene, a component of sebum, is susceptible to oxidation by oxygen and ultraviolet rays, and that squalene peroxide promotes pimple formation [26]. It has been also reported that squalene enhances the keratinization of the skin [27]. These reports suggest that squalene present in sebum and its peroxide are involved in the development of acne. Therefore, it can be inferred that JHT may improve pimples by inhibiting the oxidation of sebum via its antioxidative effect.

In the present study, the authors focused on the antioxidative effect of JHT, but antioxidative effects have also been reported for other acne treatment drugs. For example, vitamin C preparations for external and internal use and oral antibiotics such as minocycline have been revealed to have antioxidative effects [4]. Additional research is required in the future to identify the differences in the antioxidative effect of these drugs and JHT, but it can be inferred that JHT, a medicinal preparation consisting of multiple herbal components, has a unique mechanism of action, such as an ability to act against abnormally high levels of oxidative stress and to improve non-inflammatory skin rashes. Moreover, minocycline is mainly used for inflammatory skin rashes, and its administration at the pimple stage, which is the initial condition of acne, is not recommended since it can induce bacterial antimicrobial resistance of bacteria [28]. In contrast, JHT does not have any comparable problem of inducing bacterial resistance [12], and it has the advantage that its oral intake can be continued for a long time. Also, based on the findings of the present study, which revealed that a reduction of oxidative stress helps to reduce the number of pimples, JHT might contribute to a change in the constitution of treated patients towards greater resistance to acne by maintaining a normal level of oxidative stress through its continuous oral intake.

On the other hand, the present study showed a significant decrease in the number of inflammatory skin rashes following the administration of JHT, but no correlation with the decrease in oxidative stress was observed. The reasons for this are considered to be as follows. The direct cause for the development of inflammatory skin rashes is the stimulation of skin by active oxygen species and inflammatory cytokines derived from neutrophils that have migrated and been activated by *P. acnes* [4]. Therefore, the administration of an antioxidant for removing the active oxygen species is considered to be effective in improving inflammatory skin rashes. In fact, it has been reported that skin rashes were reduced when metronidazole, which has an antioxidative effect but no antibacterial effect, was administered to patients with inflammatory acne [29]. In contrast, the reason why there was no correlation between the reduction of oxidative stress in the blood due to JHT and the improvement of skin rashes is considered to be that processes such as the increased amounts of sebum secretion, lipid peroxidation, dyskeratosis, *P. acnes*, and free fatty acid occur before activated oxygen species are released from the neutrophils. JHT and its constituent herbal medicines have been reported to have various effects such as estrogen secretion enhancing effect, 5α-reductase inhibiting effect, antibacterial effect against *P. acnes*, lipase inhibiting effect, and toll-like receptor (TLR) 2 suppressing effect [12,13,30,31], in addition to the antioxidative effect revealed in this study. Therefore, it is presumed that not only its antioxidative effect, but also the various other effects of JHT comprehensively contribute to the improvement of inflammatory skin rashes.

In addition, in this study, a survey of the subjective degree of acne improvement was performed by interviewing the patients as well. The results showed a significant reduction in the mean d-ROMs value of the patient subgroup who felt that their acne was "improved" after JHT administration. This may be because a decrease in the level of oxidative stress in the blood was caused by a reduction in the patient's psychological stress, whereas there is also the possibility that the reduction in oxidative stress resulted in the improvement of acne.

The authors would like to further investigate the mechanisms of action of JHT in the future using a comprehensive digital skin image analysis system (VISIA Evolution, Canfield Scientific, Fairfield, NJ, USA).

## Conclusions

The findings of this study indicate that the Kampo medicine Jumihaidokuto can be expected to improve acne via a systemic antioxidative effect that cannot be obtained using topical acne treatment drugs, and also to alter the constitution of patients to make them less vulnerable to the development of acne.

## References

1. Nomoto M (2015) The Effect of Jumihaidokuto (Shi-Wei-Bai-Du-Tang) Containing Cherry Bark (Pruni cortex) on Refractory Acne Vulgaris: Short-term, High-Dose Administration. Nishinihon J Dermatol 77: 259-263.
2. Tohno H, Horii C, Fuse T, Okonogi A, Yomoda S (2010) Evaluation of estrogen receptor Beta binding of pruni cortex and its constituents. Yakugaku Zasshi 130: 989-997.
3. Takemura T, Tohno H, Yomoda S, Okubo T (2014) Mechanism of Action of Cherry Bark-containing Jumihaidokuto (Shi-Wei-Bai-Du-Tang) and Its Clinical Benefit in Patients with Acne Vulgaris. Nishinihon J Dermatol 76: 140-146.
4. Akamatsu H, Horio T, Hattori K (2003) Increased hydrogen peroxide generation by neutrophils from patients with acne inflammation. Int J Dermatol 42: 366-369.
5. Sarici G, Cinar S, Armutcu F, Altinyazar C, Koca R, et al. (2010) Oxidative stress in acne vulgaris. J Eur Acad Dermatol Venereol 24: 763-767.
6. Perihan O, Ergul KB, Neslihan D, Filiz A (2012) The activity of adenosine deaminase and oxidative stress biomarkers in scraping samples of acne lesions. J Cosmet Dermatol 11: 323-328.
7. Abdel Fattah NS, Shaheen MA, Ebrahim AA, El Okda ES (2008) Tissue and blood superoxide dismutase activities and malondialdehyde levels in different severities of acne vulgaris. Br J Dermatol 159: 1086-1091.
8. Adityan B, Kumari R, Thappa DM (2009) Scoring systems in acne vulgaris. Indian J Dermatol Venereol Leprol 75: 323-326.
9. Takemura T (2011) The Effect of Jumihaidokuto (Shi-Wei-Bai-Du-Tang) Containing Cherry Bark (Pruni cortex) on Female with Acne Vulgaris: High-Dose Administration study. Phil Kampo 34: 18-19.
10. Seki Y (2009) Evaluation of total oxidative stress by d-ROMs testing. J Anal Bio Sci 32: 301-306.
11. Tanaka I, Kitagawa M (2014) Changes in oxidative stress and antioxidative potency during pregnancy period. J Jpn Acad Midwif 28: 51-59.
12. Higaki S, Nakamura M, Morohashi M, Hasegawa Y, Yamagishi T (1996) Activity of Eleven Kampo Formulations and Eight Kampo Crude Drugs against Propionibacterium acnes Isolated from Acne Patients: Retrospective Evaluation in 1990 and 1995. J Dermatol 23: 871-875.
13. Tohno H, Yomoda S, Takemura T (2014) Significance of cherry bark-formulation in Jumihaidokuto (Shi-Wei-Bai-Du-Tang) for acne vulgaris treatment. BIO Clinica 3: 124-131.
14. Shinohara K, Fujita N (2016) The Effect of Jumihaidokuto (Shi-Wei-Bai-Du-Tang) and Cherry Bark (Pruni cortex) on sebum synthesis. Jpn J Med Pharm Sci 73: 579-583.
15. Hayashi N, Higaki Y, Kawamoto K, Kamo T, Shimizu S, et al. (2004) A cross-sectional analysis of quality of life in Japanese acne patients using the Japanese version of Skindex-16. J Dermatol 31: 971-976.
16. Atanackovic D, Brunner-Weinzierl MC, Kröger H, Serke S, Deter HC (2002) Acute Psychological Stress Simultaneously Alters Hormone Levels, Recruitment of Lymphocyte Subsets, and Production of Reactive Oxygen Species. Immunol Invest 31: 73-91.
17. Tochio T, Morichi E, Hirose O, Nakata S, Kuze J (2008) Makeup Inhibits Reduction of Reactive Oxygen Scavenging Enzyme Activity Induced by Mental Stress. J Soc Cosmet Chem Jpn 42: 121-127.
18. Kobayashi H, Ishii M, Takeuchi S, Tanaka Y, Shintani T, et al. (2010) Efficacy and Safety of a Traditional Herbal Medicine, Hochu-ekki-to in the Long-term Management of Kikyo (Delicate Constitution) Patients with Atopic Dermatitis: A 6-month, Multicenter, Double-blind, Randomized, Placebo-controlled Study. eCAM 7: 367-373.
19. Okahara K, Ishida Y, Hayashi Y, Inoue T, Tsuruta K, et al. (2010) Effects of Yokukansan on behavioral and psychological symptoms of dementia in regular treatment for Alzheimer's disease. Prog Neuropsychopharmacol Biol Psychiatry 34: 532-536.
20. Okamoto M, Sakakibara H, Yoshida H, Fukazawa Y, Takashima K, et al. (2010) Effects of Saireito on the ovarian function of patients with polycystic ovary syndrome. Reprod Med Biol 9: 191-195.
21. Nakanishi T, Inoue K (2011) Antioxidant Potential of Jumihaidokuto. Kampo New Ther 20: 89-91.
22. Matsumoto T, Matsubara Y, Mizuhara Y, Sekiguchi K, Koseki J, et al. (2015) Plasma Pharmacokinetics of Polyphenols in a Traditional Japanese Medicine, Jumihaidokuto, Which Suppresses Propionibacterium acnes-Induced Dermatitis in Rats. Molecules 20: 18031-18046.
23. Arican O, Kurutas EB, Sasmaz S (2005) Oxidative stress in patients with acne vulgaris. Mediators Inflamm 2005: 380-384.
24. Kurokawa I, Danby FW, Ju Q, Wang X, Xiang LF, et al. (2009) New developments in our understanding of acne pathogenesis and treatment. Exp Dermatol 18: 821-832.
25. Kurokawa I (2014) The Role of Hyperkeratinization. Pathogenesis and Treatment of Acne and Rosacea 3: 71-76.
26. Saint-Leger D, Bague A, Lefebvre E, Cohen E, Chivot M (1986) A possible role for squalene in the pathogenesis of acne. II. In vivo study of squalene oxides in skin surface and intra-comedonal lipids of acne patients. Br J Dermatol 114: 543-552.
27. Motoyoshi K (1983) Enhanced comedo formation in rabbit ear skin by squalene and oleic acid peroxides. Br J Dermatol 109: 191-198.

28. Thiboutot D, Gollnick H, Bettoli V, Dréno B, Kang S, et al. (2009) New insights into the management of acne: an update from the Global Alliance to Improve Outcomes in Acne group. J Am Acad Dermatol 60: S1-S50.

29. Oguchi M, Akamatsu H, Asada M, Kubo K, Namura S, et al. (1987) Treatment of acne with oral metronidazole. Skin Res 29: 995-1000.

30. Higaki S, Hasegawa Y, Toyomoto R, Miyazaki K, Masaaki M, et al. (1993) The Anti-lipase Activities of Jumi-Haidoku-To and Minocycline Against Propionibacterium acnes. Jpn J Dermatol 103: 33-37.

31. Kaneko A, Sekiguchi K, Osegi J, Nishimura H, Hattori T, et al. (2014) Multi Targeting Action of Jumihaidokuto (Shi-Wei-Bai-Du-Tang) against Acne Vulgaris. J New Rem Clin 63: 38-49.

# 26

# Effects of Yoga on Dysmenorrhea: A Systematic Review of Randomized Controlled Trials

**Hyun-Nam Ko**[1], **Sam-Sun Le**[2] **and Sang-Dol Kim**[3*]

[1]*Department of Nursing, Jinju Health College, Jinju, Republic of Korea*

[2]*Department of Nursing, Koje College, Koje, Republic of Korea*

[3]*Department of Nursing, College of Health Science, Kangwon National University, Samcheok-si, Republic of Korea*

[*]**Corresponding author:** Sang-Dol Kim, Department of Nursing, College of Health Science, Kangwon National University: 346 Hwangjo-gil, Dogye-eup, Samcheok-si, Gangwon-do 245-907, Republic of Korea, E-mail: nu11110@kangwon.ac.kr

## Abstract

**Objectives:** To assess the evidence for the effectiveness of yoga in the management of menstrual pain and the symptoms associated with dysmenorrhea.

**Methods:** A search was conducted using CINAHL, the Cochrane library, Embase, PsycINFO, PubMed, and KoreaMed electronic databases to identify randomized controlled trials (RCTs) reported effects of yogic intervention on dysmenorrhea published in any language between January 1966 and October 2014. Quality assessment was conducted using the Cochrane risk of bias tool.

**Results:** Two potential trials were identified of which two were included in the review. Quality critical appraisal had low or moderate risk of bias. The available data could only be included as a narrative description. A significant difference was observed between experimental and control groups in pain intensity and pain duration ($p<0.05$) and thyroid-stimulating hormone ($p<0.002$), follicle-stimulating hormone ($p<0.02$), luteinizing hormone ($p<0.001$), and prolactin ($p<0.02$) were decreased significantly in the experimental group, compared with the control group.

**Conclusions:** There is evidence from two RCTs that yoga interventions may be favorable effective for dysmenorrhea. However the findings should be interpreted with caution due to the number of small RCTs and quality limitation partly. Therefore further high quality RCTs are required to investigate the hypothesis that yoga alleviates menstrual pain and the symptoms associated with dysmenorrhea, to confirm and further comprehend the effects of standardized yoga programs in dysmenorrhea.

**Keywords:** Dysmenorrhea; Yoga; Systematic review

**Abbreviations:** CONSORT: Consolidated Standards of Reporting Trials; IUCD: Intra-Uterine Contraceptive Device; OCP: Oral Contraceptive Pills; RCTs: Randomized Controlled Trials; VAS: Visual Analogue Scale

## Introduction

Although the prevalence of dysmenorrhea varied in range from 25% of menstruating women to 90% of adolescent females or 45% to 95% of any age, dysmenorrhea seems to be the most common gynecological condition in women, regardless of age, race, or nationality [1-4]. Furthermore, dysmenorrhea is a critical global health issue in reproductive age women, as it causes school absences, poor academic performance, lost work time, and has a significantly negative affect on daily activities [5,6]. Dysmenorrhea is generally defined as difficult monthly flow and describes painful menstruation of uterine origin [2,7].

Dysmenorrhea can be classified into two subtypes. The pathogenesis of primary dysmenorrhea is commonly explained by "an abnormal increase in vasoactive prostaglandins originating in secretory endometrium and menstrual fluid, which may induce myometrial hyperactivity and uterine tissue ischemia and pain" [8,9].

In addition, various psychological problems have also been proposed [8,9]. Secondary dysmenorrhea can occur many years after menarche and is associated with identifiable pelvic pathology such as endometriosis [8,9].

Dysmenorrhea is characterized by cramping lower abdominal pain that may radiate to the lower back and upper thighs and is commonly associated with nausea, headache, fatigue, diarrhea, lethargy, breast tenderness and emotional symptoms [5-7,10].

Dysmenorrhea is usually treated with drugs such as oral contraceptive pills or non-steroid anti- inflammatory drugs [2,10]. A variety of alternatives for dysmenorrhea, such as transcutaneous electrical nerve stimulation, acupuncture, acupressure, topical heat, behavioral interventions, relaxation, and herbal and dietary therapies, are increasingly growing in attention [2,8,11,12].

A growing body of evidence supports the belief that yoga benefits physical and mental health via down-regulation of the hypothalamic-pituitary-adrenal axis and the sympathetic nervous system [13,14]. Yoga may be a safe and cost-effective intervention for managing menstrual problems [9]. Yoga plays an important role in reducing stress and sympathetic activity, increasing parasympathetic activity, improving one's quality of life, and decreasing psychological symptoms levels [3-19].

As stated, there is evidence for the benefit of yoga in reducing pain and symptoms of dysmenorrhea. However, the quality of the evidence deeds to be examined to establish whether or not we can advocate yoga as an alternative and complementary therapy for women with painful periods. Therefore, the aim of this review is to assess the evidence for the effectiveness of yoga in the management of menstrual pain and the symptoms associated with dysmenorrhea.

## Methods

### Search strategy

The review was planned and conducted in accordance with Consolidated Standards of Reporting Trials (CONSORT) guidelines for Reporting Parallel Group Randomized Trials [20]. We searched CINAHL, Cochrane Library, Embase, PsycINFO, PubMed, and KoreaMed electronic databases to identify RCTs published through October 2014. Our search terms were as follows: (1) yoga ("yoga" or "yoga nidra") and (2) dysmenorrhea ("dysmenorrhea" or "menstrual cramps" or "menstrual pain").

We manually searched the reference lists by 'footnote chasing' to identify any additional studies relevant to our analysis. Two independent investigators reviewed all the articles from the previous search based on the following selection criteria. Statistical practitioners trained these researchers in systematic review methods and meta-analytic operations. All potentially eligible studies were retrieved and the full-text articles were reviewed to determine whether they met the inclusion criteria.

To be eligible, studies had to meet the following conditions. The inclusion criteria was evaluated by two researchers independently using the criteria recommended by the Cochrane Menstrual Disorders and Subfertility Group and the Consolidated Standards of Reporting Trials [7,12,20]:

**Population:** Women in the trials had to meet all the following inclusion criteria for the trial to be included in the review: dysmenorrhea (pain affecting daily activity or with a high baseline score); dysmenorrhea in the majority (>50%) of menstrual cycles; dysmenorrhea for at least one day of menses; of reproductive age; primary or secondary dysmenorrhea. If participants in the trial met any of the exclusion criteria, the trial was not included in the review: With irregular or infrequent menstrual cycles (usually outside of the typical range of a 21 to 35 day cycle); using an intra-uterine contraceptive device (IUCD) or taking oral contraceptive pills (OCP).

**Intervention:** Randomized controlled trials were included that used yoga as an intervention to review or reduce symptoms associated with dysmenorrhea compared with no yoga.

**Comparison:** Any randomized controlled trials (RCTs) comparing yoga (as treatment) for dysmenorrhea versus no yoga;

**Outcomes:** Primary outcomes were; (1) pain relief (measured either by a visual analogue scale (VAS), other scale (menstrual disorders questionnaire), or dichotomous outcome (i.e. pain relief yes or no), (2) overall improvement in symptoms (measured by changes in dysmenorrhea symptoms, either self-reported or investigator-observed treatment effectiveness, or other similar measures), (3) pathophysiological parameters improvement (measured by change in hormone levels, serum homocysteine and nitric oxide levels etc.), (4) adverse effects from treatment (incidence and type of side effects).

Secondary outcomes were; (1) restriction of daily life activities (measured as the proportion of women who reported activity), (2) absence from work or school (measured as the proportion of women reporting absences from work or school, and also as hours or days of absence as a more selective measure), (3) requirement for medication additional to assigned treatment (measured as a proportion of requiring analgesics additional to their assigned treatment).

### Quality assessment

Two reviewers independently conducted assessments using a critical appraisal Cochrane risk of bias tool RCTs, which was recommended by the Cochrane Handbook for systematic Reviews of Interventions [21]. The Cochrane risk of bias tool is a six-item list designed to assess sequence generation, allocation concealment, blinding, incomplete outcome data, selective outcome reporting, and other potential sources of bias. Each item was rated as "yes," "no," or "unclear".

According to the Cochrane Handbook, quality of clinical trials can divided into three levels. If the study design fully met the preceding six criteria, it is considered A level, which means the low risk of bias. B level would be assigned when one or more criteria were partly met.

If one or more criteria were not met, the study would be defined as C level, implying high risk of bias. Studies rated as C level would be eliminated. Any disagreements were resolved by reviewers' discussion.

### Data synthesis

No meta-analysis was performed as only two studies were identified due to heterogeneity among the included studies. Data are presented descriptively as no usable data were available.

## Results

### Study description

A total of 1,120 titles related to our search terms were screened. Among these, there were 1,025 potential trials identified from CHINAL, 5 from the Cochrane Library, 61 from KoreaMed, 6 from PsycINFO and 23 from the PubMed databases.

After the titles were retrieved a total of 257 studies were excluded either because they were duplicates or they were newsletters, commentaries or no target concepts which mean no dysmenorrhea.

The remaining 863 abstracts were retrieved. After assessing the abstracts, 858 studies were excluded because there was no yoga intervention. Five potential trials were identified in the search conducted in October 2014.

Five potentially relevant papers were retrieved for evaluation of full text. After the five full text assessment, three studies were excluded because two of them did not meet the selection criteria and one had no randomized trial. Figure 1 depicts the literature retrieval process. Characteristics of the included studies are presented in Table 1.

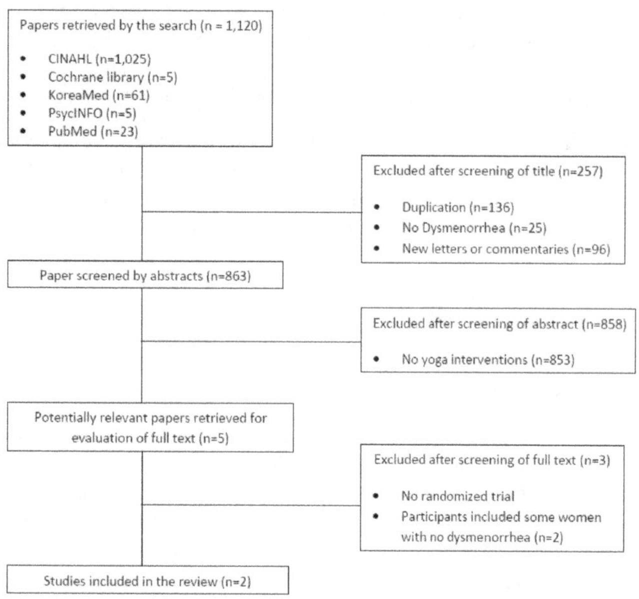


**Figure 1:** Flowchart of included studies through the literature searches.

## Participants and settings

One RCTs originated in India and another from Iran. Studies were conducted at a medical university or university midwifery department. Participants were recruited from obstetrics and gynecological departments or by interviews at a university. Sample sizes in the 2 studies ranged from 92 to 126 participants and totaled 218 participants. Participants' mean age ranged from 18.0 years to 28.5 years with a median of 23.2 years. Participants had a primary dysmenorrhea in 1 RCT and menstrual abnormalities such as pathological amenorrhea, dysmenorrhea, oligomenorrhea, polymenorrhea, menorrhagia, metrorrhagia, and hypomenorrhea in 1 RCT.

## Design and intervention

Two RCTs were identified in this review. Yoga traditions were heterogeneous between studies: 1 RCT used three poses and 1 RCT used yoga nidra. One yoga program included yoga postures such as cobra, cat and fish while the other program included resolve, rotation of consciousness, awareness of the breath, feeling and sensation, visualization, and ending the practice with resolve. Program length, frequency, and duration of one trial was one 20 min session a day for 14 days, another trial was 35 min to 40 min session a day, 5 days per week for 6 months. Yoga was performed under the guidance and supervision of yoga experts and faculty members in one trial, while another trial used a booklet with level to level explanations along with movements and breathing. One RCT compared yoga to no treatment and another RCT compared yoga nidra with conventional medication to conventional medication only.

## Outcomes

Two studies were identified that compared a control group with a yoga intervention group and evaluated the effect on dysmenorrhea. The available data could only be included as a narrative description. A significant difference was observed between experimental and control groups in pain intensity and pain duration ($p<0.05$). Thyroid-stimulating hormone ($p<0.002$), follicle-stimulating hormone ($p<0.02$), luteinizing hormone ($p<0.001$), and prolactin ($p<0.02$) were decreased significantly in the intervention group, compared with the control group. Neither included trial reported data on overall improvement in symptoms, adverse effects of treatment, restriction of daily activities, or absence from work or school etc.

## Critical appraisal of quality

Assessments on each methodological quality item for all included trials are described in Table 1. Of two trials, one trial was quality level A, another trial was quality level B.

# Discussion

The purpose of this review was to assess the evidence for the effectiveness of any yoga interventions for the primary or secondary dysmenorrhea when compared to no yoga. A meta-analysis combining results from all the trials were not feasible due to only two identified studies and heterogeneity among them. Data were reported descriptively as no usable data were available.

Only two RCTs were identified and included in this review. Interventions included yoga pose and yoga nidra to manage menstrual pain and symptoms [3,4]. Of the two, one trial reported a significant decrease in pain intensity and pain duration during the menstrual phase of the trained group. The other trial reported a significant decrease in hormone levels such as thyroid-stimulating hormone, follicle-stimulating hormone, luteinizing hormone, and prolactin in the intervention group compared to the control group. This study also stated that after yoga nidra practice, menstrual symptoms such as painful cramps, heavy bleeding, and irregular periods were relieved in participants. Wonderfully, the symptoms were also reduced in both groups. The mechanism behind yoga effectiveness for dysmenorrhea is still unclear. However, in spite of both groups having received medication, reductions of the symptoms in the yoga group were higher than in the control group. Therefore, these results support yoga practice as a positive manager of menstrual pain and dysmenorrhea symptoms.

According to the mechanism which an abnormal increase in vasoactive prostanoids in the endometrium and menstrual fluid may induce myometrial hyperactivity and tissue ischemia subsequently [2,4,8,22,23], a yoga intervention improves blood flow at the pelvic level as well as stimulating the release of B endorphine acting as non-specific analgesics [4]. In addition, another study reported that yoga poses improve spinal flexibility and strengthens muscles in the back and yoga nidra means psychic sleep which may induce deep relaxation and, subsequently decrease oxygen consumption causing pain relief [11,18,22,24].

Besides, these results support research findings demonstrating that relaxation training is an effective treatment for spasmodic dysmenorrhea or producing improvements in general measures of dysmenorrhea [25]. As stated, these reviewers identified the two RCTs in this review as having evidence for the favorable effectiveness of yoga on dysmenorrhea management.

| Study, year, location | Participants | Interventions | | Outcome measures | Main results | Adverse events | Limitations |
|---|---|---|---|---|---|---|---|
| | | Experimental group | Control group | | | | |
| | Population<br>Sample size (N;EG, CG)<br>Mean age (age range)<br>Drop out n (%) | Interventions<br>Delivery method<br>Duration<br>Interventionist | | | | | |
| Rani et al. [9],<br>India/Uttar Pradesh | University students with menstrual disorders<br>N=126 (EG: 65, CG: 61)<br>28 years (-)<br>24 (31.9) | Yoga nidra+Conventional medication<br>35 min to 40 min per day, 5 days per week in the morning<br>6 months<br>Yoga experts and faculty members | only Conventional<br>medication | Pathophysiological parameters<br>TSH<br>FSH<br>LH<br>Prolactin<br>Progesterone<br>Estradiol<br>Testosterone<br>DHEA-S | TSH ($p<0.002$), FSH ($p<0.02$), LH ($p<0.001$), and Prolactin ($p<0.02$) significantly decreased after yoga nidra practice when compared with the control group. | None | All menstrual disorders were included.<br>The sample size was not large enough to analysis hypo and hypermenorrhic subgroup separately.<br>The phase of the menstrual cycle was based on the participant's reports not on ultrasound scans. |
| Rakhshaee [11],<br>Iran/Rasht | University students with primary dysmenorrhea<br>N=92 (EG: 50, CG: 42)<br>20 years (18-22)<br>28 (30.4) | Yoga movement with cobra, Cat, and<br>fish poses<br>120 min per day,<br>14 days for menstrual cycle<br>Booklet described the yoga | Did not receive any intervention | Pain relief<br>pain intensity<br>Pain duration | A significant difference was observed between experimental and control groups in pain intensity and pain duration ($p<0.05$). | None | The obtained data is based on female adolescent participants' responses. |

**Table 1:** Characteristics of included randomized controlled trials.

| Study, year | Random allocation | Allocation concealment | Blinding | Incomplete outcome | Selective reporting | Other bias | Quality level |
|---|---|---|---|---|---|---|---|
| Rani et al. [9] | Yes | Yes | Yes | Yes | Yes | Yes | A |
| Rakhshaee [11] | Yes | Unclear | No | Yes | Yes | Yes | B |
| Yes: criteria met; No: criteria not met; Unclear, unclear whether criteria were met | | | | | | | |

**Table 2:** Methodological quality summary of all included studies.

In the two trials included in this review, they were too heterogeneous in the participants' condition (primary dysmenorrhea or all menstrual disorders), the type of yoga (three yoga poses composed of physical exercise and breathing or yoga nidra combining meditation and relaxation), interventionist (only booklet or yoga experts), duration of the intervention delivery (14 days for menstrual cycle or 6 months), outcome measures (pain intensity and pain duration or hormonal responses) etc. The rate of drop out was also high in the two RCTs. In one trial, 24 (31.9%) women were lost to the analysis for several reasons such as acute pain, family problems, transportation problems, scheduling, or being non-responsive, etc. In another trial, 28 (30.4%) participants did not complete the study because they had an irregular menstrual cycle and failed to comply.

Overall, the trials in this review had no adverse effects, stated that yoga poses are a safe and simple treatment for primary dysmenorrhea.

The quality rating of the trials included in this review had a low or moderate risk of bias. One trial was unclear about how treatment allocation was concealed. One of the two trials was single blind and the other did not mention blinding. The trials in this review had moderate or high methodological quality (Table 2). However, no strong conclusion can be made due to the number of small trials and other methodological considerations.

This strength of this systematic review includes the use of strict methodological criteria. Major strengths of this group of studies include study, the use of randomization, and the quality of measurement tools. Both studies were RCTs. This may be the first comprehensive review of yoga for dysmenorrhea.

Limitations were also identified. Menstrual disorders such as menorrhea, dysmenorrhea, oligomenorrhea, polymenorrhea, menorrhagia, metrorrhea, and hypomenorrhea were included in one trial all together. The sample size was also not large enough to analyze the hypomenorrhic group and hypermenorrhic subgroups separately. The methods of the participants' selection have the following flaws. The phase of the menstrual cycle was based on the participant's reports not on ultrasound scans. The obtained data is also based on female adolescent participants' responses. Generalizability of findings from these two studies is limited due to the number of small trials and limited quality partly. However, they provide a strong basis for future studies and suggest that yoga could provide a safe, cost-effective therapy for the growing public health issue of dysmenorrhea. There is currently a lack of available evidence to support the use of yoga in the alleviation of symptoms associated with dysmenorrhea. The broader health benefits of yoga should be discussed with women experiencing dysmenorrhea. Future research should consider these limitations. Furthermore, this review contributes to the development of knowledge in complementary and alternative medicine about how female adolescents with dysmenorrhea can manage themselves.

In conclusion, although this review has a limited number of small trials and homogeneity among them, and limited quality partly, findings from the two trials suggest that yoga practice can effectively alleviate menstrual pain and the symptoms associated with dysmenorrhea. However further high-quality RCTs are needed to confirm and further comprehend the effects of standardized yoga programs to control menstrual pain and symptoms in dysmenorrhea.

## Acknowledgement

This study was supported by 2016 Research Grant from Kangwon National University (No. 620160142).

## References


1. Osayande A, Mehulic S (2014) Diagnosis and initial management of dysmenorrhea. Am Fam Physician 89: 341-346.
2. Perry M (2012) Treatment options for dysmenorrhea. Nurs Pract 23: 195-198.
3. Shah M, Monga A, Patel S, Shah M, Bakshi H (2013) A study of prevalence of primary dysmenorrhea in young students-a cross sectional study. Healthline 4: 30-34.
4. Proctor ML, Farquhar CM (2006) Diagnosis and management of dysmenorrhoea. BMJ 332: 1134-1138.
5. Seven M, Güvenç G, Akyüz A, Eski F (2014) Evaluating dysmenorrhea in a sample of Turkish nursing students. Pain Manage Nurs 15: 664-671.
6. Cheng HF (2011) Management of perimenstrual symptoms among young Taiwanese nursing students. J Clin Nurs 20: 1060-1067.
7. Brown J, Brown S (2010) Exercise for dysmenorrhea. Cochrane Database Syst Rev CD004142.
8. Chien LW, Chang HC, Liu CF (2013) Effect of yoga on serum homocysteine and nitric oxide levels in adolescent women with and without dysmenorrhea. J Altern Complement Med 19: 20-23.
9. Rani M, Singh U, Agrawal GG, Natu SM, Kala S, et al. (2013) Impact of Yoga nidra on menstrual abnormalities in females of reproductive age. J Altern Complement Med 19: 925-929.
10. Han SH, Hur MH, Buckle J, Choi JY, Lee MS (2006) Effect of aromatherapy on symptoms of dysmenorrhea in college student: a randomized placebo-controlled clinical trial. J Altern Complement Med 12: 535-541.
11. Rakhshaee Z (2011) Effect of three yoga poses (cobra, cat and fish poses) in women with primary dysmenorrhea: a randomized clinical trial. J Pediatr Adolesc Gynecol 24: 192-196.
12. Proctor ML, Murphy PA, Pattison HM, Suckling JA, Farquhar C (2007) Behavioural intervention for dysmenorrhea. Cochrane Database Syst Rev CD002248.
13. Kanojia S, Sharma VK, Gandhi A, Kapoor R, Kukreja A, et al. (2013) Effect of yoga on autonomic functions and psychological status during both phases of menstrual cycle in young healthy females. J Clin Diagn Res 7: 2133-2139.
14. Beets MW, Mitchell E (2010) Effects of yoga on stress, depression, and health-related quality of life in a nonclinical, bi-ethnic sample of adolescents: a pilot study. Hisp Health Care Int 8: 47-53.
15. Tul Y, Unruh A, Dick BD (2011) Yoga for chronic pain management: a qualitative exploration. Scand J Caring Sci 25: 435-443.
16. Kuntsevich V, Bushell WC, Theise ND (2010) Mechanism of yogic practices in health, aging, and disease. Mt Sinai J Med 77: 559-569.
17. Ross A, Thomas S (2010) The health benefits of yoga and exercise: a review of comparison studies. J Altern Complement Med 16: 3-12.
18. Satyanada SS (2006) Yoga nidra. Yoga Publication Trust, Munger, Bihar, India.
19. Daley AJ (2008) Exercise and primary dysmenorrhea. A comprehensive and critical review of the literature. Sports Med 38: 659-670.
20. Schulz KF, Altman DG, Moher D (2010) CONSORT 2010 statement: updated guidelines for reporting parallel group randomized trials. J Clin Epidemiol 63: 834-840.
21. Higgins JPT, Green S (2011) Cochrane Handbook for Systematic Reviews of Interventions. The Cochrane Collaboration, John Wiley and Sons, New Jersey, USA.
22. Nayak NN, Shankar K (2004) Yoga: A therapeutic approach. Phys Med Rehabil Clin N Am 15: 783-798.
23. French L (2005) Dysmenorrhea. Am Fam Physician 71: 285-291.
24. Sharma M (2014) Yoga as an alternative and complementary approach for stress management: a systematic review. J Evid Based Complementary Altern Med 19: 59-67.
25. Sigmon ST, Nelson RO (1988) The effectiveness of activity scheduling and relaxation training in the treatment of spasmodic dysmenorrhea. J Behav Med 11: 483-495.

# 27

# Use of Traditional East Asian Medicine to Diagnose and Kampo Medicine Kamishoyosan to Treat Survivors of the Great East Japan Earthquake 2011

**Takashi Seki**[1*], **Keiko Sasaki**[2], **Seiichi Mori**[2] **and Kenichi Meguro**[1]

[1]*Division of Geriatric Behavioral Neurology, Tohoku University CYRIC, 6-3 Aoba, Aramaki, Aoba-ku, Sendai, Miyagi 980-8578, Japan*

[2]*Urayasu special elderly nursing home, 86-5 Shimoyoden aza Kasima, Natori, Miyagi 981-1223, Japan*

[*]**Corresponding author**: Takashi Seki, Division of Geriatric Behavioral Neurology, Tohoku University CYRIC, 6-3 Aoba, Aramaki, Aoba-ku, Sendai 980-8578, Japan, E-mail: tseki.tohoku@gmail.com

**Abstract**

Objective: In the aftermath of the Great East Japan Earthquake of March 11, 2011 and the associated tsunami, the Japanese medical system was not adequately prepared to deal with the many cases of post-traumatic stress disorder (PTSD), and commonly used pharmaceuticals were not always effective in dealing with the symptoms of PTSD. The aim of this paper is to evaluate the physical and mental condition of tsunami survivors by using traditional East Asian medicine (TEAM) principles and examine the effects of Kampo medicine (Japanese herbal medicine) Kamishoyosan (Jia-wei-xiao-yao-san) on stress-related disorders such as PTSD.

Method: The study participants consisted of 32 tsunami survivors of the Great East Japan Earthquake. Clinical records were used to analyze (1) patient complaints, (2) diagnosis, and (3) treatment with traditional Chinese medicine. The clinical records were also used for Japanese-language version of the Impact of Event Scale – Revised (IES-R-J) assessments.

Results: Thirty-two employees at the Urayasu nursing facility (7 men, 25 women; age, 40 ± 13 years) were enrolled as patients. The physical symptoms reported by the patients were insomnia, fatigue, palpitations, and shoulder discomfort; the mental symptoms included anxiety, sense of guilt, dreams, fear, anger, and irritation. Among TEAM syndromes, "liver qi stagnation" and "depressed liver qi transforming into fire" were most common. The herbal medicine Kamishoyosan was prescribed for 23 participants. The IES-R-J scores after the prescribed use of Kamishoyosan showed significant improvement compared to the pre-treatment IES-R-J scores.

Conclusions: Kamishoyosan for applicable cases can be helpful as an adjunctive therapy for treatment of stress-related disorders such as PTSD following major disasters. Further investigation of the role of Kamishoyosan in reducing the symptoms of PTSD is warranted. Follow-up for survivors and rescue workers affected by the Great East Japan Earthquake is indispensable.

**Keywords:** Post-Traumatic Stress Disorder (PTSD); Herbal medicine; Kamishoyosan; IES-R; the Great East Japan Earthquake

## Introduction

The Great East Japan Earthquake of March 11, 2011 was the fourth earthquake of its size in the world since 1900 [1] and there are many reports of post-traumatic stress disorder (PTSD) associated with it [2]. PTSD is more common than previously thought [3]; for example, 4 years after tsunami caused by the Hokkaido Nanseioki Earthquake, 16.7% of survivors reported that their life remained unsettled [4].

A total of 15,887 persons are known to have died in the Great East Japan Earthquake and the number of people still missing was 2,615 as of July 10, 2014 [5]. The number of refugees and evacuated persons living in temporary housing was 251,419 as of June 12, 2014 [6]. Of the 1,006 victims of the disaster living in the stricken areas of Iwate, Miyagi, and Fukushima prefectures, 59% reported that reconstruction had not been taking place, 53% said that the reason for the lack of reconstruction was that the location of their future residence had not yet been decided, and 24% said that they did not want to return to where they lived before the tsunami. The most common reason given for not returning to their previous home was anxiety about the tsunami [7]. Rescue workers, as well as survivors, are at risk for developing mental disorders [8,9].

Our institution and nursing facility—Tohoku University and the Urayasu special elderly nursing home—were located at the center of disaster area; there were varying responses to the tragic disaster [10-12].

One of the observations that became apparent after the earthquake was that commonly used pharmaceuticals were not always effective and often proved unsatisfactory for patients. For example, the drugs commonly used to treat PTSD were known to have side effects and could pose risks for some people [13-15]. There was also insufficient evidence to recommend Complementary and Alternative Medicine (CAM) approaches, including traditional medicine, as first-line treatments for PTSD. Nevertheless, herbal medicines have been in common use for mental care in traditional East Asian medicine

(TEAM) from ancient times [16]. Kampo medicine Kamishoyosan (Jia-wei-xiao-yao-san) is an example of one such Japanese herbal medicine currently in use [17-23]. After the Sichuan earthquake in China in 2008, Xiao-Tan-Jie-Yu-Fang, which was developed from Jia-wei-xiao-yao-san (Kamishoyosan), was used for patients with PTSD [24]. We used TEAM to treat the survivors of the Great East Japan Earthquake in 2011; 72% of patients, for whom Kamishoyosan was indicated by TEAM syndromes, were prescribed Kamishoyosan. The IES-R-J scores obtained before and after treatment were analyzed based on the medical records.

## Materials and Methods

### Study design and participants

This retrospective study was conducted in Natori City, which is located near the center of the tsunami disaster area associated with the Great East Japan Earthquake in 2011 (Figure 1). The study participants were surviving employees of the Urayasu nursing home facility, which was destroyed by the tsunami.

After the tsunami disaster, the authors visited the survivors and treated them in the facility to which they had been taken. All the patients were suffering from stress-related disorders such as PTSD. They were diagnosed according to the theories of TEAM and prescribed herbal medicines. To evaluate the effects of the herbal medicines on the patients, IES-R-J assessments were performed before and after prescription of the medicines.

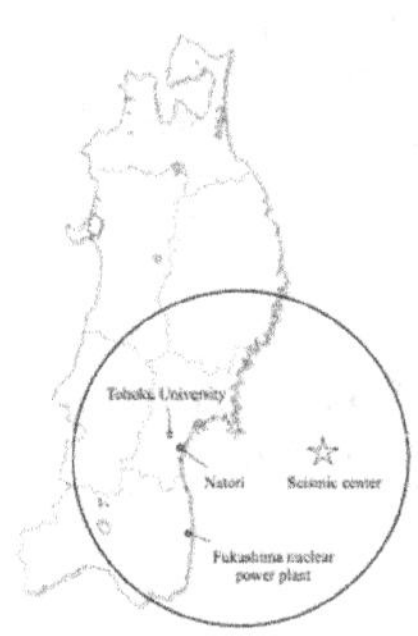


**Figure 1:** Location of Natori city

### Outcome Measures

Assessments of the damage to the patients caused by the earthquake and tsunami were carried out in three stages: (1) identifying chief complaints reported at the first examination, which took place 1 to 2 months after the disaster, (2) performing diagnosis according to TEAM theories, and (3) assessing medical records with the Japanese-language version of the Impact of Event Scale – Revised (IES-R-J) [25]. All three stages were performed using the patient's clinical records. Most of the patients completed the IES-R-J twice, as requested—before and after receiving the prescription. The IES-R-J assessments were analyzed only in patients for whom Kamishoyosan was indicated by TEAM syndromes such as "liver qi stagnation" or "depressed liver qi transforming into fire."

The IES-R-J is a short, self-reporting questionnaire with 22 questions, 5 of which were added to the original Horowitz (IES) [26] to better capture the DSM-IV (Diagnostic and Statistical Manual of Mental Disorders) criteria for PTSD [27]. This tool is an appropriate instrument to measure the subjective response to a specific traumatic event in the senior population, especially in the response sets of intrusion (intrusive thoughts, nightmares, intrusive feelings and imagery, dissociative-like re-experiencing), avoidance (numbing of responsiveness, avoidance of feelings, situations, and ideas), and hyperarousal (anger, irritability, hypervigilance, difficulty concentrating, heightened startle), as well as to produce a total subjective stress IES-R-J score.

### Preparation of herbal medicine Kamishoyosan (Jia-wei-xiao-yao-san) and dispensing of the medicine

Kamishoyosan extract is an over-the-counter (OTC) drug that was supplied for prescription to the patients by Kotaro Pharmaceutical Co., Ltd (Osaka, Japan). Kamishoyosan extract is produced by Kotaro Pharmaceutical Co., Ltd. It contains 10 herbs in the following quantities: Bupleuri Radix (1.5g), Angelicae Radix (1.5g), Poria (1.5g), Atractylodis Rhizoma (1.5g), Paeoniae Radix (1.5g), Menthae Herba (0.5g), Glycyrrhizae Radix (1.0g), Zingiberis Rhizoma (0.5g), Moutan Cortex (1.0g), and Gardeniae Fructus (1.0g). These herbs are registered in the Pharmacopoeia of Japan, 15th version. Patients who participated in the study and were approved to receive the Kamishoyosan prescription as the result of having one or more TEAM syndromes received 3 tablets of Kamishoyosan (0.75 g extract) 3 times a day. The processes involved in the production and distribution of Kamishoyosan, in compliance with Good Manufacturing Practices for Kampo products, have also been approved by the Ministry of Health, Labor, and Welfare of Japan.

### Statistical Analysis

Scores for the IES-R-J obtained before and after the prescription of Kamishoyosan were compared using paired t-test. The statistical analysis software used was JMP Pro version 11.0 (SAS Institute Inc., Cary, NC, USA). Significance levels were defined as $p < 0.05$.

## Results

### Participants

A total of 32 employees (7 men and 25 women; age, 40 ± 13 years) at the Urayasu nursing home facility were enrolled as patients in the research project.

### The damage situation for the study patients

The Urayasu nursing facility was completely destroyed by the tsunami. Forty-three of the 163 elderly residents died, along with 4 of the 62 employees. Of the 32 employees enrolled as patients in the study, 31 witnessed the death of one or more residents, or experienced a crisis in their own life. The families of 2 patients died in the disaster and the families of 2 other patients disappeared; 4 patients had their houses completely destroyed, and the houses of 2 other patients were partially destroyed. The cars of 14 patients were carried away by the tsunami.

### Chief complaints of patients at the first examination

Figure 2a shows the physical symptoms and Figure 2b shows the mental symptoms at the first examination. Among physical symptoms, insomnia, fatigue, palpitations, and shoulder discomfort were most prevalent, while anxiety, sense of guilt, dreams, fear, anger, and irritation were the most common mental symptoms. The reasons given by the patients for their anxiety were vague, relating to aftershocks, the tsunami, uncertainty about their future, and lack of employment.

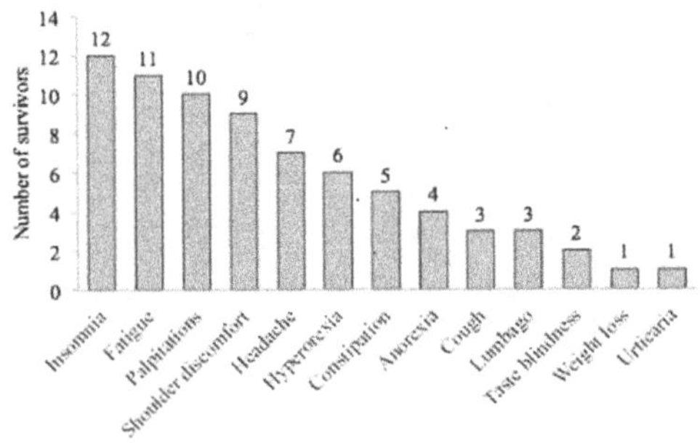


**Figure 2A:** Symptoms at first medical examination.

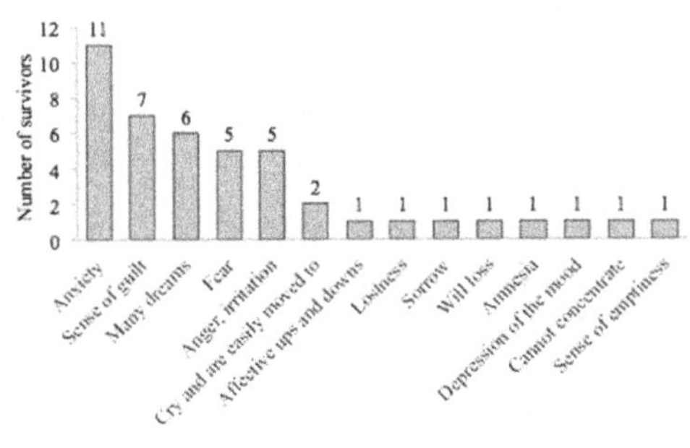


**Figure 2B:** Mental symptoms at first medical examination.

## Diagnosis according to the TEAM theories (TEAM syndromes)

The most common TEAM syndromes were "liver qi stagnation" (43%) and "depressed liver qi transforming into fire" (28%) (Figure 3).

## Treatment with herbal medicines at the first examination

Prescriptions for herbal medicine at the first medical examination were as follows: Kamishoyosan (Jia-wei-xiao-yao-san), 23 patients; Rikkunshito (Liu-jun-zi-shang), 5 patients; Keishibukuryogan (Gui-zhi-fu-ling-wan), 4 patients; Shoseiryuto (Xiao-qing-shang), 2 patients; Shin'iseihaito (Xin-yi-qing-fei-shang), 1 patient; Keigairengyoto (Jing-gai-lian-qiao-shang), 1 patient; and Rokumigan (Liu-wei-wan), 1 patient. Multiple herbal medicines were prescribed to patients, as needed.

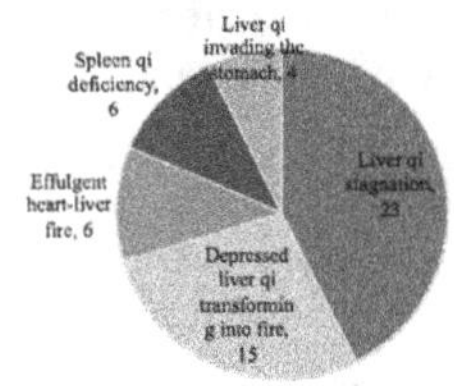


**Figure 3:** TEAM syndromes in patients

## The Impact of Event Scale – Revised Japanese-language version (IES-R-J)

Twenty-three of the 32 patients participating in the study were considered appropriate to receive Kamishoyosan; 18 of the 23 patients who were prescribed Kamishoyosan completed the IES-R-J twice (before and after receiving the herbal prescription). Table 1 shows the IES-R-J patient scores including the total IES-R-J score, the sub-totals of the intrusion factor, the hyperarousal factor, and the avoidance factor. Most of the items showed significant improvement after the patients were prescribed Kamishoyosan, except for the following: "My feelings about it were kind of numb," "I found myself acting or feeling like I was back at that time," "I tried to remove it from my memory," and "I tried not to talk about it."

The first examinations and first IES-R-J assessments were performed between April and June 2011. The length of time between the first and second IES-R-J assessments was 4 to 6 months. Sixteen of the 18 patients showed improvement in their IES-R-J scores. However, the scores for 2 patients worsened—not only the total IES-R-J score but also the scores for all other items. It should be noted that these 2 patients had experienced terrible sights when the tsunami occurred. They saw some of the elderly residents of the nursing facility drown in front of them but were unable to help. For this, they were criticized by the bereaved family of the deceased elderly residents and were told, "My father died. Why are you living?"

### Adverse events

There were no reports of adverse events associated with the use of the medicines.

## Discussion

This study showed the potential effectiveness of the herbal medicine Kamishoyosan in improving the IES-R-J scores of tsunami survivors with stress-related disorders like PTSD at 1 to 2 months after the Great East Japan Earthquake.

### TEAM treatment for PTSD and syndromes in earthquake survivors

Meng et al. used the herbal medicine Xiao-Tan-Jie-Yu-Fang to treat patients with PTSD after the 2008 earthquake in China. Xiao-Tan-Jie-Yu-Fang was modified from a classic formula, Shoyosan (Xiao-Yao-San), the basic component of Kamishoyosan that we used on the earthquake survivors in Japan. Numata et al. used

Saikokeishikankyoto, which, like Kamishoyosan, is applied when there is "liver qi stagnation." TEAM syndromes in patients with PTSD, who were recruited by posting flyers or ads in the local media, were "liver qi stagnation," "heart shen disturbance"and"kidney deficiency" in another study [28].

| Subscale | Item | Before Mean ± SD | After Mean ± SD | P value | Subscale | Item | Before Mean ± SD | After Mean ± SD | P value |
|---|---|---|---|---|---|---|---|---|---|
| Int | Any reminder brought back feelings about it | 2.5 ± 1.1 | 1.4 ± 0.7 | <.0001 | Avo | I was aware that I still had a lot of feelings about it, but I dint deal with them | 1.4 ± 1.1 | 0.7 ± 0.6 | 0.0008 |
| Int | I had trouble staying asleep | 1.8 ± 1.3 | 0.9 ± 0.9 | 0.0028 | Avo | My feelings about it were numb | 1.2 ± 1.2 | 0.9 ± 1.1 | 0.1631 |
| Int | Other things kept making me think about it | 1.6 ± 1.4 | 0.7 ± 0.7 | 0.0009 | Int | I found myself acting about it were kind of numb | 0.9 ± 1.2 | 0.6 ± 0.8 | 0.0827 |
| Hyp | I felt irritable and angry | 1.3 ± 1.0 | 0.9 ± 0.8 | 0.007 | Hyp | I had trouble falling asleep | 1.4 ± 1.2 | 0.7 ± 0.8 | 0.0043 |
| Avo | I avoided letting myself get upset when I thought about it or was reminded of it | 1.7 ± 1.0 | 0.9 ± 0.6 | 0.0007 | Int | I had waves of strong feeling about it | 2.1 ± 1.0 | 1.2 ± 0.7 | 0.0001 |
| Int | I thought about it when I dint mean to | 2.1 ± 1.1 | 1.3 ± 0.7 | 0.0134 | Avo | I tried to remove it from my memory | 0.8 ± 0.9 | 0.4 ± 0.6 | 0.069 |
| Avo | I felt as if it hadn't happened or wasn't real | 1.6 ± 1.2 | 0.9 ± 0.9 | 0.0229 | Hyp | I had trouble concentrating | 1.4 ± 1.5 | 0.8 ± 1.2 | 0.0079 |
| Avo | I stayed away from reminders of it | 1.6 ± 1.1 | 1.0 ± 1.0 | 0.0445 | Hyp | Reminds of it caused me to have physical reactions, such as sweating, trouble breathing, nausea, or a pounding heart | 1.4 ± 1.2 | 0.9 ± 1.0 | 0.0081 |
| Int | Pictures about it popped into my mind | 1.5 ± 1.0 | 0.8 ± 0.8 | 0.0018 | Int | I had dreams about it | 0.9 ± 1.1 | 0.4 ± 0.6 | 0.046 |
| Hyp | I was jumpy and easily started | 1.8 ± 1.3 | 0.9 ± 0.9 | 0.009 | Hyp | I felt watch full and on-guard | 1.9 ± 1.1 | 1.2 ± 0.9 | 0.0018 |
| Avo | I tried not to think about it | 1.3 ± 1.1 | 0.8 ± 0.5 | 0.0346 | Avo | I tried not to think about it | 0.8 ± 0.8 | 0.5 ± 0.6 | 0.0827 |
| Instruction Factor (Subtotal) | | | | | | | 14.6 ± 7.1 | 8.1 ± 3.6 | <.0001 |
| Hyperarousal Factor (Subtotal) | | | | | | | 11.3 ± 6.0 | 6.4 ± 3.9 | 0.0002 |
| Avoidance Factor (Subtotal) | | | | | | | 7.1 ± 4.0 | 4.2 ± 3.0 | 0.0008 |
| Total | | | | | | | 32.9 ± 14.5 | 18.8 ± 7.9 | <.0001 |
| Int = Instruction Factor; Hyp = Hyperarousal Factor; Avo = Avoidance Factor | | | | | | | | | |

**Table 1**: Scores of IES-R-J before and after prescription of Kamishoyosan.

In the present study, patients were diagnosed with TEAM and, where indicated, herbal medicines were prescribed. However, it was observed that all of the TEAM syndromes other than "liver qi stagnation" that were found in patients could have come from "liver qi stagnation," and the majority of patients (72%) were diagnosed as having "liver qi stagnation," for which the herbal medicine Kamishoyosan was indicated. It is known that the main cause of "liver qi stagnation" is mental stress. Thus, according to TEAM theories, it is reasonable to suggest that these patients were suffering from mental stress. The TEAM syndromes "depressed liver qi transforming into fire," "effulgent heart-liver fire"and "liver qi invading the stomach," which some patients were suffering, can show as irritable conditions [29].

## Indication and mechanisms of action of Kamishoyosan

Traditionally, Kamishoyosan has been used to treat a wide variety of mental and physical problems, including limb problems, heaviness of the head, dizziness, insomnia, irritability, burning sensation, menstrual abnormalities, and hot flashes [30], and has effects on mild-to-moderate somatization disorders [31], women's general malaise and agitation [32], affective disorders [33,34], psychological stress insomnia [17], and depression [22,35].

In the IES-R-J scores of the study patients, it was found that three avoidance factor items—"My feelings about it were kind of numb," "I tried to remove it from my memory," and "I tried not to talk about it" — plus one intrusion factor item—"I found myself acting or feeling like I was back at that time"—did not change significantly after prescription of Kamishoyosan (Table 1). This may show the limitations of Kamishoyosan in treating PTSD-like stress.

Some of the major ingredients in Kamishoyosan are known to produce a sedative effect; they include the following: Angelicae Radix has a sedative effect in rabbits [36]; Paeoniae Radix has sedative and analgesic effects in mice [37]; Bupleuri Radix affects the central nervous system, causing sleep prolongation, sedation, and analgesia [38]; and Liquiritin, a flavone compound derived from Glycyrrhizae Radix, has shown an antidepressant effect in animal studies [39].

The psychological effects of Shoyosan, the basic component of Kamishoyosan, have also been reported; they include the following: antidepressant effect on rats in metabolomics study [40], amelioration of brain cortex 5-HT and 5-HIAA content in a mouse model of depression [41], regulation effect on the expression of AMPA receptors in chronic immobilization stress [42], upregulation of AMPA receptor subunit mRNA expression in the hippocampal region CA1 and amygdala [43], maintenance of the stability of hippocampal neurons [44], inhibition of hypothalamic-pituitary-adrenocortical axis negative feedback regulation [45], and counteraction on an increase in $Ca^{2+}$ concentration in hippocampal synaptosomes [46].

### Situation of the study participants

The patients who participated in the study were employees at the nursing facility for the elderly when it was hit by the tsunami. Thus, they were both rescue workers for the elderly at the facility and victims of the disaster. When the tsunami hit, their priority was to save the elderly residents of the nursing facility rather than focusing on their own need to escape and save themselves.

Most of the patients in the study lost their cars in the tsunami, and there was little gas available for those that still had cars. As a result, these patients did not have the opportunity to visit clinics for their own health. Moreover, because of the damage to transportation networks, hospitals, and the factory that produces Kampo medicine (Japanese herbal medicine), the availability of medical supplies in the disaster-stricken area was limited. OTC herbal medicines were supplied free by Kotaro Pharmaceutical Co., Ltd (Osaka, Japan). Authors visited the study facility as medical volunteers every weekend.

The earthquake and tsunami survivors suffered psychological as well as physical damage. The earthquake occurred on March 11, 2011, but from then until April 30, 2011, there were a total of 165 aftershocks with seismic intensity of 4 or more [47]. It was said that many of the survivors were affected psychologically, and 1 to 2 months after the disaster, many had become disillusioned [48]. Eleven of the 32 patients reported anxiety about the tsunami and aftershocks. Some of the patients with insomnia refused to take the soporific, because of the fear of another tsunami coming.

The victims of the Great East Japan Earthquake will need to receive ongoing care for physical and mental health issues for some time in the future. PTSD is associated with high healthcare costs [49]. Because herbal medicines are inexpensive and have few side effects, they are being used to treat many earthquake and tsunami victims in Japan. Furthermore, a matter of urgency is the predicted "Tokai Earthquake," a giant magnitude 8 earthquake with an epicenter inland of Shizuoka prefecture (near Tokyo), from the Gulf of Suruga [50].

Further investigation is warranted to explain the mechanisms of the use of the herbal medicine Kamishoyosan in the treatment of PTSD. The strategy of using an inexpensive herbal medicine to treat PTSD is worth studying.

## Limitations

This retrospective study was limited by the fact that it included only a small number of participants (32) who survived the earthquake, and there were no controls. Second, because of the dynamics of the post-earthquake situation, the authors were unable to have the study participants diagnosed by psychiatrists. Third, the herbal medicines that were given to the study participants were OTC products because of the limited medical conditions at the time; therefore, the quantity of herbal medicine prescribed may not have been sufficient to effect the desired results in some patients.

## Conclusion

Survivors of the Great East Japan Earthquake who had limited access to medical care were diagnosed and treated according to TEAM theories and syndromes. More than 40% of the patients included in the study showed the TEAM syndrome "liver qi stagnation" 1 to 2 months after the disaster. They suffered not only stressful disorders like PTSD but also other TEAM syndromes caused by mental stress. The IES-R-J scores obtained for the patients showed improvement after administration of the herbal medicine Kamishoyosan to those for whom it was indicated by TEAM. However, the mental state of patients who had particularly violent or unpleasant experiences during or after the earthquake was exacerbated. The study suggested that the herbal medicine Kamishoyosan can be helpful in treating some stressful disorders like PTSD that result from disasters such as earthquakes.

## Acknowledgements

The authors would like to thank Kotaro Pharmaceutical Co., Ltd, which provided herbal medicine to the earthquake survivors at no cost. We also wish to thank Ms. Hiroko Kobayashi (Tohoku University Hospital, Department of Laboratory Medicine), who supported our data collection efforts. We pray for the souls of the people who died in the Great East Japan Earthquake; may they rest in peace.

## References

1. US Geological Survey Largest Earthquakes in the World Since 1900. In: U. S. Department of the Interior | U. S. Geological Survey, editor.

2. Neria Y, Nandi A, Galea S (2008) Post-traumatic stress disorder following disasters: a systematic review. Psychol Med 38: 467-480.
3. Kessler RC, Sonnega A, Bromet E, Hughes M, Nelson CB (1995) Posttraumatic stress disorder in the National Comorbidity Survey. Arch Gen Psychiatry 52: 1048-1060.
4. Wakabayashi Y (2003) Psychology of disaster and its fringe - a comunity approach fot stricken area by Hokkaido Nanseioki Earthquake. Tokyo
5. The Urgent Disaster Guard Head Quarters (2014) The damage situation and police action of the Tohoku district Pacific offing earthquake 2011. In: National Police Agency, editor. Tokyo.
6. Reconstruction Agency (2014) The number of refugees of the whole country. Tokyo.
7. NHK (2013) "Cannot have an actual feeling of the revival" 60 % in 3 Tohoku prefectures. NHK NEWS WEB.
8. Fullerton CS, Ursano RJ, Wang L (2004) Acute stress disorder, posttraumatic stress disorder, and depression in disaster or rescue workers. Am J Psychiatry 161: 1370-1376.
9. Epstein RS, Fullerton CS, Ursano RJ (1998) Posttraumatic stress disorder following an air disaster: a prospective study. Am J Psychiatry 155: 934-938.
10. Kim Y (2011) Great East Japan earthquake and early mental-health-care response. Psychiatry Clin Neurosci 65: 539-548.
11. Meguro K (2011) Local response following the Great East Japan Earthquake 2011. Neurology 77: e12-15.
12. Satomi S (2011) The Great East Japan Earthquake: Tohoku University Hospital's efforts and lessons learned. Surg Today 41: 1171-1181.
13. Schoenfeld FB, Marmar CR, Neylan TC (2004) Current concepts in pharmacotherapy for posttraumatic stress disorder. Psychiatr Serv 55: 519-531.
14. Cukor J, Olden M, Lee F, Difede J (2010) Evidence-based treatments for PTSD, new directions, and special challenges. Ann N Y Acad Sci 1208: 82-89.
15. Foa EB, Franklin ME, Moser J (2002) Context in the clinic: how well do cognitive-behavioral therapies and medications work in combination? Biol Psychiatry 52: 987-997.
16. Hoizey D, Hoizey M-J (1993) A History of Chinese Medicine. Bailey P, translator. Edinburgh: Edinburgh University Press.
17. Li Y, Xu BY, Xiao F (2009) Effect of modified xiaoyao powder for improving sleep in patients with psychological stress insomnia. Chinese journal of integrated traditional and Western medicine 29: 208-211.
18. Yu HT (2006) Clinical observation on treatment of somatic disorder with combination of Xiaoyao Powder and Wendan Decoction. Chinese journal of integrated traditional and Western medicine 26: 1114-1116.
19. Yi ZH, Zhu LP, Long B (2010) Clinical observation on treatment of major depressive disorder by paroxetine combined with chaihu xiaoyao mixture. Chinese journal of integrated traditional and Western medicine 30: 1257-1260.
20. Yang ZY, Zhang WB, Liu JL (2007) Comparative study of Modified Xiaoyao Pill combining amitriptyline on therapeutic effect and compliance in treating patients with depression. Chinese journal of integrated traditional and Western medicine 27: 642-644.
21. Yu GH, Liang SC, Sun QZ (2007) Study on Modified Xiaoyao Decoction combining Clomipramine treating depression. Chinese journal of integrated traditional and Western medicine 27: 318-320.
22. Luo HC, Qian RQ, Zhao XY, Bi J, Xin H, et al. (2006) Clinical observation on effect of danzhi xiaoyao powder in treating depression. Chinese journal of integrated traditional and Western medicine 26: 212-214.
23. Qian LQ, Wang B, Niu JY, Gao S, Zhao DY (2010) Assessment of the clinical effect of Chinese medicine therapy combined with psychological intervention for treatment of patients of peri-menopausal syndrome complicated with hyperlipidemia. Chin J Integr Med 16: 124-130.
24. Meng XZ, Wu F, Wei PK, Xiu LJ, Shi J, et al. (2012) A chinese herbal formula to improve general psychological status in posttraumatic stress disorder: a randomized placebo-controlled trial on sichuan earthquake survivors. Evid Based Complement Alternat Med 2012: 691258.
25. Asukai N, Kato H, Kawamura N, Kim Y, Yamamoto K, et al (2002) Reliability and validity of the Japanese-language version of the Impact of Event Scale-Revised(IES-R-J);Four studies on different traumatic events. J Nerv Ment Dis: 175-182.
26. Horowitz M, Wilner N, Alvarez W (1979) Impact of Event Scale: a measure of subjective stress. Psychosom Med 41: 209-218.
27. Weiss DS, Marmar CR, Wilson J, Keane T, et al (1997) The impact of event scale-revised. In: Assessing psychoogical trauma and PTSD. New York The Guilford Press Pp 399-411.
28. Hollifield M, Sinclair-Lian N, Warner TD, Hammerschlag R (2007) Acupuncture for posttraumatic stress disorder: a randomized controlled pilot trial. J Nerv Ment Dis 195: 504-513.
29. Liu G, Hyodo A (2006) Fundamentals of acupuncture & moxibustion. Huaxia publishing house Beijing
30. Otuka K, Yakazu D, Shimizu T (2001) Kanpo Shinryo Iten: Nanzando Co Ltd
31. Yamada K (2003) Application of the Kami-shoyo-san in neuropsychiatry. Kanpo to Saisin Chiryou 12: 57-60.
32. Morita H, Arita M, Ishida S, Ozaki T (1997) Kami-shoyo-san's autonomic nervous function and effects on mind and body symptoms. Kanpo Igaku 21: 177-179.
33. Zhang LD, Zhang YL, Xu SH, Zhou G, Jin SB (1994) Traditional Chinese medicine typing of affective disorders and treatment. Am J Chin Med 22: 321-327.
34. Oka T (2003) Effect of Kami-shoyo-san on antistress and stress associated diseases. Kanpo to saisin chiryo 12: 66-68.
35. Xu ZW, Wu LL, Ya VC (2003) The experimental research on anti-depression effects of xiaoyaosan decoction and danzhi xiaoyaosan decoction. Acta Chinese Medicine and Pharmacology 31: 61.
36. Saeki T (1965) Basic study on mechanism of action for the rabbit ocular tension of Angelicae Radix-effects for the blood pressure. Rinsyo Ganka 19: 647-654.
37. Takagi K, Harada M (1969) Pharmacological Studies on Herb Paeony Root. I. : Central Effects of Paeoniflorin and Combined Effects with Licorice Component FM 100. Yakugaku Zasshi 89: 879-886.
38. Takagi K, Shibata T (1969) Pharmacological Studies on Bupleurum falcatum L.I. : Acute Toxicity and Central Depressant Action of Crude Saikosides. Yakugaku Zasshi 89: 712-720.
39. Zhao Z, Wang W, Guo H, Zhou D (2008) Antidepressant-like effect of liquiritin from Glycyrrhiza uralensis in chronic variable stress induced depression model rats. Behav Brain Res 194: 108-113.
40. Dai Y, Li Z, Xue L, Dou C, Zhou Y, et al. (2010) Metabolomics study on the anti-depression effect of xiaoyaosan on rat model of chronic unpredictable mild stress. J Ethnopharmacol 128: 482-489.
41. Bao L, Chen J, Huang L, Chen W, Lin Q, et al. (2008) Effects of Xiaoyao Wan on the behavioral despair and stress depression mice. Journal of Chinese medicinal materials 31: 1360-1364.
42. Yue GX, Wang ZF, Zhang QL, Zhao X, Yue LF, et al. (2008) Expression of AMPA receptors and related protein in immobilization stressed rats and effect of Xiaoyaosan. Chinese journal of applied physiology 24: 129-132.
43. Yue GX, Wang ZF, Zhang QL (2007) Changes of central AMPA receptor subunits and related protein mRNA expression in immobilization stressed rats and effect of Xiaoyaosan on them. Chinese journal of integrated traditional and Western medicine 27: 1110-1115.
44. Xu ZW, Sun Q, Ao HQ, Wang WZ, Fu WJ (2011) Effects of Xiaoyao powder on NR1, NR2A and NR2B mRNA expression in cultured hippocampal neurons of rats under chronic stress. Journal of Guangzhou University of Traditional Chinese Medicine 28: 36–42.
45. Xu ZW, Fu WJ, Ao HQ (2009) Effect of Xiaoyaosan on HPA axis negative feedback regulation function of rats with chronic stress. Journal of Shanxi College of Traditional Chinese Medicine 10: 15–17.

46. Xu ZW, Ao HQ, Yan C, Wu LL, Wang WZ (2005) Effect of Xiaoyao powder on Ca2+ in hippocampal synaptosome of Multi-stress model rats. Journal of Guangzhou University of Traditional Chinese Medicine 22: 42–45.
47. Department of Earthquake and Volcano (2014) Number of earthquakes of Tohoku district Pacific offing earthquake 2011: maximal seismic intensity 4 or more. In: Japan Meteorological Agency Tokyo.
48. Romo D (1995) Handbook of disaster and psychological care: ASK human care inc.
49. Walker EA, Katon W, Russo J, Ciechanowski P, Newman E, et al. (2003) Health care costs associated with posttraumatic stress disorder symptoms in women. Arch Gen Psychiatry 60: 369-374.
50. Japan Meteorological Agency (2014) Urgency of occurrence of Tokai Earthquake. In: Ministry of Land Infrastructure and Transport

# 28

# Evaluation of Semi Standardized Individualized Homeopathic Treatment of 77 Women with Premenstrual Disorders: Observational Study with 9 Months Follow-Up

**Klein-Laansma CT[1,2]*, Jansen JCH[1], Van Tilborgh AJW[1] and Van Vliet M[2]**

[1]*Dutch Doctor's Association for Integrative Medicine (AVIG), The Netherlands*

[2]*Healthcare and Nutrition, Louis Bolk Institute, The Netherlands*

**Abstract**

**Background:** A large proportion (8-32%) of women in the fertile age suffers from premenstrual syndrome/ symptoms (PMS/S). Individualized homeopathy could offer relief and this should be further investigated. Semi-standardized treatment with a limited number of homeopathic medicines and strictly defined prescription criteria could minimize prescription variability and increase reproducibility of the individualized treatment.

**Objective:** In an extension of a previous pilot study, the utility of a semi-standardized algorithm with 11 medicines for individualized homeopathic treatment of women with PMS/S was further evaluated in daily practice with 9 months follow-up.

**Methods:** Women completed symptom diaries during to 2 months to confirm PMS/S. Women diagnosed with PMS/S were included, consulted a homeopathic physician and completed a questionnaire with keynote symptoms for 11 homeopathic medicines. A computerized algorithm would process the answers and indicate the first homeopathic prescription. At follow-up visits change of prescription was possible. Main outcome measures were frequencies and proportions of (non-) algorithm-based prescriptions during the study and percentage of responders (≥ 50% drop in PMS scores). Secondary outcome measures were mean changes in PMS scores over time.

**Results:** 77 women were included, 52 completed the study. The usefulness of the semi-standardized treatment protocol was confirmed. In 30 (57.5%) of the 52 analyzed women, PMS scores had dropped by ≥ 50%. For the estimated mean changes in PMS scores, it made no difference if women had used one or more of the 11 algorithm-based or also other homeopathic medicines ($p=0.765$). A significant association was found between symptom severity at baseline and changes in mean PMS scores ($p<0.001$).

**Conclusions:** A semi-standardized individualized homeopathic treatment of women with PMS/S with 11 medicines proved useful in daily homeopathic practice, with improved reproducibility of individualized treatment. This treatment could be further tested in effectiveness research.

**Keywords:** Premenstrual syndrome; Premenstrual symptoms; Homeopathy; Individualized; Personalized; Semi-standardized

## Introduction

### Premenstrual disorders

Worldwide, a meaningful proportion of fertile women (8-32%) suffer from moderate to severe physical and emotional symptoms during the luteal phase of the menstrual cycle [1]. The core premenstrual disorders are premenstrual syndrome (PMS) and premenstrual dysphoric disorder (PMDD) [2]. Premenstrual symptoms can have an adverse impact on a woman's quality of life and lead to increased direct and indirect medical costs [3]. Moderate to severe PMS and PMDD are associated with impairment of work productivity and increased absenteeism and thus pose an economic burden [4].

### Pharmacological treatments

Evidence-based pharmacological treatments for women with severe PMS or PMDD are antidepressants of the Selective Serotonin Re-uptake Inhibitor (SSRI) type and the Combined Oral Contraceptive (COC) drospirinone/-ethinylestradiol (Dros/EE) [5-7]. These treatments can effectively reduce symptoms, but have important limitations. The use of SSRIs would only be warranted for women with moderate to severe mental symptoms and not for women with mainly physical or mild mental symptoms. After discontinuation of treatment with SSRIs, relapse can occur so that long-term treatment would be required [8]. Many women suffering from PMS who were treated with SSRIs reported only minor improvements and no cure, implicating this treatment as 'effective but not enough' [9]. Also, women could object to taking antidepressants because of unwanted side effects or preference for a more 'natural and safe' treatment approach [5,10]. Women may be averse to treatment with COCs, because they want to get pregnant or have previously suffered from side effects of the drug. One of the leading researchers in the field concluded that the majority of women with PMS or PMDD would respond to any of the available treatments, but "further research to develop new therapies for the 40% of women with PMS who do not respond to the currently available treatments is needed" [11].

***Corresponding author:** Christien Klein-Laansma, Healthcare and Nutrition, Louis Bolk Institute, The Netherlands, Joubertweg 3, 6861 DM Oosterbeek, The Netherlands, E-mail: ctlaansma@planet.nl

### Homeopathic treatment of PMS

In an Israeli double-blind controlled pilot study, the effects of 5 specific homeopathic medicines were compared with placebo in 20 women with PMS [12]. The relative improvement rate of PMS symptoms in the verum group was significantly better than in the placebo group. In this study, a patient questionnaire containing questions representing so-called 'keynote' symptoms of 5 homeopathic medicines was used for the homeopathic medicine selection (keynote symptom: a specific symptom that strongly indicates the use of a particular homeopathic medicine). Women, whose symptoms did not match the profile of one of these 5 medicines, were allocated to a parallel trial. Other standardized as well as individualized homeopathic approaches have been explored in clinical studies of various design in the past [13-17]. Two more recent studies will be briefly discussed here. In a South-African double-blind placebo-controlled trial on individualized homeopathy in 39 women (27 completed the study), no statistical difference was detected between the placebo and verum group [18]. Homeopathic prescriptions were based on individual symptoms, but no details were revealed about a specific method of homeopathic medicine selection. A case series was published about individualized homeopathic treatment in 23 French women who reported premenstrual symptoms [19]. A positive impact on premenstrual symptoms and quality of life was observed in the majority of women.

### The 'Dutch approach'

Inspired by the Israeli research, a semi-standardized homeopathic treatment of women with PMS was developed in the Netherlands. The aim of semi-standardization was to optimize the reproducibility of the treatment to facilitate clinical research and yet respect the individualized homeopathic treatment. The approach comprised a patient questionnaire to identify keynote symptoms for 11 selected homeopathic medicines and a computerized algorithm to process the answers. In 2007-2008 a pilot study was conducted to evaluate the feasibility of using the questionnaire and algorithm in 20 medical homeopathic practices in the Netherlands in 38 women suffering from premenstrual syndrome/premenstrual symptoms (PMS/S), with 3 months' follow-up [20]. The use of the questionnaire and algorithm was evaluated as feasible.

### Rationale

Semi-standardized individualized homeopathic treatment could be beneficial for targeted subgroups of women with PMS. In an extension of a previous pilot study, the utility of an algorithm for homeopathic medicine selection was further evaluated with 77 women at 9 months' follow-up. The results of this evaluation, as discussed in this paper, will inform follow-up research.

## Objectives

Primary objectives were to evaluate the use of the 11 selected homeopathic medicines, identify prognostic characteristics and calculate the overall proportion of responders. The main hypotheses were that at least 50% of the women in the study population could be treated by one of the 11 algorithm-based medicines, with satisfying results. Secondary objectives were to measure short- and long-term results by estimating changes of PMS scores over time and evaluate the association between use of the 11 selected homeopathic medicines and response to treatment. This extended observational pilot study was completed in mid-2011.

## Methods

### Design

A prospective uncontrolled observational study about individualized homeopathy with semi-standardized treatment was conducted in 20 homeopathic medical practices in the Netherlands.

### Study size

The aim was to analyze data of 80 women. A sample size for this observational study was difficult to estimate, since no previous studies of similar design and follow-up duration have been carried out. In the preceding feasibility study, 38 of the 183 women who showed interest and received information were included. Based on these numbers, we would have to recruit 385 interested women.

### Approval, recruitment, information and informed consent

The Medical Ethics committee (METc) of the Vrije Universiteit Medical Center (VUMC), Amsterdam, approved the study protocol. Women were recruited by articles and advertisements in newspapers and magazines, letters to general practitioners and by launching a website about the project. Women who were interested received written information with explanation about homeopathy in general, the Israeli pilot study and the outline of the present study. We informed that treatment costs would be reimbursed, if not covered by their own insurance company. Women were invited to contact a participating homeopathic doctor, plan an intake visit and provide informed consent. We kept no records of women who, after receiving information, did not make an appointment for an interview.

### Inclusion and exclusion criteria and diagnosis

The inclusion criterion for the pre-treatment phase was a premenstrual symptom pattern as reported by women aged 18-50 years. Exclusion criteria were: a wish to get pregnant during the course of the study, use of antidepressants or hormones (except oral contraceptive pills (OCPs)), other treatment for PMS/S (except incidental use of painkillers or tranquillizers on single days) or recent homeopathic treatment for any disorder.

Before entering the treatment phase, volunteering women had to record their symptoms daily and prospectively on a 10-point scale during two months/cycles, to confirm the diagnosis PMS/premenstrual symptoms. The treating doctors confirmed or refuted the diagnosis and this was checked by the research coordinator. The 12 pre-defined premenstrual symptoms in the diaries are listed in Table 1. This diary was also used as a measurement instrument for calculation of PMS symptom scores (see below: Measurement instruments).

| Pain or swelling of breasts |
|---|
| Headache |
| Joint- or muscle-pain |
| Swelling of hands or feet |
| Bloated abdomen |
| Feeling tense |
| Craving for food |
| Thirst |
| Irritability |
| Fatigue |
| Feeling down, depressed |
| Anxious feeling |

**Table 1:** List of pre-defined symptoms in diaries.

| ICPC-code | Diagnosis | Criteria |
|---|---|---|
| X89 | Premenstrual syndrome | A cyclic occurrence in the menstrual cycle of two or more of the following symptoms during each of two consecutive cycles: peripheral oedema; breast tenderness/ swelling; headache; irritability; mood changes |
| X09 | Premenstrual symptom/ complaint | A cyclic occurrence of at least one premenstrual symptom (as stated above) during two consecutive cycles, and the criteria for X89 are not met |

**Table 2:** ICPC-2 criteria for PMS or premenstrual symptom/complaint.

| Name | Abbreviation |
|---|---|
| *Calcarea carbonica* | *Calc-c* |
| *Cimicifuga racemosa* | Cimic |
| Lac caninum | Lac-c |
| *Lachesis mutus* | Lach |
| *Lilium tigrinum* | Lil-t |
| Magnesium carbonicum | Mag-c |
| Magnesium phosphoricum | Mag-p |
| Natrium muriaticum | Nat-m |
| Phoshorus | Phos |
| *Pulsatilla pratensis* | Puls |
| *Sepia officinalis* | Sep |

**Table 3:** The 11 selected algorithm medicines in alphabetical order.

With a clear premenstrual pattern of at least one symptom and a symptom-free interval of at least 5 days in the follicular phase (=before ovulation), a woman could be included and enrolled into either the diagnosis category premenstrual syndrome or the category premenstrual symptoms. We used the International Classification of Primary Care (ICPC)-2 criteria for premenstrual syndrome (code: X89) and premenstrual symptom/complaint (code: X09). The criteria are summarized in Table 2.

## Homeopathic treatment

The participating women were treated in in various regions in the Netherlands by 20 homeopathic doctors in their own practice, all members of the Dutch Association of Homeopathic Doctors (VHAN) and trained in classical homeopathy. All treating doctors had practical experience in homeopathy of more than 5 (most with more than 10) years. Before the first visit, participating women completed a homeopathic questionnaire with 123 questions, representing keynote symptoms for 11 homeopathic medicines. The answers were transferred to the computerized diagnostic algorithm, which would present a priority list for the 11 homeopathic medicines. The doctors consulted the algorithm, followed the instructions and prescribed the first homeopathic medicine as indicated by the algorithm. At follow-up visits (after 1, 2, 3, 5, 7 and 9 months/cycles), they could continue the first (algorithm-based) prescription, or prescribe another (algorithm-based or non-algorithm-based) medicine, according to their own professional opinion. The duration of the first consultation was approximately one hour and follow-up consultations would take half an hour on average. It was not dictated what potencies could be used, but the doctors were restricted to use potencies that were considered safe according to the European Directive 2001/83/EC [21]. The study medication was dispensed and sent by regular post by the Hahnemann Pharmacy, Heiloo, The Netherlands. If registered in the Netherlands, the medicines were manufactured by VSM, Alkmaar, The Netherlands. Unregistered medicines could be manufactured by the Hahnemann pharmacy or obtained from other manufacturers.

The medicines that were selected for the algorithm are listed in Table 3. The treating homeopathic doctors would inform the women as usual about how to take the homeopathic medicines, what changes could be expected, the possibility of aggravations, etc. Women who took conventional medicines for concomitant conditions before entering the pre-treatment phase, continued to do so during the study.

## Measurement instruments

For two months before treatment and during the first three and final three months of the treatment, the women kept daily records about premenstrual symptoms, use of medication and absence from work.

Before every follow-up visit they completed a short questionnaire, with a Likert scale ranging -4 to +4 called AGOS (Adapted Glasgow Homeopathic Hospital Outcome Score), as previously described [22]. The AGOS for symptoms rated changes in premenstrual symptoms, while the AGOS for general health rated changes in general health, both compared to the start of the treatment.

## Data collection

Data were collected between October 2007 and April 2011. A study outline is presented in Figure 1. At baseline the following characteristics were recorded: age, diagnosis (X89 or X09), duration of symptoms, age of menarche, co-diagnoses, and use of conventional medicines for PMS/S, contraceptive methods, number of pregnancies and of births, history of sexual abuse, post-partum depression (PPD) and other psychiatric illness. For each woman, the baseline premenstrual symptom score (PMS score) was calculated and recorded. It was based on the diaries and defined as the sum of daily scores of the second premenstrual period (14 days) in the pre-treatment phase. Baseline premenstrual symptom scores up to and including 150 were defined as 'mild' symptoms and scores above 150 as 'moderate to severe' symptoms.

During the treatment phase, calculations of the PMS scores, use of extra medication (to a maximum of 2 different medicines) and loss of work days were based on diary reports during 14 days prior to the start of menses. Intermediate outcomes of these parameters were assessed after 3 months, 7 months and ≥ 8 months (end scores), depending on the duration of treatment for the individual participant.

Prescription reports were collected at all consultations. The sequence of homeopathic prescription types (algorithm-based or non-algorithm-based) throughout the study was evaluated in retrospect at the 5$^{th}$ follow-up visit after 7 months, because at the 6$^{th}$ follow-up the study would be completed and if women wished to continue the homeopathic treatment, problems other than PMS would also be targeted. We invited all doctors to report adverse events or worsening of symptoms.

AGOS scores were recorded just before each follow-up visit. We collected all AGOS questionnaires and evaluated the AGOS scores at the 3$^{rd}$ and last follow-up consultation. The diaries and questionnaires were collected by the treating doctors and were sent to the research coordinator. The doctors reported the details of the homeopathic prescriptions at all consultations: name, potency, dose, frequency.

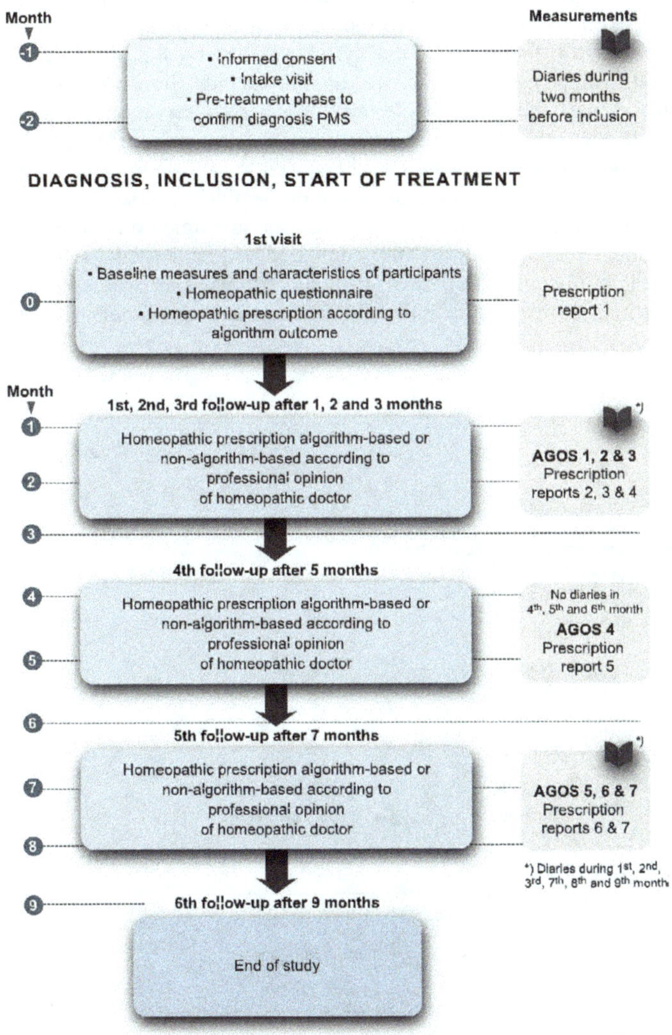


**Figure 1:** Study Outline.

## Outcome measures

Primary outcome measures were:

1a) Frequencies of actual 'algorithm-based' or 'non-algorithm-based' medicine prescriptions as measured by cross-section at the 1st visit and at the 3rd and 5th follow-up. An algorithm-based medicine was defined as a prescription according to the algorithm outcome. A non-algorithm-based medicine was defined as any other homeopathic prescription.

1b) Sequence (change/continuation) of algorithm-based and non-algorithm-based medicine prescriptions in all participants since the first visit as assessed retrospectively at the 5th follow-up visit.

1c) Frequencies of identified women in two 'overall prescription categories': those who received 'only algorithm-based' medicines versus those who received 'also non-algorithm-based' homeopathic medicines throughout the study, as assessed retrospectively at the 5th follow-up.

2) Percentage of 'responders' defined as women with a clinically relevant improvement in PMS score. PMS scores were defined as the total sum of daily scores of 12 pre-defined symptoms in the 14 days prior to the start of menstruation. Response to treatment was defined as ≥ 50% reduction in symptom ratings (PMS scores). In the literature, this is considered a clinically relevant improvement in PMS/PMDD treatment trials, 'although smaller differences may also be meaningful' [23]. We measured intermediate response after 3 months (measured in the cycle preceding the 3rd follow-up), after 7 months (measured before the 5th follow-up) and the final response after 8 months or more (the first of two cycles recorded before the last follow-up visit).

3) Association between baseline characteristics (age, use of contraceptives, severity of symptoms, psychiatric history, chronic co-morbidity) and 'response' to treatment.

Secondary outcome measures were:

4) Changes in mean PMS scores measured at consecutive visits, adjusted for 'overall prescription category' ('only algorithm-based' medicines versus 'also non-algorithm-based' medicines) and symptom severity at baseline ('mild PMS symptoms' versus 'moderate to severe PMS symptoms').

5) Association between 'overall prescription category' and 'response' to treatment at the 5th follow-up visit.

6) Self-reported changes of symptoms and general health before the 3rd and last follow-up visit as measured by the AGOS.

7) Correlation between AGOS scores and PMS scores.

## Analysis

Because of the observational nature of this evaluation study, per protocol analysis was applied for the primary and secondary outcome measures, unless otherwise stated (n=54). Incidental missing values were regarded as minor protocol violations and therefore 15 women who completed the study with incomplete intermediate reports were included in the analysis. Data were analyzed using SPSS 19.0. A two-sided p-value ≤ 0.05 was considered statistically significant.

**Analysis of primary outcomes:** 1. Descriptive statistics were used to: a) calculate frequencies of algorithm-based and non-algorithm-based medicine prescriptions, b) evaluate sequences of algorithm-based and non-algorithm-based prescriptions, c) calculate frequencies of women in the two 'overall prescription categories' as defined before.

2. Descriptive statistics were used to measure the proportion of responders.

3. Logistic regression was used to find possible associations between baseline characteristics (e.g. age, symptom severity, chronic co-morbidity, psychiatric history) and 'response' to treatment.

**Analysis of secondary outcomes:** 4. linear models were built by mixed models analysis. This method was chosen since it can deal with missing values. Mixed models analysis was used to determine the association between 'symptom severity' at baseline (mild or moderate to severe) as well as 'overall prescription category' (based on prescription reports after the 5th follow-up) and changes in PMS scores throughout the study.

5. Descriptive statistics were used to evaluate the association between the identified 'overall prescription category' and 'response' to treatment.

6. Descriptive statistics were also used to evaluate AGOS for symptoms and general health.

7. Spearman's correlation coefficient was used to calculate the correlation between the AGOS scores and PMS scores.

## Results

### Participants, dropouts and missing data

Recruitment took place between October 2007 and April 2010 and was paused between August 2008 and February 2009, for an intermediate evaluation of reimbursed treatment costs within the study budget. 77 women with premenstrual symptoms were found eligible and were included for the treatment phase. A flow chart is presented in Figure 2.

The age range was 24-49, the mean age 38.44 years. In 7 participants a major improvement of symptoms (drop of PMS scores of ≥ 50% between the first and second cycle) was observed during the pre-treatment phase. However, we did not exclude these women from further participation, considering this was an observational study. In Table 4, characteristics of women at baseline are presented, as well as associations between baseline characteristics and completers versus dropouts. The dropout rate was considerable. A relatively higher dropout rate was found in two categories: in women diagnosed with premenstrual symptoms (X09) compared to premenstrual syndrome (X89) (Chi-square test, two-sided, p=0.019) and in women with a psychiatric history (other than PPD) compared to women without a

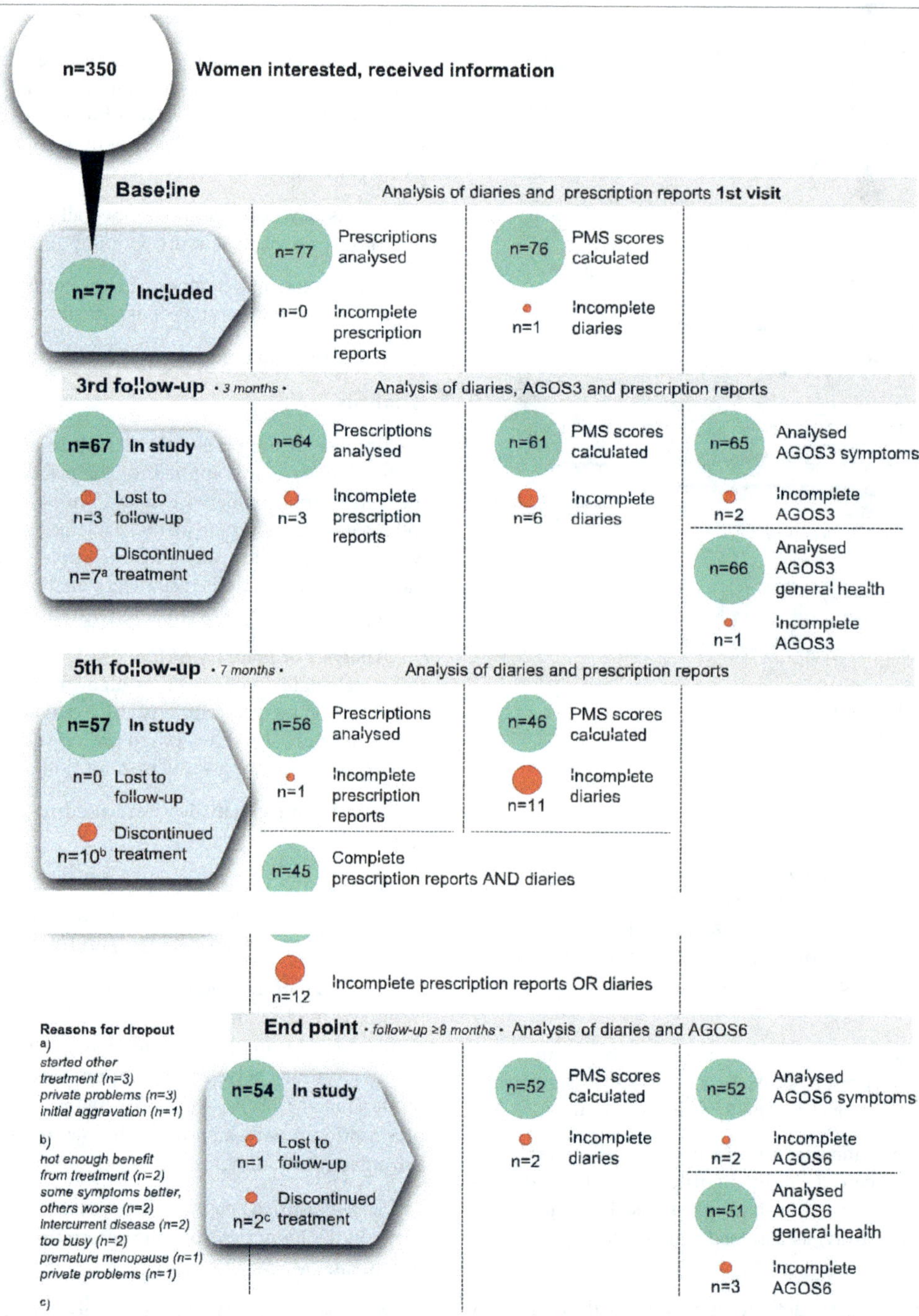


**Figure 2:** Flowchart.

| Baseline characteristics | Total (N=77) | Completed study (N=54) | Dropouts (N=23) | Significance. Pearson 2-sided chi-square test |
|---|---|---|---|---|
| *Age. 3 groups* | | | | *P=0.229* |
| 18-30 years | 7 (9.1%) | 3 (5.6%) | 4 (17.4%) | |
| 31-40 years | 41 (53.2%) | 29 (53.7%) | 12 (52.2%) | |
| 41-51 years | 29 (37.7%) | 22 (40.7%) | 7 (30.4%) | |
| *Contraceptive methods* | *(N=74)* | *(N=52)* | *(N=22)* | *P=0.790* |
| OCP | 5 (6.7%) | 4 (7.7%) | 1(4.5%) | |
| Levonorgestrel-releasing IUD | 3 (4.0%) | 2 (3.8%) | 1(4.5%) | |
| Copper IUD | 4 (5.4%) | 2 (3.8%) | 2 (9.1%) | |
| None | 62 (83.8%) | 44 (84.6%) | 18 (81.8%) | |
| *Co-morbidity* | *(N=77)* | *(N=54)* | *(N=23)* | |
| Yes | 43 (55.8%) | 30 (55.6%) | 13 (56.5%) | *P= 0.938* |
| *Diagnosis category* | *(N=74)*)* | *(N=53)* | *(N=21)* | ***P= 0.019*** |
| PMS symptoms (X09) | 9 (12.0%) | 3 (5.7.%) | 6 (28.6%) | |
| PMS syndrome (X89) | 65 (88.0%) | 50 (94.3%) | 15 (71.4%) | |
| *Psychiatric history* | *(N=69)* | *(N=49)* | *(N=20)* | ***P= 0.006*** |
| Post partum depression (PPD) | 9 (13.0%) | 8 (16.3%) | 1 (5.0%) | |
| Other psychiatric diagnosis | 10 (14.5% | 3 (6.1%) | 7 (35.0%) | |
| No psychiatric diagnosis | 50 (72.5%) | 38 (77.6%) | 12 (60.0%) | |
| *PMS scores at baseline* | *(N=76)*)* | *(N=53)* | *(N=23)* | *P= 0.721* |
| Mild symptoms | 34 (44.2%) | 23 (43.4%) | 11 (47.8%) | |
| Moderate to severe symptoms | 42 (55.3%) | 30 (56.6%) | 12 (52.2%) | |
| *Overall prescription category (whole study)* | *(N=67)* | *(N=54)* | *(N=13)* | *P= 0.455* |
| All according to algorithm | 35 (52.2%) | 27 (50.0%) | 8 (61.5.4%) | |
| Not all according to algorithm | 32 (58.2%) | 27 (50.0%) | 5 (38.5%) | |

**Table 4:** Association between baseline characteristics and completers/dropouts as well as association between baseline characteristics and 'overall prescription category'.

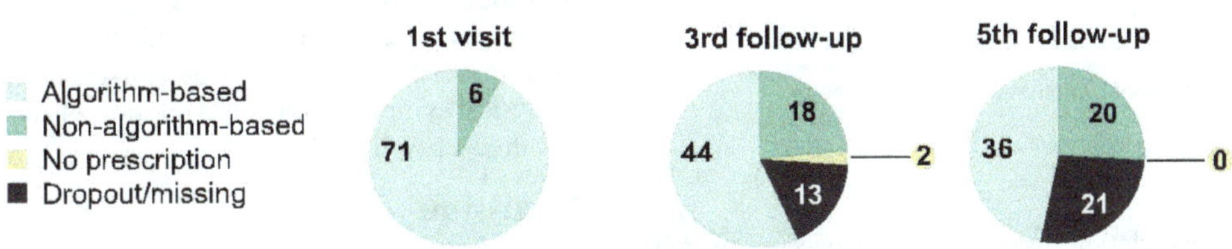


**Figure 3:** (Non)-algorithm-based prescriptions at the 1st visit, and at the 3rd and 5th follow-up.

psychiatric history (Chi-square test, two-sided, p=0.006).

Throughout the study, reports could be incomplete or missing. Numbers with complete reports could vary for diaries, AGOS questionnaires (both completed by patients), or prescription reports (completed by doctors). 39 women had complete reports and diaries at all measurement points. No influence of baseline characteristics on complete or incomplete data was found (Chi-square test, two-sided; age group: p=0.910; contraceptive method: p=0.897; co-morbidity: p=0.414; diagnosis category: p=0.072; psychiatric history: p=0.264; PMS scores at baseline: p=0.504).

## Duration of follow-up

The timing of the 3rd follow-up visit varied from 2.5 to 4 months. The final visit took place after 8 or 9 months in 38 women, after 10 or 11 months in 11 women and after 12 months or more in 5 women. The mean duration of treatment was 7.5 months and the median was 8.0 months.

## Primary outcomes

1a) The proportion of algorithm-based prescriptions declined considerably between the 1st visit and the 3rd follow up and then stabilized. At the first visit, 92.2% of the prescriptions was algorithm-based (n=71), this was 68.8% at the 3rd follow-up (n=44) and 64.3% at the 5th follow-up visit (n=36). Numbers of (non-) algorithm-based prescriptions and dropouts/missing values per visit are presented in Figure 3.

1b) In 17 of the 36 women who were using an algorithm-based medicine at the 5th follow-up, the prescription had been unchanged since the start of the study (47.2%).

1c) In total, 29 women had used only one or more algorithm-based medicines during the study (51.8%), while 27 had used also non-algorithm-based homeopathic medicines (48.2%) as measured in retrospect at the 5th follow-up.

2) At the end of the study, 57.7% (30 out of 52) of the women in the study were identified as responders (decrease of PMS scores ≥ 50%). In table 5, details are given about the percentage of responders and other result categories throughout the study.

3) In the responders group, no characteristics were found that were independently associated with a 50% drop in PMS scores.

| | 3rd follow-up | | End visit | |
|---|---|---|---|---|
| Result category | N | *Valid %* | N | *Valid %* |
| Positive response | 25 | *41.7* | 30 | *57.7* |
| Moderate improvement | 10 | *16.7* | 8 | *15.4* |
| No change/unsure | 15 | *25.0* | 8 | *15.4* |
| Deterioration | 10 | *13.0* | 6 | *11.5* |
| Analyzed | 60 | *100* | 52 | *100* |
| Dropouts, missing/incomplete reports | 17 | | 25 | |
| Total | 77 | | 77 | |

**Table 5:** Numbers and percentages of women in various result categories.

| AGOS scores | 3rd follow-up visit | | | | End visit | | | |
|---|---|---|---|---|---|---|---|---|
| | Changes in premenstrual symptoms | | Changes in general health | | Changes in premenstrual symptoms | | Changes in general health | |
| Score | N | % | N | % | N | % | N | % |
| +4 | 1 | 1.5 | 1 | 1.5 | 2 | 3.8 | 2 | 3.8 |
| +3 | 13 | 20.0 | 4 | 6.1 | 18 | 34.6 | 10 | 18.9 |
| +2 | 16 | 24.6 | 11 | 16.7 | 8 | 15.4 | 7 | 13.2 |
| +1 | 14 | 21.5 | 13 | 19.7 | 16 | 30.8 | 11 | 20.8 |
| 0 | 12 | 18.5 | 26 | 39.4 | 2 | 5.8 | 17 | 34.0 |
| -1 | 3 | 4.6 | 7 | 10.6 | 3 | 5.8 | 1 | 1.9 |
| -2 | 2 | 3.1 | 2 | 3.0 | 2 | 3.8 | 3 | 3.9 |
| -3 | 4 | 6.2 | 2 | 3.0 | 0 | 0 | 1 | 1.9 |
| -4 | 0 | 0 | 0 | 0 | 0 | 0 | 0 | 0 |
| Evaluated | 65 | 100 | 66 | 100 | 51 | 100 | 52 | 100 |
| Invalid/ missing score/ dropout | 12 | | 11 | | 26 | | 25 | |
| Total | 77 | | 77 | | 77 | | 77 | |

**Table 6:** AGOS scores for symptoms and general health.

## Secondary outcomes

4) No significant association was found between 'overall prescription category' ('only algorithm-based' versus 'also non-algorithm-based') and changes in mean PMS scores throughout the study (n=54; p=0.765). Meanwhile, an overall effect was detected: a significant association was found between symptom severity at baseline (mild or moderate to severe) and changes in mean PMS score throughout the study (n=54; p<0.001).

5) Additionally, in the group with 29 women who had received 'only algorithm-based medicines' at the 5th follow-up visit, 15 were identified as responders (51.8%), while in the group with 16 women who had received 'also non-algorithm-based medicines', 5 were identified as 'responders' (31.3%). Data of 45 women with complete diaries and prescription reports at the 5th follow-up were evaluated.

6) At the end of the study, 28 out of 51 women (36.4%) with valid scores at the AGOS for symptoms reported a score of +2 (associated with moderate improvement) or more, while 10 out of 52 reported +2 or more at the AGOS for general health (24.7%). All intermediate and final outcomes of the AGOS for symptoms and AGOS for general health are listed in Table 6.

7) We found a significant correlation between the course of PMS scores and the AGOS for symptoms (Spearman's correlation coefficient -0.4, p<0.001) as well as a borderline significance on correlation between the changes in PMS scores and the AGOS for general health (Spearman's correlation coefficient -0.12, p=0.054).

## Homeopathic medicines used

Overall, 43 different homeopathic medicines were prescribed during the study, mostly for PMS/S symptoms, sometimes for additionally treating inter-current, acute complaints or a general condition. In Table 7 details of homeopathic medicines that were used in the study are presented.

## Potency and dose

The following potencies were used: D12, C30, C200, 30K, 200K, MK, XMK, Q1, Q3, Q6, Q12 (see: List of abbreviations). Repetition varied from daily doses with D12 or low Q-potencies, to once per week, or every two, four or six weeks. Sometimes women were instructed to take a dose at a particular phase of the menstrual cycle. All medicines were dispensed as granules.

## Adverse Events/Aggravations

No unexpected or serious adverse reactions were reported that could be attributed to the homeopathic treatment. Several important events were reported during the study time, like death of family members, loss of work, serious illness, divorce, major surgery, admission to mental hospital and burnout. In some cases these events led to termination of participation (Figure 2, reasons for dropout). In 26 cases, doctors reported mild, transient aggravation of symptoms that could be explained as an initial reaction to the homeopathic medication. In 4 participants, old symptoms returned and disappeared again during the course of the treatment. Initial aggravations and return of old symptoms are commonly observed during homeopathic treatment [24]. 3 women dropped out after their symptoms had worsened: 1 suffered from a burnout and it is unclear if the aggravation of symptoms could be attributed to the homeopathic medicine; 1 had only mild symptoms that improved by 50%, but acne worsened; 1 reported improvement of physical symptoms but deterioration of mental symptoms and she consulted a psychologist.

# Discussion

In this study, the utility of a previously designed and tested questionnaire and algorithm for semi-standardized individualized homeopathic treatment of women with PMS/S with 11 medicines was confirmed in 77 women with 9 months' follow-up, with promising results. The use of this questionnaire and algorithm could be recommended to facilitate further clinical research about homeopathic treatment of women with PMS. With the non-randomized study design it was not possible to evaluate efficacy of the 11 selected medicines.

## Considerations about the semi standardized treatment

Almost half (47.2%) of the first algorithm-based prescriptions remained stable throughout the 9 months' study period in women who completed the study. This could indicate that in these women the medicine selection by the algorithm was considered accurate by the treating doctor. This finding is meaningful, because in this study, with 11 medicines and strict criteria for the first prescription, the first homeopathic medicine selection might have led to inaccurate 'individualized' homeopathic prescriptions in a considerable (beforehand unknown) proportion of the participating women. The increase in non-algorithm-based prescriptions at the 3rd follow-up visit supports this last assumption. The association between 'overall prescription category' and results was evaluated by qualitative, descriptive and by quantitative analysis. Relatively more 'responders' were found in the group who had used 'only algorithm-based

| Medicines prescribed | First visit | | Follow-up 1 | | Follow-up 2 | | Follow-up 3 | | Follow-up 4 | | Follow-up 5 | | Follow-up 6 | |
|---|---|---|---|---|---|---|---|---|---|---|---|---|---|---|
| | N | % | N | % | N | % | N | % | N | % | N | % | N | % |
| *Sepia officinalis* | 19 | 24.7 | 15 | 21.7 | 16 | 24.2 | 16 | 25.4 | 9 | 17.3 | 9 | 16.1 | 7 | 13.4 |
| *Natrium muriaticum* | 14 | 18.2 | 10 | 14.5 | 8 | 12.1 | 5 | 7.9 | 7 | 13.5 | 6 | 10.7 | 7 | 13.4 |
| *Lilium tigrinum* | 11 | 14.3 | 10 | 14.5 | 7 | 10.6 | 9 | 14.3 | 9 | 17.3 | 10 | 17.9 | 11 | 21.1 |
| *Cimicifuga racemosa* | 6 | 7.8 | 7 | 10.1 | 6 | 9.1 | 7 | 11.1 | 4 | 7.7 | 2 | 3.6 | | |
| *Lachesis mutus* | 6 | 7.8 | 5 | 7.2 | 2 | 3.0 | 3 | 4.8 | 3 | 5.8 | 2 | 3.6 | 2 | 3.8 |
| Magnesium carbonicum | 6 | 7.8 | 5 | 6.5 | 4 | 6.1 | 3 | 4.8 | 3 | 5.8 | 3 | 5.4 | 3 | 5.8 |
| Magnesium phosphoricum | 6 | 7.8 | 4 | 5.2 | 5 | 7.6 | 4 | 6.3 | 3 | 5.8 | 3 | 5.4 | 2 | 3.8 |
| Phosphorus | 3 | 3.9 | 2 | 2.6 | 2 | 3.0 | 2 | 3.2 | | | 1 | 1.8 | 1 | 1.9 |
| Calcarea carbonica | 1 | 1.3 | | | 3 | 4.5 | 3 | 4.8 | 4 | 7.7 | 3 | 5.4 | 3 | 5.8 |
| *Lac caninum* | 1 | 1.3 | 1 | 1.4 | | | 1 | 1.6 | 1 | 1.9 | 2 | 3.6 | 1 | 1.9 |
| *Pulsatilla pratensis* | 1 | 1.3 | 2 | 2.9 | 1 | 1.5 | 2 | 3.2 | 2 | 3.8 | 2 | 3.6 | 2 | 3.8 |
| *Lycopodium clavatum* | 1 | 1.3 | | | | | | | | | | | | |
| *Nux vomica* | 1 | 1.3 | 1 | 1.4 | 1 | 1.5 | 1 | 1.6 | 1 | 1.9 | 3 | 5.4 | 2 | 3.8 |
| Natrium carbonicum | 1 | 1.3 | 1 | 1.4 | 1 | 1.5 | 1 | 1.6 | 1 | 1.9 | 1 | 1.8 | 2 | 3.8 |
| Folliculinum | | | 2 | 2.9 | 2 | 3.0 | | | | | | | 1 | 1.9 |
| Tuberculinum | | | | | 1 | 1.5 | 1 | 1.6 | 1 | 1.9 | 1 | 1.8 | 1 | 1.9 |
| Chamomilla | | | | | 1 | 1.5 | 1 | 1.6 | | | | | | |
| Carcinosinum | | | | | | | 1 | 1.6 | 2 | 3.8 | 1 | 1.8 | 1 | 1.9 |
| Staphysagria | | | | | | | | | 1 | 1.9 | 1 | 1.8 | | |
| Samarium muriaticum | | | | | | | | | | | 1 | 1.8 | 1 | 1.9 |
| No medicine prescribed | 0 | | 3 | | 4 | | 1 | | 2 | | 0 | | 5 | |
| Missing/dropout | 0 | | 8 | | 11 | | 14 | | 25 | | 21 | | 25 | |
| Total analysed | 77 | | 69 | | 66 | | 63 | | 52 | | 56 | | 52 | |

**Table 7:** Homeopathic medicines used in the study.

medicines' compared to the group who had used 'also non-algorithm-based prescriptions'. However, after estimation of changes in mean PMS scores, no statistical significant differences were found between the groups with 'only algorithm-based' versus 'also non-algorithm-based' homeopathic medicines. To compare this semi-standardized treatment to 'unrestricted' individualized treatment (according to the personal analysis of the homeopath) would require a different study design.

## Dropouts

It was evaluated what proportion of the women who dropped out, had experienced no improvement or deterioration of symptoms. Of the 23 dropouts, 7 women (30.4%) reported 'improvement of symptoms' at the time of dropout (AGOS: +1, +2, +3 or +4), 6 (26.1%) reported 'no change/unsure' (AGOS=0) and 7 (30.4%) reported 'deterioration' (AGOS: -1, -2, -3 or -4). 3 women (13.0%) dropped out before the first follow-up visit and did not complete the first AGOS questionnaires.

## Duration of follow-up

In 16 women, the follow-up duration was more than 9 months. This could be due to lengthy menstrual cycles, planning problems or holidays. Several women who completed 9 months had missed at least one intermediate follow-up visit. We would define their last visit as the 6$^{th}$ follow-up and report missing data at the 5$^{th}$ follow-up (7 months). This explains why we have more missing data at the 5$^{th}$ than at the 6$^{th}$ follow-up. The lengthy follow-up may have contributed to the overall high dropout rate (22% after 3 months, 30% at the end).

## Course of individual premenstrual symptoms

The mean scores of most of the 12 individual pre-defined symptoms (Table 1) gradually declined throughout the study, except for the symptom 'pain or swelling of breasts'. The mean score of this symptom decreased, but returned to baseline levels at the end of the study. In general, without a control group, we cannot know which proportion of any symptom improvement might be attributed to regression to the mean or to specific or non-specific treatment effects.

## Use of medication and absence from work

Women also reported about use of additional (conventional) medication and loss of work days. Some women not only reported the use of medication for PMS symptoms, but also for other complaints, such as flu or post-operational pain. Based on this inadequate reporting, we can draw no conclusions about changes in use of additional medicines for PMS symptoms during the study, even where we observed a considerable decline. Neither could evaluation of loss of work days lead to conclusions, because of small numbers: only 5 women reported absence from work because of PMS symptoms at baseline.

## General health

At the end of the study, 12 women reported 'major improvement of general health' or 'cure' by the AGOS for general health, as can be observed in table 6 (23.1%; n=52). A borderline significant association was found between mean changes in PMS scores and AGOS for general health. Not all women, whose premenstrual symptoms improved, reported improvement in general health additionally. This was also observed in the previous pilot study, where several participants whose premenstrual symptoms improved, explained they had enjoyed excellent general health before the start of the study and this had not changed.

## Positioning this research

For research about individualized homeopathic interventions in specific clinical conditions, like PMS, various pieces of evidence are required. Efficacy of specified homeopathic medicines in controlled conditions as well as effectiveness of well-defined homeopathic interventions in daily practice should be evaluated. Yakir et al. explored the efficacy of specified homeopathic medicines compared to placebo in semi-standardized individualized homeopathic treatment of women with PMS in controlled conditions [14]. The Dutch research line focused on pragmatic research, to evaluate the effectiveness of a homeopathic intervention with semi-standardized medicine selection. This homeopathic treatment was as close to 'real life' homeopathic practice as possible, within the limitations of the study design. The results of pragmatic trials are more generalizable than those of explanatory trials [25].

In October 2012, as a next step, the present research group started an international pilot study in the Netherlands, Germany and Sweden, to investigate the feasibility of organizing a large pragmatic randomized controlled trial.

## Conclusions and Recommendations

A semi-standardized algorithm for individualized homeopathic treatment of women suffering from PMS/S with 11 medicines proved useful in daily homeopathic practice. Restrictions for the first prescription improved reproducibility of the treatment. The proportion of algorithm-based prescriptions declined during the study, but was still 68.8% at the 3rd follow-up and 64.3% at the 5th follow-up. At the end point (≥ 8 months follow-up), a clinically relevant improvement of premenstrual symptoms had occurred in 57.5% of the analyzed group (n=52) and in 39% of women who were included (n=77). Additionally, the mean decline in premenstrual symptoms throughout the study was statistically significant. Significantly more women with mild PMS symptoms dropped out (compared to women with moderate to severe symptoms), as well as women with a psychiatric history other than PPD (compared to women without a psychiatric history). These outcomes could have implications for inclusion or exclusion of these groups in future research.

The PMS algorithm could be used in follow-up research about PMS treatment in other settings. A shorter duration of follow-up would be recommended to limit dropout rates. To diminish the proportion of missing diaries, online diaries could be used. If the algorithm-based treatment for PMS is validated in controlled clinical trials, it could be implemented in primary care for women with premenstrual disorders. Similar semi-standardized types of homeopathic treatment could be tested for other relevant clinical conditions.

## Acknowledgement

The study was sponsored by the Dutch medical research organization ZonMw, the Dutch patients/ consumers organization Koninklijke Vereniging Homeopathie Nederland (KVHN), VSM Geneesmiddelen BV, Alkmaar, the Netherlands (who provided the registered medicines used in the study) and the Louise van Eeghen Stichting. All medicines were delivered free of postal charge by the Hahnemann Pharmacy, Heiloo, the Netherlands. We wish to thank the participating women, the participating homeopathic doctors and the (previous) Dutch Association of Homeopathic Doctors (VHAN) for secretarial and administrative support. We also thank Daniëlle van der Windt (previously at EMGO-institute for research in primary care, Vrije Universiteit Medical Center (VUMC), Amsterdam, presently at Institute for Primary Care and Health Sciences, Keele University, UK) for her expert help to set up the study, Robert Mathie (British Homeopathic Association) for his helpful critical comments on the manuscript and Annet van den Berg (independent designer) for the excellent infographics.

## References

1. Halbreich U, Backstrom T, Eriksson E, O'Brien S, Calil H, et al (2007) Clinical diagnostic criteria for premenstrual syndrome and guidelines for their quantification for research studies. Gynecological endocrinology : the official journal of the International Society of Gynecological Endocrinology. 23: 123-130.
2. O'Brien PM, Backstrom T, Brown C, Dennerstein L, Endicott J, et al. (2011) Towards a consensus on diagnostic criteria, measurement and trial design of the premenstrual disorders: the ISPMD Montreal consensus. Archives of women's mental health.14: 13-21.
3. Mishell DR (2005) Jr. Premenstrual disorders: epidemiology and disease burden. The American journal of managed care 11: S 473-479.
4. Heinemann LA, Minh TD, Filonenko A, Uhl-Hochgraber K (2010) Explorative evaluation of the impact of severe premenstrual disorders on work absenteeism and productivity. Women's health issues: official publication of the Jacobs Institute of Women's Health 20: 58-65.
5. Marjoribanks J, Brown J, O'Brien PM, Wyatt K (2013) Selective serotonin reuptake inhibitors for premenstrual syndrome. Cochrane Database Syst Rev 6: CD001396.
6. Shah NR, Jones JB, Aperi J, Shemtov R, Karne A (2008) Selective serotonin reuptake inhibitors for premenstrual syndrome and premenstrual dysphoric disorder: a meta-analysis. Obstetrics and gynecology. 111: 1175-1182
7. Lopez LM, Kaptein AA, Helmerhorst FM (2012) Oral contraceptives containing drospirenone for premenstrual syndrome. Cochrane database of systematic reviews 2: CD006586.
8. Freeman EW, Rickels K, Sammel MD, Lin H, Sondheimer SJ (2009) Time to relapse after short- or long-term treatment of severe premenstrual syndrome with sertraline. Archives of general psychiatry 66: 537-544.
9. Halbreich U (2008) Selective Serotonine Reuptake Inhibitors and Initial oral contraceptives for the treatment of PMDD: Effective but not enough. CNS Spectr 13: 566,569-572.
10. Sundstrom-Poromaa I, Bixo M, Bjorn I, Nordh O (2000) Compliance to antidepressant drug therapy for treatment of premenstrual syndrome. J Psychosom Obstet Gynaecol, 21: 205-211.
11. Freeman EW (2010) Therapeutic management of premenstrual syndrome. Expert opinion on pharmacotherapy 11: 2879-2889.
12. Yakir M, Kreitler S, Brzezinski A, Vithoulkas G, Oberbaum M, et al (2001) Effects of homeopathic treatment in women with premenstrual syndrome: a pilot study. Br Hom J 90: 148-153.
13. Lepaisant C (1995) Clinical trials in homeopathy: treatment of mastodynia due to premenstrual syndrome. Rev Fr Gynecol Obstet 90: 94-97.
14. Chapman EH, Angelica J, Spitalny G (1994) Strauss M. Results of a study of the homeopathic treatment of PMS. J Am Inst Hom 87: 14-21.
15. Komar T, Peck KS, Torline JR, Deroukakis M (2006) A qualitative study to determine the efficacy of the homeopathic simillimum in the treatment of premenstrual syndrome. Am J Hom Med 99: 196-204.
16. Fäustle R (1992) Behandlung des prämenstruellen Syndroms mit einem homoöpathischen Kombinationspräparat. Biol Med 6: 423-426
17. Martinez B (1990) Folliculinum: Efficacy in premenstrual syndrome. Br Hom J 79: 104-105.
18. Laister, C-A (2008) The efficacy of homoeopathic simillimum in the treatment of premenstrual syndrome (PMS). PhD thesis. Department of Homoeopathy, Durban Institute of Technology .
19. Danno K, Colas A, Terzan L, Bordet MF (2013) Homeopathic treatment of premenstrual syndrome: a case series. Homeopathy 102: 59-65.
20. Klein-Laansma CT, Jansen JCH, van Tilborgh AJW, Van der Windt DAWM, Mathie RT, et al (2010) Semi-standardised homeopathic treatment of premenstrual syndrome with a limited number of medicines: Feasibility study. Homeopathy 99: 192-204.

21. Directive 2001/83/EC of the European Parliament and of the Council of 6 November 2006 on the Community Code relating to the Medicinal Products for Human Use.

22. Borenstein JE, Dean BB, Leifke E, Korner P, Yonkers KA (2007) Differences in symptom scores and health outcomes in premenstrual syndrome. J Women's Health 16: 1139-1144.

23. Rossi E, Bartoli P, Bianchi A, Endrizzi C, Da Frè M (2012) Homeopathic aggravation with Quinquagintamillesimal potencies. Homeopathy 101: 112-120.

24. Thompson E, Barron S, Spence D (2004) A preliminary audit investigating remedy reactions including adverse events in routine homeopathic practice. Homeopathy 93: 203-209.

25. Witt CM (2009) Efficacy, effectiveness, pragmatic trials--guidance on terminology and the advantages of pragmatic trials. Forschende Komplementarmedizin 16: 292-294.

# 29

# Low Frequency Electro-Acupuncture and Physical Exercise Induces Menstruation in a Young Woman with Amenorrhea Related to Polycystic Ovary Syndrome

**Dongmei Huang**[1*], **Qing Wang**[1,2], **Haoxu Dong**[2], **Lina Zhang**[2] **and Yanjuan Liu**[3*]

[1]*Institute of Integrated Traditional Chinese and Western Medicine, Tongji hospital, Huazhong University of Science and Technology, China*

[2]*Department of Obstetrics and Gynecology, First Affiliated Hospital, Heilongjiang University of Chinese Medicine, China*

[3]*Department of Integrated Traditional Chinese and Western Medicine, Tongji hospital, Huazhong University of Science and Technology, China*

[*]**Corresponding author:** Dongmei Huang, Institute of Integrated Traditional Chinese and Western Medicine, Tongji hospital, Huazhong University of Science and Technology, China, E-mail: hdmjcr@qq.com

## Abstract

**Objectives**: We report a successful case in a young woman with amenorrhea related to polycystic ovarian syndrome (PCOS) following low-frequency electro-acupuncture (EA) and physical exercise.

**Subject:** A 26 year old woman had secondary amenorrhea since 2002 and was diagnosed to have PCOS in 2007. She always took medroxyprogesterone acetate (MPA) for getting withdrawal bleeding every 3 months from 2002 to 2007. She had been treated with metformin, ethinylestradiol, cyproterone acetate tablets (Dyne-35) and Chinese medicine on an irregular basis from 2007 to April in 2012. When she attended our clinic, she had suffered from amenorrhea for 4 months as she stopped taking any medicine.

**Interventions:** The patient did regular physical exercise and received two courses of acupuncture treatment separated by an interval of 5 months. Each course of acupuncture treatment included 32 sessions of low-frequency EA.

**Results:** During the first course of EA treatment, she did not have any period returned. However, in the subsequent five months without any treatment, her periods returned four times. During the second EA treatment course, the patient had period for three times. Her abnormal high serum LH/FSH ratio reduced obviously and the morphology of polycystic ovaries was not found on pelvic scanning. During the following four months after the second EA treatment course, the patient had period for three times, and her sex hormone profile and ovarian morphology still kept normal.

**Conclusion:** This case illustrated that acupuncture and physical exercise can be an effective treatment for PCOS patients with ovulatory disorder.

## Introduction

Polycystic ovary syndrome (PCOS) affects about 6-8% of reproductive age women and is the most common reproductive endocrine disorder [1]. Women with PCOS are characterized by oligo-ovulation or anovulation, hyperandrogenism, polycystic ovary, inappropriate gonadotropin secretion (elevated level of circulating luteinizing hormone) and insulin resistance accompanying with compensatory hyperinsulinemia.

Acupuncture is a kind of non-drug therapy originated from traditional Chinese medicine. It is a safe treatment with few side effects [2]. Now it has been already widely used all over the world. Previous studies have shown that acupuncture can inhibit androgen secretion, regulate gonadotropin secretion and enhance ovulation and menstruation [3]. Here, we report a successful case in a young woman with amenorrhea related to PCOS following low-frequency electro-acupuncture (EA) and physical exercise without using any other treatments including western medicine and Chinese herbs.

## Case History

In August 2012, a 26 year old single woman attended the out-patient department of integrated traditional Chinese and western medicine in Tongji hospital for the treatment of amenorrhea related to PCOS. She complained of secondary amenorrhea since 2002 and had to take medroxyprogesterone acetate (MPA) every three months for withdrawal bleeding from 2002 to 2007. In November 2007, she took an ultrasonic examination showing that there were many small follicles liking honey comb in both ovaries. She told us she was diagnosed as PCOS at that time and had ever taken metformin, ethinylestradiol and cyproterone acetate tablets (Dyne-35) and Chinese medicine on an irregular basis from 2007 to April 2012. From April to August in 2012, she stopped taking any medicine for fear of potential side effects of the drugs and she did not have period during this period. Thus, she attended our clinic and resorted to complementary therapy other than medications.

On 26 January 2011, the patient underwent Oral Glucose Tolerance Test (OGTT) and Insulin Release Test (IRT), showing that Fasting

Plasma Glucose (FPG) and insulin (FIns), 1 h, 2 h and 3 h postprandial plasma glucose and insulin were all normal. But the insulin secretion peak was postponed to 3 h postprandial.

On 10 March 2012 (the third day of menstruation, D3), serum levels of sex hormones were examined as the following: Luteinizing Hormone (LH) level was 18.78 IU/L, follicle-stimulating hormone (FSH) level was 4.67 IU/L, prolectin (PRL) level was 10.59 μg/L, progesterone (P) level was 1.89 nmol/L, Estradiol (E2) level was 156.6 pmol/L and Testosterone (T) level was 2.02 nmol/L.

On 3 August 2012, the patient undertook an ultrasonic examination, showing that there were over 12 follicles with diameter <10 mm in both ovaries.

Before our intervention, the patient is 155 cm high and 60 kg weight. Her body mass index (BMI) is 25.

## Materials and Methods

### Life style intervention

The patient was informed of benefits of regular physical exercise for PCOS [4]. Since August 2012 until now, she has kept on physical exercise including jogging, cycling and kick boxing regularly, 4-5 times a week and each time lasting for about 2 hours. Physical exercise was self-monitored by counting her pulse rate to ensure a heart rate of 120 beats/min.

### Acupuncture treatment

The patient received two courses of low-frequency EA treatment with a maximum of 32 treatment sessions in each course. The low-frequency EA treatment was performed twice a week and each treatment session lasting for 30 minutes was separated by an interval of 2-4 days. EA treatment was stopped during menstruation. The acupuncture was conducted by two qualified acupuncturists with over 3 years of clinical experience.

Acupuncture protocol was as same as that used in reference [5]. Two sets of acupoints were used alternatively. The first set consisted of conception vessel (CV) 3, CV 6, governor vessel (GV) 20 and bilateral stomach (ST) 29, spleen (SP) 6, SP 9, large intestine (LI) 4 (Figure. 1). Disposable, single-use, sterilized needles (Size: 0.25×40 mm and 0.30×40/50 mm; Lot: 251226; Wuxi Jiajian Medical Instrument, Wuxi, China) made of stainless steel were inserted into a depth of 15–35 mm and stimulated manually to evoke needle sensation (de qi). CV 3, CV 6, ST 29, SP 6 and SP 9 were thereafter connected to electrical stimulator (Export Abteilung, Schwa-Medico GmbH, Wetzlarer Str. 41-43; 35630 Ehringshausen) and stimulated with low-frequency EA of 2 Hz, 0.3 ms pulse. The length and intensity were adjusted to produce local muscle contractions without pain or discomfort. Needles which were not connected to the electrical stimulator were manually stimulated to evoke needle sensation every 10 min, in total 4 times. The second set of acupoints consists of ST 25 and ST 29 bilaterally (electrical stimulation), SP 6 and liver (LR) 3 bilaterally (electrical stimulation), CV 3 and CV 6 (manual stimulation), pericardium (PC) 6 bilaterally and GV 20 (both manual stimulation) (Figure 2). The method of electrical stimulation is the same as the first set.

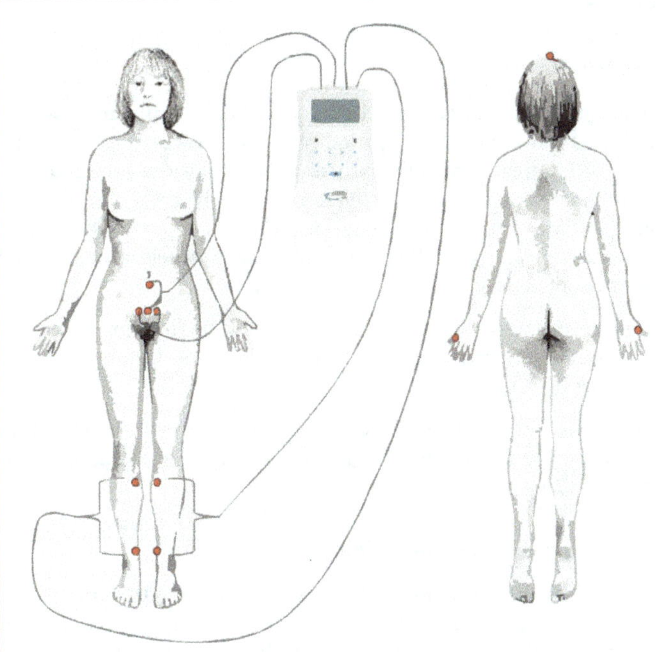

**Figure 1:** Location of the first set of acupuncture points

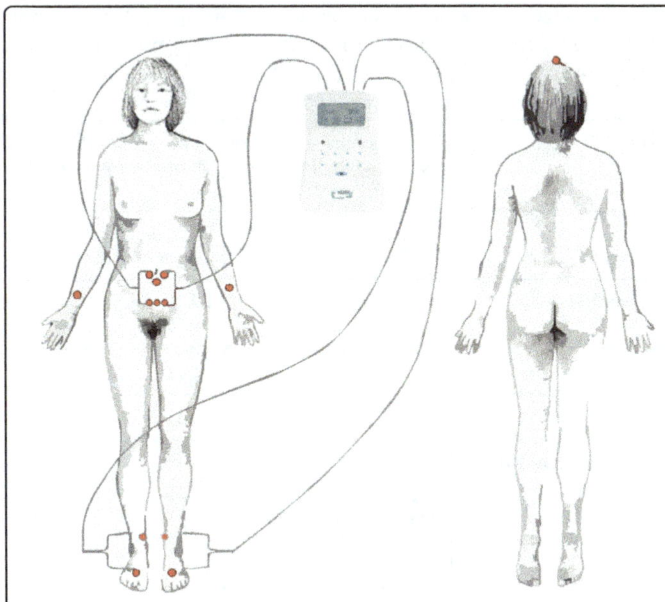

**Figure 2:** Location of the second set of acupuncture points

From August 2012 to January 2013, the patient received the first course of EA treatment which started shortly after a withdrawal bleeding following progestin? Because of the return of periods after the first course of EA treatment, she asked for another course of EA treatment. Thus, from July to December 2013, the patient received the second course of EA treatment and the protocol of EA was the same as the first course.

## Results

### Menstruation

During the first course of EA treatment (32 acupuncture sessions), the patient did not have any period returned. However, after the first course of EA treatment was finished, from January to June 2013, the patient had periods for four times respectively on 7 February, 27 March, 26 May and 26 June of 2013. During this period, the patient just went on jogging, cycling and kick boxing as before without any other treatments.

During the second course of EA treatment, the patient got periods for 3 times respectively on 11 September, 19 October and 23 November of 2013.

After she finished two courses of acupuncture in December 2013, the patient got periods for 3 times respectively on 31 Juanuary, 14 March and 20 April, of 2014.

### Ultrasonography examination

On 4 June, 2013 (the tenth day of menstruation, D10), the patient underwent a color Doppler ultrasonography(CDU) examination, showing that there were 5-6 follicles in the right ovary with a 19×14 mm dominant follicle and 6-7 follicles in the left ovary.

On 7 November, 2013 (the 20$^{th}$ day of menstruation, D20), the patient received ultrasonic examination, showing that there were about 10 follicles in both ovaries with a 18×17 mm dominant follicle in the right ovary.

On 3 April, 2014 (the twenty-first day of menstruation, D21), ultrasonic examination showed that there was a 1.6×1.5 cm dominant follicle in the right ovary.

### Serum levels of sex hormones

On 28 June, 2013 (the third day of menstruation, D3), serum levels of sex hormones of the patient was observed showing LH level 0.34 IU/L, FSH level 1.18 IU/L, PRL level 7.35 μg/L, P level 2.45 nmol/L (0.77 ng/ml), E2 level 77.1 pmol/L (21.00 pg/ml) and T level 0.60 nmol/L (0.19 ng/ml).

On 13 September, 2013 (the third day of menstruation, D3), serum levels of LH, FSH and T were 0.11 IU/L, 0.87 IU/L and 0.96 nmol/L, respectively.

On 16 March, 2014 (the third day of menstruation, D3), serum levels of sex hormones were detected as: LH level 4.73 IU/L, FSH level 3.41 IU/L, E2 level 84.4 pmol/L (23.00pg/ml) and T level 0.98 nmol/L (0.31ng/ml).

### OGTT and IRT

On 5 November, 2013, the patient took an OGTT and IRT once again. The results showed that 3 h postprandial plasma glucose (3hPG) was lower than normal and 1 h postprandial insulin (1hIns) was higher than normal, whereas the other criteria were all normal.

The weight of the patient was always about 60 kg without obvious change during the total intervention (EA and/or physical exercise). All the results are showed in Table 1.

| **Period** | **4 months before acupuncture treatment** | **First course of acupuncture treatment** | **6 months after the first course of acupuncture treatment** | **Second course of acupuncture treatment** | **The following 4 months** |
|---|---|---|---|---|---|
| **Time** | from April to August, 2012 | from August, 2012 to January, 2013 | from January to July, 2013 | from July to December, 2013 | From December, 2013 to April, 2014 |
| **Intervention** | no intervention | EA plus physical exercise | physical exercise | EA plus physical exercise | physical exercise |
| **BMI** | 25 | 25 | 25 | 25 | 25 |
| **Menstruation** | zero | zero | 4 times | 3 times | 3 times |
| **Ultrasonic examination** | 2012.08.03:<br>>12 follicles in both ovaries; without follicle larger than 10×10 mm | no | 2013.06.04(D10):<br>5-6 follicles in the right ovary with a 19×14 mm dominant follicle; 6-7 follicles in the left ovary | 2013.11.07(D20):<br>About 10 follicles in both ovaries; with a 18×17 mm dominant follicle | 2014.4.3 (D21):<br>there was a 1.6×1.5 cm dominant follicle in the right ovary |
| **Serum levels of sex hormones** | 2012.03.10(D3):<br>LH: 18.78 IU/L<br>FSH: 4.67 IU/L<br>PRL: 10.59 μg/L<br>PROG: 1.89 nmol/L<br>E2: 156.6 pmol/L<br>T: 2.02 nmol/L | no | 2013.6.28(D3):<br>LH: 0.34 IU/L<br>FSH: 1.18 IU/L<br>PRL: 7.35 μg/L<br>PROG: 2.45 nmol/L<br>E2: 77.1 pmol/L<br>T: 0.60nmol/L | 2013.9.13(D3):<br>LH: 0.11 IU/L<br>FSH: 0.87 IU/L<br>T: 0.96 nmol/L | 2014.3.16 (D3):<br>LH: 4.73 IU/L<br>FSH: 3.41 IU/L<br>E2: 84.4 pmol/L<br>T: 0.98 nmol/L |
| **OGTT** | 2011.01.26 :<br>FPG: 4.91 mmlo/L<br>1hPG: 4.99 mmlo/L<br>2hPG:6.22 mmlo/L | no | no | 2013.11.05:<br>FPG: 4.78 mmlo/L<br>1hPG: 7.14 mmlo/L<br>2hPG:6.35 mmlo/L | no |

| | 3hPG: 3.63 mmlo/L | | | 3hPG: 2.60 mmlo/L | |
|---|---|---|---|---|---|
| **IRT** | 2011.01.26 :<br>FIns: 9.40 uIU/L<br>1hIns: 21.50 uIU/L<br>2hIns:36.20 uIU/L<br>3hIns: 5.90 uIU/L | no | no | 2013.11.05:<br>FIns: 9.67 uIU/L<br>1hIns: 80.51 uIU/L<br>2hIns:44.24 uIU/L<br>3hIns: 5.21 uIU/L | no |

**Table 1:** Treatment and progress, BMI-Body Mass Index; LH-Luteinizing Hormone; FSH- Follicle-Stimulating Hormone. PRL- Prolactin; P-Progesterone; E2-Estradiol; T-Testosterone

## Discussion

PCOS is the most common endocrinopathy in women of reproductive age. Women with PCOS may complain of various clinical manifestations including oligomenorrhea or amenorrhea, hirsutism, acne, and infertility. Oligomenorrhea or amenorrhea is usually the biggest problem disturbing young PCOS girls who have no immediate fertility wish and also usually the primary reason for them to see a doctor for the first time. Those methods such as clomiphene citrate, exogenous gonadotropin therapy, and laparoscopic ovarian drilling which are commonly used to induce ovulation [6] are not suitable for this part of PCOS patients.

In this case, before the patient received the intervention of physical exercise and acupuncture treatment, she had suffered from secondary amenorrhea for about 10 years and just took progestin or Dyne-35 for withdrawal bleeding. Her serum T level was normal and she had no acne and hirsutism. However, her LH/FSH ratio was 4.02, much higher than normal and there were over 12 small follicles with diameter <10 mm in both ovaries. According to the Rotterdam's criteria [7], the patient conformed to the diagnosis of PCOS.

It is uncertain why she did not have periods returned during the first course of acupuncture treatment. But after she finished the first course of acupuncture treatment, she had periods for 4 times in the following 6 months without any medication and further 3 times during the second course of acupuncture treatment. We deduced that maybe acupuncture produce effect only when acupuncture treatment achieves a certain quantity, and it has a post-treatment effect for a long time, which has been observed in animal experiments [8,9]. In 5α-dihydrotestosterone-induced PCOS rats who received 2 Hz EA five times per week for 4-5 weeks, 88% of them had oestrous cycle change only during the last 2 weeks of EA treatment [8].

At the end of interval between two courses of acupuncture treatment, her LH level on the third day of menstruation decreased markedly from 18.78 IU/L before treatment to 0.34 IU/L, whereas her FSH level also decreased from 4.67 IU/L to 1.18 IU/L and her T level decreased from 2.02 nmol/L to 0.60 nmol/L. During the second course of acupuncture treatment, her LH level continued to decrease from 0.34 IU/L to 0.11 IU/L and FSH level decreased from 1.18 IU/L to 0.87 IU/L, whereas T level increased from 0.60 nmol/L to 0.96 nmol/L. It seemed that acupuncture plus physical exercise inhibited the secretion of LH, FSH and T and this effect became much more obvious on LH and FSH with the prolongation of intervention.

The influence of acupuncture on sex hormones also has been found by other investigators. Johansson et al. [10] found that acupuncture decreased testosterone, free testosterone, estradiol, dehydroepiandrosterone, dehydroepiandrosterone sulfate and androstenedione accompanied by a higher ovulation frequency, but with no effect on LH secretion. Pastore et al. [11] had a different conclusion. They observed that acupuncture decreased LH/FSH ratio from 1.9 ± 1.4 at baseline to 1.4 ± 1.4 (P=0.039) after 12 sessions of acupuncture and further to 1.3 ± 0.7 (P=0.001) post three-month follow-up, also lowered free testosterone and fasting insulin, and improved ovulation even they did not find a difference between true and sham acupuncture. Acupuncture may alter the release of GnRH and CRH through influencing hypothalamic β-endorphin secretion, and then further produce an effect on LH and FSH secretion [12]. Furthermore, excessive physical exercise can inhibit LH and FSH secretion [13]. For this patient, EA combined with physical exercise had a very obviously inhibitory effect on LH, FSH and T secretion, especially on LH and FSH secretion.

Because the levels of LH and FSH decreased too much and had already been lower than normal, we ever advised the patient to stop EA treatment. But the patient insisted on finishing the second course of acupuncture treatment. We also advised the patient to reduce the strength and duration of exercise and monitor the serum levels of sex hormones in six months. Her serum levels of LH and FSH showed normal on 16 March, 2014 when she had already stopped EA treatment and reduced the strength and duration of the exercise for nearly three months. We has not yet known the accurate reason why her serum levels of LH and FSH recover to normal, which may be related to both the cease of EA and the reduction of physical exercise. Therefore, we should monitor the serum levels of sex hormones and then regulate the frequency of EA treatment and the intensity of physical exercise according to the change of sex hormone levels in the treatment of PCOS.

Before our intervention, the ovaries of the patient showed as typical polycystic change with over 12 small follicles in both ovaries. However, the patient took ultrasonic examination for three times respectively at six months after the first course of acupuncture treatment, during the second course of acupuncture treatment and five months after the second course of acupuncture treatment, which all found a dominant follicle (19×14 mm, 18×17 mm and 16×15 mm, respectively) and no more than 12 follicles in both ovaries. Acupuncture combined with physical exercise was effective in inducing the production of dominant follicle and ovulation. It has been observed that EA and exercise improved ovarian morphology in PCOS rats, maybe through modulation of sympathetic outflow to the ovaries [9].

About 42% of PCOS patients have insulin-resistance, and 48% have hyperandrogenism. Insulin-resistance is commonly associated with hyperinsulinemia, and the latter enhances androgen production by theca cells and leads to hyperandrogenism [14]. Therefore, insulin-sensitizing drugs are used to inhibit or limit testosterone production, and improve spontaneous ovulation and regular menstrual cycles in PCOS patients. Lifestyle modification including physical exercise can reduce body weight and improve insulin resistance, which are beneficial to PCOS [15]. Before the patient came to us, she had normal glucose tolerance and insulin sensitivity. During the total intervention, her weight and BMI did not change at all. Except that 1hPG and 1hIns after 15 months of intervention were nearly 1.5 and 4 times those before intervention respectively, there was no obvious change in FPG, FIns, 2hPG, 2hIns, 3hPG and 3hIns after intervention. Therefore, for this patient, it seemed that physical exercise did not produce effect on PCOS through improving insulin resistance or reducing hyperinsulinemia. However, we cannot deny the beneficial influence of physical exercise on PCOS [16], which may through regulating the secretion of LH, FSH or Tt.

In conclusion, after the intervention of physical exercise and two courses of acupuncture treatment, the patient's menstruation improved markedly, her abnormal high LH/FSH ratio dropped down greatly and the morphology of the polycystic ovaries was not found on pelvic scanning. Our result is similar to aother study [17] which showing that either Low-frequency EA or physical exercise improved hyperandrogenism and menstrual frequency more effectively than no intervention in women with PCOS or Low-frequency EA was superior to physical exercise. In this case, we combined EA with physical exercise to treat PCOS, which showed much more inhibitory effects on LH, FSH and T secretion. Now our research team is doing a randomized controlled clinical trial about the effect of EA on PCOS (United States National Institutes of Health Clinical Trials Registry : NCT 01812161). It will disclose the effectiveness of acupuncture as a treatment for PCOS women. We think it necessary to commit a clinical trial to investigate the role of acupuncture combined with physical exercise, and to compare the effect of both acupuncture and physical exercise with either one. It will be an excitement If we can find a kind of non-medical treatment for oligo-/amenorrhea, hyperandrogenism and ovulation dysfunction in PCOS.

## Conclusions

This case illustrated that acupuncture and physical exercise can achieve return of menstruation in PCOS patients with amenorrhea. Acupuncture integrated with physical exercise may be a good substitute for medication in the treatment of PCOS.

## Acknowledgements

All authors are very grateful to Dr. Ernest Hung Yu Ng (department of obstetrics & gynecology, university of Hong Kong, Hong Kong) for proofreading this manuscript.

## References

1. Azziz R, Woods KS, Reyna R, Key TJ, Knochenhauer ES, et al (2004) The prevalence and features of the polycystic ovary syndrome in an unselected population. Journal of Clinical Endocrinology and Metabolism 89: 2745-2749.
2. Witt CM, Pach D, Brinkhaus B, Wruck K, Tag B, et al (2009) "Safety of acupuncture: results of a prospective observational study with 229,230 patients and introduction of a medical information and consent form." Forschende Komplementärmedizin 16: 91-97.
3. Johansson J1, Stener-Victorin E (2013) Polycystic ovary syndrome: effect and mechanisms of acupuncture for ovulation induction. Evidence-Based Complementary and Alternative Medicine Epub.
4. Stener-Victorin E, Jedel E, Janson PO, Sverrisdottir YB (2009) Low-frequency electro-acupuncture and physical exercise decrease high muscle sympathetic nerve activity in polycystic ovary syndrome. American Journal of Physiology Regulatory, Integrative and Comparative Physiology 297: 387–395.
5. Kuang H, Li Y, Wu X, Hou L, Wu T, et al (2013) Acupuncture and clomiphene citrate for live birth in polycystic ovary syndrome: study design of a randomized controlled trial. Evid Based Complement Alternat Med.
6. The Thessaloniki ESHRE/ASRM-Sponsored PCOS Consensus Workshop Group: Consensus on infertility treatment related to polycystic ovary syndrome (2008) Hum Reprod 23 :462–477.
7. Rotterdam ESHRE/ASRM-Sponsored PCOS consensus workshop group (2004) Revised 2003 consensus on diagnostic criteria and long-term health risks related to polycystic ovary syndrome (PCOS). Hum Reprod 19: 41-47.
8. Feng Y, Johansson J, Shao R, Manneras-Holm L, Billig H, et al. (2012) Electrical and manual acupuncture stimulation affects estrouscy clicity and neuroendocrine function in a DHT-induced rat polycystic ovary syndrome model. Exp Physio l97: 651-662.
9. Manneras L, Cajander S, Lonn M, Stener-Victorin E (2009) Acupuncture and exercise restore adipose tissue expression of sympathetic markers and improve ovarian morphology in rats with dihydrotestosterone-induced PCOS. Am J Physiol Regul Integr Comp Physio l296: 1124–1131.
10. Johansson J, Redman L, Veldhuis PP, Sazonova A, Labrie F, et al (2013) Acupuncture for ovulation induction in polycystic ovary syndrome: a randomized controlled trial. Am J Physiol Endocrinol Metab 304: E934-943.
11. Pastore LM, Williams CD, Jenkins J, Patrie JT (2011) True and sham acupuncture produced similar frequency of ovulation and improved LH to FSH ratios in women with polycystic ovary syndrome. J Clin Endocrinol Metab 96: 3143–3150.
12. Johansson J, Stener-Victorin E (2013) Polycystic ovary syndrome: effect and mechanisms of acupuncture for ovulation induction. Evid Based Complement Alternat Med.
13. Orio F, Muscogiuri G, Ascione A, Marciano F, Volpe A, et al. (2013) Effects of physical exercise on the female reproductive system. Minerva Endocrinologica 38: 305-319.
14. Abbott DH, Bacha F (2013) Ontogeny of polycystic ovary syndrome and insulin resistance in utero and early childhood. Fertil Steril 100: 2-11.
15. Haqq L, McFarlane J, Dieberg G, Smart N (2014) Effect of lifestyle intervention on the reproductive endocrine profile in women with polycystic ovarian syndrome: a systematic review and meta-analysis. Endocr Connect 3: 36-46.
16. Domecq JP, Prutsky G, Mullan RJ, Hazem A, Sundaresh V, et al (2013) Lifestyle modification programs in polycystic ovary syndrome: systematic review and meta-analysis. J Clin Endocrinol Metab 98: 4655-4663.
17. Jedel E, Labrie F, Odén A, Holm G, Nilsson L, et al (2011) Impact of electro-acupuncture and physical exercise on hyperandrogenism and oligo/amenorrhea in women with polycystic ovary syndrome: a randomized controlled trial. Am J Physiol Endocrinol Metab 300: E37-45.

# Changing Pattern of Complementary and Alternative Medicine in Tikapur Nepal: A Hope for Future Health

**Ranabhat Chhabi[1*], YA Do[2], DW Ahn[3], KJ Lee[3,4] and CB Kim[1]**

[1]*Department of Preventive Medicine, Wonju College of Medicine Yonsei University, Wonju, Republic of Korea*
[2]*Management Support Team, Management Support Department, Korea International Cooperation Agency 825 Daewangpangyo-ro, Sujeong-go, Seongnam-si, Gyeonggi-do, 461-833 Republic of Korea*
[3]*Institute for Poverty Alleviation and International Development, Yonsei University Wonju, Republic of South Korea*
[4]*Department of Environmental Medical Biology, Wonju College of Medicine Yonsei University, Wonju, Republic of Korea*

**Abstract**

Primitive Medicines; Ayurvedic Herbal and other treatment therapy are the oldest way of treatment in eastern philosophy and now it is classified Complementary and the Alternative Medicine (CAM). In Nepal they have been very famous since last century. There was high utilization in mid and far western region of Nepal in the past. So it is necessary to explore their use in that territory.

**Objectives:** The main objective of this study was to explore the available herbs product and their utilization as therapeutic.

**Methodology:** A cross sectional study was done within Kailali district in Nepal.The respondents were selected in systematic random sampling and the clusters were selected in PPS having 27% in household base. Pretested questionnaire were used for the study. Ethical Approved was taken from Nepal health research council and informed consent was taken from respondents. Epi data 3.1 version was used to entry the data and SPSS 20 was used for the data analysis. Chi Square test was used to show the association between different variable and CAM utilization.

**Results:** During the study 24 types of herbs were found in practice. About 1/4th (23.7%) used the herbs as therapeutic use, Narayanpur used least proportion (10%), and the people who had misconception of food used the herbs. More than 1/3rd (37%) used those herbs for cough and respiratory symptoms. The person who had information about the cause of disease and the knowledge of preventive ways with the application of herbs were statistically significant ($p<0.0001$).

**Conclusion:** The behavior of using CAM is very old practice and very effective of some illness even now. The utilization of therapy is done together with current allopathic treatment system and there is limited research of CAM utilization with comparative study. A comparative study should be necessary to find the implication of herbs with the modern allopathic system and economic aspects. If their application can be updated and used with research, it will have good result for the treatment.

**Keywords:** Ayurvedic; Herbal; Jadibuti; CAM; Palliative care

## Introduction

Alternative medicine was defined late in the 20th century as a type of medicine or treatment other than conventional medicine or health care [1]. Alternative medicine was named because of its use as an alternative to conventional medicine, which is practiced by medical doctors in western culture. Complementary and Alternative Medicine was introduced to the western world through immigrants from other countries.As an example of this, after the Vietnam war, many refugees sought a new life in America, incorporating the cultures and beliefs of that part of the world with those of America [2]. The origin of CAM is in Asia like, Japan Korea, India, Nepal, China etc. and there is still practice of Yoga, Ayurvedic Medicine, Herbal Medicine, Naturopathy, Acupuncture, Amchiand other local and cultural type of therapy. During the war period and world migration the practice of such therapy has been global [3]. As a therapy the almost source are the plants.

Complementary and alternative medicine (CAM) interventions are popular among consumers and are widely employed to treat diverse physical and mental health conditions [4]. The application of CAM use is estimated at 25% among residents of the United Kingdom, [5] 50% among German, French, and Australian population [5,6], and 42% to 69% among residents of the United States [6,7]. CAM is a major growth industry in Europe [8,9]. A summary of 26 surveys across 13 countries concluded that the prevalence of CAM use by cancer patients overall 31.4% [10]. The results of a recent national survey show that nearly 38 percent of U.S. adults use CAM approaches to manage a range of physical and emotional health concerns, including pain, anxiety, and depression [11,12]. Recent studies in the United States [13] and abroad support the current use of alternative health care. For example, a 1994 survey of physicians from a wide array of medical specialties (in Washington State, New Mexico, and Israel) revealed that more than 60% recommended alternative therapies to their patients at least once in the preceding year, while 38% had done so in the previous month [14,15]. Herbal resources are other form of Ayurvedic wealth.

In 1999, the first national survey on CAM use among the general population in the Republic of Korea reported that 29% of the

***Corresponding author:** Ranabhat Chhabi, Department of Preventive Medicine, Wonju College of Medicine, Yonsei University, Wonju, Gangwon 220-701, Republic of Korea, E-mail: chhabir@gmail.com population, as determined by telephone interview, had used CAM within the preceding 12-month period [16]. In 2006, another surveys showed that the 3,000 subjects, 2,244 (74.8%) reported using CAM in the previous 12-month period [17]. The application of the use of CAM was disease prevention, health promotion, anti-ageing beauty and weight reduction, stress management and stamina [17]. Similarly the application of CAM has been used to treat the cancer patients in Korea [18].

The application of use of the CAM with top 5 problems listed wereback problems (19.7%); allergies (16.6%); sprains/muscle strains (15.7%); digestive problems (14.5%); and lung problems, pneumonia, or respiratory infections (13%) respectively [13]. The same study shows that the top 4 treatment categories were chiropractic (15.7%); lifestyle diet (8.0%); exercise/movement (7.2%); and relaxation (6.9%). The most frequently cited health problems treated with alternative therapies were chronic pain (37%); anxiety, chronic fatigue syndrome, and "other health condition" (31% each); sprains/muscle strains (26%); addictive problems and arthritis (both 25%); and headaches (24%) [13]. Two-thirds of women in this study followed conventional treatment for breast cancer with one or more CAM therapies, which, they believed, that they could prevent cancer recurrence, cosmetic use, tonic, reduce the fat and ageing and/or improve their quality of life [19]. The geographical structure and advanced bio-diversity has made it possible for the Himalayan country to grow different valuable medicinal plants. The Medicinal and Aromatic database of Nepal covers 1624 species of plants found in wild state or cultivated or naturalized or imported belonging to 938 genera and 218 families [20]. These are known to be used as medicine in Nepal.

The World Health Organization (WHO) estimates that 4 billion people, 80 percent of the world population, presently use herbal medicine for some aspect of primary health care [21]. Herbal medicine is a major component in all indigenous peoples' traditional medicine and a common element in Ayurvedic medicine. WHO notes that of 119 plant-derived pharmaceutical medicines, about 74% are used in modern medicine in ways that correlated directly with their traditional uses as plant medicines by native cultures [22]. Major pharmaceutical companies are currently conducting extensive research on plant materials gathered from the rain forests and other places for their potential medicinal value.

CAM utilization rate vary, depending on the particular geographic region and the ways in which "alternative/complementary medicine" is defined. Although some studies suggest that CAM use is greatest among those between the ages of 35 and 50 [23], a recent multivariate analysis found no significant effect of age on CAM utilization [24].

As described in Ayurveda, the Himalayan Jadibuti is used for healthy body and happy mind. These are used in different means such as toiletries and cosmetics; incense and aromas; health promoting agents, supplements and medicines; natural manures, pesticides; environmental cleaning and protection; food, food additives and drinks etc.

Traditional medicine, Ayurvedic medicine, herbal medicine, alternative medicine etc. are using as same term in most of the study. Some of the studies have been published in international journals too. Most of the researches are focused to explore the existing herbal product of Nepal but they are silent about the proportion of using herbal product in different sets of community as a therapy. It will be extra important that such plants can be linked with different set of demographic variables. On the other hand current practices of herbal products really alternative therapy with allopathic model are or not.

Such study is helpful to conduct further study in the area of different utilization practice with focusing confined area. Because previous studies have highlighted that limited people are using such treatment system, whereas herbal therapy activist clam that it is sufficient to cure many diseases and illness. Even most of the allopathic medicines are abstracted form herbal abstract. Finding the proportion of the CAM and is application is the first steps and then it is necessary to do research more specific and precise. The main focus of the study was to find out the current pattern of CAM and changing pattern of that use in other specific purpose. Globally, the importance of CAM in general illness because of the replacement of western medicine but as cosmetic, tonic, palliative care etc. their important is more famous.

## Methodology

### Study design and sampling

It was a cross sectional study conducted in Kailali District, the far western Regional of Nepal. Kailali district was selected purposively having one Municipality Tikapur and the surrounding 4 VDCs namely, Dhansingpur, Narayanpur, Durgauli and the Pathariya. Each VDC was stratified in 9 cluster and Municipality in 3 clusters on Population Propionate sampling (PPS) about 27% which was 4204 House hold and the head of the family were the respondent of the research. Pre tested household questionnaire. The training was provided to the enumerators and the supervisor.

### Data analysis

Data entry were completed to the Epi data 3.1 and analyzed by SPSS 20 version. The data were cleaned and verified by statistician for the data quality. The data were analyzed with univariate and bivariate analysis with Pearson chi square test in 95% confidence interval and probability 0.05. The quality of data was maintained tool design, pilot study, and preparation of the guidelines for the supervisor, respondent and data entry personnel by parallel data entry with SPSS and Epi data software. After finalization of the draft peer review was done by the experts.

Another complementary study was done about the use of herbal product in different disease in 2 clusters having the 500 sample size randomly. For that purpose, pre tested questionnaires were used. For Ethical consideration, Nepal Health research council was followed, permission was taken from local VDC and Municipality, and there was valid agreement to conduct research from Ministry of Health and Population of Nepal. Informed consent was taken from household respondent.

## Result

The availability of local herbs was asked to the respondents during the study. During that time they had replied about the use for their health problems since their practice in before the availability of modern allopathic medicines but most of the respondents (75%) were not currently used. The study showed that the utilization of the CAM was 24% (10-29%). Among the occupation, the service holders used the CAM 42% where unemployed household used only 20%.

Most of the available herbs were used in gastro intestinal problems like diarrhoea, loose motion, stomachache, worms, gastritis etc. Similarly, easily available herbs like Basil (Tulashi), Amala, Pipala were used in respiratory problems especially in children. Few people (≤ 15%) used herbs for fever and Diarrhoea but more than 1/3$^{rd}$ (37%)

People used those for in respiratory diseases. Even they have little bit knowledge for the therapeutic use by about half population (46%) (Table 1).

Table 2 shows, 3/4th (75%) people use the CAM with allopathic medicine, more than half (58%) apply as a medicine at initial stage of the illness and more interestingly, more than half (51%) belief that CAM is the good way to promote sexual health.

## Distribution and association of herbs application with different variables

Statistical test was used to show the association between the variables.The following table 3 shows that, there is no any statistical significant (p value >0.05) between the herbs use and with occupation, resident id status and the head of household during the research. Similarly, there is association between family type and knowledge about the cause of diseases and the preventive ways of disease with the application of herbs. Nowadays, people who have broad knowledge about the disease and illness are using the CAM (p=<0.001) (Tables 1-3).

## Discussion

The application of primitive medicine is worldwide and it was the main treatment therapy before 18th century where the allopathic medicine was alternative medicine. Now the situation is vice versa and the previous treatment practice is used as complementary and alternative medicine which includes several types of treatment practice [2]. Nepal is one of the great sources of herbal products and so many treatment practices [25]. The Kailali, a district of far western region was similar to other hilly district of Nepal. Of the 48 species from 46 genera and 40 families were displayed about the application of their in the study, indigenous uses of about 70% species resembled to the earlier ethno medicinal reports [26]. Such application coincides with this result. The prevalence of the local herbs to use for the therapeutic application is only 24.7% as a complementary use not as full treatment approach. Such research is not sufficient to prove their application it needs another clinical trial to prove exact application. There are 83% people live in rural area [27] and the modern allopathic system is not accessible to all grass root level. If facts prove about the therapeutic application of locally endemic disease, obviously these people could be benefited. Traditional herbal medicine renders primary health care needs of two thirds of the rural population of the Nepalese, represents a largely unexplored source for potential development of new drugs [26,28,29].

Medicinal plants play vital roles in the Nepalese livelihood [30] and the use of medicinal plants is frequent in several Nepalese regions [26,31]. It is estimated that only 15-20% of the population of Nepal -living in and around urban areas-has access to modern medicinal facilities, whereas the rest depend on traditional medicines [32]. Nepal is a natural storehouse of medicinal plants [33,34]. Each year thousands of tons of raw material are exported, mostly to India, but also to Asia, Europe and America [35]. The government of Nepal aims to promote medicinal plant use and conservation programs for livelihood improvement and poverty alleviation through various policies. However, the contribution of this sector to the national economy is still nominal.

Protection and preservation, development and commercialization of indigenous knowledge and herbal resources have become an issue. Herbal resources have been over exploited as usual and indigenous

| Herbs Name | Application as herbal tea and other paste | Category | Frequency | % |
|---|---|---|---|---|
| Neem, Gurje Pomegranate, Guava leaf, Dhade, Raktamul, Pepper mint (Pudina), Bark of Jamun tree, Leaf of lemon tree, Bark of mango tree, Raw banana skin | Diarrhoea and gastro intestinal problems | Yes | 53 | 8 |
| | | No | 457 | 92 |
| Jatropha (Rithha), Dodder (Aakashbeli), Mugwort (Titepati) Bark of papal tree Barmuda grass | Fever, jaundice, wounds, boils etc | Yes | 75 | 15 |
| | | No | 425 | 85 |
| Basil (Tulasi), Myrobalans (Amala), Long pepper (Pipala), Batul pate | Respiratory disease, fever, common cold, poisoning etc | Yes | 185 | 37 |
| | | No | 315 | 63 |

**Table 1:** Utilization of herbs use for general illness (N= 500).

| Practice and attitude | Response | Category | Frequency | % |
|---|---|---|---|---|
| **Practice** | Practice of Herbs as treatment last year | Frequently | 73 | 15 |
| | | Seldom | 201 | 40 |
| | | None | 226 | 45 |
| | Use of the herbal therapy in illness | Single | 54 | 11 |
| | | With allopathic medicine | 375 | 75 |
| | | With traditional healers | 71 | 14 |
| | Time for herbs consumption | Starting of illness | 280 | 56 |
| | | During the illness | 140 | 28 |
| | | As a tonic | 80 | 16 |
| | Specific use of CAM | Chronic Disease and illness | 162 | 32 |
| | | Cancer and Palliative care | 83 | 17 |
| | | Sexual tonic | 255 | 51 |
| **Attitude** | Attitude of herbs towards therapeutic use | Very useful | 47 | 9 |
| | | Little bit | 231 | 46 |
| | | Not useful | 8 | 2 |
| | | Don't know | 214 | 43 |

**Table 2:** Changing pattern of CAM (n=500).

| Variables | | Crosstab Utilization of herbal plant | | p value (95% CI) |
|---|---|---|---|---|
| | | No | Yes | |
| Occupation having agriculture | No | 1699 | 584 | 0.8 |
| | | 74.4% | 25.6% | |
| | Yes | 77 | 25 | |
| | | 75.5% | 24.5% | |
| Residence status | Temporary | 154 | 53 | 0.74 |
| | | 74.4% | 25.6% | |
| | Permanent | 3013 | 984 | |
| | | 75.4% | 24.6% | |
| Head of household | Female | 885 | 260 | 0.07 |
| | | 77.3% | 22.7% | |
| | Male | 2282 | 777 | |
| | | 74.6% | 25.4% | |
| Family type | Single | 1770 | 543 | 0.004 |
| | | 76.5% | 23.5% | |
| | Extended | 358 | 157 | |
| | | 69.5% | 30.5% | |
| | Joint | 1039 | 337 | |
| | | 75.5% | 24.5% | |
| Known cause of diseases | Poor knowledge | 490 | 74 | <0.001 |
| | | 86.9% | 13.1% | |
| | Good knowledge | 2677 | 963 | |
| | | 73.5% | 26.5% | |
| Know how to prevent diseases | No knowledge | 482 | 64 | <0.001 |
| | | 88.3% | 11.7% | |
| | Correct knowledge | 2685 | 973 | |
| | | 73.4% | 26.6% | |

**Table 3:** Association between herbs application with different variables (n=4204).

knowledge either humiliated or under threat of piracy. It has been estimated that four out of five medicinal plants utilized by human beings are collected currently from the wild. Since herbal resources are one of the most reliable sources of income for a majority of the people living in rural areas, competition for harvest begins before the right season.

Locals do not have scientific knowledge or technology and tools to harvest. Probability of regeneration, therefore, becomes lesser by the year and finally reaches extinction. There are two urgent steps required to check this: First, the local people who rely on such natural resources for their lives must be trained; second, encourage them to cultivate these herbs commercially. Research has found that due to change in socio-psychological factors and educational patterns, the present generations of traditional healers do not follow the old methods. This is a threat to indigenous knowledge

It has been estimated that around 119 pure chemical substances extracted from some 90 species of higher plants are used in medicines throughout the world. Over 21,000 plant names that have medicinal uses are reported by WHO (1992). In Nepal, more than 1,600 species of wild plants are used in traditional medicinal practice and majority of which await proper documentation [36]. Currently, people are using the allopathic medicine and herbs as a complementary even though the people who have wider knowledge are more attractive to use with scientific clarification. ($p \leq 0.001$)

Previously, when there was no practice of allopathic medicine there was highly applicable of herbs in Nepal. Every people were compulsion to search and use in every day practice but when allopathic system interrupted in health system, the previous practice is near to disappear that the above findings shows. The young generation is indifferent with this system. Now there is going to be failure some of the chronic disease by allopathic system scientist have attention for the herbs application and exploration. For this new scientific research should be done more with comparative ways with the failure of the allopathic drugs.

## Limitation of the Study

Previously the CAM was the leading approach of treatment in Nepal but now a day it is going to be disappeared. So the first step could be to find out the utilization ratio in the community. Later on the research should be focused on treatment efficacy, other aspects of herbal products and direct to the industrialization. There are very few articles in this area and it is necessary to find more and more in coming days. This article just explores the possibility of complementary and alternative medicine in the community and local area. In the survey the Information about the diseases was the perception of the respondents. It was not from any clinical diagnosis or checking their medical history or record. Therefore, the distribution of the disease may not reflect the true disease morbidity in the survey population.

### Acknowledgements

This work was supported by the National Research Foundation of Korea Grant funded by the Korean Government (NRF-2013-S1A5B8-A01055336). It is because the publication was accomplished in 2013.

## References

1. Zollman C, Vickers A (1999) What is complementary medicine? BMJ 319: 693-696.
2. Levin J, Chatters LM, Taylor RJ (2005) Religion, health and medicine in African Americans: implications for physicians. J Natl Med Assoc 97: 237-249.
3. Alter JS (2005) Asian medicine and globalization.Univ of Pennsylvania Press.
4. Rafferty AP, McGee HB, Miller CE, Reyes M (2002) Prevalence of complementary and alternative medicine use: state-specific estimates from the 2001 Behavioral Risk Factor Surveillance System. Am J Public Health 92: 1598-600.
5. Molassiotis A, Fernadez-Ortega P, Pud D, Ozden G, Scott JA, et al. (2005) Use of complementary and alternative medicine in cancer patients: a European survey. Ann Oncol 16: 655-663.
6. MacLennan AH, Myers SP, Taylor AW (2006) The continuing use of complementary and alternative medicine in South Australia: costs and beliefs in 2004. Med J Aust 184: 27-31.
7. Astin JA, Pelletier KR, Marie A, Haskell WL (2000) Complementary and alternative medicine use among elderly persons: one-year analysis of a Blue Shield Medicare supplement. J Gerontol A Biol Sci Med Sci 55: M4-9.
8. Moenkhoff M, Baenziger O, Fischer J, Fanconi S (1999) Parental attitude towards alternative medicine in the paediatric intensive care unit. Eur J Pediatr 158: 12-17.
9. Fisher P, Ward A (1994) Complementary medicine in Europe. BMJ 309: 107-111.
10. Ernst E, Cassileth BR (1998) The prevalence of complementary/alternative medicine in cancer: a systematic review. Cancer 83: 777-782.
11. Barnes PM, Bloom B, Nahin RL (2008) Complementary and alternative medicine use among adults and children: United States, 2007. US Department of Health and Human Services, Centers for Disease Control and Prevention, National Center for Health Statistics.
12. Unützer J, Klap R, Sturm R, Young AS, Marmon T, et al. (2000) Mental disorders and the use of alternative medicine: results from a national survey. Am J Psychiatry 157: 1851-1857.
13. Astin JA (1998) Why patients use alternative medicine: results of a national study. JAMA 279: 1548-1553.
14. Ernst E, Resch KL, White AR (1995) Complementary medicine. What

physicians think of it: a meta-analysis. Arch Intern Med 155: 2405-2408.

15. MacLennan AH, Taylor AW, Wilson DH, Wilson D (2000)The prevalence of pelvic floor disorders and their relationship to gender, age, parity and mode of delivery. BJOG107: 1460-1470.
16. Lee SI, Khang YH, Lee MS, Koo HJ, Kang W, Hong CD (1992) Complementary and alternative medicine use in Korea: prevalence, pattern of use, and out-of-pocket expenditures. Korean J Prev Med 32: 546-555.
17. Ock SM, Choi JY, Cha YS, Lee J, Chun MS, et al. (2009) The use of complementary and alternative medicine in a general population in South Korea: results from a national survey in 2006. J Korean Med Sci 24: 1-6.
18. Kim MJ, Lee SD, Kim DR, Kong YH, Sohn WS, et al. (2004) Use of complementary and alternative medicine among Korean cancer patients. Korean J Intern Med 19: 250-256.
19. Henderson JW, Donatelle R (2004) Complementary and alternative medicine use by women after completion of allopathic treatment for breast cancer. Altern Ther Health Med 10: 52-57.
20. Biziou B (2006) The Joy of Ritual: Spiritual Recipies to Celebrate Milestones, Ease Transitions, and Make Every Day Sacred: Cosimo, Inc.
21. Wootton JC (2006) WHO global atlas of traditional, complementary and alternative medicine. Journal of Alternative & Complementary Medicine12: 93-94.
22. Bodeker G, Ong CK (2005) World Health Organization Global Atlas of Traditional, Complementary, and Alternative Medicine: World Health Organization.
23. Kessler RC, Soukup J, Davis RB, Foster DF, Wilkey SA, et al. (2001) The use of complementary and alternative therapies to treat anxiety and depression in the United States. Am J Psychiatry 158: 289-294.
24. Healthcare L (1998) The Landmark report on public perceptions of alternative care. Sacramento, Calif: Landmark Healthcare.
25. Singh MP, Malla SB, Rajbhandari SB, Manandhar A (1979) Medicinal plants of Nepal-retrospects and prospects. Economic Botany 33: 185-198.
26. Kunwar RM, Shrestha KP, Bussmann RW (2010) Traditional herbal medicine in far-west Nepal: a pharmacological appraisal. J Ethnobiol Ethnomed 6: 35.
27. Statistics CBo (2011) National Population and Housing Census.
28. Uprety Y, Asselin H, Boon EK, Yadav S, Shrestha KK (2010) Indigenous use and bio-efficacy of medicinal plants in the Rasuwa District, Central Nepal. J Ethnobiol Ethnomed 6: 3.
29. Kunwar RM, Bussmann RW (2008) Ethnobotany in the Nepal Himalaya. J Ethnobiol Ethnomed 4: 24.
30. Bhattarai KR, Ghimire M (2006) Commercially important medicinal and aromatic plants of Nepal and their distribution pattern and conservation measure along the elevation gradient of the Himalayas. Banko Janakari 16: 3-13.
31. Shrestha K, Tiwari N, Ghimire S (2000) Medicinal and aromatic plants database of Nepal (MAPDON). Proceedings of Nepal-Japan Joint Symposium on Conservation and Utilization of Himalayan Medicinal Plant Resources 53-74.
32. Sharma U, Malla K, Uprety R (2004) Conservation and management efforts of medicinal and aromatic plants in Nepal. Banko Janakari 14: 3-11.
33. Manandhar NP (2002) Plants and People of Nepal Timber Press. Oregon 192.
34. Baral SR, Kurmi PP (2006) A compendium of medicinal plants in Nepal: Rachana Sharma Maijubahal, Kathmandu.
35. Popescu R, Kopp B (2013) The genus Rhododendron: an ethnopharmacological and toxicological review. J Ethnopharmacol 147: 42-62.
36. Uprety Y, Boon EK, PoudelRC, Shrestha KK, Rajbhandary S, et al. (2010) Non-timber forest products in Bardiya district of nepal: indigenous use, trade and conservation. Journal of Human Ecology 30: 143-158.

# 31

# Islamic Wet Cupping and Risk Factors of Cardiovascular Diseases: Effects on Blood Pressure, Metabolic Profile and Serum Electrolytes in Healthy Young Adult Men

**Bassem Refaat[1]*, Adel Galal El-Shemi[1,2], Anwar Abdelgayed Ebid[3], Ahmed Ashshi[1] and Mohammad A BaSalamah[4]**

[1]*Laboratory Medicine Department, Faculty of Applied Medical Sciences, Umm Al-Qura University, Al Abdeyah, Makkah, PO Box 7607, KSA*
[2]*Department of Pharmacology, Faculty of Medicine, Assiut University, Egypt*
[3]*Physiotherapy Department, Faculty of Applied Medical Sciences, Umm Al-Qura University, Al Abdeyah, Makkah, PO Box 7607, KSA*
[4]*Pathology Department, Faculty of Medicine, Umm Al-Qura University, Al Abdeyah, Makkah, KSA*

## Abstract

**Background:** Wet cupping (Hejamah) has been used as alternative treatment for several diseases.

**Objectives:** To measure the effects of hejamah treatment for 2 consecutive months in healthy young adult men on blood pressure, blood glucose, lipid profile, serum sodium and potassium.

**Materials and methods:** 16 participants were treated with hejamah for 2 consecutive months. Blood pressure was measure before and 30 minutes after the treatment. Blood samples were collected from all participants before and 48 hours after hejamah and all participants were fasting for 12 hours before sample collection.

**Results:** Diastolic blood pressure, but not systolic, was significantly decreased following therapy ($P<0.05$). Fasting blood glucose was significantly decreased before the treatment in the second month only. The levels of serum triglycerides significantly decreased after the first treatment and remained low in the 2nd month. There was no significant difference between the different time points in total cholesterol except for the 48 hours of the second month compared to the samples collected before the procedure of the same month. There was a significant decrease in LDL and significant increase in HDL following hejamah therapy ($P<0.05$). Significant decrease in sodium and significant increase in potassium 48 hours following treatment with hejamah was observed in the 2 months ($P<0.05$).

**Conclusions:** The performance of hejamah during fasting state could represent a useful complementary method for the regulation of diastolic blood pressure and prevention/treatment of risk factors associated with cardiovascular diseases. Further studies are required to explore the role of hejamah in controlling blood pressure and prevention of cardiovascular diseases.

**Keywords:** Wet cupping; Hejamah; Cardiovascular diseases; Blood pressure; Lipid profile; Sodium; Potassium

## Introduction

Cardiovascular Diseases (CVDs) are major health problems and they are associated with mortality and morbidity. Several risk factors have been associated with the pathogenesis of CVDs, including metabolic disorders (e.g. hyperlipidaemia, diabetes mellitus, etc.) and increase salt intake that are major etiological factors for hypertension (HTN), coronary heart disease (CHD) and stroke [1-3]. The World Health Organization (WHO) has reported that CVDs are responsible for 30% of all deaths, which is equivalent to the combined death rates associated with several other medical conditions [4]. The estimated number of death due to CVDs by the WHO is 17.3 million people per year and the number is expected to increase to 23.3 million/year in 2030 [4,5].

Several benefits for Complementary Medicine (CM)/Alternative Medicine (AM), also known as traditional medicine, have been shown and it is effective in the prevention of disease, treatment of non-communicable diseases, and improvement of the quality of life for persons living with chronic diseases [6]. The WHO has been encouraging the implementation of traditional medicine since many patients are not satisfied by the outcomes of modern medicine particularly those related to chronic diseases [7].

Several CMs and AMs have been suggested for the control/treatment of HTN [8]. Blood-letting/leeching by phlebotomy significantly decreased the Blood Pressure (BP) compared to triple therapy in resistant hypertension [9]. Similar results were also seen in patients suffering from erythropoietin-induced malignant HTN [10] and post-transplant HTN associated with erythrocytosis [11].

Hejamah is a traditional Islamic treatment and a part of the prophetic medicine recommended by the prophet Mohammed, Peace Be Upon Him (PBUH), and it is used for the treatment of a variety of medical conditions [12]. Hejamah is a form of cupping therapy, also known as wet-cupping, blood leach or blood-letting therapy [12-16]. According to the prophetic medicine, hejamah should be performed at specific times during the odd days of full moon (day 17, 19 and 21) in the lunar months (Islamic calendar) and the patients should be fasting [17].

Cupping has been recommended by several physicians for CVDs [18-20]. A recent meta-analysis has reported that using cupping therapy is beneficial in controlling and lowering BP [21]. Similar

***Corresponding author:** Bassem Refaat, Laboratory Medicine Department, Faculty of Applied Medical Sciences, Umm Al-Qura University, Makkah, PO Box 7607, KSA, Ext: 4242; E-mail: Bassem.refaat@yahoo.co.uk results were also reported on mean arterial pressure [22]. However, a recent study by Zarei et al. [23] failed to show beneficial effects on anthropometric and BP compared to diet treatment in patients with HTN [23]. Additionally, acupuncture combined with cupping therapy could improve clinical symptoms, enhance tolerance of exercise, and reduce angina frequency, duration and consumption of nitrates of the patients with stable exertional angina with fewer side effects [20,24]. Furthermore, cupping has been used in stroke rehabilitation with potential benefits. However, evidence for the effectiveness of cupping in this area is not strong due to the lack of randomized controlled trials [21,25,26].

Increase in blood cholesterol level is a major risk factor for HTN and CVDs. Blood donation has been shown to significantly reduce the levels of serum cholesterol and thus decreasing the risk for CVDs among blood donors [27-30]. Blood donation significantly decreased Low Density Lipoprotein (LDL) compared to the patients treated with gemfibrozil only [27]. Phlebotomy has been recommended to reduce serum lipoprotein levels [28,30]. Wet cupping has also been shown to decrease the levels of total cholesterol and LDL and increases the level of High Density Lipoprotein (HDL) [31,32]. Additionally, blood-letting has been shown to increase the insulin sensitivity, which is a major risk factor for metabolic syndrome [33].

Our study objectives were to measure the effect of performing Islamic hejamah for two consecutive months in healthy young adult men on their blood pressure, serum sodium and potassium, serum cholesterol, triglycerides, LDL and HDL and blood glucose levels.

## Materials and Methods

### Ethical approval

The study was approved by the institutional review board and ethics committee of Faculty of Applied Medical Sciences (AMSEC10-15-03-2013). All samples were collected following obtaining informed written consent from all the participants.

### Study design

This was a prospective analytical study. Sixteen healthy young adult men aged between 18 and 25 years were recruited into the study according to the inclusion and exclusion criteria (Table 1). Wet cupping was performed on the study subjects for 2 consecutive months according to the Islamic protocol. All participants were asked to be fasting for at least 12 hours and blood pressure and a blood sample were obtained before the initiation of the procedure. At the end of the session, another measurement of blood pressure was obtained 30 minutes after the termination of wet cupping. A second blood sample was obtained from the participants 48 hours later and they were all fasting for 12 hours. The same procedures were followed in the second month of the study.

| Principal inclusion criteria | Principle exclusion criteria |
|---|---|
| Patient age ≥ 18 and <30 years. | Patient age <18 years or ≥ 30. |
| No chronic disease (e.g. HTN, diabetes mellitus, renal failure, etc.) | Chronic disease (Renal failure, coronary heart disease, etc.) |
| Not using any drug on regular basis during the previous 3 months prior to the study (e.g. antibiotics, analgesics, etc.) | Using medical drugs on regular basis |
| Willing to comply with the required fasting state and the full duration of the study | Not willing to comply with the study protocol |

**Table 1:** Principles inclusion and exclusion criteria.

### Types of samples

Five ml of blood was collected before the initiation and 48 following the termination of wet cup therapy in each month. A total of 64 samples were collected and the serum was separated by centrifugation for 15 minutes at 15000 RPM and it was stored in -20°C freezer till processed.

### Wet cupping protocol

The 16 participants were divided into 3 groups as follow: Group1 included 6 participants and they were requested to attend fasting for cup therapy on the morning of the 17th of lunar month (Islamic calendar). The second and third groups included 5 participants each and they were requested to attend on the 19th and 21st day of the lunar month, respectively. Before the initiation of cup therapy, the participants were given instructions on the procedure and the planned steps of the protocol. Blood pressure was measured and 5ml of venous blood was obtained before the commencement of the procedures.

Cupping therapy were performed using six points on the back of each participants and they were as follow: a) two cups for the lower end of the neck cervical vertebrate (C7) and thoracic vertebrate (T2), b) two cups on each scapula and c) two cups lateral to the lumbar vertebrate (L3). The sites of cupping were identified on the back of the participants and they were sterilized using alcohol swabs. The wet-cupping procedures lasted 15 minutes per participant and the steps were as follow:

**Primary sucking:** The cups were placed on the designated sites and a negative pressure was created by manual suction using the provided pump with the kit. The cups were left for a period of 5 minutes after ensuring their firm attachment to the skin.

**Incision:** The cups were removed and 10-12 superficial incisions were made on each designated area of the skin using sterile surgical blades.

**Blood-letting:** After soaking the cups, they were replaced back on the designated areas of the skin and negative pressure was created as previously described. The cups were left on the skin till they were filled with blood from the capillary vessels.

**Removal:** The cups were removed approximately after 3 minutes and new cups were placed on the same areas as previously mentioned. The used cups were socked in betadine for sterilization.

**Blood-letting:** The process of blood-letting was repeated for 3 times in total.

**Clean and sterilise:** The cupping areas were cleaned using betadine followed by placement of clean dressing.

Following the termination of cupping therapy, each participant was offered 125 ml of fruit juice and blood pressure was recorded 30 minutes later. Same procedures were followed for the other 2 groups and during the 2 months duration of the study. Another 5 ml blood samples were collected from each participant 48 hours following the termination of cupping therapy and all the participants were also fasting for 12 hours.

### Measurement of blood pressure, metabolic parameters and serum electrolytes

Blood pressure was measured using conventional sphygmomanometer and a stethoscope (Welch Allyn Inc, NY, USA). All serum samples were processed using Cobas 6000 analyzer (Roche Diagnostics, IN, USA) to measure blood levels of glucose, triglycerides, total cholesterol, HDL, LDL, sodium and potassium.

### Statistical analysis

Statistical analysis of the results was performed using SPSS version 16. Normality and homogeneity of data were assessed with the Kolmogorov and Smirnoff test and Levene test, respectively. Paired-samples T test was used to compare between the different time points of the study (before and after the intervention). P value<0.05 was considered significant.

## Results

### Effects of hejamah on Metabolic Profile

Overall, the results showed significant alterations in the levels of fasting blood glucose, total cholesterol, triglycerides, HDL and LDL following 2 months of wet cup therapy compared to the results obtained before the initiation of the procedure.

**Fasting blood sugar:** Although a slight increase in Fasting Blood Sugar (FBS) was detected 48 hours after therapy in the first month, there was no significant difference between samples collected before and 48 hours later during the first month (P>0.05). However, a significant decrease was detected in samples collected before the initiation of the procedure in the 2nd month compared to the two collected samples during the first month (p=0.002 and 0.0005, respectively). Still, a significant increase in FBS level was observed in the 2nd month in samples collected 48 hours following therapy (p=0.001) compared to those obtained before the initiation of the treatment in the same month. There was no significant difference between samples of 48 hours (2nd months) and the two samples collected at the first month (Figure 1).

**Lipid profile:** Serum triglycerides decreased significantly 48 hours after the commencement of the therapy during the first month (p=0.003) and it remained significantly lower in the two collected samples in the second month compared to the 2 samples of the first month. However, there was no difference between the 48 hours of the first month, before and 48 hours of the second month (Figure 1).

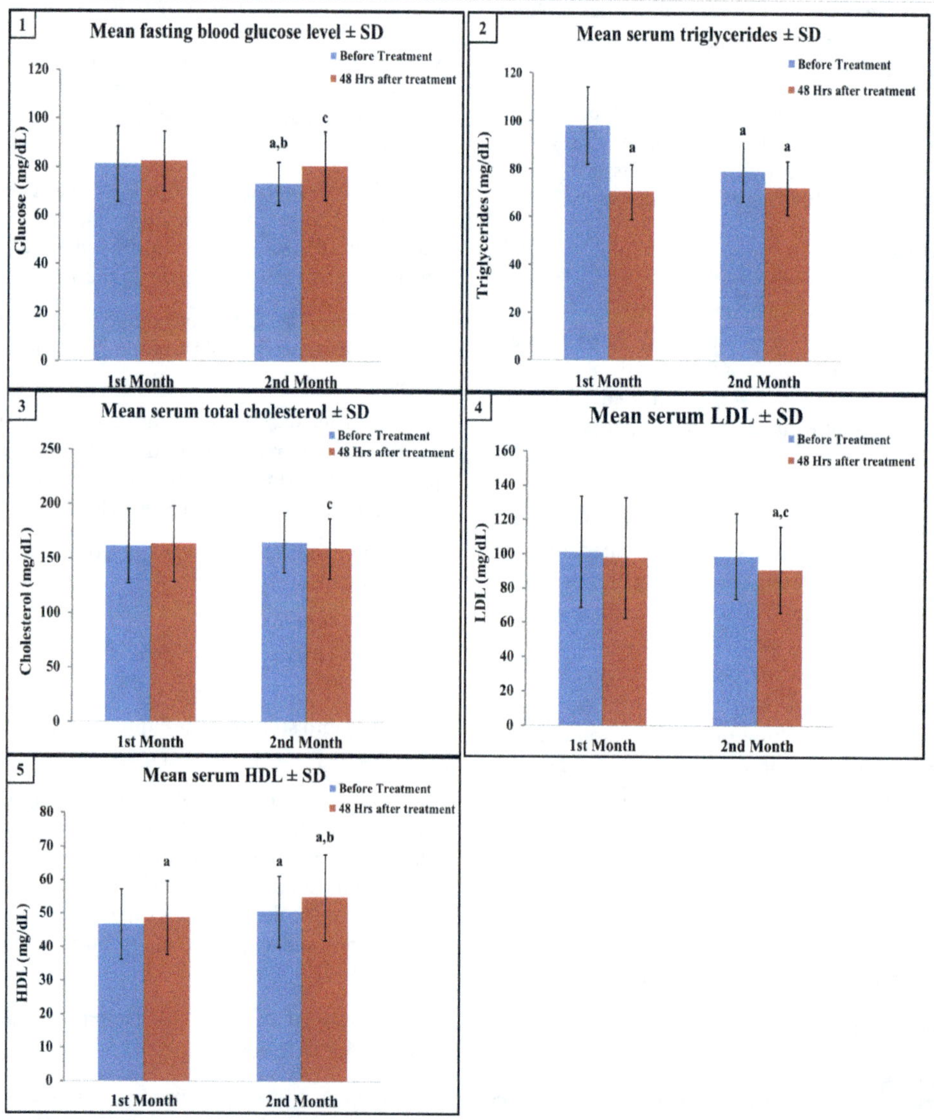


**Figure 1:** Mean ± SD of (1) fasting blood glucose, (2) triglycerides (3) total cholesterol (4) LDL and (5) HDL in the different times of the study. (a=p<0.05 compared to before 1st month, b=p<0.05 compared to 48 hours of 1st month and c=p<0.05 compared to before of the 2nd month).

There was no significant difference between the different time points in total cholesterol except for the 48 hours of the second month compared to the samples collected before the procedure of the same month (Figure 1). LDL significantly decreased in samples collected 48 hours after the procedure in the second month compared to the initial sample (before) of the 1st and 2nd month of therapy. However, there was no significant difference between the two 48 hours samples collected in the 1st and 2nd month (Figure 1). HDL was significantly elevated 48 hours after the commencement of the treatment during the 1st month and it reached its peak at the end of the study in the 48 hours samples of 2nd month, which was significantly higher compared to the other time points of the study (Figure 1).

## Effect of cup therapy on blood pressure

There was no significant change in systolic blood pressure during the different times of the study ($p>0.05$). However, a significant decrease in diastolic pressure was detected 48 hours after treatment during the first month compared to before treatment ($p = 0.002$), and between 48 hours after treatment in the 2nd month compared to before treatment of 1st month ($p=0.006$) and before treatment of the 2nd month ($p=0.0003$) (Table 2 and Figure 2).

| | 1st Month | | 2nd Month | |
|---|---|---|---|---|
| | Before | 30 minutes after | Before | 30 minutes after |
| Systolic pressure (mmHg) | 115.3 ± 10.08 | 113.6 ± 7.1 | 116.9 ± 7.3 | 117.5 ± 4.8 |
| Diastolic pressure (mmHg) | 77.3 ± 5.31 | 69.7 ± 10.8$^{a}$ | 76.18 ± 5.4 | 71.2 ± 6.7$^{a,c}$ |

**Table 2:** Mean ± SD of systolic and diastolic pressures during the different time points of the study (a=p<0.05 compared to before of 1st month, c=p<0.05 compared to before of the 2nd month).

## Effect of cup therapy of blood sodium and potassium

Sodium levels varied during the study. Sodium decreased significantly 48 hours after therapy during the first month compared to the collected sample before treatment ($p<0.001$). However, a significant increase was detected before the initiation of therapy in the 2nd month compared to the 48 hours of the first month ($p=0.004$). Interestingly, the levels of sodium decreased once more 48 hours after treatment in the 2nd month compared to the 3 previous time points (Table 3) (Figure 3).

Potassium levels were opposite to sodium, where a significant increase was observed 48 hours following treatment in the 1st month ($p=0.0002$). This was followed by a significant decrease in the sample collected before the initiation of therapy in the second month compared to the previous time point ($p=0.04$). The second cup therapy resulted in a significant increase in potassium levels 48 hours following the treatment compared to 3 previous time points (Table 3 and Figure 3).

## Discussion

Both bleeding and cupping belong to the oldest medical procedures practiced in the human history and the therapeutic potential of cupping therapy is unlimited and the secrets of its mechanisms still mysterious. Wet cupping/hejamah are part of the traditional medicine in the Arab and Islamic world as the Prophet Mohammad (peace be upon him) said: "If there is a benefit in any of your treatment modalities, benefit

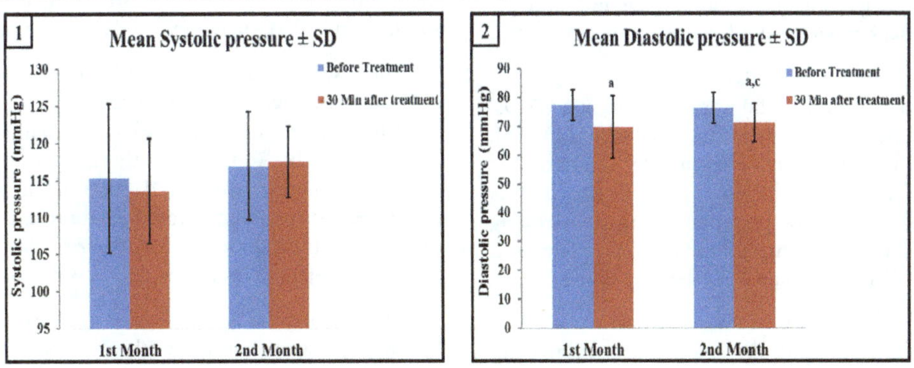


**Figure 2:** Mean ± SD of (1) systolic and (2) diastolic blood pressure in the different times of the study. (a=p<0.05 compared to before 1st month, b=p<0.05 compared to 30 minutes of 1st month and c=p<0.05 compared to before of the 2nd month).

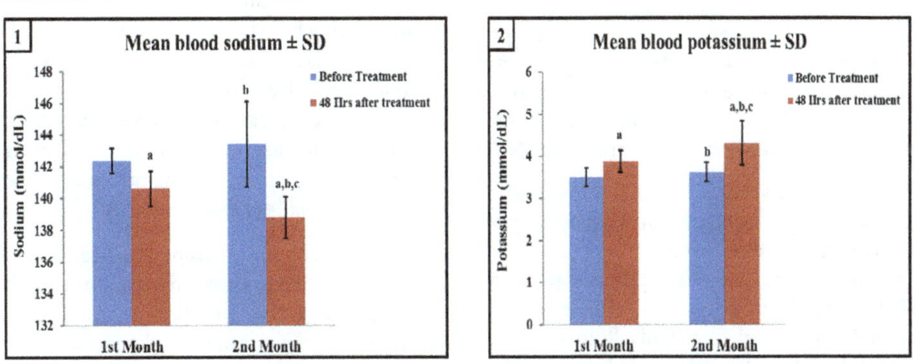


**Figure 3:** Mean ± SD of blood levels of (1) sodium and (2) potassium in the different times of the study. (a=p<0.05 compared to before 1st month, b=p<0.05 compared to 48 hours of 1st month and c=p<0.05 compared to before of the 2nd month).

| | 1st Month | | 2nd Month | |
|---|---|---|---|---|
| | **Before** | **48 hours after** | **Before** | **48 hours after** |
| Fasting Blood Sugar (mg/dL) | 81.36 ± 15.5 | 82.5 ± 12.4 | 73.1 ± 8.9[a,b] | 80.5 ± 14.2c |
| Triglycerides (mg/dL) | 98 ± 16.1 | 70.3 ± 11.4[a] | 78.9 ± 12.6[a] | 72.05 ± 11.3[a] |
| Total Cholesterol (mg/dL) | 161.4± 33.9 | 163.09 ± 34.7 | 164.4 ± 27.5 | 159.1 ± 23.4[c] |
| LDL (mg/dL) | 101.04 ± 32.4 | 97.6 ± 35.2 | 98.8 ± 25.07 | 91 ± 25.1[a,c] |
| HDL (mg/dL) | 46.76 ± 10.5 | 48.7 ± 11[a] | 50.51 ± 10.6[a] | 54.8 ± 12.8[a,c] |
| Sodium (mmol/dL) | 142.37 ± 0.8 | 140.6 ± 1.1[a] | 143.4 ± 2.7[b] | 138.8 ± 1.3[a,b,c] |
| Potassium (mmol/dL) | 3.6 ± 0.22 | 3.88 ± 0.25[a] | 3.62 ± 0.23 | 4.31 ±0.52[a,b,c] |

**Table 3:** Mean ± SD of fasting blood sugar, blood triglycerides, total cholesterol, LD, HDL, sodium and potassium levels during the different time points of the study (a=p<0.05 compared to before of 1st month, b=p<0.05 compared to 48 hours of 1st month and c=p<0.05 compared to before of the 2nd month).

will be in the blade puncture in cupping therapy" [12,17,18,34].

The current study aimed to evaluate the effects of cupping therapy on BP, lipid profile and sodium/potassium blood levels, as well as on FBS. Our results showed significant decrease in end of the study period in diastolic BP accompanied by a significant decrease in serum sodium and significant increase in serum potassium. Additionally, there was a significant increase in HDL, and a significant decrease in LDL and triglycerides. Finally, FBS was variable and inconsistent during the study.

There are several drawbacks to our study. First, the sample size is small and the study included only healthy subjects. However, several other reports were conducted on similar participant number and our results showed significant difference before and after the treatment [9-11]. Another limitation is that we did not measure hormones (e.g. aldosterone, cortisol, etc.) that are known to play an important role in the regulation of metabolic parameters, sodium, potassium and BP. However, this is a preliminary report and a large randomised control trial has been planned.

Elevated BP and hypertension are major risk factors for CVDs, especially CHD, stroke and heart failure, as well as renal failure [35,36]. It has been estimated that high BP is involved in 49% of all chronic heart diseases and 62% of all stroke incidences [37-39]. Nearly 50% of adults worldwide are estimated to be hypertensive or experiencing episodes of raised BP [35,36]. More importantly, all currently used antihypertensive drugs, without exception, have several dose-dependent side effects [35,36].

CM has been suggested for the control/treatment of hypertension [8]. A recent meta-analysis that included tow randomized controlled trials using wet and dry cupping in the treatment of hypertension has reported that using cupping therapy is beneficial in controlling and lowering BP [21]. Similar results were also reported by another study on 15 healthy men and the authors have shown a significant decrease in the mean arterial pressure following wet cupping therapy [22]. In the present study, application of cupping therapy resulted in a significant decrease in the diastolic BP at 30 minutes after cupping. Therefore, hejamah is a potential therapy that could be used as prophylactic and/or complementary treatment for the prevention and control of HTN.

Sodium is essential nutrient that is involved in several homeostatic processes [38,40]. There is a compelling body of evidence that that hypernatremia or a high salt intake strongly contribute to the development of HTN and CVDs, whereas reduced sodium consumption decreases BP [41-43]. Also, potassium is an essential nutrient that is needed for maintenance of total body fluid volume, acid and electrolyte balance, and normal cell function [37]. Previous systematic reviews have suggested that increased potassium intake lowers blood pressure in adults with and without hypertension [37]. A recent 11 cohort studies reported an inverse association between blood potassium level and risk of hypertension and stroke [44]. Also, in a more recent systemic review that included 22 randomised controlled trials in adults confirm that increased potassium intake reduces systolic and diastolic BP as well as improve the prevention and control of the stroke [37].

Our results correlate with the previous studies as they showed a significant decrease in diastolic BP accompanied by a significant decrease in serum sodium and significant increase in serum potassium at the end of the study. Taken together, our findings suggest that hejamah decreases the BP by modulating the blood concentrations of sodium and potassium. However, despite that the observed significant alteration in serum electrolytes in the present study were within the normal range, measuring the concentrations of adrenal cortex hormones, blood and urine pH would exclude pathological causes of hyponatremia such as hypoadrenalism and/or type 4 renal tubular acidosis. Therefore, further research are necessary to reveal the mechanism(s) by which hejamah regulate BP and serum electrolytes.

Increase in blood cholesterol levels is a major risk factor for CVDs. Blood donation and phlebotomy have been shown to significantly reduce the levels of serum cholesterol and thus decreasing the risk for CVDs [30]. Rukzan et al. [45] conducted a study to evaluate the effect of cupping therapy on serum lipid profile concentration in 31 men (35 to to 55 years old), with hyperlipidaemia and who were not using diet or drug therapy. The serum levels for total cholesterol, LDL, triglyceride, and HDL were determined before cupping and then once a week for two weeks after cupping. Cupping significantly decreased total cholesterol, LDL, and LDL/HDL ratio compared to before cupping [45]. Moreover, similar results have been reported by other studies [31,32].

The results of the current study are in agreement with the previous observations. There was a significant decrease observed in triglycerides after the first treatment and the levels remained significantly low till the end of the study. Additionally, there was a significant decrease in LDL and significant increase in HDL observed in samples collected 48 hours of the second treatment. However, there was no significant change in the levels of total cholesterol. Further studies are required to illustrate the role of hejamah in the regulation of the lipid profile.

Bloodletting has been shown to increase the insulin sensitivity [33], which is a major risk factor for the development of metabolic syndrome if impaired. In a constant line, Ranaei-siadat and his colleagues measured the venous blood concentrations of several molecules before and after five times of cupping (one time per month) in young healthy males (20-27 years). Interestingly, their results showed that cupping can regulate cholesterol, HDL, LDL and FBS. However, in the present study the effect of cupping on fasting glucose level was variable and not constant. This could be due to the difference in study design or the small sample size between our study and the previous reports. Additionally, the observed increase in FBS 48 hours following treatment could be due to an increase in the production of glucocorticoids, which are known to be released during stress and they are potent inducers of hyperglycaemia [46].

Though cupping therapy has been used for thousands of years as a traditional therapy for various ailments, the underlying mechanism that mediates its beneficial effect is still obscure. Many questions arise from time to time about the exact role of cupping in treating diseases and to explain benefits of cupping therapy. It was suggested that cups produce hyperaemia or haemostasis which results in a therapeutic effect [13]. Michalsen et al. [47] postulated that cupping gathers and removes harmful blood [47], which also has been discussed and suggested in the 'Taibah Theory' by El-Sayed et al. [12] and, by the findings of Bilal et al. [48] and Ranaei-siadat et al. [46]. Rukzan et al. [45] demonstrated that cupping therapy enhances blood circulation, treats congestion, stops the inflammatory extravasations from the tissues, affect the autonomic nervous system, and reduces pain [45]. It was also reported that injury to the skin leads to the release of β-endorphin and adrenocortical hormones into the systemic circulation [49].

Therefore, the observed significant variations in BP, lipid profile and serum electrolytes could be due to the removal of harmful substances and the induction of several other molecules that are involved in the modulation of lipid metabolism and body water content. However, future research is mandatory to explore the mechanism(s) by which hejamah regulates the blood pressure.

In conclusion, hejamah/wet cupping could represent a potential beneficial line of therapy used as a prophylactic and/or complementary for lowering blood pressure by modulating serum sodium and potassium. It also could provide protection against CVDs by decreasing LDL and increasing HDL. However, large randomised control trials using Islamic protocol of wet cupping in patients with HTN and hyperlipidaemia are required. Furthermore, measuring the effect of Islamic wet cupping on the serum levels of aldosterone, cortisol, adrenaline and thyroid hormones could provide a better understanding on the underlying mechanism(s) by which it could affect the metabolic parameters.

## References

1. Labarthe DR (2012) From cardiovascular disease to cardiovascular health: a quiet revolution? Circ Cardiovasc Qual Outcomes 5: e86-92.
2. Whelton PK, Appel LJ, Sacco RL, Anderson CA, Antman EM, et al. (2012) Sodium, blood pressure, and cardiovascular disease: further evidence supporting the American Heart Association sodium reduction recommendations. Circulation 126: 2880-2889.
3. Labarthe DR, Dunbar SB (2012) Global cardiovascular health promotion and disease prevention: 2011 and beyond. Circulation 125: 2667-2676.
4. Rehm J, Mathers C, Popova S, Thavorncharoensap M, Teerawattananon Y, et al. (2009) Global burden of disease and injury and economic cost attributable to alcohol use and alcohol-use disorders. Lancet 373: 2223-2233.
5. Ng N, Johnson O, Lindahl B, Norberg M (2012) A reversal of decreasing trends in population cholesterol levels in Västerbotten County, Sweden. Glob Health Action 5.
6. Burge SK, Albright TL (2002) Use of complementary and alternative medicine among family practice patients in south Texas. Am J Public Health 92: 1614-1616.
7. WHO (2002) WHO Traditional Medicine Strategy 2002-2005: World Health Organization, Geneva, Switzerland.
8. Nahas R (2008) Complementary and alternative medicine approaches to blood pressure reduction: An evidence-based review. Can Fam Physician 54:1529-1533.
9. Zidek W, Tenschert W, Karoff C, Vetter H (1985) Treatment of resistant hypertension by phlebotomy. Klin Wochenschr 63: 762-764.
10. Fahal IH, Yaqoob M, Ahmad R (1992) Phlebotomy for erythropoietin-induced malignant hypertension. Nephron 61: 214-216.
11. Barenbrock M, Spieker C, Rahn KH, Zidek W (1993) Therapeutic efficiency of phlebotomy in posttransplant hypertension associated with erythrocytosis. Clin Nephrol 40: 241-243.
12. El Sayed SM, Mahmoud HS, Nabo MMH (2013) Methods of Wet Cupping Therapy (Al-Hijamah): In Light of Modern Medicine and Prophetic Medicine. Altern Integ Med 2:1-16.
13. Cao H, Li X, Liu J (2012) An updated review of the efficacy of cupping therapy. PLoS One 7: e31793.
14. Cao H, Hu H, Colagiuri B, Liu J (2011) Medicinal cupping therapy in 30 patients with fibromyalgia: a case series observation. Forsch Komplement Med 18:122-126.
15. Cao H, Zhu C, Liu J (2010) Wet cupping therapy for treatment of herpes zoster: a systematic review of randomized controlled trials. Altern Ther Health Med 16: 48-54.
16. Cao H, Han M, Li X, Dong S, Shang Y, et al. (2010) Clinical research evidence of cupping therapy in China: a systematic literature review. BMC Complement Altern Med 10: 70.
17. Mahmoud HS, Abou-El-Naga M, Omar NAA, El-Ghazzawy HA, Fathy YM, et al. (2013) Anatomical Sites for Practicing Wet Cupping Therapy (Al-Hijamah): In Light of Modern Medicine and Prophetic Medicine. Altern Integ Med 2: 1374-1378.
18. Hajar Albinali HA (2004) Chairman's Reflections: Blood-letting. Heart Views 5: 74-85.
19. Shaikh BT, Hatcher J (2005) Complementary and Alternative Medicine in Pakistan: Prospects and Limitations. Evid Based Complement Alternat Med 2: 139-142.
20. Shekarforoush S, Foadoddini M (2012) Cardiac effects of cupping: myocardial infarction, arrhythmias, heart rate and mean arterial blood pressure in the rat heart. Chin J Physiol 55: 253-258.
21. Lee MS, Choi TY, Shin BC, Kim JI, Nam SS (2010) Cupping for hypertension: a systematic review. Clin Exp Hypertens 32:423-425.
22. AL-Shamma YMH, Abdil Razzaq A (2009) Al-Hijamah Cupping Therapy. Kufa Med Journal 12: 49-56.
23. Zarei M, Hejazi S, Javadi SA, and Farahani H (2012) The efficacy of wet cupping in the treatment of hypertension. ARYA Atherosclerosis Journal 8: 1-4.
24. Yin LH, Miao BH, Chen J, Chai TQ (2009) Clinical study about acupuncture combined with cupping therapy for treating stable exertional angina pectoris in the middle-age or old patients. Chinese J Clin Healthcare 12: 465-467.
25. Lee MS, Choi TY, Shin BC, Han CH, Ernst E (2010) Cupping for stroke rehabilitation: a systematic review. J Neurol Sci 294: 70-73.
26. Lee MS, Kim JI, Ernst E (2011) Is cupping an effective treatment? An overview of systematic reviews. J Acupunct Meridian Stud 4: 1-4.
27. Kumar H (1994) Repeated blood donation effective in treating hyperlipidemia. J Assoc Physicians India 42: 468-469.
28. Salonen JT, Tuomainen TP, Salonen R, Lakka TA, Nyyssönen K (1998) Donation of blood is associated with reduced risk of myocardial infarction. The Kuopio Ischaemic Heart Disease Risk Factor Study. Am J Epidemiol 148: 445-451.
29. Tuomainen TP, Punnonen K, Nyyssönen K, Salonen JT (1998) Association between body iron stores and the risk of acute myocardial infarction in men. Circulation 97: 1461-1466.
30. Meyers K, Falkner B (2009) Hypertension in children and adolescents: an approach to management of complex hyper-tension in pediatric patients. Curr Hypertens Rep 11: 315-322.
31. Niasari M, Kosari F, Ahmadi A (2007) The effect of wet cupping on serum lipid concentrations of clinically healthy young men: a randomized controlled trial. J Altern Complement Med 13: 79-82.
32. Mustafa LA, Dawood RM, Al-Sabaawy OM (2012) Effect of Wet Cupping on Serum Lipids Profile Levels of Hyperlipidemic Patients and Correlation with some Metal Ions. Raf J Sci 23: 129-136.
33. Equitani F, Fernandez-Real JM, Menichella G, Koch M, Calvani M, et al. (2008) Bloodletting ameliorates insulin sensitivity and secretion in parallel to reducing liver iron in carriers of HFE gene mutations. Diabetes Care 31: 3-8.

34. Parapia LA (2008) History of bloodletting by phlebotomy. Br J Haematol 143: 490-495.

35. WHO (2012) Guideline: Sodium intake for adults and children.

36. WHO (2013) A global brief on hypertension Silent killer. Global Public Health Crisis 82.

37. Aburto NJ, Hanson S, Gutierrez H, Hooper L, Elliott P, et al. (2013) Effect of increased potassium intake on cardiovascular risk factors and disease: systematic review and meta-analyses. BMJ 346: f1378.

38. Aburto NJ, Ziolkovska A, Hooper L, Elliott P, Cappuccio FP, et al. (2013) Effect of lower sodium intake on health: systematic review and meta-analyses. BMJ 346: f1326.

39. Yusuf S, Hawken S, Ounpuu S, Dans T, Avezum A, et al. (2004) Effect of potentially modifiable risk factors associated with myocardial infarction in 52 countries (the INTERHEART study): case-control study. Lancet 364: 937-952.

40. He FJ, Li J, Macgregor GA (2013) Effect of longer term modest salt reduction on blood pressure: Cochrane systematic review and meta-analysis of randomised trials. BMJ 346: f1325.

41. Chobanian AV, Bakris GL, Black HR, Cushman WC, Green LA, Izzo JL, Jr, et al. (2003) Seventh report of the Joint National Committee on Prevention, Detection, Evaluation, and Treatment of High Blood Pressure. Hypertension 42: 1206-1252.

42. He FJ, Jenner KH, Macgregor GA (2010) WASH-world action on salt and health. Kidney Int 78: 745-753.

43. He FJ, MacGregor GA (2010) Reducing population salt intake worldwide: from evidence to implementation. Prog Cardiovasc Dis 52: 363-382.

44. D'Elia L, Barba G, Cappuccio FP, Strazzullo P (2011) Potassium intake, stroke, and cardiovascular disease a meta-analysis of prospective studies. J Am Coll Cardiol 57: 1210-1219.

45. Rukzan LM, Al-Sabaawy DO (2012) Effect of Wet Cupping on Serum Lipids Profile Levels of Hyperlipidemic Patients and Correlation with some Metal Ions. Raf J Sci 23: 128-136.

46. Ranaei-siadat SO, Kheirandish H, Niasari, Adibi K (2004) The effect of cupping (hejamat) on blood biochemical and immunological parameters. IJPR 3: 31-32.

47. Michalsen A, Bock S, Ludtke R, Rampp T, Baecker M, et al. (2009) Effects of traditional cupping therapy in patients with carpal tunnel syndrome: a randomized controlled trial. J Pain 10: 601-608.

48. Bilal M, Khan AR, Ahmed A, Afroz S (2011) Partial Evaluation of Technique Used In Cupping. Journal of Basic And Applied Science 7: 65-68.

49. Han JS (2004) Acupuncture and endorphins. Neurosci Lett 361: 258-261.

# 32

# Golden Ratio and the Fibonacci Series in the Homeopathy Theory and Practice

**Bela Tőkés[1]* and Attila Tőkés[2]**

[1]University of Medicine and Pharmacy in Targu Mures, Romania
[2]Angio-Center Targu Mures, Romania

**Abstract**

Homeopathy is the medicine of the third millennium. According to homeopathy the only remedy that assure a real remission of te patient is his constitutional chronic one. Potentiation, reached by high dilution and succusion, is the way that eliberates the healing energy of the remedy. In this process are delineated as general laws: the golden ratio and the Fibonacci potency series. The authors explain how the water structure keeps in its "memory" the properties (inclusive the pharmacologcal ones, also) of the active ingredient, and what is the role of the basic dynamisation steps in this mechanism. The Fibonacci potencies series was introduced by Rozencwajg to correctly choose the homeopathic data ("Removing the guesswork from potency selection"). Is demonstrated that succussion might be responsible for creating nano-bubbles. The trituration and succusion process generates shockwaves in a transient localized region of high pressure (10,000-15,000 atmospheres) which is powerful enough to trigger fundamental changes in the structure and properties of the carrier media. "Weak Quantum Theory" (a version of Quantum Mechanics) predicts a generalised form of entanglement-a concept established by Schrödinger in 1935. The organism receptors receive and process the information in the remedy according to its state: (1) The raw material for the preparation of a homeopathic remedy is the information matrix. (2) The solvent (water or water-alcohol) employed in the homeopathic preparation is the information carrier: "imprint"- through succession-or "erase"- through electromagnetic fields-the information contained in it. Homeopathy is now FDA regulated.

**Keywords:** Homeopathy; Golden ratio; Fibonacci series; Potency; Ultradilution; Succussion

Homeopathy in contrast to conventional medicine (allopathy) offers no cure symptoms but shows the way how the patient suffering from the disease may help himself [1-3]. Theoretically it contains even more controversial aspects. The paper outlines a few thoughts on the exact and correct interpretation.

A number of fundamental scientific discoveries of last decades considered homeopathic research milestones are shown below [1-6].

1988: the water structure memory is presented

1990: description is given how the water molecules create structures able to store electromagnetic signals

1991: emphasized that the potentiation creates molecular clusters in water

1999: described that the potentiation changes the properties of water

2001: pointed out that in the water "nanogrouping" are formed

2003: the quantum macro entanglement model is created

2007: found that the succussion creates colloidal nanoparticles

2008: Indicated that homeopathic medicines are stable, clathrate-type water structures, of nano-heterogeneous particle dimensions, which can be described by measurable properties

2008: proved that the dilution determines the density of nano-bubbles

2009: described that the nano-structures are created by the potentiation

2011: proved that the potentiation of the water molecules creates domains of nanoscale dimensions or nanocrystals

2012: it is shown that the nanoparticles remain stable below the Avogadro limit

Perhaps the scientific recognition of the homeopathy is the fact that the alternative Nobel Prize (Right Livelihood Award) in 1996 was awarded Georgios Vithoulkas, Greek homeopath [4,5,7], for his contribution in the application of classical homeopathy.

Homeopathy is now FDA (U.S. Food and Drug Administration) regulated.

The main operations of the homeopathic practice are the serial high dilution, and the succussion of the (liquid or solid solution) preparation. These operations are jointly termed potentiation. Not enough dilution required succussion, too.

A serial dilution proposed by Hahnemann [8] and other schools [9-11], can be feasible in various ratios, of which the most usual are the decimal (D: 1/10, and this continued for a further 1/10 with dilution on every new sequence term) and the centesimal (C: same, but now 1/100 scale serial dilutions) technique. For example, using the latter series, the molar concentrations will be reduced in the following ratios: $10^{-2}$, $10^{-4}$, $10^{-6}$, $10^{-8}$, $10^{-10}$ M, etc. Here, for the sake of simplicity, it is assumed that we started from a 1 M stock solution ("mother tincture"). Highest

***Corresponding author:** Bela Tőkés, Professor Emeritus, University of Medicine and Pharmacy in Targu Mures, Romania, E-mail: belatokes@yahoo.com concentrations are already of the solubility rare, but if the dilution is desired, it would be meaningless. Easy to see that solution of 12C no longer contains a single molecule. In case of homeopathy the main point of attack is connected with the increasingly high dilution. Question is usually that why can act a solution, wherein the active substance is not present nor in a single molecule? At first glance this appears to be well founded objection [12-14]. Really it does not contain a single molecule of the active substance, either, of course, on average, if the fluctuations are taken into account. Even Hahnemann himself felt that in ordinary causal relationships cannot rely on. He assumed that the solvent (usually water or alcohol-water mixture) preserves the memory of the properties ("fingerprints") of the substance (pharmacological ones too) and passes them on your body (of course, receptors does not imply the existence of). It is worth recalling that when Benveniste (1988) also "trusted" the transmission of information to the memory of water [15-18], his colleagues mocked him, but they also, later, when it did not have a Nobel Prize Award to Benveniste excluded, flattered their former irony target.

It is interesting that the "memory effect" more often is detected in different areas, over time. e.g. in electrode reactions [19,20] the deposition potential depends also on if the depolarizer molecule is directly introduced into the reaction space, or as a product of a previous process it "born" in the electrode force field, and its spatial orientation and further fate are predetermined. In the latter case, the intermediate product already includes some information, they define the character of the next stages, and which are absent in the case of compounds introduced from outside. The electrode is actually the source of electrons entering in and out of depolarizer agent. The transmission of information to the electrode/electron system is easy to see. It is worth noting: the memory effect is also established by a field of force (energy transfer).

Also known the role of the structure of liquid water forming hydrogen bridge bonds [21,22]. The existence of molecule association groups were already known in the first half of the last century. Examining the hydrogen bonds in the context of an universal relation comes in sight the law of the golden ratio (golden-mean) [23]. It describes a (very often recognizable and considered as universal) relationship according to which from two quantities ($a$ and $b$, $a>b$) the larger one is proportional to the smaller parts such as the lesser extent to their difference, that is, $b$ is the geometric mean of theses latter quantities:

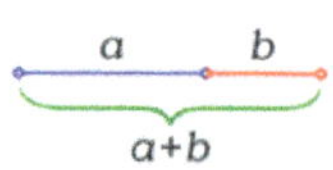


$$\frac{a}{b} = \frac{b}{a-b},$$

that is

$$b^2 = a \cdot (a - b)$$

The golden ratio numerically is described by an irrational number: $\Phi \approx 1.618$. Its inverse is $\varphi \approx 0.618$. Figure 1 shows the case of the hydrogen bridge

The hydrogen bridges present a tetrahedral space structure of water molecules, with a relatively rigid hexagonal conformation. This means a more or less energetically stable state can be developed, separated by energy barriers. Due to the relatively low activation energies (several kJ/mol) quasi-continuous transition is achieved between the stable and

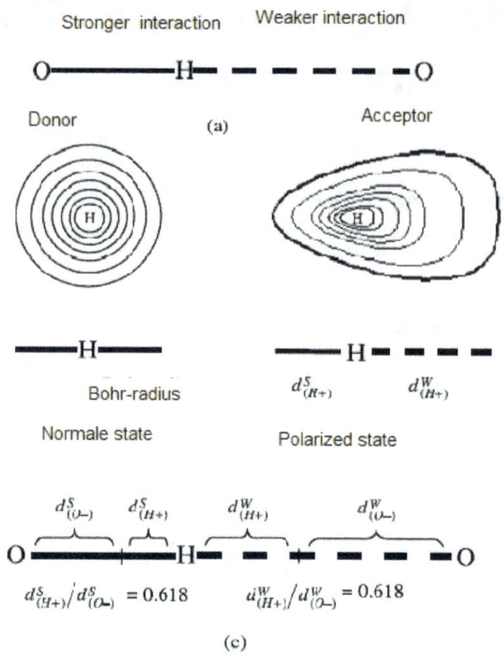


**Figure 1:** The golden ratio at the H-bond.

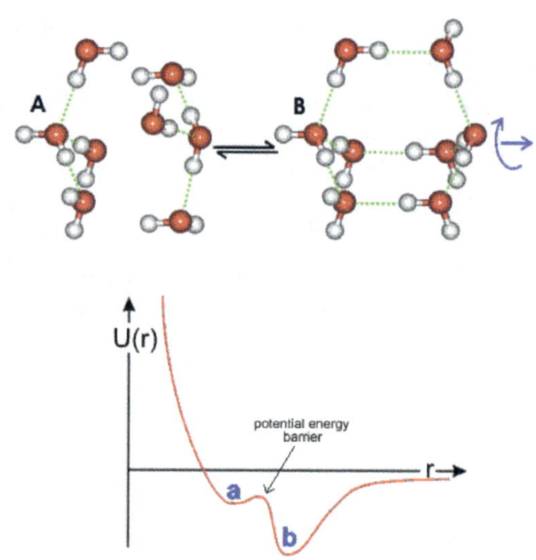


**Figure 2:** The water conformation and the potential energy variation.

metastable states. The golden mean may immediately be observed in Figure 2. Certainly other examples can be cited as well.

According to the above, the water conformational associations are determined by their related energy field.. Energy fields can also be created by molecules, ions, free radicals-actually also by molecules of active pharmaceutical ingredients, and the independent water structures themselves can interact with other molecules. In order to exert an effect the active constituents are linked to proteins (receptors). The force fields generated by the active particles and the corresponding water cluster structures play a decisive role in the behavior of the partner molecules.

Emoto [http://www.is-masaru-emoto-for-real.com] has shown

that water ice-in a globally ordered crystalline structure-will create different geometric shapes, depending on the crystallization conditions. These conditions are influenced by solutes, by different energy fields, -including music-, just as by mental control. Some apparently absurd example may be quoted in Figure 3.

The Kirlian spectra (auras) of water in Figure 4 and the dissolved substances (drugs) [24] may lead to similar conclusions. It seems evident the water models different structures in various energy fields and conditions, respectively various water structures generate different energy fields.

Chaplin in his critical analysis [25-27] showed the stability of the clusters increases with the dilution. This interpretation is in accordance with the Arndt Schulz's rule (1888), as substances (drugs) which are toxic in large amounts present a curative effect when diluted.

As it was already noticed, the medium is often a mixture of water and ethanol. According to a nice story an international team observed differences in hydrogen-bonding strength in vodkas using H-NMR, FT-IR, and Raman spectroscopy. It was suggested differences in taste are given by clathrate structure. The story goes, that the Nobel Prize winner Linus Pauling believed the clathrates give alcohol a narcotic effect.

It is to emphasize, in the potentiation the shaking has a decisive effect [3,11,25,26]. This explanation should lay in the instant pressure effect of ten or fifteen thousand atmospheres causing the structural changes the in water associations (respectively in other molecular clusters). It seems, it is a "necessary and sufficient" condition. The dilution itself

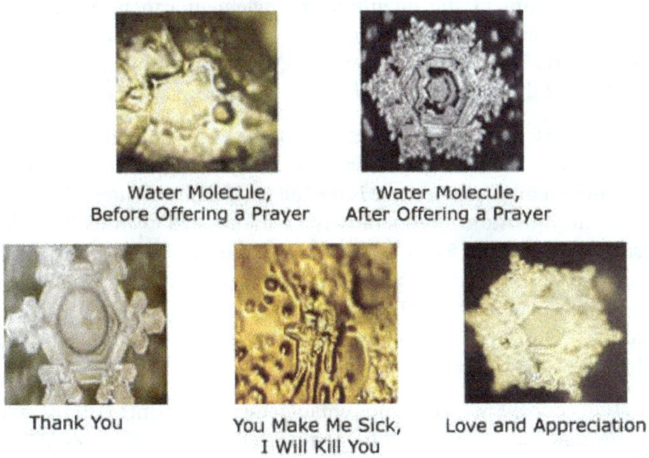


**Figure 3:** Water crystals images.

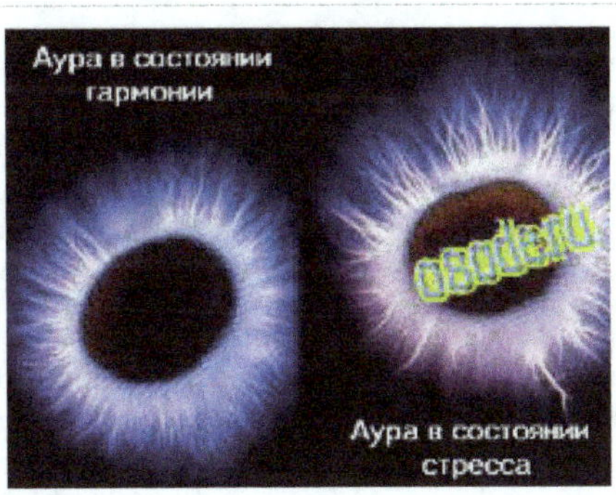


**Figure 4:** Kirlian's auras in harmonic and stressed states.

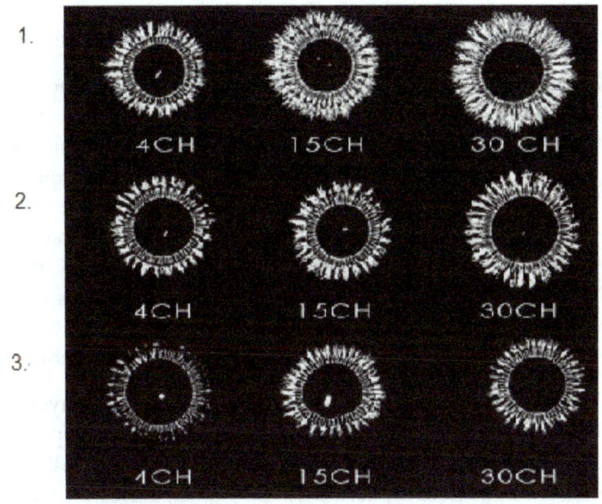


**Figure 5:** Kirlian's auras in different homeopatic conditions:
1. seriea: 4C–15C–30C dilutions with manual succusion
2. series: 4C–15C–30C dilutions with mechanic succusion
3. series: 4C–15C–30C solutions, no succusion

is necessary for storaging and transmission of information. In fact the two operations together satisfy the "necessary and sufficient condition" (Figure 5).

The same effect as by a homeopathic drug may also be achieved if the energy is transmitted by other means to the (biological) system, (e.g. by light-interference devices).

Energy transmitted by the succussion is accumulated and causes fast mechano-chemical effects provoked by free radicals and other mechanisms (it occurs in femtosecond of time, 1 fs=$10^{-15}$ s) generating different structures (clusters, domains).

Between the ultrasonic chemistry [28] and the succussion an analogy can be perceived The ultrasound can be divided into active and passive range, which-by convention-the power is considered passive under 1W/cm$^2$ (10 kW/m$^2$), and active above this value. Passive ultrasounds are used for testing materials, while the active ones are applied to alter their properties.

In the 1930s German chemists observed that dispersed substances in aqueous solution will react when exposed to ultrasonic effect even if normally they would not react with one another. The explanation is that the ultrasounds create bubbles, and by collapse these bubbles-due to the Casimir effect-release an impact with so much energy as a significant local heating occurs (The reaction space may be heated to thousands of degrees Kelvin). This sonochemical effect was soon forgotten, because the practical application proved to be too expensive [29]. However in the 1990s, as more advanced measurement techniques were available, it was noticed that the collapsing bubbles sometimes generate an energy with several orders of magnitude higher than expected by normal physical reasons Due to the high energy the collapsing bubbles can flash, so this phenomenon is also known as sonoluminescence. After a long time of searching for an explanation, the answer was finally found by the Nobel Prize-winner physicist Julian Schwinger as that the vacuum energy is responsible for the significant temperature raise [30].

The behavior of homeopathic preparations may be explaind based on the quantum entanglement phenomenon [1,23,31,32]. This concept, described in 1935 by Erwin Schrödinger, the Austrian Nobel laureate, was originally known in the 1930s, as Einstein-Podolsky-

Rosen paradox. The entangled particles are not separate units, but they should be seen as a complete system [http:/www.newscientist.com/article/mg20927952.900scorn-over-claim-of-teleported-dna.html].

Nobel Prize-winner Montaignier et al. [33] has shown that organized water clusters (nanoparticles, domains) are able to transmit electromagnetic signals between each other and with the outside world. This is a special case of resonance, and satisfies the requirements of quantum entanglement. The phenomenon has been modelled in 2003. Certainly the quantum theory has to be applied to the bonds, the electrons involved in bonding must be characterized by the particle-wave duality, reflecting the principle of Heisenberg's uncertainty, and the bondones have to present quantum nature [23]. In fact all these theories, show a strong correlation with the rule of golden ratio.

Concerning the Montagnier experiments, J. Reimers, says, "If the results are correct, these would be the most significant experiments performed in the past 90 years, demanding re-evaluation of the whole conceptual framework of modern chemistry" [ http://en.wikipedia.org/wiki/Luc_Montagnier].

Montagnier produced biologically active "aqueous nanostructures" like in homeopathic medicine, using the serial agitated dilution in water. His research on detection of electromagnetic signals in the plasma from patients with Alzheimer's and Parkinson's disease, multiple sclerosis and rheumatoid arthritis confirms what the homeopaths have been telling the scientific world for many years [1,2,11,30,33-36].

Montagnier found that in the stimulation of the dilute an electromagnetic background of very low frequency was essential. The background was either produced by natural sources (the Schumann resonances which start at 7.83 Hz) or by artificial ones. Homeopaths considered these studies as a further proof, that homeopathic remedies have distinct supramolecular structural features emitting electromagnetic signals that can affect biological entities. It is also providing further insight into the physics of homeopathy.

Montagnier have proved the major point of contention in favor of homeopathy, respectively the memory of water, which is biologically specific.

The sinusoidal wave is a common graph for results in almost all homeopathic studies, no matter are they physical, *in vivo* or *in vitro*. As dilutions increase changes in amplitude and frequency may occure. The most commonly used dilutions in available homeopathic remedies OTC are 6C, 12C and 30C. A keen mathematical eye might spot what the relationship is between those three numbers: they fall upon an advanced Fibonacci scale, mathematically defining the spiral (Figure 6).

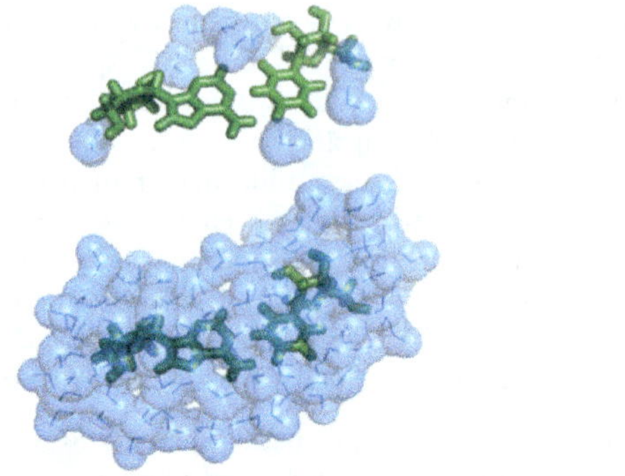

**Figure 6:** The clathrate, homeopathy's missing link. RNA with solvation shell.

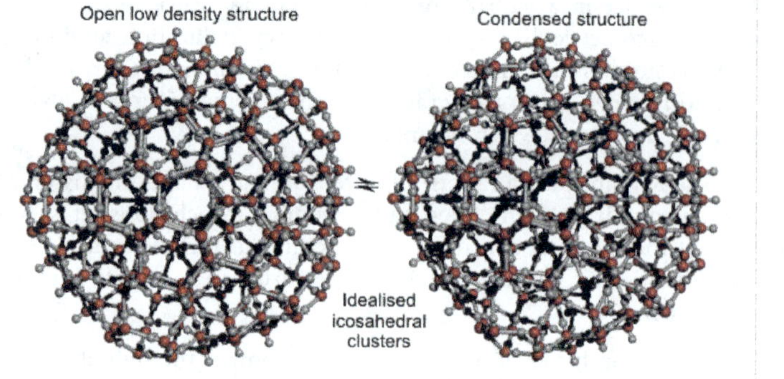


**Figure 7:** Structure variations and quantum cooperation in water.

Richard Bartlett [31] introduced the energy concept describing the state of being (using an energy matrix) and the concept how to control the disease. In his view, all energy species, including the human energy field-known as the morphogenetic field-are under concious control. Actually the forerunner of this idea is the Jungian collective unconsciousness. The morphogenetic field is the blueprint of life-the source of information for DNA.

Physicists have only recently demonstrate that an electron or a photon may appear in multiple spatial locations at a time, which is an unusual perception and rather exciting in itself. It might also offer a new dimension to notions regarding teleporting. Perhaps even more astonishing is that any change in the status of the particle pairs of "twins" can lead to a change-wihout delays of any kind and regardless of distance (the speed of light is not a limit). Now, in the extremely noisy environment the quantum entanglement can be experienced (eventually even investigated) in a biological medium, at room temperature. These findings put a new light on understanding the coordinated thinking and action of the twins from a singel ovum.

Going back to the quantified state of the water domains, Mae-Wan Ho [http://www.i-sis.org.uk/QuantumJazz.php] suggested in 1990, that the water quantum-coherence is the life itself (*Life is Water's Quantum Jazz*). The quantum co-operativity is manifested by the H-bridges formed between the water molecules, i.e. the interaction between the local units conducting to global effects resulting in the formation of supramolecular clusters. The icosahedral shapes of $(H_2O)_{280}$ are an example. This assumption was later proved by quantum chemical calculations as well (Figure 7).

The concept of quantum entanglement and interactions (and increasingly its practice) is consistent with the torsional waves of Tesla (1900), [http://www.fractalfield.com/fractalalchemy] later extended ( 1970) by Kozyrev to various systems (including the structure of the water domains).

The Fibonacci series should also express (besides the golden ratio), an universal law (applicable to water domains as well) and with a closely related other natural law. This is originally described by a specific progression, wherein each member is the sum of the two previous ones: (0), 1, 1, 2, 3, 5, 8, 13, 21, 34, 55, 89, 144, 233, etc. Later, more general series (Lucas, Binet, etc.) were also developed with members deducted from Pascal's triangle (Figure 8).

The formula and the figures illustrate the method of calculation, the relationship with the golden ratio, their graphic illustration and derivation from the Pascal's triangle. Taking into account as the golden ratio itself may be considered a progression wherein any of the members is the geometric mean of the previous and the next members

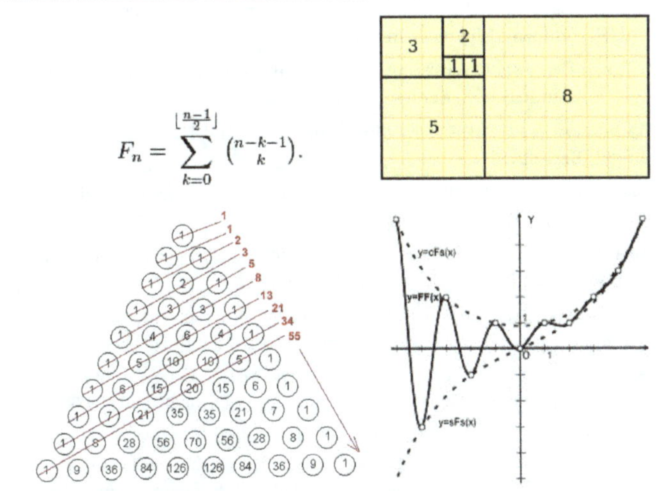

**Figure 8:** Relations between the golden rate and the Fibonacci series.

| Fibonacci Series | Starting potency (3C) and the dilution series | Starting potency (5C) and the dilution series | Starting potency 8C) and the dilution series |
|---|---|---|---|
| **1** | 3C | 5C | 8C |
| **5** | 15C | - | - |
| **8** | 120C | 40C | - |
| **13** | 1.5 M | 520C | 104C |
| **21** | 33 M | 11 M | 2 M |
| **34** | 1 MM | 370 M | 74 M |
| **55** | 61 MM | 20 MM | 4 MM |
| **89** | 5.5 MMM | 2 MMM | 363 MM |
| **144** | 78 MMM | 262 MMM | 52 MMM |
| **233** | 180 MMMM | 61 MMMM | 12 MMMM |

**Table 1:** Often used potency scales as function of Fibonacci series.

(in the same time the coefficient a/b=$\Phi\approx1.618$ that is $\varphi\approx0.618$, universal constant expressed by an irrational number). Compared to the Fibonacci terms, it will be observed that the numbers of the two series coincide. At the beginning the graphical image is a waveform curve with decreasing amplitudes. The oscillation is also a common (perhaps universal) natural phenomenon, manifesting, in the biological systems, both in organic and inorganic world (e.g. in chemical processes).

Fibonacci series seem to be omnipresent. It can be observed in nature, as the mathematical proportion of shapes of flowers, cacti, vegetables like Brassica, Pineapple, Nautilus Shell, Butterfly, inner and external human ears etc. It is also used in many mathematical formulas for accounting and trading. It is even present in art and music. The rhythm found in nature led to use the same one in homeopathic potencies and such series of centecimal potencies are called the Fibonacci Potencies.

Rozencwajg examined the logic between the different potency scales (The title of his paper is significant: "Removing the Guesswork from potency selection"). He observed initially a linearity between the series, but the nature of the relationships is rarely linear. The regularity became more evident when he reached the examination of the golden ratio and Fibonacci series [http://hpathy.com/homeopathy-papers/the-fibonacci-potencies-series-update-discussion-and-conclusions].

For practical homeopathic purposes, the Fibonacci series begin with the lowest potencies. On a centesimal scale, depending on the agent, these are 3C or 5C. Starting with 3C, the following members of the series are 5C, then 8C (3+5), followed by 13C (5+8), 31C, 34C, 55C, 89C, 233C etc.

Rozencvaig feared that these relatively low potencies do not produce the desired effect. Howevert he found that they grow further exponentially and lead to excellent results. For example, starting with a 5C potential dose and continuing later the administration with the same medication of 8C potency, the effect was equivalent with 40C (5×8), and if the next dose was 13C, their overall effect became equivalent to 520C (13×40), a.s.o.. Looking in more details on the evolution of the frequently used initial potencies (Table 1) seems to be useful. Starting potencies are considered: 3C, 5C or 8C.

**3C:** This is the so-called "low potency", the starter potency for non-toxic plants and non-toxic materials. Its actual concentration-or rather dilution-is one part per million (1 ppm), still detectable with regular laboratory techniques. Without taking into account the factor of dynamisation, 1 ppm still has physiological effects and therefore may not be used with toxic substances, poisons, venoms etc.

It is to be emphasized these potencies are not a simple succession of weird ones, but they have a multiplying, exponential effect, allowing to reach extraordinary high potency levels which otherwise should be unattainable.

**5C:** This level of dilution is equivalent to ten parts per billion (10 ppb). 5C is used as the starter potency for toxic plants, poisons, metals and minerals in general. Some of these are not available in a lower dilution.

**8C:** It is a starting potency for the nosodes.

Currently, preparations of the Fibonacci-type homeopathic potency series are produced only by a few pharmaceutical companies, often up to 33C, The customized values can be obtained by anyone "at home" from the accessible preparations of intermediate potency.

As the mother tincture is more toxic, it is preferable to use dilutions until the probability of an atom or molecule of drug entering the patient body during the treatment is reduced close to zero. No matter what the dilution is, the probability never drops to zero can only approach it. It is understandable, the higher the dilution, the more time, energy, carrier agent are necessary for the preparation of the drug solution. To improve the situation, the active ingredient will only be diluted until the information is transcribed. For this purpose adequate instruments are necessary for measuring or-at least to estimate-the information content. When these are not available the only possibility remains optimizing the succussion.

Usually drug molecules have been removed from the information carrier substrate by dilution. Alternatively, a variety of careful screening procedures may be used. These may be: molecular sieve, osmosis filter, fine centrifugation or sedimentation. The point is that the screening process may not compromise the information content of the carrier.

Carrier of distilled water is recommended as the presence of dissolved minerals change the structure clusters of the water molecules. The cleaner-physically and "informatically"-the carrier is, the noiseless will be the drug made of it.

For the transcription of information two ways are considered:

- Primary (direct) transcription encountering a drug particle to a carrier molecule.

- Secondary or repeated transcription which encounters a transcribed substrate molecule with a pure one.

As it might be expected the primary way is more efficient. The first potentiation has the best effect, and the least number of successions is required. The more diluted the drug (or the higher dilution is used), the more succussions are necessary for a successful transcription. (A single drug molecule must collide with several carrier molecules for a primary transcription). It is necessary to insert a rest between each succession for satisfactory mixing the molecules. Before the succession it is efficient to apply a good mixing of the mother tincture with the carrier.

In case the symptoms induced by the active ingredient are more similar to those of the disease, a more dilute agent must be used. The reason is that the "injected" information will stimulate the body, but in the absence of the toxic drug the antibodies produced by the immune system, cannot attack its molecules, and they will concentrate on the disease carrier (the patient body). Essentially, the body was "misguided" and it is switched over to natural control.

Low dilutions of substances are effective in physical sicknesses whereas high ones in the psychlogic ones as well. The reason lies in the information content. The psyche and the body are in permanent information contact and interact with each other. The principle of "sound mind in a sound body" applies. The sick soul makes sick its body and the sick patient's body cripples the soul. Improving the general feeling of body can improve the state of mind. This dynamic feedback and self-perpetuating, self-protective process may interfere with various substances (like toxins, drugs, aphrodisiacs a.o.) or psychological factors (learning, habituation, hypnosis, suggestion, meditation, etc) just as energetic actions as well (acupuncture, earth radiation, etc.). The highly diluted substances have to be administered rarely, as they maintain the stimulatory effect for a longer time. Potentiation is done manually with 10 succussions at each stage.

In summary, once the drug is selected; the most important operation is its potentiation. Rozencwajg, a sailant personality of modern homeopathy, an excellent knowner and tiller of acupuncture, homeopathy, TCM (Traditional Chinese Medicine), food sciences, herbs, aromatherapy, natural medicine, Reiki, and other areas, developed more potency scales [37]. These studies, highlighting the need for homeopathy, launched a tremendous progress-on the bases of the Fibonacci potency scale-both from theoretical and practical (operational) point of view.

From all those outlined it seems clear (and that's only the tip of the iceberg !) that homeopathy is studied by the most prominent experts and huge volume of facts and results are processed (a real Mount-Blac of data). Modern research methods and high-tech achievements have been launched in the battle. It's enough to notice the modern spectrometry, various forms of modern diffraction techniques, the thermometric, chemical equipment, electrical, magnetic, and optical devices.

## References


1. Bellavite P, Signorini A (2002) The Emerging Science of Homeopathy. North, Atlantic Book, Berkeley.
2. Dobrescu D (2011) Farmacologie Homeopata Ecologica. Farmacologie generala. (3rdedn). Universitara, Bucureti.
3. Ernst E (1997) Homoeopathy: past, present and future. Br J Clin Pharmacol 44: 435-437.
4. Vithoulkas G (1880) The Science of Homeopathy. Grove Press, New York.
5. Vithoulkas G (2000) Homeopathy: Medicine for the New Millennium. IACH, California Hypnosis Institute.
6. Ullman D (1991) Discovering Homeopathy: Medicine for the 21st Century. North Atlantic Books, Berkely.
7. Vithoulkas G (1892) A New Model for Health and Disease. North Atlantic Books, Berkeley.
8. Hahnemann S (1960) Organon of medicine. (6thedn). Calcutta: M. Bhattacharyya & Co.
9. Elia V, Niccoli M (1999) Thermodynamics of extremely diluted aqueous solutions. Ann N Y Acad Sci 879: 241-248.
10. Khuda-Bukhsh AR (2003) Towards understanding molecular mechanisms of action of homeopathic drugs: An overview. Mol Cell Biochem 253: 339-345.
11. Khuda-Bukhsh AR, Pathak S (2008) Homeopathic drug discovery: theory update and methodological aspect. Expert Opin Drug Discov 3: 979-990.
12. Anagnostatos GS, Pissis P, Viras K, Soutzidou M (1998 ) Theory and experiments on high dilutions. In: Homoeopathy-a critical appraisal. Butterworth-Heinemann, Reed Educational and Professional Publishers Ltd.
13. Berkowitz CD (1994) Homeopathy: keeping an open mind. Lancet 344: 701-702.
14. Berwin TH (1995) What's wrong with complementary medicine? The Sceptic 8: 6-9.
15. Benveniste J, Ducot B, Spira A (1994) Memory of water revisited. Nature 370: 322.
16. Benveniste J (1994) Further Biological Effects Induced by Ultra High Dilutions: Inhibition by a Magnetic Field. Kluwe Academic Press, Dordrecht.
17. Benveniste J, Aïssa J, Guillonnet D (1999) The molecular signal is not functional in the absence of "informed" water, FASEB Journal 13: A163.
18. Benveniste J (2005) Ma vérité sur la 'mémoire de l'eau' (Préface du professeur Brian D. Josephson, Prix Nobel de Physic). Albin Michel, Paris.
19. Donáth-Nagy G, Buchwald P, Vancea S, Croitoru M, Tokés B (2008) The quantitative characterization of free radical sources and traps by electromigration applications. J Biochem Biophys Methods 70: 1317-1323.
20. Tókés B, Suciu G, Nagy G (2002) Interdependent chemical-electrochemical steps in retrometabolism-based drug and safer chemical design. Pharmazie 57: 122-126.
21. Elia V, Napoli E, Germano R (2007) The 'Memory of Water': an almost deciphered enigma. Dissipative structures in extremely dilute aqueous solutions. Homeopathy 96: 163-169.
22. Prokop O, Hopff W (1992) Erklarung zur Homöopathie. Dtsh Apotheker Zeitung 132: 1630-1632.
23. Putz M V (2012) Valence atom with bohmian quantum potential: the golden ratio approach. Chemistry Central Journal 6: 135-157.
24. Opalinski J (1979) Kirlian-type images and the transport of thin-film materials in high-voltage corona discharges. Journal of Applied Physics 50: 498-504.
25. Chaplin MF (2000) A proposal for the structuring of water. Biophys Chem 83: 211-221.
26. Chaplin MF (2007) The Memory of Water: an overview. Homeopathy 96: 143-150.
27. Chaplin MF (2008) Reply to Comment on 'The memory of water; an overview'. Homeopathy 97:43-44.
28. Silvo M, Arnaldo P (1990) Ultrasonographic study of homeopathic solutions. Br Homeopathic J 179: 212.
29. Bordag M, Mohideen U, Mostepanenko VM (2001) New Developments in the Casimir Effect. Phys Rep 353: 1-205.
30. Jack Ng Y (1996) Julian Schwinger J The Physicist, the Teacher, and the Man. Singapore: World Scientific.
31. Bartlett R (1998) Matrix Energetics: The Science and Art of Transformation, Ed. Adevar Divin, Brasov.

32. Feynman RP (1985) Introduction in QED: the strange theory of light and matter. Princeton University Press, Princeton, NJ 1-20

33. Montagnier L, Aïssa J, Ferris S, Montagnier JL, Lavallée C (2009) Electromagnetic signals are produced by aqueous nanostructures derived from bacterial DNA sequences. Interdiscip Sci 1: 81-90.

34. Benveniste J (1993) Molecular signaling at high dilution or by means of electronic circuitry. Journal of Immunology 150: 146A.

35. Khuda-Bukhsh AR (1986) Some homeopathic drugs as radio-protective agents in X-irradiated mice. Perspectives in Cytology and Genetics 5: 407-412.

36. Benveniste J (1994) Transfer of the molecular signal by electronic amplification, FASEB Journa 8: A398.

37. Rozencwajg J (2009) The Potency: Advanced Prescribing in Homeopathy. Emryss Haarlem.

33

# The Amen Anti-Addiction Intervention: Theoretical Foundations of an Alternative Protocol for the Prevention and Treatment of Addiction

**Nun Sava-Siva Amen-Ra***

*The Amen Institute of Ascetic Psychology, Maryland, USA*

**Abstract**

The Amen Anti-Addiction Intervention (AAI) is an austere intervention intended to eradicate addictive impulses and behaviors. The theoretical and empirical foundations of this intervention are explicated herein. The AAI entails daily cyclic fasting, chronic caloric restriction, supplementation with specific neutraceutical agents, rigorous exercise, and minimalist meditation. The physiological focus of the AAI is twofold: the augmentation of neurogenesis in a manner analogous to the effect of psychotropic drugs and the activation of areas in the brain involved in the regulation of emotional arousal and reward. The psychological focus of the AAI is similarly twofold: the attenuation of anxiety and/or impulsivity and the cultivation of mental mastery and/or self-control. It shall be argued that the AAI, by virtue of its explicit integration of biological, psychological, and sociological elements—each of which evidently influence addiction—will plausibly be an improvement over existing interventions aimed at the treatment of addiction.

**Keywords:** Amen Anti-Addiction Intervention (AAI); Addiction; Neutraceuticals

## Introduction

There is evidence extant in extensive scientific literature that addiction to various agents and behaviors share common molecular mechanisms. Further, there is considerable scientific support for the supposition that biological, psychological, and sociological factors influence the propensity of individuals to succumb to addiction [1]. As such, it would seem that the most effective interventions should emanate from the integration of these three domains—biology, psychology, and sociology. In short, the most prudent theoretical perspective for the prevention and treatment of addiction is ideally bio-psycho-social in its overall orientation. Such is the case with the protocol proposed herein. The Amen Anti-Addiction Intervention (AAI) is an outgrowth of the Amen Optimal Health Protocol (AOHP). The aim of the AOHP is to incorporate into a single practical system every intervention that has proven to extend maximum longevity and/or optimize health in model organisms [2,3]. In accordance with scientific data amassed over nearly a century, the AOHP entails the following physiological elements: cyclic fasting amounting to 23+ hours per day; dietary restriction amounting to 25-50% reductions in customary caloric intake consumed in a single span of an hour or less; a fixed, virtually invariant, schedule of feeding consonant with the solar day; vigorous daily exercise; and supplementation with select nutrients and neutraceuticals (i.e. natural compounds with defined bioactive agents). The AOHP entails a single psychological element: *minimalist meditation* aimed at attenuating anxiety and instilling a state of psychic equanimity. Lastly, the AOHP entails a sociological element-specifically, social support conferred by the small community of committed practitioners of the analogous Amen protocols.

## Exposition of the Amen Anti-Addiction Intervention

In the course of exploring the biological bases of drug addiction, it became clear to the Author that the same neurological systems involved in drug addiction are also altered by intermittent fasting, caloric restriction, and scheduled feeding. Additionally, the Author found evidence for the efficacy of exercise in the excitation of reward systems in the brain—systems acted upon by various drugs of abuse. The Author apprised himself of evidence that impulsivity and anxiety influence the propensity for addiction. This revealed the relevance of meditation as a means of attenuating impulsivity and anxiety, thereby supporting its suitability in the prevention and mitigation of addiction. Social support is crucial in the adoption of an intervention as rigorous as the AOHP. Adherents invariably find the support provided by fellow practitioners to be particularly valuable. Given the evidence that social environs influence addictive behaviors, it is plausible that the social support extant in the community of AOHP/AAI adherents could counterbalance the deleterious social signals which promote and sustain illicit substance use. This realization prompted the Author to consider other elements of the AOHP that are potentially conducive to the attenuation of addiction.

Arguments have been advanced that much substance abuse is intended to "self-medicate" symptoms of mental disorders, particularly depression and anxiety [1]. According to this line of thought, drug abuse is driven by the desire to modulate mood, particularly depressive or anxious states. Thus, illicit drugs are "intended" to exert the same effect as licit psychotropic drugs—that is, to elevate mood. The molecular mode of action of common classes of psychotropic drugs used to treat depression and anxiety is incompletely understood. However, experiments in animals suggest that one such molecular modality may be the induction of endogenous neurotrophic factors in the brain. Neurotrophic factors include peptides or proteins such as Brain-Derived Nerve Growth Factor (BDNF), which promote the growth and development of neurons in the brain. Diverse classes of psychotropic drugs including non-selective antidepressants (e.g. imipramine), norepinephrine-selective reuptake inhibitors (e.g. desipramine) and serotonin-selective reuptake inhibitors (e.g. fluoxetine) increase the generation of new neurons in the brain—that is, they induce

***Corresponding author:** Nun Sava-Siva Amen-Ra, The Amen Institute of Ascetic Psychology, 25101 Chimney House Court, Damascus, Maryland, USA, E-mail: Amen-Ra@AmentaEliteAthlete.com neurogenesis [4]. Thus, neurogenesis is thought to mediate the mood elevation that commonly accompanies pharmacotherapeutic treatment of mood disorders. An intervention that is able to induce increased neurogenesis in relevant regions of the brain known to modulate mood could likely exert an effect—preventative or therapeutic—on illicit drug use and other addictive behaviors potentiated by affective impairments. Caloric restriction is such an intervention. It has been demonstrated that cyclic fasting and/or chronic caloric restriction (CF/CR) increase the expression of BDNF, resulting in enhanced generation of neurons in such regions as the hippocampus, neocortex, and striatum of experimental mammals [5]. Conversely, it has been shown that several drugs of abuse impair the proliferation of new neurons in the brain, particularly in the hippocampus. Such drugs include alcohol [6], opiates [7], and stimulants [8,9]. We herein hypothesize that CF/CR can conceivably counter addiction by attenuating impaired neurogenesis engendered by several classes of commonly abused drugs.

Complementing the evidence that fasting and caloric restriction may improve psychological well-being by mimicking the neurogenic effects of psychotropic drugs is evidence that exercise acts in a similar manner. This effect was established by Huang et al. [10], who found that daily voluntary exercise in experimental mice was as effective as the antidepressant drug fluoxetine in inducing an antidepressant effect. The molecular mechanisms underlying this effect in both the fluoxetine and exercise intervention groups was found to be an induction of neurogenesis and increased dendritic spine density in hippocampal neurons. Other empirical investigations have substantiated this experimental finding [11].

Stress is known to induce neuronal loss in specific regions of the adult brain [12]. Interventions that successfully alleviate stress have the potential to antagonize addiction by inducing an antidepressant, anxiolytic (i.e. anxiety reducing) effect. Meditation is one such intervention that has been shown to diminish depression, stress, and anxiety [13]. Meditation, moreover, has been applied as an intervention in the treatment of drug addiction. Witkiewitz et al. [14] found that a type of meditative technique termed Mindfulness-Based Relapse Prevention (MBRP) was able to reduce drug cravings and substance use in an efficacy trial. A randomized, controlled pilot study by Brewer et al. [15] found meditation to be as effective as cognitive behavioral therapy (CBT) in reducing stress among groups of clients undergoing substance abuse treatment. It has been found, moreover, that meditation of the MBRP variety increased unilateral hippocampal thickness in a group of practitioners as established by magnetic resonance imaging [16].

Certain natural substances are known to promote neurogenesis in particular regions of the brain, such as the hippocampus. Among such agents is the polar compound choline. Glenn et al. [17] demonstrated that administration of choline to adult rodents augmented expression of BDNF and consequently induced increased neurogenesis in the hippocampus. Administering this agent to developing rats exerted antidepressant like effects therein. Several studies have demonstrated the capacity of ginseng (*Panax* species) to induce neurogenesis in the hippocampus via induction of neurotrophic factors. A study by Jiang et al. [18] found that a chemical constituent of ginseng (Rg1) augmented neurogenesis in the hippocampal regions of mice via BDNF induction. The effect attenuated various indices of depression and stress in the experimental subjects, an effect that was comparable to the antidepressant imipramine, which the investigators employed as a positive control. Constituents of coffee (inclusive of caffeine) have equivocally been found to exert a protective effect on neurological function and this has been attributed to increases in hippocampal neurogenesis [19]. These and other non-toxic neutraceuticals are common constituents of the Amen Apothecary. Though the Amen Apothecary was originally formulated to advance the aim of lifespan extension, several of the substances contained in the formulary are known to be neurogenic. In addition to those already indicated, blueberry extract [20], cocoa [21], grape seed extract [22] the unicellular autotroph spirulina [23] garlic [24] soy [25], and conventional tea (*Camellia senensis*) [26], have each been found to induce neurogenesis. Indeed, it has been determined that diets rich in plant polyphenols may generally promote hippocampal neurogenesis [27]. The Amen Diet as such is substantially soy-based, containing significant amounts of spirulina and garlic and therefore theoretically capable of heightening the neurogenic effect of the supplements constituting the Amen Apothecary proper. Though soy has been consumed for centuries, especially in Asiatic countries, it is known to contain estrogen-analogues—chemicals comparable in their effects to the female sex hormone. Although this has caused some theorists to question the propriety of its consumption in males, there is suggestive evidence that soy reduces the risk of prostate cancer [28], a malignancy responsible for considerable morbidity and mortality in male populations of the West. Importantly, the Amen Diet is thoroughly vegetal, containing no meat or other animal products. There is complementary evidence that dietary cholesterol compromises hippocampal neurogenesis [29] and, conversely, that cholesterol-lowering drugs (i.e. *statins*) promote neurogenesis in a manner analogous to antidepressants [30]. Given that animal products are the sole sources of naturally occurring cholesterol, a diet devoid of meat accommodates heightened hippocampal neurogenesis relative to omnivorous diets inclusive of meat.

It has been found that extracts of the South African herb, *Aspalathus linearis* (also known as Rooibos or red tea) inhibits the age related reduction in hippocampal thickness [31], an effect which may plausibly be related to enhanced neurogenesis. Tea—both traditional tea and red tea—is imbibed throughout the lengthy Amen Fast and this practice may further promote neurogenesis, potentially providing a protracted state of neurotrophic stimulation during the diurnal period.

It is evident that each element of the AAI plausibly possesses the potential to attenuate addictive behavior via an empirically established ability to induce regionally specific neurogenesis in a manner similar to psychotropic drugs. Six separate components serve this salutary end—cyclic fasting, caloric restriction, exclusively vegetal nutriment, exercise, neutraceuticals, and meditation. The multifaceted nature of the AAI, combined with its manifest molecular mimicry of the psychotropic medication modality and its absence of artificiality (and presumably deleterious pharmacologic side-effects) may make it inherently more effective than alternative preventative/therapeutic interventions.

Though there is no current consensus on the etiology of drug addiction, there is substantial support for the role of molecularly mediated motivation [32]. More specifically, drugs of abuse are thought to alter the actions of neurotransmitters in particular regions of the brain associated with reward and motivation [33]. As explained in a review by McCarthy et al. [34], dopamine serves a central role in regulating reward:

"A major CNS dopaminergic pathway is the mesolimbic pathway. In this pathway, dopamine synthesized in the ventral tegmental area (VTA) of the mid brain is transported to the nucleus accumbens (NAc), amygdala, hippocampus, and prefrontal cortex (PFC) in the forebrain. The mesolimbic dopaminergic pathway is also referred to as the 'reward pathway' because of its critical involvement in mediating rewarding effects of drugs such as cocaine (p. 439)".

Additionally, impulsivity and impaired self-control are common, compelling, explanatory elements of theories and models of addictive behaviors [35-37]. According to such theories, addiction entails an inability to control impulses impelling engagement in drug use and the consistent failure to control such impulses ultimately eventuates in the compulsion of chronic drug use. If, indeed, excessive impulsivity potentiates drug abuse and addiction, it would seem that an intervention aimed at extinguishing addiction should endeavor to attenuate impulsivity in order to enable the acquisition of self-control. Such is the case with the AAI.

It is herein hypothesized that cyclic fasting/caloric restriction (CF/CR) may be effective in the treatment of addiction insofar as it is operative in the two dimensions discussed above—that is, CF/CR may modulate molecularly mediated motivation and it may plausibly inhibit impulsivity. Evidence indicates that feeding restriction alters the chemistry of the brain such that pleasure centers (principally limbic structures) are activated [38]. This activation apparently enhances the pleasurability of hedonic stimuli such as food and illicit drugs. Fang et al. [39] found that electrical stimulation of specific limbic nuclei in recovering heroin addicts induced a state of euphoria comparable to the drug. Dopaminergic (dopamine sensitive) neurons play a prominent part in the perception of pleasure; heightened dopamine signaling accompanies the ingestion of food (especially after an extended interval of fasting) as well as certain psychoactive drugs [40]. Hypothetically, an extended (23-hr) period of food deprivation followed by a brief (1-hr) period of feeding should partially mimic the effect of drug administration on the dopaminergic system. This hypothesis is substantiated by an investigation by Yamamoto et al. [38] which explored the expression of genes in reward-related regions of the brain (prefrontal cortex, amygdala, and hypothalamus) in rodents subjected to fasting and restricted feeding. Analyses indicated that the most substantial alteration of expression was an upregulation of dopamine receptor signaling indicative of increased dopaminergic activity. The Author speculates that the similarity between the chemical cascade catalyzed by temporal food restriction and that induced upon drug ingestion may enable one to substitute the reward engendered by feeding for the reward which ordinarily accompanies intoxication. In the analogous context of alcohol addiction and exercise, Ozburn [41] has termed this concept "hedonic substitution". Given the hedonic enhancement associated with feeding restriction, it is possible that individuals ingesting illicit agents may experience an intensification of euphoria. Conceivably, this could incline some individuals to increase or sustain their substance abuse instead of attenuating or eliminating it. In this respect it is important to acknowledge that an intervention such as the AAI is likely to be less effective in persons lacking a considerable cognitive commitment to disavow deleterious drug usage and eschew addiction.

Fasting entails self-imposed control over the impulse to eat. Foregoing feeding for 23 hours daily and partaking of a single evening meal of moderate energy density facilitates (and indeed constitutes) self-control. Appetitive impulses are suppressed during extended fasting and such suppression serves to strengthen one's psyche thereby enabling the attenuation of addiction according to the hypothesis advanced herein. The feasibility of fasting for 23 hours daily is experientially established by the Author's personal practice of the protocol for a period exceeding a decade and his assistance in aiding patients in the successful adoption of the AOHP in the context of his private practice. The feasibility of fasting consistently for spans of 24+ hours has been empirically established by several clinical trials. In a review of caloric restriction studies in humans, Varady [42] compared the reported weight-loss efficacy of daily caloric restriction versus intermittent fasting (feeding on alternating days for 24 hours). Varady [42] identified 11 conventional caloric restriction trials (entailing 15-60% CR), 5 published intermittent fasting trials, and 2 theretofore unpublished trials conducted in his laboratory. Such studies (which ranged in duration from 4-24 weeks) suggest that consistent CR and fasting can be well tolerated for moderate periods whereas the Author's anecdotal experience and that of clients counseled in the implementation of the AOHP, illustrates the tolerability of combined CR and daily fasting for an extensive, decade-long period without noticeable negative effects and considerable perceived positive effects (e.g. increased mental and physical energy, maintenance of ideal body weight and body composition, etc.).

Anxiety is among the effects of drug withdrawal [43]. Attenuating the anxiety associated with drug withdrawal may increase the odds that addicts undergoing treatment will abstain from drug abuse. Meditation has demonstrated some efficacy in the attenuation of anxiety [44]. The inclusion of meditative techniques in the AAI may thereby aid in drug rehabilitation via anxiety reduction. Further, meditation may mitigate impulsivity, which (as discussed above) is implicated in addiction. The Author [45] has developed and practiced a form of meditation that may be especially effective at attenuating the impulsivity allegedly underlying addictive behaviors. In contrast to such meditative techniques as Mindfulness (the anti-addiction efficacy of which has indeed been established in short-term follow-up of 2-4 months) [46], Amen Meditation (AM) is 'contentless', involving no imagery, verbal guidance or prolonged facilitation. These factors—namely, no necessity for facilitation after inconsiderable initial instruction—may make AM more effective insofar as it can be initiated more rapidly and executed independently by the practitioner/patient. Briefly, AM entails an attempt to expurgate ideas, images, and emotions from the mind and suppress awareness of sensation in the body—it is an intentional inhibition of the impulse to think, feel, and move, an intentional imposition of insipidity or ataraxy. Amen meditation adopts the Jainist posture of *kayotsarga* (connoting in Prakrit "forgetting the body" [47] or the Yogic posture of *savasana* (denoting in Sanskrit "corpse posture"). Kayotsarga is a relaxed, standing, statuesque posture. Alternatively, AM practitioners may adopt an immobile recumbent, horizontal posture—such is savasana. Merely maintaining such postures (for 10-20 minute intervals as the protocol prescribes) requires impulse control—control of the urge to ambulate. Can the conscious control of thought and posture that AM entails be applied to addictive behavior; is it generalizable? Such is what we hypothesize—that AM is able to eliminate or attenuate chemical and behavioral addiction owing to its antagonism of impulsivity.

## Future Research

Preliminarily, the Author proposes to conduct a feasibility study, the intent of which is to ascertain the capacity of persons in an addiction treatment facility to comply with the elements of the AAI. The Author endeavors to execute the investigation in an outpatient addiction clinic over a 3-month period. Participants will be recruited from incoming clients seeking treatment for alcohol and drug addiction and randomly assigned to the standard or alternative (AAI) treatment groups. The standard treatment group shall consist of incoming clients assigned to conventional treatment—specifically, weekly individual and group psychotherapy sessions employing CBT as the primary treatment technique. The alternative treatment group shall be instructed in the implementation of the AAI, asked to record their food intake, be provided with select neutraceutical agents included in the Amen Apothecary (specifically, the two types of tea—traditional and red), asked to indicate the time and duration of fasting and exercise, and record the frequency and duration of meditation. Clients in the alternative group will not be counseled to consume a certain quantity of calories, as it is likely that the limitation of feeding to a 1-hour interval will result in substantial caloric restriction relative to the pre-intervention period [3]. Individuals in the alternative group will be encouraged to exercise twice daily, ideally in the morning and evening, for 15-minute intervals or more. Instruction shall be provided to clients concerning the performance of aerobic and resistance exercises which require no equipment and entail moderate physical exertion. The intensity and duration of exercise shall be tailored to the fitness level of the participant. Patients will be instructed to engage in meditation immediately after the twice-daily exercise sessions for a period of 10 minutes or more. Individuals in the alternative group will be encouraged and expected to abstain from illicit drug use. Any participants in the alternative group desirous of availing themselves of pharmacotherapeutic treatment will be transferred forthwith and treated conventionally. Given the co-morbid conditions that commonly characterize clients seeking treatment for substance abuse, the conduct of the proposed study shall be closely monitored by trained medical personnel in the employ of the agency. Subsequent studies shall be aimed at integrating all elements of the AAI over increasingly lengthy intervals of investigation.

## References


1. Abadinsky H (2010) Drug Use & Abuse: A Comprehensive Introduction. (7th edn). Belmont, CA: Cenage Learning.
2. Amen-Ra N (2013) The Amen Optimal Health Protocol: An Exposition On the Experimental, Theoretical & Practical Underpinnings of Lifespan Extension & Optimal Health Promotion, A Discourse on the Method of Gerostasis, Amenta Press.
3. Amen-Ra N (2007) The Optimal Human Diet: Theoretical Foundations of the Amen Protocol. Diet Therapy Research Trends, Nova Science, New York.
4. Pechnick RN, Zonis S, Wawrowsky K, Cosgayon R, Farrokhi C, et al. (2011) Antidepressants stimulate hippocampal neurogenesis by inhibiting p21 expression in the subgranular zone of the hipppocampus. PLoS One 6: e27290.
5. Duan W, Guo Z, Mattson MP (2001) Brain-derived neurotrophic factor mediates an excitoprotective effect of dietary restriction in mice. J Neurochem 76: 619-626.
6. Herrera DG, Yague AG, Johnsen-Soriano S, Bosch-Morell F, Collado-Morente L, et al. (2003) Selective impairment of hippocampal neurogenesis by chronic alcoholism: protective effects of an antioxidant. Proc Natl Acad Sci U S A 100: 7919-7924.
7. Eisch AJ, Harburg GC (2006) Opiates, psychostimulants, and adult hippocampal neurogenesis: Insights for addiction and stem cell biology. Hippocampus 16: 271-286.
8. Sudai E, Croitoru O, Shaldubina A, Abraham L, Gispan I, et al. (2011) High cocaine dosage decreases neurogenesis in the hippocampus and impairs working memory. Addict Biol 16: 251-260.
9. Teuchert-Noodt G, Dawirs RR, Hildebrandt K (2000) Adult treatment with methamphetamine transiently decreases dentate granule cell proliferation in the gerbil hippocampus. J Neural Transm 107: 133-143.
10. Huang GJ, Ben-David E, Tort Piella A, Edwards A, Flint J, et al. (2012) Neurogenomic evidence for a shared mechanism of the antidepressant effects of exercise and chronic fluoxetine in mice. PLoS One 7: e35901.
11. Curlik DM 2nd, Shors TJ (2013) Training your brain: Do mental and physical (MAP) training enhance cognition through the process of neurogenesis in the hippocampus? Neuropharmacology 64: 506-514.
12. Esch T, Stefano GB, Fricchione GL, Benson H (2002) The role of stress in neurodegenerative diseases and mental disorders. Neuro Endocrinol Lett 23: 199-208.
13. Marchand WR (2013) Mindfulness meditation practices as adjunctive treatments for psychiatric disorders. Psychiatr Clin North Am 36: 141-152.
14. Witkiewitz K, Lustyk MK, Bowen S (2013) Retraining the addicted brain: a review of hypothesized neurobiological mechanisms of mindfulness-based relapse prevention. Psychol Addict Behav 27: 351-365.
15. Brewer JA, Sinha R, Chen JA, Michalsen RN, Babuscio TA, et al. (2009) Mindfulness training and stress reactivity in substance abuse: results from a randomized, controlled stage I pilot study. Subst Abus 30: 306-317.
16. Hölzel BK, Carmody J, Vangel M, Congleton C, Yerramsetti SM, et al. (2011) Mindfulness practice leads to increases in regional brain gray matter density. Psychiatry Res 191: 36-43.
17. Glenn MJ, Adams RS, McClurg L (2012) Supplemental dietary choline during development exerts antidepressant-like effects in adult female rats. Brain Res 1443: 52-63.
18. Jiang B, Xiong Z, Yang J, Wang W, Wang Y, et al. (2012) Antidepressant-like effects of ginsenoside Rg1 are due to activation of the BDNF signalling pathway and neurogenesis in the hippocampus. Br J Pharmacol 166: 1872-1887.
19. Costa MS, Botton PH, Mioranzza S, Ardais AP, Moreira JD, et al. (2008) Caffeine improves adult mice performance in the object recognition task and increases BDNF and TrkB independent on phospho-CREB immunocontent in the hippocampus. Neurochem Int 53: 89-94.
20. Casadesus G, Shukitt-Hale B, Stellwagen HM, Zhu X, Lee HG, et al. (2004) Modulation of hippocampal plasticity and cognitive behavior by short-term blueberry supplementation in aged rats. Nutr Neurosci 7: 309-316.
21. Fernández-Fernández L, Comes G, Bolea I, Valente T, Ruiz J, et al. (2012) LMN diet, rich in polyphenols and polyunsaturated fatty acids, improves mouse cognitive decline associated with aging and Alzheimer's disease. Behav Brain Res 228: 261-271.
22. Yoo DY, Kim W, Yoo KY, Lee CH, Choi JH, et al. (2011) Grape seed extract enhances neurogenesis in the hippocampal dentate gyrus in C57BL/6 mice. Phytother Res 25: 668-674.
23. Bachstetter AD, Jernberg J, Schlunk A, Vila JL, Hudson C, et al. (2010) Spirulina promotes stem cell genesis and protects against LPS induced declines in neural stem cell proliferation. PLoS One 5: e10496.
24. Nam SM, Yoo DY, Kim W, Yoo M, Kim DW, et al. (2011) Effects of s-allyl-L-cysteine on cell proliferation and neuroblast differentiation in the mouse dentate gyrus. J Vet Med Sci 73: 1071-1075.
25. Pan M, Li Z, Yeung V, Xu RJ (2010) Dietary supplementation of soy germ phytoestrogens or estradiol improves spatial memory performance and increases gene expression of BDNF, TrkB receptor and synaptic factors in ovariectomized rats. Nutr Metab (Lond) 7: 75.
26. Wang Y, Li M, Xu X, Song M, Tao H, et al. (2012) Green tea epigallocatechin-3-gallate (EGCG) promotes neural progenitor cell proliferation and sonic hedgehog pathway activation during adult hippocampal neurogenesis. Mol Nutr Food Res 56: 1292-1303.
27. Dias GP, Cavegn N, Nix A, do Nascimento Bevilaqua MC, Stangl D, et al. (2012) The role of dietary polyphenols on adult hippocampal neurogenesis: molecular mechanisms and behavioural effects on depression and anxiety. Oxid Med Cell Longev 2012: 541971.
28. van Die MD, Bone KM, Williams SG, Pirotta MV (2013) Soy and soy isoflavones in prostate cancer: a systematic review and meta-analysis of randomised controlled trials. BJU Int .
29. Kim IY, Hwang IK, Choi JW, Yoo KY, Kim YN, et al. (2009) Effects of high cholesterol diet on newly generated cells in the dentate gyrus of C57BL/6N and C3H/HeN mice. J Vet Med Sci 71: 753-758.
30. Can OD, Ulupinar E, Ozkay UD, et al. The effect of simvastatin treatment on behavioral parameters, cognitive performance, and hippocampal morphology in rats fed a standard or a high-fat diet. Behav Pharmacol 2012; 23(5-6): 582-92.
31. Inanami O, Asanuma T, Inukai N, Jin T, Shimokawa S, et al. (1995) The

suppression of age-related accumulation of lipid peroxides in rat brain by administration of Rooibos tea (Aspalathus linearis). Neurosci Lett 196: 85-88.

32. Vetulani J (2001) Drug addiction. Part II. Neurobiology of addiction. Pol J Pharmacol 53: 303-317.
33. Blum K, Liu Y, Shriner R, Gold MS (2011) Reward circuitry dopaminergic activation regulates food and drug craving behavior. Curr Pharm Des 17: 1158-1167.
34. McCarthy DM, Brown AN, Bhide PG (2012) Regulation of BDNF expression by cocaine. Yale J Biol Med 85: 437-446.
35. Gardner EL (2011) Addiction and brain reward and antireward pathways. Adv Psychosom Med 30: 22-60.
36. Orford J (2001) Addiction as excessive appetite. Addiction 96: 15-31.
37. Sussman S, Sussman AN (2011) Considering the definition of addiction. Int J Environ Res Public Health 8: 4025-4038.
38. Yamamoto Y, Tanahashi T, Kawai T, Chikahisa S, Katsuura S, et al. (2009) Changes in behavior and gene expression induced by caloric restriction in C57BL/6 mice. Physiol Genomics 39: 227-235.
39. Fang J, Gu JW, Yang WT, Qin XY, Hu YH (2012) Clinical observation of physiological and psychological reactions to electric stimulation of the amygdaloid nucleus and the nucleus accumbens in heroin addicts after detoxification. Chin Med J (Engl) 125: 63-66.
40. Carr KD (2002) Augmentation of drug reward by chronic food restriction: behavioral evidence and underlying mechanisms. Physiol Behav 76: 353-364.
41. Ozburn AR, Harris RA, Blednov YA (2008) Wheel running, voluntary ethanol consumption, and hedonic substitution. Alcohol 42: 417-424.
42. Varady KA (2011) Intermittent versus daily calorie restriction: which diet regimen is more effective for weight loss? Obes Rev 12: e593-601.
43. Rothwell PE, Thomas MJ, Gewirtz JC (2009) Distinct profiles of anxiety and dysphoria during spontaneous withdrawal from acute morphine exposure. Neuropsychopharmacology 34: 2285-2295.
44. Chen KW, Berger CC, Manheimer E, Forde D, Magidson J, et al. (2012) Meditative therapies for reducing anxiety: a systematic review and meta-analysis of randomized controlled trials. Depress Anxiety 29: 545-562.
45. Amen-Ra N (2011) Mind, Matter, Mathematics, & Mortality: Meditations on a Momentous Metaphysical Theory, Damascus, MD: Amenta Press.
46. Bowen S, Chawla N, Collins SE, Witkiewitz K, Hsu S, et al. (2009) Mindfulness-based relapse prevention for substance use disorders: a pilot efficacy trial. Subst Abus 30: 295-305.
47. Jacobi H. Jaina Sutras (1895) The Sacred Books of the East. Oxford, UK: Oxford University Press.

# Permissions

All chapters in this book were first published in A&IM, by OMICS International; hereby published with permission under the Creative Commons Attribution License or equivalent. Every chapter published in this book has been scrutinized by our experts. Their significance has been extensively debated. The topics covered herein carry significant findings which will fuel the growth of the discipline. They may even be implemented as practical applications or may be referred to as a beginning point for another development.

The contributors of this book come from diverse backgrounds, making this book a truly international effort. This book will bring forth new frontiers with its revolutionizing research information and detailed analysis of the nascent developments around the world.

We would like to thank all the contributing authors for lending their expertise to make the book truly unique. They have played a crucial role in the development of this book. Without their invaluable contributions this book wouldn't have been possible. They have made vital efforts to compile up to date information on the varied aspects of this subject to make this book a valuable addition to the collection of many professionals and students.

This book was conceptualized with the vision of imparting up-to-date information and advanced data in this field. To ensure the same, a matchless editorial board was set up. Every individual on the board went through rigorous rounds of assessment to prove their worth. After which they invested a large part of their time researching and compiling the most relevant data for our readers.

The editorial board has been involved in producing this book since its inception. They have spent rigorous hours researching and exploring the diverse topics which have resulted in the successful publishing of this book. They have passed on their knowledge of decades through this book. To expedite this challenging task, the publisher supported the team at every step. A small team of assistant editors was also appointed to further simplify the editing procedure and attain best results for the readers.

Apart from the editorial board, the designing team has also invested a significant amount of their time in understanding the subject and creating the most relevant covers. They scrutinized every image to scout for the most suitable representation of the subject and create an appropriate cover for the book.

The publishing team has been an ardent support to the editorial, designing and production team. Their endless efforts to recruit the best for this project, has resulted in the accomplishment of this book. They are a veteran in the field of academics and their pool of knowledge is as vast as their experience in printing. Their expertise and guidance has proved useful at every step. Their uncompromising quality standards have made this book an exceptional effort. Their encouragement from time to time has been an inspiration for everyone.

The publisher and the editorial board hope that this book will prove to be a valuable piece of knowledge for researchers, students, practitioners and scholars across the globe.

# List of Contributors

**Hegyi Gabriella, Csütörtöki Krisztina, Pfeifenróth Anna and Göbölyös Ildiko**
Department of Dietetic and CAM, Pecs University, Hungary

**Roberti di Sarsina Paolo**
Observatory and Methods for Health, University of Milano-Bicocca, Italy

**Lia Hafiyani, Satoru Yokoyama, Sherif Abdelhamed, Yoshihiro Hayakawa and Ikuo Saiki**
Division of Pathogenic Biochemistry, Institute of Natural Medicine, University of Toyama, Toyama, Japan

**Jing Zheng Song and John WS Ho**
Biochemistry Programme, School of Life Sciences, The Chinese University of Hong Kong, Shatin, Hong Kong

**Maja Petrič, Renata Vauhnik and Miroljub Jakovljević**
Cesta v log 24, Ljubljana, Slovenia

**Tibor Hajtó, András Adámy, Lilla Baranyai, Monika Kuzma and Perjési Pál**
Institute of Pharmaceutical Chemistry, Medical University Pecs, Hungary

**Zoltán Langmár**
Semmelweis University, 2nd Department of Gynecology, Budapest

**Angelika Kirsch**
Private practice, Arlesheim, Switzerland

**Lajos Ábrahám**
Surgical Department of Szent János Hospital Budapest, Hungary

**Mohammed E Grawish and Ahmed Ragheb Zaher**
Department of Oral Biology, Mansoura University, Egypt

**Mathias Wagner**
Department of Pathology, Saar State University, Homburg Campus, Homburg Saar, Germany

**Benjamin Vicinus**
Department of General, Visceral, Vascular and Paediatric Surgery, Saar State University, Homburg Campus, Homburg Saar, Germany

**Michael J Jack**
Competence Centre for Complementary Medicine and Naturopathy, Technical University Munich, Munich, Germany

**Tereza Richards**
Medical Library, University of the West Indies, Mona Campus, Kingston, Jamaica, W.I.

**Chen Xi**
Department of Applied Biology and Chemical Technology, Hong Kong Polytechnic University, Hong Hom, Kowloon, Hong Kong

**Margherita Ciano**
Department of Experimental, Diagnostic and Specialty Medicine (DIMES), University of Bologna, Italy
Section of Molecular Medicine, National Heart and Lung Institute, Imperial College London, UK

**Fernando Ferretti, Anna Ferretti and Gianluigi Veronesi**
Institute of Human Physiology, University of Bologna, Italy

**Stefano Iotti**
Professor of Biochemistry, Department of Pharmacy and Biotechnology, University of Bologna, Italy
National Institute of Biostructures and Biosystems, Rome, Italy

**Pierluigi Lenzi**
Institute of Human Physiology, University of Bologna, Italy
Former professor of Physiology, Faculty of Medicine, University of Bologna, Italy
National Institute of Biostructures and Biosystems, Rome, Italy

**Silvia Canaider and Federica Facchin**
Department of Experimental, Diagnostic and Specialty Medicine (DIMES), University of Bologna, Italy
National Institute of Biostructures and Biosystems, Rome, Italy

**Ganesh Chandra Jagetia and Ravikiran PB**
Department of Zoology, Mizoram University, India

**Liudmila B Boldyreva**
The State University of Management, Moscow, Russia

**Aamer AA**
Department of Animal Medicine, Faculty of Veterinary Medicine, Assiut University, Assiut, Egypt

**Abdul-Hafeez MM and Sayed SM**
Animal Health Research Institute, Assiut Lab, Assiut, Egypt

**Burkhard Kloesch, Elisabeth Dietersdorfer and Silvia Loebsch**
Ludwig Boltzmann Institute for Rheumatology and Balneology, Cluster Rheumatology, Balneology and Rehabilitation, Vienna, Austria

**Guenter Steiner**
Ludwig Boltzmann Institute for Rheumatology and Balneology, Cluster Rheumatology, Balneology and Rehabilitation, Vienna, Austria
Division of Rheumatology, Department of Internal Medicine III, Medical University Vienna, Austria

**Lingling Yang, Wenxiao He, Changkai Jia and Yao Wang**
Shandong Provincial Key Lab of Ophthalmology, Shandong Eye Institute, Shandong Academy of Medical Sciences, Qingdao, China

**Huihua Qu and Dongmin Liu**
Department of Human Nutrition, Foods and Exercise, Virginia Tech, Blacksburg, USA

**Yiqiang Wang**
Shandong Provincial Key Lab of Ophthalmology, Shandong Eye Institute, Shandong Academy of Medical Sciences, Qingdao, China
University Research Center, Beijing University of Traditional Chinese Medicine, Beijing, China

**Mohammad Akram Randhawa**
Department of Pharmacology, College of Medicine, Northern Border University, Arar, Saudi Arabia

**Shehab Ahmed Alenazi**
Department of Pediatrics, College of Medicine, Northern Border University, Arar, Saudi Arabia

**Sohel MDD and Sultana T**
Department of Pharmacy, State University of Bangladesh, Dhanmondi, Dhaka-1205, Bangladesh
Incepta Pharmaceuticals Ltd, Dewan Idris Road, Zirabo, Savar, Dhaka, Bangladesh

**Kawsar MDH**
Incepta Pharmaceuticals Ltd, Dewan Idris Road, Zirabo, Savar, Dhaka, Bangladesh

**Sumon MDHU**
Department of Pharmacy, University of Asia Pacific, Dhanmondi, Dhaka-1209, Bangladesh

**Sulaiman Abdullah Al Shammari**
Department of Family and Community Medicine, Chair of Health Education and Health Promotion, King Saud University, Saudi Arabia

**Saleh Abdullah Alhaidar, Mazen Ayidh Alotaibi, Abdullah Alrayed Alanazi, Waleed Khalid Al Shammari, Abdulaziz Mashuj Alanazi, Hossam Khalid Alsahabi and Abdulmajeed Fahad Altammami**
College of Medicine, King Saud University, Saudi Arabia

**Talal Mohammed Thaher**
King Khalid General Hospital, Al Majmaah, Saudi Arabia

**Shabnam Zahid, Aysha Raza and Fahmida Kousar**
Department of Ilmul Qabalat wa Niswan wa Atfal, Ayurvedic & Unani Tibbia College, Karol Bagh, New Delhi

**Hina Rehman**
Research officer, Central research institute of Unani Medicine, Hyderabad, Telangana

**Sachin A Shah, Ji Hyun Jamie Lee and Frank Son**
Thomas J Long School of Pharmacy and Health Sciences, University of the Pacific, Stockton, CA, USA

**Gloria St John**
Thomas J Long School of Pharmacy and Health Sciences, University of the Pacific, Stockton, CA, USA
Parhar Health Systems, Roseville, CA, USA

**Narinder Singh Parhar**
Parhar Health Systems, Roseville, CA, USA

**Louisa MT Silva, Mark Schalock, Kristen R Gabrielsen and Gretchen HD**
Teaching Research Institute, Western Oregon University, USA
Associate Research Professor, Teaching Research Institute, Western Oregon University, USA
MPH, Project Director, Consultant for Teaching Research Institute, Western Oregon University, USA
Consultant/Project Manager, Teaching Research Institute, Western Oregon University, USA

**Samiha A. Mourad**
Prophetic Medicine Research Clinic, King Abdulaziz University, Jeddah, Saudi Arabia

**Soad K. Al-Jaouni**
Department of Hematology, Faculty of Medicine, King Abdulaziz University, Jeddah, Saudi Arabia

**Matthew Kutch**
Department of Economics, Ohio Northern University, USA

**Danish Jahan**
National Institute of Unani Medicine, Kottigepalya, Bengaluru, Karnataka, India

**Wajeeha Begum and Mariyam Roqaiya**
Luqman Unani Medical College, Hospital & Research Centre, 12 Naubag, Bijapur, Karnataka, India

**Yousuf Khalil Hussaini**
Jamia Tibbiya Deoband, Uttar Pradesh, India

**Tadele Girum**
Department of Public Health, Arba Minch College of Health Sciences, Arba Minch, Ethiopia

**Di Pierro Francesco**
Velleja Research, Milan, Italy

**Campana Andrea, Panatta Maria Laura, Antenucci Valeria and De Vincentiis Giovanni**
Ospedale Pediatrico Bambino Gesù, Rome, Italy

**Ilaria Giangrandi, Monica Dinu, Giuditta Pagliai and Alessandro Casini**
Department of Experimental and Clinical Medicine, University of Florence, Italy
Unit of Clinical Nutrition, University Hospital of Careggi, Florence, Italy

**Francesco Sofi**
Department of Experimental and Clinical Medicine, University of Florence, Italy
Unit of Clinical Nutrition, University Hospital of Careggi, Florence, Italy
Don Carlo Gnocchi Foundation Italy, Onlus IRCCS, Florence, Italy

**Mayumi Nomoto**
Nomoto Mayumi Skincare Clinic, 1-3-7 Bandai, Chuo-ku, Niigata-shi, Niigata-ken, Japan
Department of Clinical Pharmacology, Faculty of Pharmaceutical Sciences, Niigata University of Pharmacy and Applied Life Sciences, 265-1 Higashijima, Akiha-ku, Niigata, Japan

**Hyun-Nam Ko**
Department of Nursing, Jinju Health College, Jinju, Republic of Korea

**Sam-Sun Le**
Department of Nursing, Koje College, Koje, Republic of Korea

**Sang-Dol Kim**
Department of Nursing, College of Health Science, Kangwon National University, Samcheok-si, Republic of Korea

**Takashi Seki and Kenichi Meguro**
Division of Geriatric Behavioral Neurology, Tohoku University CYRIC, 6-3 Aoba, Aramaki, Aoba ku, Sendai, Miyagi 980-8578, Japan

**Keiko Sasaki and Seiichi Mori**
Urayasu special elderly nursing home, 86-5 Shimoyoden aza Kasima, Natori, Miyagi 981-1223, Japan

**Jansen JCH and Van Tilborgh AJW**
Dutch Doctor's Association for Integrative Medicine (AVIG), The Netherlands

**Klein-Laansma CT**
Dutch Doctor's Association for Integrative Medicine (AVIG), The Netherlands
Healthcare and Nutrition, Louis Bolk Institute, The Netherlands

**Van Vliet M**
Healthcare and Nutrition, Louis Bolk Institute, The Netherlands

**Dongmei Huang**
Institute of Integrated Traditional Chinese and Western Medicine, Tongji hospital, Huazhong University of Science and Technology, China

**Qing Wang**
Institute of Integrated Traditional Chinese and Western Medicine, Tongji hospital, Huazhong University of Science and Technology, China
Department of Obstetrics and Gynecology, First Affiliated Hospital, Heilongjiang University of Chinese Medicine, China

**Haoxu Dong and Lina Zhang**
Department of Obstetrics and Gynecology, First Affiliated Hospital, Heilongjiang University of Chinese Medicine, China

**Yanjuan Liu**
Department of Integrated Traditional Chinese and Western Medicine, Tongji hospital, Huazhong University of Science and Technology, China

**Ranabhat Chhabi and CB Kim**
Department of Preventive Medicine, Wonju College of Medicine Yonsei University, Wonju, Republic of Korea

**YA Do**
Management Support Team, Management Support Department, Korea International Cooperation Agency 825 Daewangpangyo-ro, Sujeong-go, Seongnam-si, Gyeonggido, 461-833 Republic of Korea

**DW Ahn**
Institute for Poverty Alleviation and International Development, Yonsei University Wonju, Republic of South Korea

**KJ Lee**
Institute for Poverty Alleviation and International Development, Yonsei University Wonju, Republic of South Korea
Department of Environmental Medical Biology, Wonju College of Medicine Yonsei University, Wonju, Republic of Korea

**Bassem Refaat and Ahmed Ashshi**
Laboratory Medicine Department, Faculty of Applied Medical Sciences, Umm Al-Qura University, Al Abdeyah, Makkah, KSA

**Adel Galal El-Shemi**
Laboratory Medicine Department, Faculty of Applied Medical Sciences, Umm Al-Qura University, Al Abdeyah, Makkah, KSA
Department of Pharmacology, Faculty of Medicine, Assiut University, Egypt

**Anwar Abdelgayed Ebid**
Physiotherapy Department, Faculty of Applied Medical Sciences, Umm Al-Qura University, Al Abdeyah, Makkah, KSA

**Mohammad A BaSalamah**
Pathology Department, Faculty of Medicine, Umm Al-Qura University, Al Abdeyah, Makkah, KSA

**Bela Tőkés**
University of Medicine and Pharmacy in Targu Mures, Romania

**Attila Tőkés**
Angio-Center Targu Mures, Romania

**Nun Sava-Siva Amen-Ra**
The Amen Institute of Ascetic Psychology, Maryland, USA

# Index

www.ingramcontent.com/pod-product-compliance
Lightning Source LLC
LaVergne TN
LVHW060539210926
848485LV00005B/1227